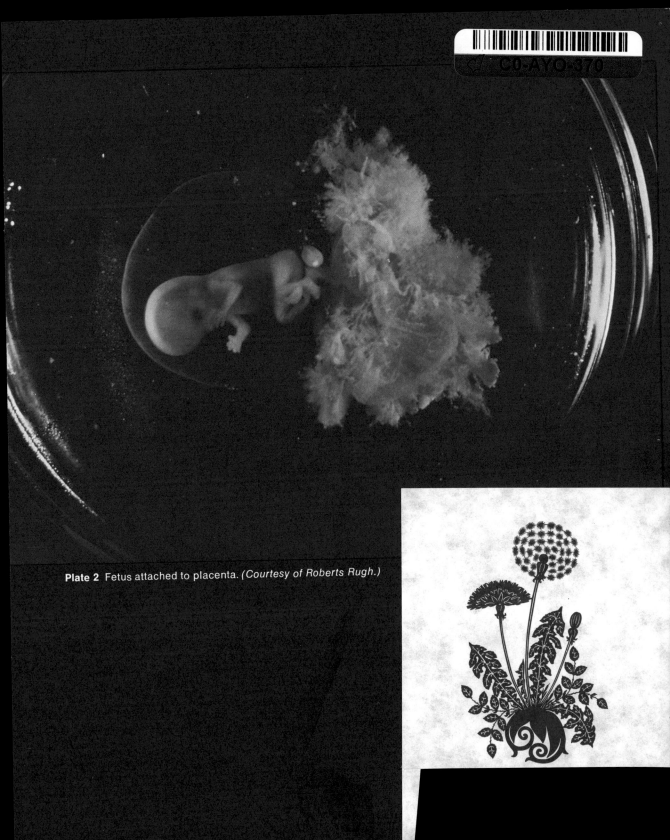

Plate 2 Fetus attached to placenta. *(Courtesy of Roberts Rugh.)*

MATERNAL AND INFANT CARE
a text for nurses

McGraw-Hill
Book Company

A Blakiston Publication

New York
St. Louis
San Francisco
Auckland
Düsseldorf
Johannesburg
Kuala Lumpur
London
Mexico
Montreal
New Delhi
Panama
Paris
São Paulo
Singapore
Sydney
Tokyo
Toronto

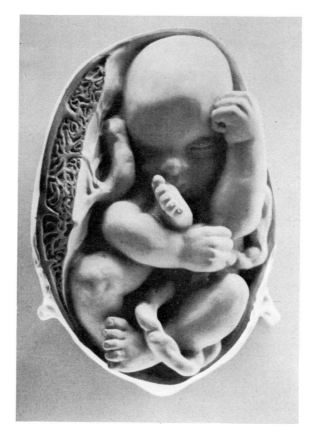

MATERNAL AND INFANT CARE
a text for nurses

Edited by

Elizabeth J. Dickason
R.N., M.A.

Martha Olsen Schult
R.N., M.A.

Assistant Professors of Nursing
Queensborough Community College

NOTICE

Medicine is an ever-changing science. As new research and clinical experience broaden our knowledge, changes in treatment and drug therapy are required. The editors and the publisher of this work have made every effort to ensure that the drug dosage schedules herein are accurate and in accord with the standards accepted at the time of publication. The reader is advised, however, to check the product information sheet included in the package of each drug he plans to administer to be certain that changes have not been made in the recommended dose or in the contraindications for administration. This recommendation is of particular importance in regard to new or infrequently used drugs.

MATERNAL AND INFANT CARE
a text for nurses

1 2 3 4 5 6 7 8 9 0 V H V H 7 9 8 7 6 5

This book was set in Helvetica Light by Black Dot, Inc. The editors were Cathy Dilworth, Sally Barhydt Mobley, and Carol First; the designer was Jo Jones; the production supervisor was Dennis J. Conroy. New drawings were done by Jane Leverich and by J & R Services, Inc.
Von Hoffmann Press, Inc., was printer and binder.

Library of Congress Cataloging in Publication Data

Dickason, Elizabeth J
    Maternal and infant care.

    "A Blakiston publication."
    Includes index.
        1.   Obstetrical nursing.   2.   Pediatric nursing.
I.   Schult, Martha Olsen, joint author.   II.   Title.
[DNLM: 1.   Obstetrical nursing.   2.   Pediatric nursing.
WY157 D547m]
RG951.D52   610.73'678   74-19365
ISBN 0-07-016787-7

CONTENTS

2 the high-risk mother and infant

LIST OF CONTRIBUTORS

Nancy Thoms Block, M.D.
Staff Psychiatrist,
Children's Outpatient Services
New Jersey Medical College
Community Mental Health Center
and
Instructor in Psychiatry,
New Jersey Medical College
Newark, New Jersey

Marvin L. Blumberg, M.D.,
Director,
Department of Pediatrics
The Jamaica Hospital
Queens, New York

Evert A. Bruckner, M.D.
Assistant Professor of Medicine
Department of Internal Medicine
Division of Hematology and Medical Oncology
Emory University School of Medicine
Atlanta, Georgia

Märretje Jelles Buhrer, R.N.
Assistant Head Nurse
Labor and Delivery
and
Childbirth Education Instructor
Booth Memorial Medical Center
Flushing, New York

Constance R. Castor, R.N., B.S.
Childbirth Education Specialist
Associate Director
Council of Childbirth Education Specialists
and
formerly President and Chairman
of National Accreditation Committee
American Society for Psychoprophylaxis in Obstetrics
New York, New York

Margaret Dean, R.N., M.S.
Doctoral Student,
Teacher's College, Columbia University
and
Principal,
College of Nursing
Postgraduate Institute of Medical Education and
Research
Chandigarth, India

Elizabeth J. Dickason, R.N., M.A.
Assistant Professor
Department of Nursing
Queensborough Community College
Bayside, New York

M. Christine Dobson, R.N., M.A.
Assistant Education Coordinator
Community and Social Pediatrics
Harlem Hospital Center
New York, New York

Herbert S. Heineman, M.D.
Associate Professor of Medicine
Division of Infectious Diseases
Hahnemann Medical College and Hospital
and
Chief,
Division of Clinical Microbiology
Philadelphia General Hospital
Philadelphia, Pennsylvania

Hilda Koehler, C.N.M., M.S.
Parent Educator
St. Luke's Hospital
New York, New York

Dolores Lake, R.N., M.S.N.
Associate Professor
Bucks County Community College
Newtown, Pennsylvania

Dorothea M. Lang, C.N.M., M.P.H.
Director,
Nurse-Midwifery Service Program
Maternal and Infant Care and
Family Planning Projects
New York City Department of Health
New York, New York

Beatrice Lau Kee, R.D., M.P.H.
Instructor
Department of Nursing
Queensborough Community College
Bayside, New York

James H. Lee, Jr., M.D.
Professor of Obstetrics and Gynecology
and
Acting Chairman of the Department
The Jefferson Medical College of
Thomas Jefferson University
Philadelphia, Pennsylvania

Jean C. Metzger, R.N., M.A.
Instructor
Department of Nursing
Queensborough Community College
Bayside, New York

Joyce Hanna Nave, R.N., B.S.
formerly Public Health Nurse
Visiting Nurse Service
New York, New York

Janet S. Reinbrecht, C.N.M., M.Ed.
Community Consultant–Parent Educator
Maternity Center Association
New York, New York

Arlene Ritz, R.N., M.A.
Associate Professor
Department of Nursing
Queensborough Community College
Bayside, New York

Jane Corwin Reeves, R.N., P.N.P.
formerly Pediatric Nurse Practitioner
Martin Luther King Community Health Center
Bronx, New York

Roberts Rugh, Ph.D.
formerly Professor of Radiology (biology)
College of Physicians and Surgeons
Columbia University
New York, New York

Martha Olsen Schult, R.N., M.A.
Assistant Professor
Department of Nursing
Queensborough Community College
Bayside, New York

Sister Theresa Thomas, R.N., M.S.
Associate Professor
Department of Nursing
Vermont College Division
Norwich University
Burlington, Vermont

Jane Wilson, R.N.
formerly Charge Nurse
Pediatric and Well Baby Clinic
The Polyclinic Hospital
New York, New York

Philip E. Wilson, C.S.W.
Windham Child Care
and
Affiliated Psychotherapist
Training Institute for Mental Practitioners
New York, New York

Lois D. Young, R.N., M.A.
Learning Disabilities Consultant
John Witherspoon School
Princeton, New Jersey

PREFACE

Pregnancy is neither an illness nor a disease. It is simply a temporary change in a woman's body for the purpose of nourishing and housing the baby until the time for its birth arrives. Like any growth process, it is an orderly sequence of events which can be described and observed. When students understand this growth process, they are better equipped to apply their knowledge of nursing principles so that mother and infant are both benefited.

Maternity nursing does, of course, involve more than just the mother and her baby; it also concerns the family and the community to which they both belong. By understanding the growth processes of pregnancy, caring families are able to help the mother avoid unnecessary hardship. For this reason, the nursing student can expect families to function better when health care professionals respect the family's need for information. The nurse promotes the family's sense of well-being by expressing complete willingness to answer questions which naturally arise during the mother's pregnancy period. Thus the nurse must be an educator in addition to performing the more traditional functions.

The editors have prepared this book to encourage nursing students by "telling it like it is." They recognize the frustration many students feel when confronted by hospital policies which appear insensitive and unresponsive to the patient's needs. While change is often slow in coming about—sometimes for very good reasons—innovation must eventually take place in order for nurs-

ing care to remain effective. Community health centers, maternal care clinics, and family planning programs are but a few of the settings in which competent, enthusiastic nurses are urgently needed. The editors will feel their efforts have been successful if nurses renew their sense of dedication and commitment as a result of using this text.

The content of this book has been arranged in two parts. Part 1 describes all aspects of normal, healthy pregnancy. Various themes are emphasized, including (1) physiologic and anatomic changes in the mother; (2) psychosocial aspects of pregnancy and parenthood; (3) fetal growth and development; (4) family education and support during the childbearing cycle; (5) evaluation, feeding, and care of the infant during its first year of life; and lastly, (6) family planning. A separate unit covers the pharmacologic factors affecting the mother and her infant during the prenatal and perinatal periods.

The organization of the material in Part 2 is unique. Complications affecting the cardiovascular, hematologic, metabolic, and immunologic systems are discussed in relation to the body system involved, rather than the trimester with which the problem is usually associated. The editors feel that this method of organization is a more logical approach because complications in pregnancy often extend throughout the pregnancy and recovery periods and are not limited to one trimester. Furthermore, this approach should be particularly helpful to those students who may not have a background in medical-surgical nursing. Though all major complications are identified, the editors have emphasized those which occur most often among high-risk urban and rural poor mothers, allowing the instructor to call special attention to those problems which concern the community in which she teaches. A separate unit deals with complications affecting the high-risk infant. Because students may not often have the chance to participate in this aspect of maternity nursing, the editors have used the preterm infant to illustrate the complex problems found in neonatal intensive care.

The editors are grateful for the assistance of the many people who helped to bring this work to completion. Deep appreciation is gratefully accorded to each contributor for his part in formulating this text—and to our colleagues in nursing education for their encouragement.

Special thanks is expressed to Dr. Susan Williamson of the Presbyterian Hospital of the City of New York for her encouragement and assistance in developing the content of the book and suggesting resources to us; to Dr. Marion Laird for reviewing the manuscripts; to Dr. Virginia Apgar for her assistance with illustrations.

Finally, the editors wish to thank Elsie Downey, Penelope Anderson, Gladys Burkhardt, and Myra Alvoord for providing generous help in the preparation of the manuscript.

Elizabeth J. Dickason

Martha Olsen Schult

MATERNAL AND INFANT CARE
a text for nurses

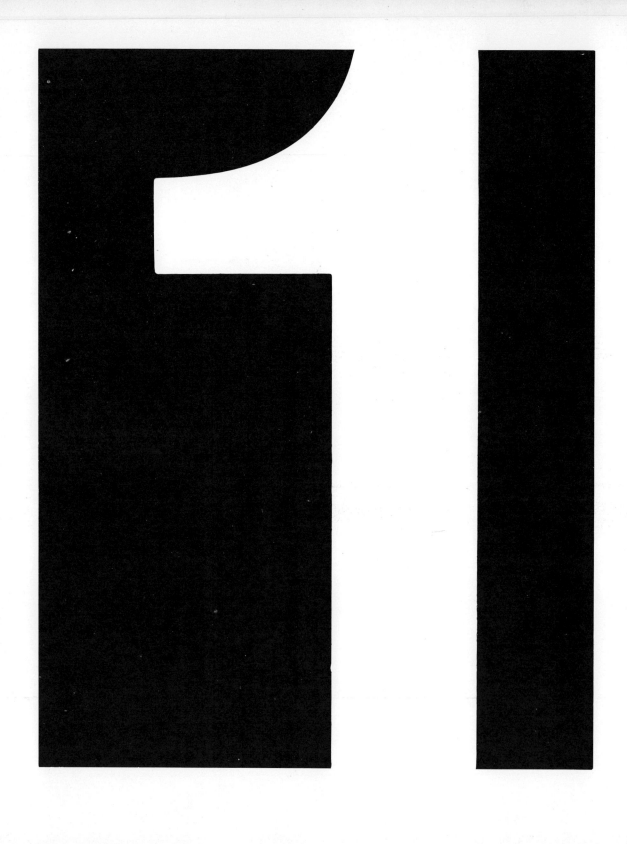

the healthy mother and infant

Society is changing. People's needs and ideas are changing. This is not a new thought by any means, but what may be new to many nursing and medical personnel is that modes of delivering health care are not as they used to be. Men and women today want more information and knowledge about the functioning of their bodies, and they are demanding that institutions be more responsive to their needs.

Traditions are being examined and challenged. The role of what could be considered the oldest institution, the family, is being questioned and redefined. The family in the traditional sense referred to either the *nuclear family* (husband, wife, and children) or the *extended family*, which might include grandparents, great-grandparents, uncles, aunts, and cousins. These two types of family arrangement are still the most common. But today the family may be defined much more loosely. One definition of a family could be two or more persons living together (or in separate facilities) who feel bound together, through legal means or not, for mutual sharing, caring, comforting, support, companionship, and pleasure. They may feel related in body and/or in spirit. Another definition of a family could be almost any group of persons who care about one another, have a commitment to one another, and think of themselves as a family. Obviously, we all have our own ideas about what constitutes a family.

What, then are the purpose and function of the family? Traditionally and historically the family was established for the continuation of the human race. Childbearing and child rearing were its primary functions. Transmission of traditions and beliefs, companionship, discipline, instilling of morals and values, providing of affection and security, tending to the physical, emotional, and psychologic needs of its members were, and in many instances still are, the functions of the family.

Many of these traditional functions and roles have been modified or changed over the years. Churches and schools have assumed some of the functions originally filled by the family. Health-care facilities have taken over others. Increasing mobility has had a hand in the changing of society and the altering of the family picture. New or modified functions are being considered. Duvall states, "The new image of family life is that of the nurturing center for human development," and then goes on to describe six emergent, nontraditional functions: (1) affection . . . ; (2) personal security and acceptance of each family member for the unique individual he is . . . ; (3) satisfaction and a sense of purpose; (4) continuity of companionship and association; (5) social placement and socialization; (6) establishing limits . . . and a sense of what is right . . ." (1).

Young people and older people today are questioning the old established institutions, including marriage, family, child rearing, and male-female roles. When so many couples divorce or separate, young people are dubious of the need, value, and purpose of marriage as their parents and grandparents experienced it. As a result they are deciding that they want neither the finality of marriage nor the trauma of divorce should the marriage bonds disintegrate. And so, many alternative styles and forms of "togetherness" are being tried and tested and are proving satisfactory for those involved. Take a look at some of the alternative styles discussed below.

Some men and women live together without marrying. They desire the closeness of a relationship with a member of the opposite sex without the limitations and finality of ties and bonds. Children may or may not be involved.

Even some older widowed people are living together without marrying lest they lose pensions and social security benefits from their former mates. For both economic reasons and companionship they live together without marrying.

Many couples or groups of the same sex live together for a variety of reasons such as economic, social, and emotional factors and companionship.

Communal living for mutual sharing and for the rearing of children is expanding throughout the country. Couples, singles, marrieds, separated people are gathering together in single or multiple dwellings to share chores, tasks of rearing and educating children, companionship, fellowship, sorrows and joys. For many, communal living is an attempt to get back to basic living off the land. They raise their own food, build their own structures, teach one another, and sometimes confine themselves to their acreage, literally shutting out the world. This way of living may be an attempt to simplify life, to gain peace and serenity of body and soul, and to counteract a materialistic society that fosters competition and the gaining of more and more material possessions. Those who have chosen to live

in communes are very often involved in the home delivery experience.

Another family arrangement, that of the single parent with child or children, is a result of separation, divorce, widowhood, or the desire of a single person to raise a child without being married or having a mate. Today single men and women who may or may not have been previously married are able to adopt children or take in foster children. The out-of-wedlock pregnant girl may also fit in this category if she decides to keep her baby and raise it without a partner.

Along with traditions and institutions, the roles of family members have changed drastically over the past 75 years. With the liberation of people from "role-assigned" tasks, women are emerging into a new life style. Some of them are no longer content to be limited to a life of domesticity. They want to prove to themselves and society that they are intellectually, socially, and economically capable.

The role of men is also changing. More and more men, having attended childbirth classes, are sharing in the joys and experience of childbirth, and from the moment of birth are sharing in the responsibilities and pleasures of caring for their children. "This surge of paternal involvement comes in part from the fading of traditional, rigidly separated sex roles. Another cause is that in an increasingly impersonal society, men have greater emotional need of their families" (2). In some settings the man has even reversed roles with his mate. He stays home and she goes to work. In some instances both parents work.

In turn little girls are encouraged to participate more in physical education and activities which were formerly limited to boys, and boys are being liberated from the roles that limited them to physical activities and contact sports; they are now allowed to enjoy playing with dolls, sewing, cooking, and baby-sitting. It is no longer considered babyish or effeminate for a boy to express tender feelings or to cry when he is hurt.

Along with these changes, nursing and medical care are also changing, slowly becoming more community-centered, less hospital-oriented. In the past, hospitals have appeared to function primarily for the convenience of doctors, nurses, laboratory technicians, and other staff workers, with the patient being required to fit into their plans and schedules. If a thoughtful person should ask why this situation continued, a typical response might be, "It works most efficiently this way."

Recently some hospitals have begun to take a look at their policies and to ease the divisions between themselves and the communities. Clinics are being established out in the communities, where people can receive treatments and minor surgery without having to be away from the family overnight.

A radical reorientation of health delivery is needed in maternity care. There are some evidences on the horizon that changes are happening. Visiting hours and privileges on maternity floors are slowly changing. Some hospitals are allowing children of all ages to visit their mother; others are permitting fathers to feed and care for their babies in the hospital.

Many couples, however, have turned their backs on hospital-centered maternity care and have decided to do-it-themselves at home.[1] Because of the increased desire for home deliveries, the entire question of providing services for these deliveries will have to be reevaluated. Whether a patient delivers at home, with skilled assistance and with a stand-by emergency squad, or in the hospital, competent prenatal care should be available to all if we are to improve the infant

and maternal morbidity and mortality rates in our country.

Working more closely with visiting nurse associations and public health agencies and clinics, nursing must move its focus beyond the hospital doors and out into the community.

Nurses may have to alter the focus of their care from doing to teaching others to do. Some hospitals, with the consent of the doctor, are relinquishing to the patients themselves the sacred task of dispensing medications (3). This is allowing the nurse more time to spend with the patient and her family in teaching them various aspects of child and maternal care.

Today's nurse can become involved in promoting optimum maternal and infant health by encouraging her neighbor to get prenatal care, teaching a friend about the prevention of pregnancy, talking with a young unwed teen-ager about the options open to her, and referring families to services they may need.

This is an exciting time for nurses and nursing. The challenges and changes in our society are being reflected in health-care trends. The changing focus of maternal and infant services in our country will give the nurse a greater opportunity than ever before to participate in the shaping of the future health and goals of our society.

---

references

1. Evelyn Millis Duvall, *Family Development*, 4th ed., J. B. Lippincott Company, Philadelphia, 1971, pp. 4–7.
2. "The New Fathers," *Life Magazine*, **73**(2):69, 1972.
3. Karen Herman, "Self-administration of Medication; A Plus for the Patient," *Journal of Gynecology and Neonatal Nursing*, **3**(1):27–30, 1974.

---

[1]At the Seventh Biennial Convention of the International Childbirth Education Association held in Milwaukee in May 1972 it was reported by Lester Hazell that there were more than 100 home deliveries per month in northern California.

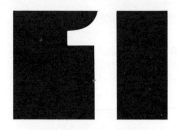

preparation for parenthood

Elizabeth J. Dickason
M. Christine Dobson
Lois D. Young

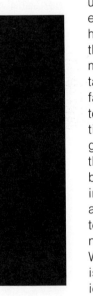

the healthy family

The birth of a baby is the exciting highlight in maternal and infant nursing. This event is unique for each mother and baby. Every expectant mother, whether the pregnancy is her first or tenth, has an experience special to the context of her own life and family. What it means to be a parent, to have a baby, and to take care of that baby, differs widely from family to family and from the birth of one child to another within the same family. The relationships among mother, father, siblings, and grandparents affect this experience, as does the family's social, religious, and ethnic background. The mother, of course, is vitally important in the childbearing process, but so are the other members of the core or extended family, because they supply the needed support for the mother and infant. When studying maternal and infant nursing, it is important, therefore, to place the experience of childbearing within this larger context.

Just as there is a medical diagnosis of pregnancy, there should be a diagnosis of the factual and emotional understanding of the pregnancy and the meaning it has for the mother and her family. Where there are gaps or misconceptions, education must be provided. Thus there is a larger dimension to the role of the nurse or whoever takes the responsibility for family education during the period of childbearing.

Each pregnant woman who comes for medical care brings with her various concepts, formed by a variety of experiences through the years of her growing up, about sex, motherhood, the birth process, family relations, and child care. Some of her understandings may be incorrect, mixed with fantasy or anxiety, and highly colored by her prior experiences. Examples of misconceptions that hinder a healthy pregnancy or labor are those connected with food taboos during pregnancy and those that aggravate fear and tension during labor.

How can we discover the specific questions, fears, misconceptions of each mother? How do we learn the context that an individual person represents? Where would assessment have to be done in order to provide her with supportive, clarifying information for the pregnancy, infant care, or family planning between pregnancies? Cohen suggests some simple questions that can elicit facts on which to base information-giving at the level of the particular person's concerns or needs (1). As you, the nursing student, study this text, you will learn some ways of assisting a mother after listening to her responses to these questions.

1. How long have you lived in this immediate area, and where does most of your family live?
2. How often do you see your mother or other close relatives?
3. Has anything happened to you in the past, or do you currently have any conditions which cause you to worry about the pregnancy or the baby?
4. What was your husband's reaction to your being pregnant?

5. What other responsibilities do you have outside the family?

It would also help the educator to know how the patient was mothered—whether she was neglected or deprived in childhood, or grew up in a warm, intact family. Supporting this need is a study which showed that women deprived of adequate parenting before age eleven had greater difficulty assuming the maternal role with their own infants (2).

The pregnant woman needs the understanding support of the maternal health professionals whom she encounters. Assessment of her situation is needed but is not often adequately included in prenatal care. Sometimes it is done within a formal series of classes in a prenatal clinic as general questions are asked to elicit the concerns of the group. Many times it is squeezed into a regularly scheduled checkup. In this case, if the mother can see the same physician for each pregnancy, she may develop a good rapport and be able to discuss problems and questions. Many women, however, go through clinics where a different person sees them at each visit and someone else cares for them at the time of delivery. Often, then, the only place where a woman may verbalize her concerns is in the hospital when she is ready to deliver. By then the task of teaching and assessment is difficult and arbitrary. Consequently, much attention is being given these days to formalizing education on family life and sex so that people will face childbearing with more adequate preparation in the biologic, social, and psychologic aspects of parenting.

some aspects of family life and sex education based upon developmental levels

The most natural and effective place for beginning and continuing preparation for parenthood is within the family itself. The attitudes of parents are most influential in a child's understanding of his or her sexual identity, the basic foundation underlying the child's future ability to parent. We know that when family relationships have disturbed the basic establishment of masculine and feminine identity in children, formal education is often ineffective.

As Wilbur and Aug so aptly stated: "The most important aspect of sex education is preparing the child to receive sexual knowledge. Planning formal sexual education for children is a secondary force in the development of the sexual life: parental attitudes remain the primary one" (3).

Unfortunately for many in our population, basic education to assume adult parental roles with confidence and pleasure is not adequately taking place in the family context. In some situations, schools, churches, community centers, medical and adolescent pediatric services, and maternal and infant care services are trying, with difficulty, to bridge the gap. Nurses are becoming involved in each of these areas.

A nursing curriculum emphasizes certain aspects of the basic content needed for teaching parents and children, but other related courses, such as human growth and development, and child psychology, contribute to the comprehensive viewpoint of the nurse-teacher. Because the need for education in family life and sex appears to be so widespread, the task of educating parents in this area, and of helping them to communicate more freely with their children on these subjects, has become part of the role of maternal and child health workers (4).

Whatever is done in education for parents or children must be guided by the principles stated by Fraiberg:

Sex instruction per se is successful whenever it has served the purpose of strengthening the child's satisfaction in his own sexual role and his destiny in this sexual role, and when it has dealt with the facts of procreation, of anatomy, of sexual feelings in such a way that the child's guilt and anxiety are reduced, and his confidence and love of his parents are deepened. (5).

"I don't want my child to be taught about sex at such an early age. She's too young!" This objection from a parent is typical and shows a lack of perception of child development. It may also reflect some fears of the parent about this area of life. A recognition of some of the basic concepts about development in young children would help parents to have a much greater understanding and provide for a more open relationship with their own children in the area of family relationships and sex education. Following are some concepts to keep in mind when working with parents or children:

1. Development is a process, and every variable changes with age. The growth tasks of the first years of life are repeated in adolescence on a different level. The child's needs, awareness, and struggles will change as he develops physically and psychologically.

2. Readiness to learn is a guiding principle in all education. Children retain only what they are ready for at a given age. Children are very open, when allowed to be, with their questions and feelings. Their own understandings should be explored before information or explanations are given. Children's questions about sex need to be answered openly in a matter-of-fact manner as any other questions are answered, simply and without long, complex explanations.

3. Sexuality is more than sex. All human beings from infancy have sexual responses that should be recognized. Some of the ways these responses are demonstrated are by loving and receiving love,

by being able to perceive and enjoy sensations, touch, smell, color, taste, by enjoying exploring and being playful.

4. Sex education for young children deals with sex not as eroticism but as a normal body function. Early direction is in establishing masculine and feminine identity as the child works through the struggle of "Who am I?"

When parents are aware of the developmental stages of their children, their own communication may become more meaningful, since the children give clear signals as to where they are in their growth. Parents may need reassurance that there is no danger in a child's learning more than he is ready for. Generally, children will not show interest in or retain what is beyond their level. If there is, however, covert anxiety about giving information, the child will retain the anxiety that is engendered in him and will become secretive and noncommunicative with the parent. Anxiety may be reduced by treating the subject as normally as if discussing why it rains. It is especially helpful to the child in dealing with normal fantasies to elicit his thoughts first. A simple factual explanation can then follow. The facts are the same at each interest level, but the detail of presentation varies with the growth process. At each level there can be emphasis appropriate to the developmental stage of the child.

INFANCY

From birth to three or three and one-half years, the child moves from being totally dependent on the parent for all his basic needs toward independence. He works through three basic developmental tasks, first establishing basic *trust* in a completely dependent, symbiotic relationship with one or more mothering persons. The second major step in development, *autonomy*, is learning to survive independently of these key persons. This is a gradual process, with the child separating from the parent at first for short moments, later for longer lengths of time. Negative behavior begins at about age two, when development of his own strengths leads to the realization, "I can do it myself!" Toilet training is another step in independent functioning at this age.

During this period parents can learn to foster healthy attitudes in their children, particularly through accepting a child's exploration of his body and his environment, through accepting and responding naturally to bowel movements, urinary functions, and food, using correct names for body parts, setting limits of behavior, and encouraging the child's expression of his feelings about himself.

CHILDHOOD

Between the ages of three and six, a child will continue working on the third task, *individuation*, exploring roles to decide who he or she will be. "Will I be like mommy or daddy, be a doctor, a dog, a cowboy, a kitten?" Children at this age find it hard to distinguish between thoughts, feelings, and actions. They move easily from one "play role" to another at home. Many children begin to have preschool experience by three and one-half to four years of age in head-start or preschool programs. They will act out many of their concerns in everyday play situations. A great deal of time is spent in the doll corner playing mommy and daddy (usually taking interchangeable roles), imitating whatever they have seen at home.

Some Aspects of Teaching Emphasis for Preschoolers Since a difference between sexes is recognized during this period, any preschool education in family life and sex is directed toward focusing on and reinforcing an awareness of relationships within the family. Recognition of the composition of families, understanding the immediate and extended family, and seeing how families differ within the group, may be focal points of teacher-child discussions. Simple concepts of life, death, growth, and learning are introduced by realistic examples from families. Most birth- and sex-related questions are answered within the framework of simple factual answers without elaboration. It is important to give proper names to body parts and to realize that there is considerable curiosity, and some anxiety, at this age about why a boy has a penis and a girl does not.

Three- to four-year-olds are unable to conceptualize how a baby got inside the mother. Like the child who asked his mother to open her mouth and called down her throat, "Hi, baby," they may fantasize that the baby is in the stomach and can hear them. Thus, when asked where the baby grows, it is not helpful to say, "In mommy's stomach." An adequate factual answer would be, "The baby grows inside the mother," holding more explanation until the child asks further questions.

Between the ages of five and six, there is a keen desire to be "big." There is more clear identification with the parent of the same sex, as well as a diminishing of the rivalry that has been experienced in attachment to parent of the opposite sex.

Some Aspects of Teaching Emphasis for Primary School From the ages of six to twelve, the child has no additional psychologic steps to master. Children are in a rest period psychologically, and if development has been successful, they can concentrate on school and play. They will acquire a great deal of their knowledge of concepts and skills during this time. The child will have many questions about all subjects as he goes about acquiring knowledge. Questions pour forth, interest flowing from animals to plants to human beings: how things come from seeds or cells, why human beings are mammals, how human mammals and other mammals

feed and protect their young, what babies look like inside the mother. What about multiple births, hospitals, doctors? Curiosity about abnormalities, monsters, siamese twins, and cross-species fertilization might mislead the parent or teacher into thinking that the child is more sophisticated in his knowledge than he is. He may be merely checking out his own fantasies or clearing up misinformation.

GRADES 1 TO 3 (AGES SIX TO NINE) Teaching objectives at level of grades 1 to 3 are related to reducing anxieties and fantasies of the prepubertal child. Giving factual information can help to correct misconceptions from peer information. The exchange of sex information among children goes on and is the child's chief source of information and anxiety when families or schools do not assume their responsibilities.

All children have to learn self-control and discipline. These developmental tasks can be emphasized in the first three grades as the child learns the responsibilities of being a family member, helping with household tasks, looking out for younger children, contributing to the smooth functioning of his own home.

Emphasis is on developing wholesome attitudes toward the body, use of correct terms, and an active vocabulary in reference to the body. The child learns to speak openly in an appropriate setting. His curiosity about how things work predominates. He learns avidly, likes to start and complete projects and to have a sense of accomplishment. A strong motive in conversation is the need to excel: to be the wittiest or the fastest, to exaggerate knowledge—all in order to ward off failure.

GRADES 4 TO 6 (AGES TEN TO TWELVE) Each year the child shows more distinct needs than in earlier years. In the fourth grade, objectives are directed toward preparation for puberty, and the teacher can start giving basic information on menstruation on a co-ed basis. Personal hygiene, friendship, and family relationships continue to be discussed as questions arise.

The beginning of secondary sexual characteristics precedes the start of *menstruation* (menarche) in the adolescent by at least 2 years. Breast budding and pubic hair will have begun to develop before the puberty growth spurt which takes place about 1 year before menarche. The growth spurt results in unfamiliarity with body movements, size, and shape, and makes some girls appear awkward and uncoordinated. Others appear to bloom suddenly, surprising everyone around them, as did one teen-ager who grew 9 in and 25 lb in the 7 months after her eleventh birthday. This growth spurt varies in when it occurs, of course, but invariably as it slows, menstruation occurs (6).

Semmens (7) has suggested a timetable to alert physicians and those who work with children. Puberty preparation can be made interesting and nonthreatening for the child if puberty is presented as a biologic time clock that follows a regular normal pattern. Girls can anticipate puberty as the sign of growing up with the same pleasure and anticipation as the five- and six-year-old looks forward to "being big enough to go to school."

In the United States, a recent study showed that menarche occurs at 12.7 ± 1.2 (SD) years. Better nutrition appears to be associated with an earlier menarche (8). Boys mature at an average of 6 to 12 months later than girls (9).

By the fifth grade, because the body gets ready physically for parenthood long before emotional readiness occurs, there should be discussion of the principle that sexual experimentation carries with it a responsibility which a child may not be able to handle. Human reproduction is taught in more detail. Discussion of the normality of friendships between the same sex at this age is important, because peer group anxieties, produced by pressure from older children (or parents), often move ten- to twelve-year-olds

into precocious heterosexuality. The objective is to make the child aware of and comfortable with the developmental tasks of his own age group.

ADOLESCENCE

Beginning at about twelve years of age, the child is thrown into a tremendous whirl as he faces physical and psychologic changes. "The rapid growth in height and weight creates an unfamiliarity with his body. Development of secondary sexual characteristics not only adds to this unfamiliarity but also forces adulthood on him" (10).

The adolescent, in a sense, retraces all his earlier psychologic steps, needing to establish basic trust, autonomy, and individuation again for himself. This is a replay of infancy and early childhood development in a new way which will allow the individual to operate as a person in the world.

Much has been written about the developmental tasks and needs during adolescence. The nurse working with this age group should become familiar with the classic literature (7, 11).

Some Aspects of Teaching Emphasis for Junior High School (ages 13 to 14) At this age level, all information given earlier in relation to sexual development and sexuality is reiterated with more complex explanations. Problems specific to this group include inherent tensions in the early teen years, rapid uneven growth, heterosexual urges without enough emotional security and maturity to deal with all the changes that occur. Some discussion is needed of appropriate defenses against unhealthy sexual approaches from adults to teen-agers.

That their decisions and behavior will always have results begins to become a reality for teen-agers. Some suggested areas for discussion in keeping with their interests are the meaning of peer approval, self-image, choices of friends, choices of recreation. Parent-child relationships are being strained by the changes of these years; frequently children in the early teens welcome adult, non-parental counsel.

Discussions should anticipate and emphasize positive explanations rather than give negative warnings regarding pubertal changes. The discussion leader needs to be careful not to get too deeply into the "feelings" to be anticipated, thus cutting off the spontaneous and discovering quality of personal experiences in this stage of adolescent development.

At this level teen-agers are also curious about details of sex, including conception, the meaning of family planning, fetal development, and homosexuality. Social issues in which they may have intense interest are drug addiction, abortion, pornography in films and literature, marriage and divorce, and communal living. Their interest is not in the detailed aspects, as it will be later, but in the moral aspects.

The important question is, "What is right for me?" Children during these years seem to be asking for leadership from adults on "which way to go," yet they often reject parental guidance. Indecision or ambivalence seems to typify the age. Coupled with indecision might be marked anxiety centered around how masculine or feminine they appear. The changing body image is often reflected in popularity; those who develop earlier look on those who are slower to mature with some pity. Popularity is extremely important, peer approval critical, and failure devastating.

Emphasis in family life and sex education would be well placed on developmental expectations and moral issues, with discussion about choices and their results. Some understanding can be imparted of independence vs. dependency needs to the extent that the struggle is part of the difficulty with parents. Seeking parental guidance somehow implies to the adolescent, "I am still a child," yet he needs and wants guidance. Adults who understand this dilemma can be supportive role models.

Some Aspects of Teaching Emphasis for High School (ages 15 and over) Emphasis in family life and sex education on the high school level is placed on preparation for adult tasks and roles. Sexual identity is completed during this period. Discussions now become far more sophisticated in relation to cultural, religious, and socioeconomic problems. Education is continued toward making choices for specific careers, family structures, and methods of child spacing. Toward the end of this period, parental relationships take on new meaning, and exchanges may begin again, with opinions from both sides beginning to emerge more positively.

Consideration of sex, sexuality, and sensuality takes on new dimensions. Discussion of these topics perhaps is preparation for the next task of finding a partner for adult relationships. Preparation, then, for the next step reflects more sophisticated interest in discussion related to the political aspects of issues such as ecology, population, housing, and implications of the changing roles in society.

By the time this age level is reached there should be thorough knowledge of human reproduction. Interest may now be focused on specific health aspects and ways of obtaining health care, with some discussion of the rights of patients. The task of beginning a family may be anticipated, as well as the more complex tasks of maintaining family responsibilities and relationships. Preparation for pregnancy, delivery, and child care can be included in discussions at this level. Now the teen-ager's own family situation is viewed more objectively and can be used in general discussions freer of the earlier fears of disapproval.

By the end of high school, the task of individuation has progressed. The adolescent's problems have become more personalized, and counseling is increasingly sought on a more individualized basis. Discussions remain a lively source of exploring, testing, and defining his own values as his own philosophy emerges.

For many adolescents, finishing high school marks the end of their formal education. Many women, or couples, attending clinics for prenatal care will have reached the end of education in the area of family life and sex. The fact is that many schools in the country give much less attention to preparation for the future than is discussed above. Therefore it becomes the responsibility of the medical personnel in community education, family crises clinics, and pediatric and maternal care services to continue as is possible what seems to be essential preparation for parenting.

Today, thorough preparation for parenthood, then, includes knowledge of the reproductive functions, conception and contraception, and the process of growth and development of children. Information given in this text concerning sex education, family planning, and abortion may not necessarily be acceptable to all who use the book. The material, however, is presented factually, for the information of students, for nurses must know the trends in society in order effectively to help patients find resources for their lives.

All the information in the chapters to follow is available to help the nurse who becomes involved in the education of the family during the time of preparation for or during the childbearing years.

planned parenthood

Faced with the inescapable fact of an uncontrollable world population, we have few years left to us for choices about fertility levels, food supplies, and natural resources. Responsible health professionals in maternal and child services will find themselves inevitably involved in the issues surrounding the fertility of human beings.

Guttmacher has stated that in 12 generations, from 1650 to 1972, the world population rose from 1.5 billion to about 3.7 billion (12). Because of the radical drop in death rates (basically, death control) due to greater control over diseases and better health and nutrition, population figures in most countries have risen spectacularly. The intricate interdependence of population, production, ecology, and natural resources is finally being widely recognized. Few, if any, would advocate euthanasia to reduce population, yet many theoretically would allow people to die slowly from starvation rather than have them taught forms of contraception. Preventive health appears a more sane choice, and in spite of the innumerable obstacles of custom, ignorance, opposition, and indifference, the trend is toward government-supported voluntary fertility planning.

Guttmacher (13) has indicated four ways to control population:

1. Postponement of marriage to more advanced age (as in mainland China today)
2. Use of contraception
3. Use of postconceptional control
4. Use of sterilization

These avenues are unevenly followed in the world today. The first usually can be enforced only in a tightly controlled social system, but abstinence is, of course, the most effective means of preventing births.

The second, contraception, has been practiced more widely in Western countries among middle and upper income groups. Inadequate health services and dissemination of information to lower income groups was responsible for their high birth rate in this country. Since 1965, when information became more available to those served by public clinics in New York City, for instance, the birth rate among mothers on welfare has gradually dropped until it now approximates that of middle and upper income women. It would appear that given a choice, most women do not want to conceive each year.

New and more effective methods of contraception have led to more widespread acceptance. It is estimated that the majority of couples in the United States now use some form of child-spacing method, not necessarily effectively.

The third method includes voluntary abortion as the most widely practiced form of postconceptional control in the world today. Menstrual extraction and postconceptional vaginal suppositories or oral tablets which precipitate an overdue menstrual period are all methods which in reality are abortive techniques.

The fourth method, sterilization, is gaining in acceptance in the world. Permanent for the most part, tubal ligation and vasectomy methods are being simplified so that they can be more readily available to more persons.

methods of family planning

MENSTRUAL CYCLE

A basic knowledge of anatomy and cyclic hormonal change in the woman is necessary to understand how conception can occur or can be prevented (Fig. 1·1).

The phases of the menstrual cycle coincide with changes in hormonal output from the hypothalamus, pituitary, ovaries, and the adrenal glands. The cycle is divided into *preovulatory* and *postovulatory* phases, for each of which specific terms describe the functions that are occurring in the ovary or uterus and concurrently in hormonal secretion.

Preovulatory Phase The primary changes during the preovulatory phase are the development of the graafian follicle (named for de Graaf, who described its function), the build-up of the endometrium (the lining of the uterus) to receive the fertilized ovum; and the rise in the levels of estrogen, the dominant hormone of the phase. The preovulatory

phase may therefore be called, in reference to ovarian function, the *follicular* or *estrogenic* phase, and in reference to the uterus, the *proliferative* phase. This period of time is one of few overt bodily changes; estrogen levels are low at first, gradually reaching a peak just before ovulation (Fig. 1·2).

The menstrual cycle ranges from 22 to 35 days in length for most women, but a number of women have a longer or shorter cycle. The preovulatory phase will vary in length (depending on the total length of the cycle) from about 7 to 8 days in the 22-day cycle to about 20 to 21 days in the 35-day cycle. Although most women average between 26 to 29 days in a cycle, menstrual cycles may vary in interval by as much as 3 or 4 days within 1 year. Women also may have different amounts of hormone production from cycle to cycle and thus may be irregular or have stretches of amenorrhea or anovulatory cycles, especially when adolescent, premenopausal, or under stress. The average adult woman (age twenty-two to forty-five) has the least variation and the fewest anovulatory cycles (about 15 percent each year). In contrast, the young teen-ager (age twelve to fourteen) may ovulate during only 15 percent of her cycles (14).

Since in every woman, ovulation usually occurs 14 days ± 2 *before* the next menstruation, if a cycle varies in length, it does so during the preovulatory phase. One of the reasons for this regularity of the postovulatory phase is that the life span of the corpus luteum is only 12 to 16 days in any cycle without fertilization.

Ovulation Ovulation is triggered by the rapid peaking of the leutinizing hormone (LH) plus a slight drop in estrogen (Fig. 3·11). Ovulation is thought to occur the day after the peak in LH is reached (15). Symptoms of the ovulatory period are minimal and usually are undetectable unless the woman is taught to look for them. A very few women feel an abdominal sensation at the time of ovulation, a midcycle pain, *mittelschmerz.*

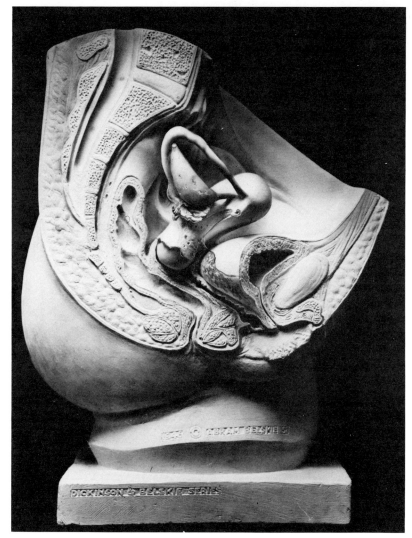

fig. 1·1 Three-dimensional view of female reproductive organs. Note how the uterus tips forward (i.e., is anteflexed), causing the cervix to enter the vagina at an angle. (*Reproduced with permission from* A Baby Is Born, Maternity Center Association, New York, 1964.)

The most apparent sign of approaching ovulation is the distinctive change in the cervical mucus. Women can observe this sign at home for 2 to 3 days just before ovulation (days 11 to 14 of a 28-day cycle).

During the preovulatory period, cervical mucus has been yellowish and viscid. Two to three days before ovulation, it changes markedly to a clear, colorless liquid, with a stringy consistency and a stretchability that can be measured. An applicator is inserted into the vagina to the cervix and mucus removed and applied to a slide. The mucus can then be stretched out with a cover glass

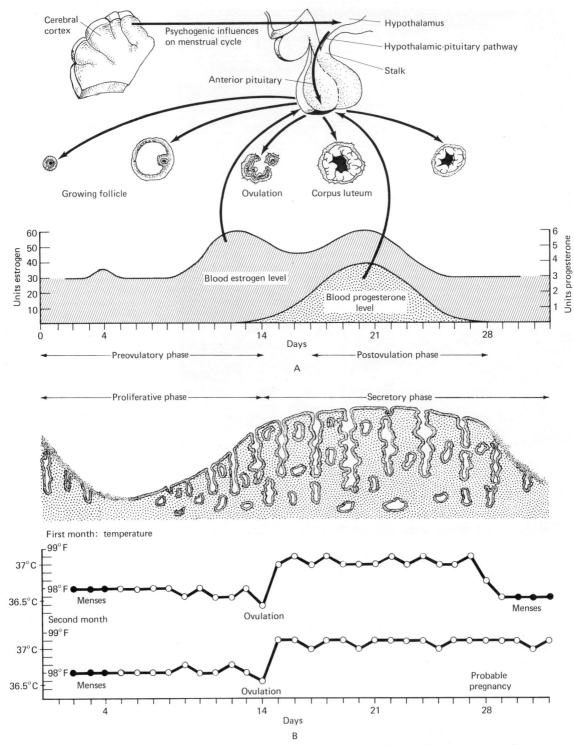

fig. 1·2 Hormonal control of the menstrual cycle. A Hormonal changes paralleling follicular changes. B Endometrial changes correlated with body temperature. (*From R. C. Benson*, Handbook of Obstetrics and Gynecology, 4*th ed., Lange Medical Publications, Los Altos, Calif.,* 1971.)

or a wooden spatula to more than 6 cm and up to 15 cm (16). Termed *spinnbarkheit*, this sign indicates the marked changes in mucus intended to "welcome" the sperm. The changes favor sperm survival and motility by providing a more alkaline environment with a higher saline and glucose content and fewer leukocytes. The mucus pattern itself changes to allow penetration by the sperm, as indicated by dried mucus on a slide observed under a microscope. During the preovulatory period, it will be granular; during ovulation it will have crystallized to a distinct "fern pattern"; and after ovulation it will again have a viscous, impenetrable quality.

Basal Body Temperature (BBT) The growth of the corpus luteum from the ruptured graafian follicle causes a sudden rise in progesterone, which causes several of the indications useful in determining when ovulation has occurred. The thermogenic action of progesterone raises the body temperature during the postovulatory phase. About the time of ovulation there is a drop of 0.1 to 0.2°C (0.2 to 0.4°F) below the base-line temperature, with an elevation of 0.5 to 0.6°C (0.8 to 1.0°F) above the lowest point by the next morning (Fig. 1·2). The temperature stays elevated until corpus luteum function diminishes. If pregnancy ensues in the cycle, the temperature remains elevated instead of dropping back to its preovulatory range.

Postovulatory phase The corpus luteum secretes large amounts of progesterone, the hormone which sustains the secreting, thick endometrium to receive and nourish the fertilized ovum. If fertilization does not occur, about 8 days after ovulation the corpus luteum begins to shrink; thus the progesterone level drops slowly, reaching a very low level by 1 to 2 days before the next menstruation begins again. The postovulatory phase is therefore called the *secretory* phase when referring to uterine function, and the *luteal* or *progestational* phase when referring to ovarian function.

During this phase some women experience extracellular edema (fluid retention), which sometimes causes a weight gain of up to 10 lb. Muscle irritability, an increase in pelvic blood supply (bloated feeling), and an increased capillary fragility (easier bruising) may be experienced by others. Tender, enlarged breasts (mastalgia) may indicate to others that the ovulatory period has passed and that they are well into the postovulatory phase.

Menstruation The sloughing of the endometrium is a result of the inhibiting action of progesterone on the oxidation of estrogen products. Without oxidation the production of LH and LTH (luteotropic hormone) is prevented, and without these supportive hormones the corpus luteum regresses. Thus, there is a true cycle of interdependent effects. Inhibition of hormonal function leads to *ischemia* (a reduction of blood supply to the thick endometrium). Bleeding begins, carrying with it glandular and tissue fragments and the two superficial layers of the uterine lining, leaving the basal layer next to the endometrium (Fig. 3·12). Flow lasts 3 to 5 days, with a volume of 60 to 80 ml as an average. The blood usually does not contain many clots; it does contain cellular debris, leukocytes, endometrial secretions, cervical mucus, and blood plasma. Menstruation is a definite point ending the cycle; therefore the first day of the last menstrual period is noted in calculating the interval of cycles.

THE RHYTHM METHOD

A couple choosing to use the natural body cycle as a guide to the time of fertility will have to learn about the phases of the cycle, the signs of approaching ovulation, and the body-temperature changes.

The first rule for calculation of the beginning of the abstinence period, using the calendar, is based on the woman's having kept a record of the interval of her menses for 3 to 6 months. She then counts the number of days in her shortest menstrual cycle and the number of days in the longest. She figures:

Day *A* = the number of days in the shortest cycle *minus* 18

Day *Z* = the number of days in the longest cycle *minus* 11

For example, a woman's cycle varies from 27 to 30 days. Day $A = 27 - 18$, or *day 9*. Day $Z = 30 - 11$, or *day 19* of her cycle. The fertile period for this person, then, is from *day A to day Z,* i.e., day 9 through day 19. These days are called the "unsafe" days. During this time she should take her basal body temperature and record it on a graph, looking for the checkpoint of the ovulation day. The end of the unsafe period can be modified by the BBT, for when three full days of temperature elevation have elapsed, even though the calendar count is incomplete, the couple may resume intercourse with little fear of pregnancy. Figure 1·2 indicates that during the first month, the woman could consider the evening of day 18 to be the beginning of the safe part of the postovulatory phase for that month.

EFFECTIVENESS If the couple are willing to follow the exact guidelines and be abstinent during the "fertile" period, the rhythm method is comparable in preventing conception to use of the diaphragm or condom alone. The failure rate is about 12 to 14 pregnancies per 100 women-years of use.[1] If basal body temperature is added correctly, the effectiveness rises to 2 to 3 pregnancies per 100 woman-years (17). (One hundred women-years of use = 50 women using a method for 2 years, or 100 women using a method for 1 year, or 25 women using a method for 4 years.) These rates are only generally comparable and include the pregnancies of those who may have

forgotten to follow the procedure. A highly motivated couple may find rhythm to be a successful contraceptive method for their life style.

The following factors influence effectiveness:

1. Without deliberate recording of cycle interval, few women can be sure that they have absolutely regular cycles.
2. Since ovulation can occur 14 days ± 2 before the next menstrual flow, the 4-day variation reduces the *predictive* value of the calendar method.
3. In some instances, ova and sperm are viable for longer than traditionally supposed (ovum, 24 h+; sperm, 48 h+).
4. Errors in temperature measurement can be made if infection or stress alters body metabolism or hormone production.
5. A tremendous amount of self-control and mutual agreement is needed to follow the rhythm method with BBT.

ADVANTAGES There are no side effects since the method is physiologic and part of a rhythm of life. Understood as such it can be a very effective method. There is no cost, other than for a thermometer, and no chemicals are needed.

WITHDRAWAL (COITUS INTERRUPTUS)

Coitus interruptus is an ancient technique of preventing conception. Before ejaculation, the male withdraws from the vagina so that semen is not deposited in or near the vagina.

This method takes skill since if any pre-ejaculate semen is deposited near the cervix, there may be enough sperm present to cause pregnancy. Withdrawal limits sexual satisfaction but is as effective a means of contraception as mechanical or chemical barriers. It has long been in use, and is of benefit to

[1]All rates of effectiveness are from "Methods of Birth Control in the United States," Planned Parenthood. New York 1972.

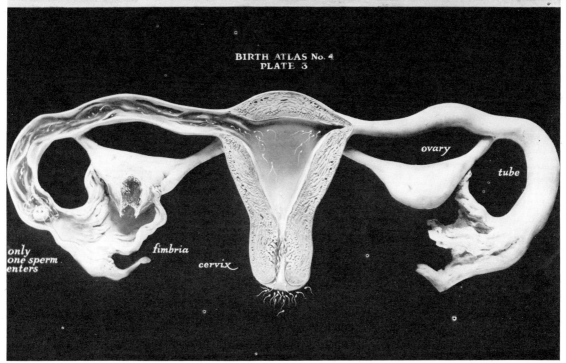

INSEMINATION : OVULATION : MEETING OF SPERM AND OVUM

BIRTH ATLAS No. 4
PLATE 3

ovary

tube

only
one sperm
enters

fimbria

cervix

fig. 1·3 Insemination, ovulation, fertilization. Chemical and mechanical barrier techniques of contraception would prevent sperm from entering the cervical opening. (*Reproduced with permission from* A Baby is Born, *Maternity Center Association, New York,* 1964.)

those who are accustomed to it or have no other method available.

CHEMICAL BARRIERS

Chemical barriers act to prevent sperm from moving up into the cervical canal and to reduce sperm motility; in varying degrees they are spermicidal. These barriers are produced in the form of jelly, cream, foam, or tablets; they have a similar mode of action, and each has its own degree of effectiveness and precautions based on the physiology of sperm function and motility. Sperm move most effectively and survive longest in an environment with a pH between 8.5 and 9.0,

i.e., much more alkaline than the normal vaginal pH. Motility is halted at a pH of 6 and destroyed below 4 (Fig. 1·3). The vagina normally has a pH of 4 to 5, being maintained in this acidic state by the Döderlein bacilli, which produce lactic acid. The preovulatory period supplies hormonal stimulus to change the vaginal pH gradually toward a more alkaline environment during the ovulatory phase, in order to "welcome" sperm. Vaginal chemical contraceptives act to turn the pH back toward 4, besides containing a spermicidal agent.

EFFECTIVENESS There are varying degrees of effectiveness among the different preparations. The Margaret Sanger Research Bureau has tested a wide variety of agents and can recommend certain preparations. A list of these is available from Planned Parenthood, 810 Seventh Avenue, New York 10019. Currently, there are about 24 different preparations, each with its own trade name and effectiveness rating.

Used alone as directed on the package insert, vaginal foam is considered more effective than jellies or creams. These chemical agents are much better than no protection, but are not as effective a mechanical barrier as a condom or diaphragm.

The following factors influence effectiveness:

1. Any chemical agent must be inserted close to the time of intercourse since the duration of effect is only about 1 h. It follows, then, that reapplication is necessary with repeated intercourse.
2. Used alone after pregnancy and delivery until full recovery, a double application is necessary because of the stretched vaginal and cervical tissue.
3. No douching is required as the preparations are hygienic and partially absorbed by the vaginal wall. No douche should take place within 6 h of intercourse, since douching would remove the barrier and the chemical effect, leaving some sperm to survive and enter the uterus.
4. A few users experience discomfort from chemical agents, either from a burning sensation or because of overlubrication of the vagina.

These agents do not need medical prescription and are available in any drug store. Purse-size unit kits are available for the mobile woman. For the person who is afraid to go to a physician for a variety of reasons, chemical contraception offers some protection. (Often a teen-ager will be more likely to use foam than to go for family planning counsel.) Some women feel that the method suits them best because it is so simple; its use parallels

insertion of a tampon and does not require manipulation of a device or change body physiology (Fig. 1·4).

MECHANICAL BARRIERS

Mechanical barriers that prevent access of sperm to the cervical opening have long been in use throughout the world. Until the recent development of hormonal contraception and the intrauterine device, mechanical barriers were the most widely used methods in the United States. Each takes manipulation or insertion just prior to intercourse and for that reason is considered a "bother" by many couples.

Diaphragm A curved rubber dome over a spring ring is inserted to cover the cervix, providing a mechanical barrier to sperm movement. Used with a spermicidal foam or jelly, the diaphragm effectively prevents sperm transport into the cervical opening. A diaphragm must be fitted by a physician, midwife, or other qualified person and checked every 2 years for fit; it must be refitted after each delivery and after marked weight gain or loss.

EFFECTIVENESS When the diaphragm is correctly fitted and used in combination with a spermicidal agent its failure rate is very low—2 to 3 pregnancies per 100 women-

fig. 1·4 Types of foam, jelly, and cream to be used with diaphragm for chemical contraception.

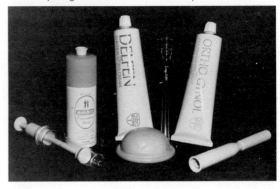

years (18). When used alone without chemical spermicide, its failure rate is equal to that of the condom used alone (12 to 14 percent).

The following factors influence effectiveness of a diaphragm:

1. About 2 in of jelly is squeezed out into the inner curved cup, and a ribbon of jelly is placed around the outer edges. The woman either lies down or stands with one leg up on a chair. The diaphragm, stretched longitudinally with an applicator, is then inserted into the vagina as far as the posterior fornix to cover the cervix. The anterior edge of the diaphragm should fit just behind the symphysis pubis. Placement should be checked by a finger. Once in place it should not be able to be dislodged, nor should it be felt by either partner during intercourse, but with unusual coital positions, there may be some chance of moving it out of place.
2. A diaphragm may be inserted within 6 h of intercourse. It must be left in place at least 6 h after intercourse for effectiveness.
3. Extra cream or jelly should be added if the diaphragm is inserted early or if intercourse is repeated.
4. A douche must not be used in this interval and is not necessary afterwards.

ADVANTAGES For the woman with a stable environment, the diaphragm is a satisfactory method. The device requires manipulation each time, but this is an easily learned technique and soon becomes routine. It does not affect body functioning in any way, and usually does not affect sensation during intercourse.

Condom The condom has been in use throughout the world since the sixteenth century. A rubber sheath placed to cover the erect penis, the condom prevents semen from entering the vagina.

EFFECTIVENESS Efficiency of the condom used alone parallels that of the diaphragm when used alone (12 to 14 pregnancies per 100 women-years of use.) For excellent protection, equal to that of the diaphragm with a spermicide, the woman can use foam or cream in addition to her partner's use of a condom.

The condom is a protection against venereal disease; its use is recommended to prevent reinfection when either partner is being treated for a genital infection such as *Trichomonas vaginalis* (Fig. 1·5).

The following factors influence effectiveness of the condom:

1. Several types include a small pouch at the end of the condom for the semen. If a pouch is not present, the man should leave about 1 in loose over the glans.
2. The condom is applied by rolling the rubber over the erect penis. Lubricated condoms should be warmed to body temperature. Nonlubricated ones may need extra lubrication with a water-soluble jelly before insertion if the woman is not sufficiently stimulated.
3. The penis must be removed from the vagina before erection diminishes in order to prevent the condom from slipping off and spilling semen into the vagina.
4. Some men state that the condom diminishes sensations. It must be put on during foreplay, before penetration into the vagina; thus it may interrupt foreplay if there is any difficulty in getting it in place.

ADVANTAGES Condoms are available everywhere in the world without prescription and are quite inexpensive. (Government-subsidized programs in some countries make condoms available for about a few pennies each.) Their use places some of the responsibility for contraception on the male partner. Women who may not have planned for contraception can insist that a condom be used if they do not wish to risk pregnancy. One study discovered that teen-agers would use condoms readily if they knew where to obtain them (19).

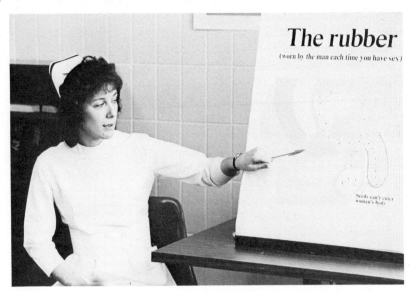

The rubber
(worn by the man each time you have sex)

Seeds can't enter woman's body

fig. 1·5 Nurse teaching class about the use of a condom. (*Photo by Nancy Goodman.*)

Cervical Cap A third type of mechanical barrier, similar to the diaphragm, is widely used in Europe but rather uncommon in the United States. A cervical cap must be fitted by the physician, and the woman must be well instructed in the method of placement and removal. One made of plastic can be left in place for several days and is sometimes left in place throughout the entire period between the menses. It *must* be left in place for at least 6 h after intercourse. The position of the cap should be checked, and, as with the diaphragm, a spermicidal agent should be inserted into the vagina prior to intercourse.

INTRAUTERINE DEVICE

Much has been written about the IUD, historically one of the oldest methods in use. Used in every country in some manner, the IUD has become since the 1960s one of the chief methods for effective, low-cost contraception. Population councils of every country facing a rising, uncontrollable birth rate have accepted the IUD as a device which can work toward lowering birth incidence.

Method of Action The method of action is still incompletely understood. Tubal and uterine motility are not significantly changed (after the first adjustment period), and ova travel freely down the tubes. It appears that the IUD has a local effect on the uterine environment. Being a foreign body, it calls forth a response of extra leukocytes and macrophages in the endometrial tissue.

There is a premature accumulation of glycogen granules in glandular tissue epithelia, thus putting the endometrium 'out of phase' with the developing ovum and preparing a hostile environment for implantation. As in experimental animals there is also an increased number of inflammatory cells in the endometrium and the uterine fluid. These observations form the basis of the present leading hypothesis linking the antifertility effect of the IUDs to a non-

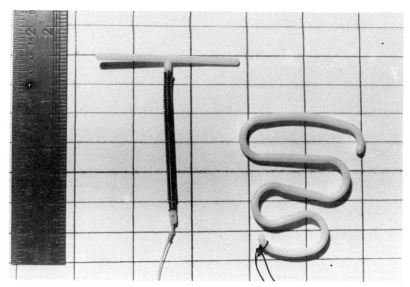

fig. 1·6 Copper T (300L) and the Lippes Loop. T Cu (300L) appears to have an effectiveness rating of 2 pregnancies per 100 women-years, an expulsion rate of 10 percent, and a removal rate of 16 percent, with a continuation rate of 71.4 percent. (*From Population Council, August,* 1973.) The Lippes Loop has an effectiveness rating of about 2 pregnancies per 100 women-years, with a continuation rate of 75 percent. (*From Family Planning Digest, March,* 1973.)

specific inflammatory cell reaction in which the IUD acts as a foreign body. (20)

This response to a noninfectious stimulus may change the endometrium so that implantation is faulty, or may somehow be toxic to the sperm as they travel up to the tubes. Metals, particularly copper, are now being added to IUDs because as they are slowly dissolved, they are spermicidal.

Whatever the process involved, it may be overridden and a pregnancy may take place; some implantations do occur. Should this happen, there is a rather high rate of spontaneous abortion (40 percent). In those pregnancies that continue to term, there is no effect on fetal development, since the IUD usually becomes part of the maternal side of the placenta and is rarely found within the amniotic sac (Fig. 1·6).

Insertion Insertion requires a medical examination, including a Papanicolaou smear for cancer cells and a culture for diagnosis of gonorrhea. Any chronic uterine or cervical infection would be an indication not to insert the IUD. It is done during the last few days of menses to ensure that there is no early pregnancy. Easier insertion is possible at this time because the cervix is more relaxed. Some physicians insert an IUD after a voluntary abortion or just after a delivery, but the rate of spontaneous expulsion is increased in these two cases (Fig. 1·7).

Side Effects There is a natural expulsive uterine reaction to the IUD which is most marked just after insertion. This reaction may continue through three or more cycles and is sensed by the woman as increased cramping and bleeding, particularly noticeable at the time of menstruation. IUD design affects the

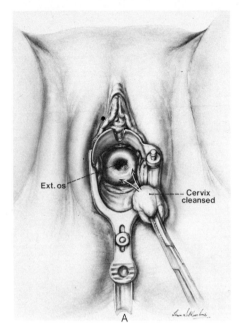

Ext. os

Cervix cleansed

A

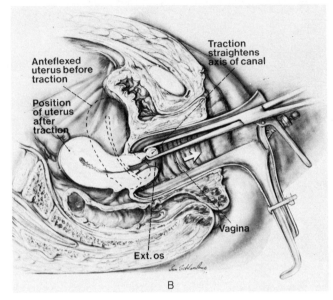

Anteflexed uterus before traction

Position of uterus after traction

Traction straightens axis of canal

Vagina

Ext. os

B

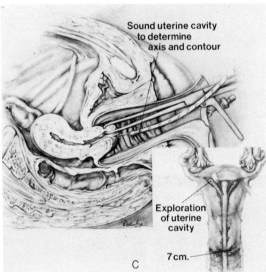

Sound uterine cavity to determine axis and contour

Exploration of uterine cavity

7 cm.

C

fig. 1·7 Preparation for IUD insertion. A Speculum in the vagina. B Traction on the cervix to straighten the uterus. C Sounding the uterus, a most critical step prior to insertion to check on the dimensions of the endometrial cavity. (*Courtesy of the H. H. Robins Company.*)

rate of expulsion, and much of the recent research has been centered on finding a shape that will stay in the uterus through this first reaction period. It is possible for an expulsion to go unnoticed; therefore women are asked to check the position of the "strings," the tiny nylon threads, attached to the IUD, which protrude from the cervix. Expulsion may occur during menstruation. The rate of expulsion varies with the type of IUD and is affected in each case by the age of the woman and the number of prior pregnancies. The younger woman who has had fewer pregnancies has more difficulty retaining an IUD. In addition to the IUDs that are expelled, numbers are removed voluntarily because of extra bleeding and cramping and, rarely, endometritis. Finally, a very few women experience a migration of the IUD to another site in the abdomen. Perforation of the uterus by the IUD may or may not be felt; if it occurs, it usually does so during the process of insertion. Every IUD is radioopaque, so that should this happen, an x-ray could indicate the location. If the IUD is found outside the uterus, the usual procedure is operative removal.

EFFECTIVENESS For those women who *can retain* the IUD without difficulty, the rate of effectiveness is high. The most effective IUDs appear to be those with added fine copper wire and the Lippes loop (21). The overall failure rate is between 2 to 3 pregnancies per 100 women-years.

The following factors influence effectiveness of the IUD (Fig. 1·8):

1. Tampons and douching can be used. The patient should be instructed to check vaginal pads during menstruation for the possibility of IUD expulsion.

2. Most physicians advise an overlapping of contraceptives during the first few months when expulsion rate is highest.

3. Women must return in 6 months for a checkup and again in 12 months. Thereafter, yearly checkups are recommended.

4. Couples should be informed of the action of the IUD in case some of them have strong feelings about the possibility of the IUD's causing an early abortion.

ADVANTAGES Once inserted, no other equipment is necessary (after the first few months of overlapping contraception). Use of the IUD does not require any foresight or preintercourse preparation. Nor does it interfere with sexual pleasure and stimulus. If inserted in a clinic, it may be virtually cost-free (the cost of the IUD is the cost of inserting it and of the necessary revisits, as the IUD itself costs very little).

HORMONAL SUPPRESSION OF OVULATION

Suppression of ovulation is the most effective means of contraception, having a failure rate of 0.5 to 1.5 pregnancies per 100 women-years of use. Varying combinations of progestogens and estrogens in tablet form are the most usual agents. Fertility can also be lowered by minidoses of progestogens alone.

Sequential Regimen Doses of hormonal agents were first planned to mimic normal 28-day body cycles. The pattern of sequential administration is the use of an estrogenic agent in the first part of the cycle (for 21 days) to inhibit ovulation. Beginning at day 11 or 15, a small amount of progestogen is added to the tablets to ensure withdrawal bleeding. The last 6 to 9 days (days 22 to 28), an inert tablet (a placebo) or a tablet containing iron, is taken to complete the cycle. Ovulation is inhibited by estrogen because the FSH and LH levels are suppressed. The endometrium is built up to a degree somewhat similar to that in the proliferative phase. However, the volume of menstrual flow is diminished.

Since the body's own hormonal levels are

fig. 1·8 Explaining IUD action. (*Photo by Nancy Goodman.*)

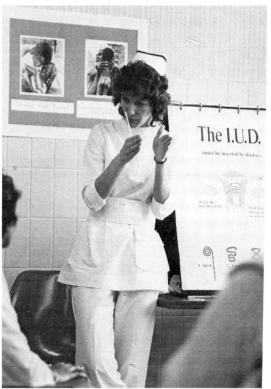

mimicked, if the woman forgets to take even one pill, ovulation may occur. Because the endometrium is in a ready state to receive the fertilized ovum, implantation can take place. Cervical mucus changes under the influence of estrogen during the first part of the cycle, as it does normally, to "welcome" the sperm. Therefore, a few pregnancies from "user failure" (forgetfulness) may occur with the sequential method. If she misses any pills, another method of birth control should be instituted for the rest of the cycle as she is unprotected for that cycle.

Low-dose Progestogens If progestogens are used alone in low doses, ovulation is not usually inhibited but fertility appears to be lowered. Progestogens initiate the normal cervical changes after ovulation; i.e., the mucus is returned to a thick, impenetrable character. Used alone, they also prevent the buildup of the endometrium to receive the ovum. These two effects, caused even by low doses of progestogens, are sufficient to prevent implantation of a fertilized ovum, even if some sperm should be able to penetrate the unfavorable cervical mucus.

Menstruation may be lighter (scanty) with use of progestogens alone, because of the lesser degree of endometrial proliferation.

Combined Regimen Tablets containing estrogen and progestogen combined are taken each day for 20 to 21 days, beginning on the fifth to seventh day. Some manufacturers include five to seven placebos in a 28-day package so that that patient does not have to remember which day to take pills. The combination tablet regimen inhibits ovulation and reduces menstrual flow by lowering endometrial buildup in the proliferative phase of the cycle. The gonadotropins FSH and LH are suppressed by the combination tablet. The progestogens affect the endometrial quality and cervical mucus penetrability during the proliferative phase.

EFFECTIVENESS Tablets containing both estrogen and progesterone provide almost 100 percent safety against conception.

Side Effects of Hormonal Contraceptives Because steroid hormones are normally present in the female body, additional doses cause side effects if not adjusted to the normal hormonal output of a particular woman. One of the key responsibilities of the prescribing physician is to determine the most likely response of an individual woman to the specific ratio of hormones in a particular tablet.

Body Types Estrogen is the basic hormone causing development of secondary sex characteristics in the female. Estrogen levels vary widely in different women and also vary during the menstrual cycle. In contrast, progestogen levels are almost the same in every woman. Therefore, the key factor to consider is the average estrogen production in a particular person's body. The so-called "estrogen profile," based on body build, history of menstrual cycles, energy and libido levels, and age, gives some indication of hyperestrogenic or hypoestrogenic states. Table 1·1 contrasts hypoestrogenic states with a balanced profile (76 to 80 percent of all women). Tests on a vaginal smear can indicate fairly accurately whether estrogen levels are high or low.

When the right balance is achieved, the woman should not experience any marked side effects, although she may take 2 to 3 months to become adjusted to the prescribed dosage. Estrogen-dominant tablets are prescribed for hypoestrogenic women, progesterone-dominant for hyperestrogenic women. Progestogen is in this case considered to be an "antiestrogen." The aim, of course, is to balance hormonal levels in the body. To this end, in normal cases, most physicians prescribe pills of no more than $50 \mu g$ of estrogen. Table 1·2 gives the results of estrogen and progestogen excess. These kinds of side effects would be noted by the physician and

table 1·1

ESTROGEN LEVELS

HYPERESTROGENIC, 10–12%	BALANCED, 76–80%	HYPOESTROGENIC, 10–12%
Heavy menstrual flow	Normal menses	Scanty menses at longer intervals
Large breasts	Normal contours	Small breasts
Tendency to gain weight	Normal weight	Boyish look
Premenstrual syndrome:		
Fluid retention		Lower libido
Emotional lability		Thinner vaginal lining
Increased libido		More vaginitis, pruritus
Increased vaginal secretion	Normal vaginal cytology and secretions	
Mastalgia		
Tendency toward fibroids		

Source: Adapted from J. Nelson, "Clinical Evaluation of Side Effects of Current Contraceptives—Oral: Combined, Sequential," *Journal of Reproductive Medicine*, **6**:2, 1971.

the dosage changed or the tablet discontinued.

Every patient begun on the hormonal tablet regimen is given a booklet describing the effects and side effects, the reportable symptoms, and the risks of taking oral contraceptives. Nurses should encourage each woman to read this information and should answer any questions she might have. This procedure is part of "informed consent," considered important in using any therapy of which there are known side effects or complications.

Women with underlying chronic disease, such as thrombophlebitis, which may be aggravated by excess hormones are not given "the pill."

Newer Methods of Hormonal Contraception The search for other ways to administer safe doses of steroids has led to injectables and implants.

The intramuscular injection of medroxyprogesterone acetate (Depo-Provera, 150 mg) provides an effect for 3 months. Side effects (of course dependent on the particular woman) are erratic bleeding patterns, plus prolonged amenorrhea and anovulatory cycles after discontinuation. This method has

been researched for almost 10 years and has had good acceptance by patients. It is now approved for *limited use* by "women who do not plan to have more children," because of the possibility of anovulatory cycles continuing long after the drug is discontinued (22).

A method still being researched is the substitution of the slow-release capsule for oral intake. Slow-release capsules are implanted into the subcutaneous tissue and may last up to 1 year. The rate of release is steady and appears to be without side effects, but implants are not yet approved by the Food and Drug Administration (FDA).

Postovulatory contraception Administration of estrogen in large amounts just after ovulation will change the tubal and endometrial function so that the fertilized ovum is not implanted. Diethylstilbestrol (DES) has recently been approved by the FDA for limited use as a "morning-after" preventive of pregnancy; however, the FDA does not consider DES to be safe for repeated use (23). Its use should be limited because large doses of estrogen are not considered physiologic. Therefore, for prevention of implantation, DES is used when midcycle, unprotected intercourse has taken place; it is

table 1·2

RESULTS OF AN EXCESS OF ESTROGEN AND PROGESTOGEN

ESTROGEN	PROGESTOGEN
GASTROINTESTINAL	
Nausea, bloated feeling	Increased appetite, real weight gain
VASCULAR AND RENAL SYSTEMS	
Fluid retention, venous capillary engorgement	
Occasional occurrence of spider nevi	
Headaches [migraine] and perhaps some elevation of blood pressure (?)	Depression, nervousness, fatigue
A slight chance of thrombo-embolism in high-risk patients	
UTERUS	
Hypermenorrhea, myoma growth	Scanty menses
	Dysmenorrhea usually improved; sometimes break-through bleeding
VAGINA	
Mucorrhea, excess secretion	Reduction in lining thick-ness and secretions; more *Candida*, pruritus
BREASTS	
Mastalgia; possible enlargement of benign cysts	Regression of breast tissue
SKIN	
Chloasma (darkening of skin over nose and cheeks	Possible occurrence of acne
GLUCOSE METABOLISM	
Increased levels in fasting state	
Decreased glucose tolerance increased insulin response to glucose	

Source: Adapted from J. Nelson, "Clinical Evaluation of Side Effects of Current Contraceptives—Oral: Combined, Sequential", *Journal of Reproductive Medicine,* **6**:2, 1971.

most often used in cases of rape. When given in the large doses needed to prevent implantation, DES has side effects which include nausea and vomiting. Taken immediately after rape, without consideration of the degree of fertility, i.e., the time in the cycle, DES will only cause uncomfortable side effects.

The effects of DES have been discovered to be toxic to a growing fetus; therefore, the drug would not be used, as it was in the early 1960s, as a way of supporting an already existing pregnancy (preventing miscarriage). Some 12 to 16 years later, some girl children of these mothers developed vaginal or cervical cancer.

Prostaglandins Prostaglandins are naturally occurring substances in the body which are especially effective in the control of human fertility because of their menstruation-inducing and labor-inducing action. They stimulate uterine activity. (Prostaglandin F_2 may also have a depressive effect on the corpus luteum.)

Prostaglandin E_2 and F_2 have the widest research use at present. Intravenous use is limited because of generalized side effects of nausea and vomiting, diarrhea, and fever. Intraamniotic or intrauterine administration appears to be most effective for abortion after the twelfth week of pregnancy. Oral tablets can effectively begin labor at term.

For contraceptive use, prostaglandins are being developed as a once-a-month antifertility agent. These substances are found to occur normally in menstrual fluid and may contribute to the cramping sensations many women experience during menstruation. Research is directed toward developing a menstruation-inducing dose without unpleasant side effects which could be used to begin a delayed menses (24).

SURGICAL STERILIZATION

Surgical sterilization permanently prevents passage of sperm or ova to their respective destinations. The term is applied to all surgical procedures that prevent conception. Sterilization, at this time, must be considered a permanent procedure and thus requires the informed consent of the person involved. The objective in current research is to find a method of sterilization simple enough to be performed as an office procedure, effective enough to eliminate future pregnancies, and yet reliably reversible so that the man or

woman would be in a state of "suspended fertility." No method to date meets these criteria completely (25).

Tubal Ligation The best time for performance of tubal ligation is just after delivery when the uterus is still enlarged in the abdomen and the tubes are near the anterior surface of the abdomen. Laparotomy allows easy visualization of the tubes for the classic procedures of tying and cutting them. General anesthesia is required, and a small scar is left at the area of the umbilicus. If a laparotomy is performed 6 weeks after delivery or when the woman is not pregnant, the incision is just above the symphysis pubis. Vaginal (culdoscopic) or abdominal (laparoscopic) instruments have been adapted which make it possible to visualize the tubes and, with attachments, to crush, cut, or clamp them. Culdoscopy leaves no visible scar; laparoscopy leaves a small incision in the abdomen which can be covered by a Band-Aid. Tubal ligation does not change regular ovulation and menstrual cycles. The ovum drops into the peritoneal cavity and is reabsorbed.

Vas Ligation (Vasectomy) Vasectomy is a legal technique for male sterilization in all states of the United States and may be performed on any adult male who consents. Although some vas deferens have been repaired after ligation, with restoration of fertility, no one should agree to a vasectomy with the expectation of complete return to fertility, for the incidence of such return is unpredictable (about 25 percent success). The sperm quality and quantity may not return to adequate fertility levels.

Temporary occlusion with various kinds of metal or plastic plugs is being tested. Sperm banks in large cities are becoming available for storage of semen for those men who request a vasectomy and yet may have a desire to father a child in the future. Sterilization is considered by families who have reached their desired fertility; as a contraceptive technique it is becoming increasingly popular in the United States.

NURSING ROLE

Wherever the nurse is, the subject of child spacing may arise. Therefore, she may consider knowledge of methods to be part of the basic preventive health care given by nurses.

In maternity services, family planning information is most commonly given after delivery. Some introductory material regarding child-spacing methods may be given during prenatal education, although patients are not usually able to focus intently on methods until after delivery. Almost universally, at this time, women are highly motivated to learn how to delay the next pregnancy. Classes should be planned for a time which is free of concern about infant feeding or visitors. Taped discussions of methods can be used for mothers who for one reason or another cannot come to group discussion. Some hospitals have film cassettes or video cassettes set up for basic information-giving to mothers, after which the skilled nurse-teacher can use group time for clarification of matters about which there are questions and problems (Fig. 1·9).

The postdelivery period may provide an excellent opportunity to talk with the adult woman about aspects of sexuality, as she will have many questions at this time (26). Bedside conferences can be set up to discuss a particular method, after the woman has had the opportunity to learn about all the methods. Whether counseling is on a one-to-one basis or in a small group, the nurse must first assess the background knowledge of each woman. Because of wider dissemination of knowledge, levels of understanding may vary. The nurse should ascertain whether patients have a working knowledge of the function of male and female reproductive systems before going into details about each

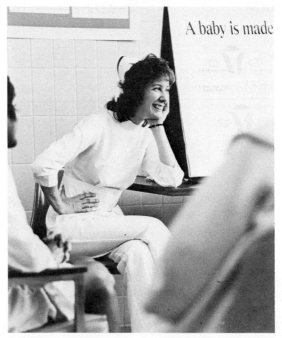

fig. 1·9 Assessment of a person's knowledge of anatomy must accompany teaching about contraceptive methods. (*Photo by Nancy Goodman.*)

method. Some sessions might be by formal presentation; others may be informal question-and-answer periods on specific areas which the group requests.

It is important to help patients understand why a family and personal medical history is essential for the physician as the best choice of method is sought.

The nurse counselor must keep in mind that the choice of a child-spacing method is highly personal. The nurse will give information free of personal convictions so that the patient is able, without pressure, to consider her own life situation.

If the newly delivered mother has not chosen a method before leaving the hospital, the opportunity is offered her at her first postdelivery checkup.

references

1. R. Cohen, "Some Maladaptive Syndromes of Pregnancy and the Puerperium," *Obstetrics and Gynecology*, **27**:562, 1966.
2. Earl Siegal and Naomi M. Morris, "Family Planning: Its Health Rationale," *American Journal of Obstetrics and Gynecology*, **118**(7):995, 1974.
3. Cornelia Wilbur and Robert Aug, "Sex Education," *American Journal of Nursing*, **73**(1):88, 1973.
4. Ibid., p. 89.
5. Selma H. Fraiberg, *The Magic Years*, Charles Scribner's Sons, New York, 1959, p. 211.
6. Edward O. Reiter and Howard E. Kulin, "Sexual Maturation in the Female," *Pediatric Clinics of North America*, **19**(3):583, 1972.
7. J. P. Semmens and K. E. Krantz, *The Adolescent Experience, a Counseling Guide to Social and Sexual Behavior*, The Macmillan Company, New York, 1970.
8. R. E. Frisch and R. Revelle, "Height and Weight at Menarche and a Hypothesis of Menarche," *Archives of Diseases of Children,* **46**:695, 1971.
9. W. A. Marshall and J. M. Tanner, "Variations in the Pattern of Pubertal Changes in Boys," *Archives of Diseases of Children,* **45**:13, 1970.
10. James P. Semmens and Jane H. Semmens, "Sex Education of the Adolescent Female," *Pediatric Clinics of North America*, **19**(3):769, 1972.
11. Helene S. Arnstein, *Your Growing Child and Sex: A Parent's Guide to the Sexual Development, Education, Attitudes and Behavior of the Child from Infancy through Adolescence*, The Bobbs-Merrill Company, Inc., New York, 1967.
12. Alan P. Guttmacher, "Progress and Failure in Population Control," *Journal of Reproductive Medicine,* **8**(4):159, 1972.
13. Ibid., p. 161.
14. Harry W. Rudel, Fred A. Kincl, and Milan R. Henzl, *Birth Control*, The Macmillan Company, New York, 1973, p. 79.
15. Ibid., p. 60.
16. Melvin R. Cohen, "Methods of Determination of Ovulation," *Journal of Reproductive Medicine*, **1**(2):182, 1968.
17. Melvin R. Cohen, *Methods of Birth Control in the United States*, The Medical Committee of Planned Parenthood, New York, 1972, p. 21.
18. Ibid., p. 23.
19. C. B. Arnold and B. E. Cogswell, "A Condom Distribution Program for Adolescents: The Findings of a Feasibility Study," *American Journal of Public Health*, **61**:739, 1971.
20. Rudel, et al., op. cit., p. 180.
21. ———"Copper IUD Protects the Never-pregnant," *Family Planning Digest*, **3**(1):11, 1974.
22. ———"FDA Okays Limited Depo-Provera Use," *Family Planning Digest*, **3**(1):16, 1974.
23. ———"FDA Approves DES, Urges Limited Use," *Family Planning Digest*, **2**(3):12, 1973.
24. Sultan M. M. Karim, "Prostaglandins in Fertility Control," chap. 8 in Malcolm Potts and Clive Wood (eds.), *New Concepts in Contraception*, University Park Press, Baltimore, 1972, p. 136.
25. Robert A. Erb et al., "Device and Technique for Blocking the Fallopian Tubes," *Contemporary OB/GYN*, **3**(2):92, 1974.
26. Ruth Wilcox, "Counseling Patients about Sex Problems," *Nursing '74,* November 1974, p. 44.

bibliography

American Academy of Pediatrics: "Counseling Opportunities in Human Reproduction," Report of the Committee on Youth, *Pediatrics,* **50**:492, 1972.

Arnold, E.: "Individualizing Nursing Care in Family Planning," *Nursing Outlook,* **15**:12, 1967.

Arnstein, Helene S.: *Your Growing Child and Sex: A Parent's Guide to the Sexual Development, Education, Attitudes and Behavior of the Child from Infancy through Adolescence,* The Bobbs-Merrill Company, New York, 1967.

Blout, J. H., W. W. Darrow, and R. E. Johnson: "Venereal Disease in Adolescents," *Pediatric Clinics of North America,* **20**(4):1021, 1973.

ACSAA Book Review Committee: *Sex Education: Recommended Reading, Annotated Bibliography,* Child Study Association of America, New York.

Child Study Association of America: *What to Tell Your Child about Sex,* Child Study Association of America—Wel-Met, Inc., Child Study Press, New York, 1974.

Emands, E.: "Nursing," in M. S. Calderone (ed.), *Manual of Family Planning and Contraception Practice,* 2d ed., The William & Wilkins Company, Baltimore, 1970, pp. 53–61.

Erickson, E. H.: *Identity: Youth and Crisis,* W. W. Norton & Company, Inc., New York, 1968.

Fischman, S.: "Choosing an Appropriate Contraceptive," *Nursing Outlook,* **15**:12, 1967.

Kogut, M. D.: "Growth and Development in Adolescence," *Pediatric Clinics of North America,* **20**(4):789, 1973.

Lebfeldt, Hans: "Psychology of Contraceptive Failure," *Medical Aspects of Human Sexuality,* May, 1971.

Maier, H. W.: *Three Theories of Child Development,* Harper and Row, Publishers, Incorporated, New York, 1965.

Manisoff, M.: *Nurse's Guide to Family Planning,* Planned Parenthood, New York, 1971.

Penfield, A. J.: "Counseling the Woman about Sterilization," *Contemporary OB/GYN,* **1**(4):29, 1972.

Rauh, J. L., L. B. Johnson, and R. L. Burket: "The Reproductive Adolescent," *Pediatric Clinics of North America,* **20**(4):1005, 1973.

Roberts, S. O.: "Some Mental and Emotional Health Needs of Negro Children and Youth," in R. Wilcox, (ed.), *The Psychological Consequences of Being a Black American,* John Wiley & Sons, Inc., New York, 1971.

Wiedenback, E.: "The Nurse's Role in Family Planning," *Nursing Clinics of North America,* **3**(2):355, 1968.

Wood, H. C.: "The Changing Trends in Voluntary Sterilization," *Contemporary OB/GYN,* **1**(4):31, 1972.

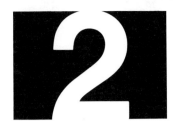

genetics

Dolores Lake

Each person is unique, different from anyone else who has ever lived. Yet, as human beings belonging to the species of Homo sapiens, we all have certain common features. The question that has puzzled scientists and anthropologists for centuries is what the natural forces are that interact to give all members of mankind a general likeness as a species and at the same time such distinct differences.

More personally, this question puzzles and perhaps worries every expectant family as they patiently await the arrival of their newborn infant. Almost from the time the child is conceived, parents cannot help but wonder what it will be like. Will it be a boy or a girl? Will it have brown or blue eyes? And will it look like father or more like mother? More important, will it be all right, or by some odd fate will it be defective or malformed? If there is a history of seizures, mental retardation, cystic fibrosis, cancer, diabetes, alcoholism, or mental illness in the family, how might this affect the unborn child? No family, if its history is examined carefully enough, is entirely free of some type of inherited disease. What are the chances that disease or defect, rather than health, will be inherited?

These questions and many others like them are asked frequently, with the expectation that the nurse will be able to provide satisfactory answers. Wherever the nurse works, patients will want to know answers to questions regarding the heredity of their children. More likely than not, she is confronted with even more intimate and demanding questions and explanations from friends and relatives who confide in her during her "off-duty" hours. The lay public expects a nurse to know and to give appropriate answers and guidance toward preventive health resources.

A basic understanding of the laws of heredity and the nature of hereditary material is a good place to begin. Environmental factors which help to promote genetic endowment or influence genetic change must also be considered, since man, like all living things, is a product of both his heredity and his environment. Often it is the interaction of heredity and environment, rather than either one separately, which determines the outcome of any one situation.

The idea that characteristics are inherited has been present for thousands of years. However, Darwin's theories of evolution (1) and Mendel's observations of hereditary traits in plants (2) were among the first contributions to modern genetics. Since 1955, man's knowledge of molecular biology has rapidly expanded the horizons of genetics. This knowledge will become a major aspect of family health care in the future. As a nurse, you may be surprised to find that though your knowledge of genetics can be applied most directly in maternal and child health nursing, there will be many other instances in which it can also be utilized. Caring for many other kinds of patients, such as those who have diabetes, heart disease, and cancer, will entail at least a basic understanding of the genetic concept so that supportive family health care may be given.

the nature of heredity

GENES: CARRIERS OF HEREDITARY TRAITS

A gene is a unit of hereditary material, *deoxyribonucleic acid* (DNA), which has a specific function. Sometimes this specific function is to determine a certain trait, such as eye color. More often the specific function is to determine a particular step in some complex process of the body's chemistry. Genes control protein synthesis, the formation of enzymes and antibodies, and the structure of hormones; they influence almost every chemical process in the body. Some of these activities are dictated directly by the genes. Other actions are made possible through the indirect genetic regulation of feedback responses. In some instances, two or more genes work together to determine precisely how the molecules of the body, such as hemoglobin, are made. There are also *operator* genes and *regulator* genes which start and stop the release of hormones and enzymes. Interacting with processes in the endocrine system through feedback signals, operator and regulator genes help to maintain homeostasis in the body. Thus, through gene action, the various enzymes and hormones can be turned on or off as needed.

If you recall how the egg and sperm are formed during gametogenesis (see Chap. 3) and how they unite when fertilization takes place, you will remember that half the genetic material comes from the mother's 23 chromosomes and half from the father's. The hereditary characteristics of the new infant are determined by the genes strung together in beadlike chains along these chromosomes. Within the chromosomes, each gene has its own particular place, or *locus*. Just as the chromosomes each have a matched partner, so the genes within them occur in pairs. One member of the pair occupies its locus on one chromosome while its partner, or *allele*, occupies the corresponding place on the matched chromosome.

The alleles in a gene pair may be identical or slightly different. The slight difference in one allele as compared with its partner in the pair is one factor accounting for differences between parents and their children. If a person has both members of a gene pair ab-

solutely alike, he is a *homozygote*. On the other hand, sometimes the genes in a pair might be slightly different because the one inherited from one parent may be slightly different from the one inherited from the other parent. The person who has two genes in a pair which are slightly different from each other is called a *heterozygote*.

Sometimes one of the alleles in a gene pair is more dominant, while its partner is recessive. The type of gene (genotype), whether dominant or recessive, influences the overt characteristics (phenotype) of the individual according to Mendel's laws. See Table 2·1 and note that the first two examples are homozygotes, while the last one is a heterozygote.

Eye color is but one of the thousands of examples illustrating Mendel's laws of heredity (Table 2·2). By applying these laws, one can see how dominant or recessive genes can influence body chemistry and metabolism. If one is lucky enough to inherit a well-operating body chemistry he will not have the problem of an inborn error in metabolism such as occurs in the child with phenylketonuria (PKU). If he has inherited a defect in gene action involving body chemistry, he has a metabolic problem which is inborn. PKU, Tay-Sachs disease, and muscular dystrophy are a few of the many hundreds of these kinds of problems.

In summary, the genes control body chemistry because they contain within them the specific instructions necessary for the

table 2·1
MENDEL'S LAWS OF DOMINANCE

GENOTYPE		
GENE	ALLELE	PHENOTYPE EXPRESSION
Dominant (*D*)	Dominant (*D*)	Dominant (*DD*)
Recessive (*r*)	Recessive (*r*)	Recessive (*rr*)
Dominant (*D*)	Recessive (*r*)	Dominant (*Dr*)

table 2·2

INHERITANCE OF EYE COLOR*

PARENT	PARENT	CHILDREN
Brown (*B, B*)	Brown (*B, B*)	Brown (*B, B*)
Blue (*bl, bl*)	Blue (*bl, bl*)	Blue (*bl, bl*)
Brown (*B, B*)	Blue (*bl, bl*)	Brown (*B, bl*) Brown (*B, bl*)
Brown (*B, bl*)	Blue (*bl, bl*)	Brown (*B, bl*) Blue (*bl, bl*)
Brown (*B, bl*)	Brown (*B, bl*)	Brown (*B, B*) Brown (*B, bl*) Brown (*B, bl*) Blue (*bl, bl*)

*According to Mendel's laws, brown (*B*) is dominant and blue (*bl*) is recessive.

body to build molecules of protein, to utilize energy, to grow, to change, and to carry on all of life's processes. How the body receives the vastly complex information about how to maintain itself is determined largely by the nature of the genetic material DNA (deoxyribonucleic acid). DNA governs all living things. The code by which DNA operates is truly the code of life itself. Life is passed on from one generation to the next through the DNA in the genes, just as chromosomes are passed on from parent to child. Life maintains itself after birth as old cells wear out, die, and are replaced by new cells with the ability to function as they should because of the remarkable DNA within them.

DNA: THE MOLECULE OF LIFE

Considering that DNA possesses all the hereditary information necessary to maintain life, it is a remarkably simple molecule. Coiling around itself, the molecule forms a double helix which looks like a twisted ladder. It has two side chains held together by cross rungs. The side chains are long, alternating links of sugar, or *deoxyribose*, bound to alternating

phosphates. The chain is bent in such a way that the sugars lean inward while the phosphates lie along the outermost parts of the helix. The cross rungs are formed by nitrogen bases called *nucleic acids*. There are four nucleic acids: *adenine, thymine, guanine,* and *cytosine*. Thus, DNA is *deoxyribonucleic acid* formed by sugar (deoxyribose) and base (nucleic acid). Sugar is always the sides of the ladder, and nucleic acids make up the rungs (see Fig. 2·1).

Base-pairing Laws The Watson-Crick base-pairing laws state that adenine (A) al-

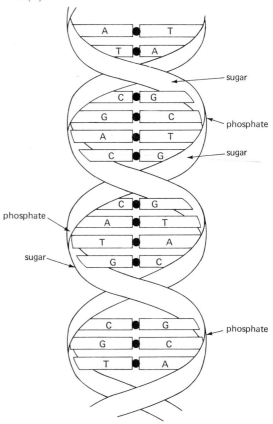

fig. 2·1 The DNA molecule is shaped like a ladder that is twisted into a helix. The sides consist of alternating phosphate bonds (outside) and sugar molecules (inner twists). The rungs are composed of nucleic acids: adenine (A), thymine (T), guanine (G), and cytosine (C).

ways pairs with thymine (T), while guanine (G) always pairs with cytosine (C) (Fig. 2·2). The reason why the nucleic acids pair in this manner is that this is the only way in which they fit together chemically. (A more detailed, but readable, explanation can be found in *The Genetic Code* by Isaac Asimov.)

The Watson-Crick base-pairing laws are universal. Whether applied to a plant, bug, cow, cat, elephant, mouse, or man, these base-pairing laws hold true. Life everywhere has within it the same structure in its DNA. You might ask, then, "If the basic structure of DNA is the same for all life, how is it possible for living things to take so many forms and for individuals in the same species to be so different from one another?" The answer to this difference among the various species of plants and animals is that the *ratio* of the base pairs differs (not the pairs themselves). The amount of guanine must equal the amount of cytosine, and the amount of adenine must equal the amount of thymine, but the ratio of the former group to the latter is species-specific. Some animals have more adenine

and thymine; other animals have more guanine and cytosine.

In addition to the ratio of base pairs from the four nucleic acids found in their DNA, animals (and human beings) differ from one another in the nature of the specific kinds of protein which form their body structure. DNA acts as an instructional pattern for making proteins. The information in the DNA map is in coded form. It is often called the genetic code, or the code of life.

RNA: THE MESSENGER

Information in DNA regarding how to make body protein and carry on all life processes remains useless if it does not have some way of getting out of the helix to the ribosomes of the cell where proteins are made. DNA itself does not go directly to the ribosomes. Instead, RNA *(ribonucleic acid)* reads the information in DNA, interprets it, takes the message to the ribosomes, and supervises the making of the proteins in the proper manner.

There are several kinds of RNA. First there is messenger RNA (mRNA), which reads the message in DNA and carries the message to the ribosomes. When the information is needed by the cell, mRNA moves to DNA and lines up along the one helix so that the bases of RNA pair up with the bases in DNA. RNA contains adenine, guanine, and cytosine, but uracil replaces thymine: A, G, C, U. They line up thus:

RNA			DNA
Uracil	U	A	Adenine
Guanine	G	C	Cytosine
Cytosine	C	G	Guanine
Adenine	A	T	Thymine

After having matched up with DNA, the bases are ready to read the DNA message. Always, three RNA bases work as triplets. The triplets are called *codons*. Thus, UGC in the example above forms a codon. In all, there

fig. 2·2 Watson-Crick base-pairing laws. Adenine always pairs with thymine (A-T); guanine always pairs with cytosine (G-C).

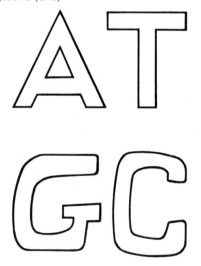

are 64 codons. Each codon specifies the message for making an amino acid. Since there are only about 20 amino acids, several codons can carry instructions for one amino acid. Some codons give the signals to start and stop, since RNA cannot begin just anywhere. It must have specific instructions about where and when to begin to read which amino acids are needed. It also must know when to stop working. The codons form the genetic code, or the code of life. For all living things, the code for making amino acids is the same.

The sequence of amino acids along a protein chain is what determines the nature of the protein molecule. Proteins are made by stringing together hundreds of amino acids in proper sequence. After mRNA takes the message to ribosomes, soluble RNA (sRNA) sees that the proper amino acid is gotten and placed in correct position on the ribosome as the links of amino acids are hooked together. When all links are finished, the new protein falls off the ribosome and goes to the spot where it is needed in the cell.

Throughout all the cells in the body, thousands of protein molecules are constantly being made in this way. Each minute of life from conception onward, thousands of DNA molecules become active at the appropriate second they are needed. RNA reads the message in the DNA coded form and oversees the manufacturing of protein to maintain life. Each step in the links required to make protein requires a particular enzyme, without which that step cannot take place. At the exact moment needed, the correct enzyme must arrive to act as a catalyst in order for the step to occur. Genes carry the information for making and releasing those enzymes. The one gene–one enzyme theory was first proposed by Beadle (3). He states that so many genes are packed into the 46 chromosomes of each cell that the information would fill 500 volumes of encyclopedias if it were typed out on an ordinary typewriter. All this information

operates through the genetic code to produce billions of precisely made complex molecules, properly arranged and structured into appropriate tissue forms composing a newborn 7-lb bundle of healthy baby! Think how many times a molecule of DNA must duplicate itself to grow, by mitosis, the millions of cells needed to form each organ. How many messages RNA has to carry and how many molecules of protein are made on the cytoplasmotic ribosomes in 9 months of gestation! By the same genetic code, the baby grows into a toddler, grade-school child, adolescent, and adult who, in time, reproduces his own offspring through marriage with his selected partner.

MUTATIONS

Considering all this, it is quite remarkable that genetic mistakes are rarely made. Mutations, or genetic changes, do occur, however, from time to time. Sometimes the mutations are produced spontaneously; at other times, they are caused by environmental factors. How often mutation occurs remains unknown, since we see only the result of mutation, not the molecular change in the DNA directly. Naturally, then, if the mutation produces no observable change, it goes unrecognized. Since our powers of observation are limited, there are probably many changes which we do not see. Helpful mutations especially are unrecognized. Harmful genetic changes are the ones upon which we tend to focus, because they are the most recognizable of natural changes in man.

Harmful mutations in human beings have been found in several types of disorders. *Point mutations* involve a single nucleotide or gene; therefore, each point mutation in the affected homozygote produces a specific inborn error in metabolism. Two examples of point mutations are sickle-cell anemia and PKU. *Chromosomal abnormalities* involve more than a single pair of genes. They involve either an entire chromosome or at least a major part of a chromosome.

the chromosomes

Genes are carried in the chromosomes. The arrangement of genes and chromosomes is very precise. It was not until 1959 that the correct number of chromosomes in human beings was known to be 46 in each living normal cell except the egg and the sperm, which have 23. Since chromosomes occur in matched pairs, there are 22 pairs of autosomes and two X chromosomes (sex chromosomes) in the female. The chromosomal pattern is called a *karyotype*. The normal female karyotopy is 44XX. The normal male has only one X chromosome, but he also has a Y chromosome. The normal male karyotype, shown in Fig. 2·3, is 44XY. Figure 2·4 gives a schematic representation of sizes and shapes of chromosomes.

Chromosomes are classified according to their size and shape and the position of the *centromere* (4). Those most alike are grouped under the same letter, according to the Denver classification, an international system for designating normal as well as abnormal chromosomes so that medical men everywhere will have a standard approach to communication in genetics. The Denver classification is shown in Table 2·3.

Although almost any tissue of the body may be used for determining the karyotype of that body, skin cells or leukocytes are usually used. The entire process is too complex to be discussed fully; in brief, the cells are put under the microscope, the laboratory technician looks for a cell in metaphase when all the chromosomes are lined up at the equator, and that cell is stained and photographed. Later, the photograph is enlarged, and the chromosomes are cut out and pasted on a sheet of paper according to their size and shape. More precise methods for determining

karyotype are available with the aid of the computer (5) (Fig. 2·5).

CHROMOSOMAL ABNORMALITIES

About once in every 1000 live births, an infant arrives in the world with a chromosomal abnormality. For the rest of his life, which may be either very short or long depending upon the specific abnormality, he must live with some sort of problem.

Many types of chromosomal disorders are known. Only part of a chromosome may be

fig. 2·3 Male karyotype. (*From Ian Porter,* Heredity and Disease, *McGraw-Hill Book Company, New York,* 1968.)

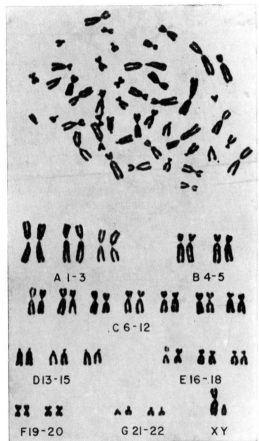

table 2·3

CLASSIFICATION OF CHROMOSOMES

GROUP	AUTOSOMES	SEX CHROMO-SOMES	CHARACTERISTICS OF CHROMOSOMES	No. OF CHROMOSOMES MEN	WOMEN
A	1–3		Large with median or slightly submedian centromere	6	6
B	4–5		Large with submedian centromere	4	4
C	6–12	X	Medium with submedian and median centromere	15	16
D	13–15		Medium, acrocentric	6	6
E	16–18		Short with median or submedian centromere	6	6
F	19–20		Short with median centromere	4	4
G	21–22	Y	Short, acrocentric	5	4
Total				46	46

Source: From Ian Porter, *Heredity and Disease*, McGraw-Hill Book Company, New York, 1971.

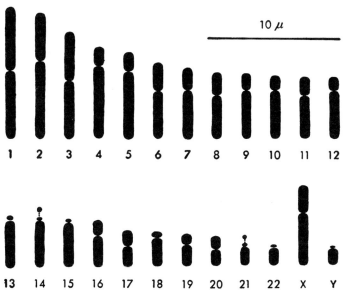

fig. 2·4 Configuration of one member of each autosomal pair and of the X and Y chromosomes in man. (*From B. M. Patten,* Human Embryology, *3d ed., McGraw-Hill Book Company,* 1968.)

passed on, as in chromosomal *deletion*. A piece of one chromosome may be improperly hooked to another so that there is a *translocation* of chromosomal material. The two ends of a chromosome may reach around and "grab hold" of each other (like a dog chasing its tail), resulting in a *ring* formation. Probably the most common chromosomal error that can

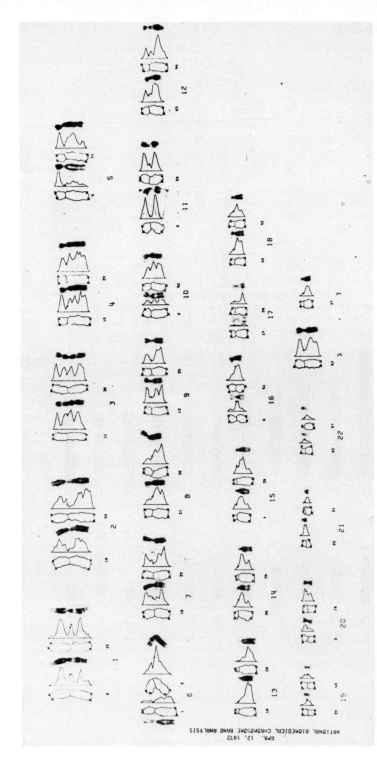

fig. 2·5 Computer printout of a karyotype. (*From H. A. Lubs and M. L. Lubs*, New Cytogenetic Techniques Applied to a Series of Children with Mental Retardation, *Nobel Symposium XXIII, Academic Press, Inc., 1973.*)

be compatible with life is the presence of an extra chromosome in one of the pairs, or a *trisomy.*

Trisomy 21 The characteristics of the person with trisomy 21 were described by Down many years before Lejeune discovered in 1959 that three chromosomes 21 appeared in all the cells of an infant with this condition (6). The syndrome (formerly called mongolism) is now called Down's syndrome or trisomy 21 (7).

NONDISJUNCTION The extra chromosome in trisomy 21 usually results from an error in meiosis called *nondisjunction.* You will recall that the normal mature ovum has 23 chromosomes and that the immature oogonia from which they are derived have 46 chromosomes. Meiosis is the process by which this *reduction division* takes place. During meiosis, one member of each of the chromosome pairs goes to form the mature ovum. The matched partner in the pair is discarded in the polar body, which is nonviable. In this way the mature ovum ends up with 23 chromosomes and, if fertilized by a sperm cell, will produce a zygote with 46 chromosomes, which is characteristic of the human race. In nondisjunction, however, both members of the twenty-first pair of chromosomes go to the ovum. (*Nondisjunction* means that the chromosome partners fail to disjoin, or separate, so that instead of one going to the polar body and one to the ovum, both go to the ovum.) When the sperm fertilizes the ovum, it contributes the third chromosome 21, resulting in trisomy 21 (Fig. 2·6).

In the female, meiosis begins during her own fetal life long before she herself is born. Then the process of meiosis stops before reaching completion, and a long resting stage takes place from before birth to puberty. During ovulation the ovum finishes its final stages of maturity. The older a woman is, the longer the resting stage of any particular ovum will have been before it becomes ready for fertilization during the normal female ovarian cycle. The long resting stage appears to have something to do with the incidence of trisomy 21 (8). There is a 50 times greater chance of an infant's being born with trisomy 21 if his mother is over forty years of age than if she is in her twenties. In fact, 95 percent of all children with Down's syndrome (Table 2·4) are born to older mothers.

TRANSLOCATION In contrast to the nondisjunction type of trisomy 21, a rare form of Down's syndrome is found among young mothers. This is *translocation,* in which part of chromosome 21 sticks to another chromosome before the ovum is mature. In addition, there is also a fully normal chromosome 21 in the ovum. The sperm brings in the third, so that there are still three chromosomes at 21. This type of Down's syndrome is found in teen-age mothers whose chromosomal patterns show by karyotype that they themselves are carriers of the problem. Translocation trisomy is extremely rare (9). Since these children are usually born to younger parents and because the disorder is familial and may therefore affect other siblings, genetic counseling is of high priority.

PHYSICAL CHARACTERISTICS The child with Down's syndrome has a characteristic appearance (10) whether his condition is of the translocation or of the nondisjunction type (see Fig. 2·7 with description). Because an entire chromosome is involved in Down's syndrome, malformations have been found in almost every organ and enzyme system (Fig. 2·8). Not every child has all of them, but each affected child has many. Cardiac defects and a tendency to develop rheumatic fever are common. Children with Down's syndrome have a genetic intolerance to atropine (11). The nurse who works with such a child must take special precaution to look for unusual effects produced by medications and anesthesia (Fig. 2·9A, B).

The single most universal characteristic of

table 2·4

RISK OF TRISOMY 21 RESULTING
FROM NONDISJUNCTION, IN RELATION TO
MOTHER'S AGE

MOTHER'S AGE, yr	RISK
Less than 29	1 in 3000
30–34	1 in 600
35–39	1 in 280
40–44	1 in 70
45–49	1 in 40

Source: From Ian Porter, *Heredity and Disease,* McGraw-Hill Book Company, New York, 1968.

Down's syndrome is mental retardation. Usually, the degree of retardation is severe enough to prevent the child from learning beyond elementary-school-level skills (if even this much can be accomplished). An occasional child has the ability and the opportunity to reach fifth- or sixth- grade levels in some areas of learning. Inherited potential is only one of the factors involved in determining how much any given child will be able to achieve. Motivation, attention span, level of anxiety, parental attitude, community facilities, and proper guidance are extremely important to the retarded child, just as they are to the normal child. Simple tasks which the normal child learns quickly will often be major accomplishments for the child with Down's syndrome. Self-help skills, such as toilet training and learning to dress, may take years to learn as each task is broken down into specific, clearly defined steps programmed into a pattern of learning responses. Routine, structure, and clear expectations are vital to learning. Love, patience, consistency in expectations and in limit setting are essential to the success and happiness of the child with Down's syndrome.

At best, the child with this disorder can be expected to work under the close supervision of an understanding adult when he is given clear, simple, repetitive tasks to perform. As an adult, he may become employable in a sheltered, workshoplike setting. He may be semi-independent, but he will require some outside supervision all his life. In view of this, the question of institutionalization or residential placement will probably arise at some time in his infancy or childhood as his family tries to decide what is best to do. No quick answer can be given. Usually, the longer the child is able to be with his natural family in a home situation, the greater advantage he has of feeling loved, wanted, and part of a family. In some situations where family tension is great, where there are other pressures of additional children or relatives, poor community facilities, or other problems, foster care or residential placement may be the best answer. Each child's situation must be handled on an individual basis.

COMMUNITY RESOURCES Community agencies, parents' groups, and the local chapter of The American Association for Retarded Children can provide considerable support and guidance. The local school system in almost every county can make arrangements for school attendance in special classes within the community. Special education teachers trained in working with retarded persons are often available for consultation. The nurse, whether in the doctor's office, in the hospital,

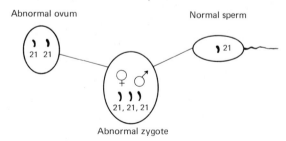

fig. 2·6 Nondisjunction of chromosomes. The abnormal zygote has an overdose of chromosome 21, which causes Down's syndrome. *(Courtesy of The National Foundation–March of Dimes.)*

Abnormal ovum   Normal sperm

21 21   21

♀ ♂
21, 21, 21

Abnormal zygote

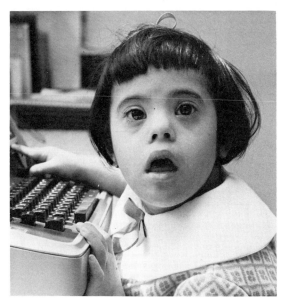

fig. 2·7 Girl with Down's syndrome. Note the small round head with a flat broad face and flat nasal bridge. Epicanthic folds at the corner of the eyelids give a slanting appearance to the eyes, resulting in the misnaming of the syndrome "mongolism." (*Courtesy of The National Foundation–March of Dimes.*)

op at the same period in embryonic life, frequently kidney abnormalities are also noted. Extra fingers, overlapping fingers, and rocker-bottom feet are very typical of children with trisomy 18.

The nurse working in the newborn nursery is sometimes the first person to discover a chromosomal abnormality such as trisomy 18. It may be possible to miss the clues to abnormality in the initial delivery room check of the newborn infant. In the nursery, the infant may fail to suck well, may have a peculiar cry, or may be hypotonic. Since not all newborn infants with trisomy 18 appear grossly deformed, this condition could possibly go undetected without alert observation. Babies

fig. 2·8 Boy with Down's syndrome. Sometimes light speckles in the iris, called Brushfield's spots, can be seen. The child's vision is often poor because of eye-muscle imbalance or because of a refractory error. (*Courtesy of The National Foundation–March of Dimes.*)

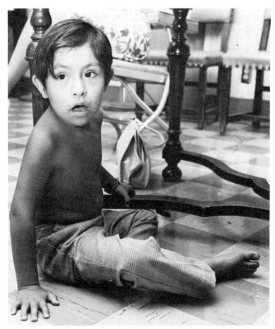

or in the home, can provide considerable help to the family because of her knowledge of growth and development and her communication skills.

Trisomy 18 About one in 3000 infants born alive has trisomy 18 (12). The karyotype shows either a complete or partial extra chromosome 18, making three rather than two chromosomes 18 and resulting in a total chromosomal count of 47, rather than the normal 46. Babies with trisomy 18, like those with trisomy 21, tend to be born to older mothers. Infant girls seem to be affected by this syndrome more than boys. Low birth weight, hypotonia, weak cry, a severely receding chin (which makes sucking difficult), and low-set, malformed ears are characteristic. Because the ears and the kidneys devel-

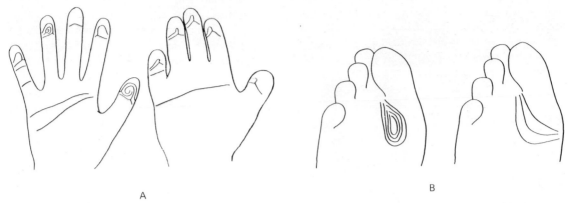

A   B

Fig. 2·9 Comparison of handprints and footprints. A The left-hand print of a normal child shows whorls on the thumb, a radial loop on the index finger, and ulnar loops on the ring and little fingers. There are two flexures in the little finger and two palmar creases. Hands of children with Down's syndrome show many more ulnar loops, and most of them have a single ("simian") palmar crease. The hands of patients with Down's syndrome are often short and stubby, with little fingers curving inward. B The left foot of a normal child shows characteristic whorls or loops in the "ball" of the foot, called the hallucal area. The foot of a child with Down's syndrome shows tibial arches instead of whorls or loops in the same area. (*Courtesy of The National Foundation–March of Dimes.*)

with trisomy 18, like all infants with genetic and congenital abnormalities, present difficult nursing-care problems. Intake of nourishment poses a problem because sucking is poor and the infant tires before he has eaten enough. Intravenous administration of fluids is frequently necessary. Respiratory failure is also likely, because of hypotonia. The nurse must also cope with her own feelings about the birth of an atypical infant who is doomed to have lifetime problems. The life expectancy of babies with trisomy 18 is usually short. Most infants with this condition die before reaching their first birthday. Some live through the first few years of life but require residential placement because of severe mental and physical retardation.

Trisomy 13 to 15 Another chromosomal disorder is trisomy 13 to 15, so named because chromosomes 13, 14, and 15 look so much alike that it is hard to distinguish one from another. In trisomy 13 to 15, there is an extra chromosome of this group, so that the total chromosomal count is 47 rather than 46, but just which one is present in triplet form is

uncertain. Infants with this syndrome are frequently severely deformed, with gross abnormalities involving the eyes, head, or any of the major organs (13).

Two-thirds of these infants have severe cleft palate and cleft lip (Fig. 2·10). The nurse must recognize that cleft palate does not always mean that the infant has a trisomy of this type. On the other hand, she must also remember that a trisomy cannot be ruled out because the cleft palate is not present.

Most often infants having trisomy 13 to 15 die in the first few months of life because so many major organs are abnormal. Should the infant live, medical and ethical problems sometimes arise about what treatment measures should be undertaken, especially whether surgical intervention and cosmetic reconstructions should be attempted. Is it morally right to go to great length to attempt to perform plastic repairs and organ transplants, for example, on an infant who is destined to be severely retarded and deformed? On the other hand, is it humane to allow an infant, no matter how different from normal, to survive with difficulty in eating or some other major discomfort when intervention could relieve the distress? Such questions as these come to mind and must be carefully considered. In most circumstances, if medical or surgical intervention promotes comfort or helps the parents to feel less anxiety without creating false hope, it is undertaken.

NURSING SUPPORT OF THE MOTHER In years gone by, it frequently was the practice not to allow mothers to see their newborn infants if they were deformed. Nurses and physicians thought it was kind to spare the mother. This practice has changed in recent years after recognition that not permitting a new mother to see her deformed infant may create greater anxiety than she would have if she had seen him. The imagination is sometimes much more cruel than the reality. Careful preparation and support are necessary before bringing such a baby to his awaiting parents. It is important to listen with quiet empathy and to accept their reactions and feelings, no matter what they may be. The nurse must be careful not to impose her own feelings and values on the already burdened parents. She must pro-

fig. 2·10 Severe cleft lip and palate. (*Courtesy of The National Foundation–March of Dimes.*)

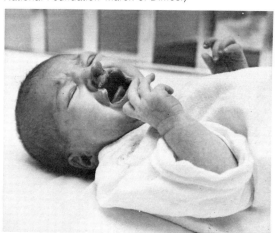

vide reassurance when it is realistic to do so. She should not give false hope. With the permission of the physician, referral can be made to agencies such as the National Foundation, local parent groups, and other resources, including religious affiliations. An understanding of the parents' reaction to the birth of a defective child, as well as an understanding of the grief and mourning process, is essential to the nurse who works with parents and their handicapped children or who in any way is involved with genetic counseling.

Cri-du-chat Syndrome In 1963, several infants and children were found to have been born with severe psychomotor retardation, small head, hypertelorism (widely separated eyes), small face, and low-set ears. The cry of such a child is a characteristic meowing like the sound of a hungry lost kitten. Hence the name *cri-du-chat* (French for "cry of the cat") is given to this syndrome, which results from a missing part (deletion) of chromosome 5 (14). Although cute at birth and in early childhood, these children often grow to become less attractive or even severely enough handicapped in appearance by facial disproportions to require later surgery for cosmetic purposes. The catlike cry is lost after a year or two, but mental retardation persists throughout life.

CHROMOSOMAL ABNORMALITIES INVOLVING THE SEX CHROMOSOMES

Turner's Syndrome So far, all the major chromosomal problems we have discussed have involved autosomal chromosomes. Changes in the sex chromosomes have different effects. The normal female karyotype is 44XX, and the normal male is 44XY. An error involving the X or Y chromosomes results in a sex chromosomal abnormality. *Turner's syndrome* is a chromosomal disorder in which one of the X chromosomes is missing (see

Fig. 2·11). Total chromosomal count is therefore only 45 instead of 46. The affected female is short, squat, and obese, with a thick neck, shieldlike chest with widely-spaced nipples, and very poor breast development (Fig. 2·12). The ovaries, if present, are poorly formed and usually do not function normally, so that usually the patient is not fertile. These little girls generally grow into adults unless they have a cardiac defect, which sometimes accompanies Turner's syndrome. Mental retardation is lifelong, and most persons with Turner's syndrome are found in institutions by the time they become adults. This trend may change in the future as better community facilities for special education become available and as the public becomes more informed about and tolerant of individuals who

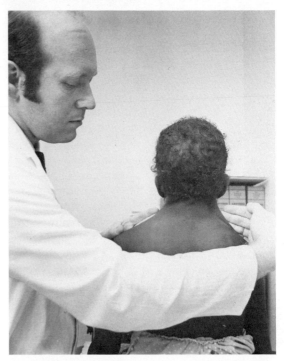

fig. 2·12 Turner's syndrome, in an eleven-year-old child, showing webbed neck. (*Courtesy of The National Foundation–March of Dimes.*)

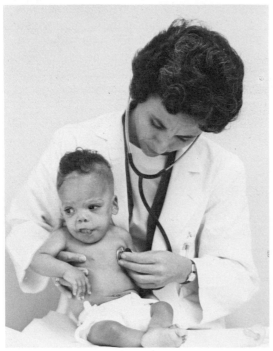

fig. 2·11 Turner's syndrome in a seven-month-old child. (*Courtesy of The National Foundation–March of Dimes.*)

are atypical or in need of special guidance at some point in their lives. Other atypical forms of Turner's syndrome exist but will not be discussed here.

Klinefelter's Syndrome About one in 200 boys are born with an extra X chromosome, so that their karyotype is 44XXY (15). Normally the male, if you recall, has only a single X chromosome. The 44XXY karyotype is called *Klinefelter's syndrome* (16). This condition is usually not very apparent until puberty, when the boy begins to develop breast enlargement along with other secondary female sex characteristics such as wide hips, high-pitched voice, and absence of hair with typical male distribution (Fig. 2·13). His penis remains small, and the testes remain undeveloped. Mental retardation is frequent but not severe; often such boys are in school but do poorly or are placed in a special class. The youth with Klinefelter's syndrome has a lanky appearance with long arms and legs but poor muscle development. Although the male with Klinefelter's syndrome may be somewhat retarded, he may live a fairly normal life within the community. Many of these young men have entered the military service, passed the physical and psychological exams, and contributed to military duty. Their

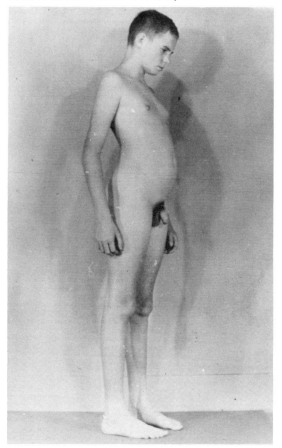

fig. 2·13 Klinefelter's syndrome. *(Courtesy of the National Foundation–March of Dimes.)*

fertility rate is low, and they often suffer slanderous remarks because of their genital and gonadal underdevelopment. Hormones may improve general male appearance but of course will not alter the underlying chromosomal abnormality in karyotype.

XYY Syndrome Recently an extremely interesting and highly controversial disorder of the male sex chromosomes has been discovered: the XYY syndrome, or the "Superman" syndrome. These males are tall—well over 6 ft 4 in—muscular, well coordinated, and highly aggressive. The first individuals found with the XYY syndrome were criminals, all serving sentences for highly aggressive crimes. Their personal histories showed accounts of repeated criminal offenses. There has very recently been speculation that criminal behavior might be produced by the extra Y chromosome. This question remains unsolved.

GENETIC DISORDERS OF MOLECULAR ORIGIN

An increased understanding of molecular biology and the genetic code has led to current knowledge and discovery of hundreds of disorders which result from failure to inherit particular genes required to make specific enzymes, or from irregularities in the enzyme function itself. These disorders, called *inborn errors in metabolism* (or disorders of molecular origin), are all transmitted by the *autosomal recessive* mode of Mendel's laws of inheritance.

Autosomal recessive transmission means that both parents are carriers (heterozygotes) of the disorder but appear normal themselves. Since they have one of the genes in a given pair, they have enough of the genetic information necessary for making a particular enzyme. Hence, phenotypically, they themselves have no overt signs of disease. With-

table 2·5

CHROMOSOMAL DISORDERS AND THEIR CHARACTERISTIC SYMPTOMS

CHROMOSOMAL DISORDER	CHARACTERISTIC SYMPTOMS
Trisomy 21 (Down's syndrome)	Flat, round face Depressed nasal bridge Protruding tongue Epicanthal folds and Brushfield's spots Short neck Thick trunk and short stature Broad hands with simian crease Hypotonia Mental retardation
Trisomy 18 (Edwards's syndrome)	Failure to thrive Difficulty in sucking Small face, receding chin Low-set, malformed ears Kidney or cardiac abnormalities Overlapping fingers Rocker-bottom feet Hypotonia Mental retardation
Trisomy 13-15 (Patau's syndrome)	Failure to thrive Microphthalmia Cerebral dysgenesis Cleft palate and lip Congenital heart condition Polydactyly Deformed extremities (Note: Symptoms vary; gross deformities are common.)
Deletion of short arm of chromosome 5 (cri-du-chat)	Failure to thrive Round face with low-set ears Hypertelorism Microencephaly Mental retardation "Cat cry" Sucking difficulty
Turner's syndrome (XO)	Often not detected until puberty Short stature Lack of secondary female sex characteristics Shield chest Web neck Infertility Mental retardation (mild)
Klinefelter's syndrome (XXY)	Often not detected until puberty Secondary female characteristics in male Infertility Poor development of male characteristics Mild mental retardation

table 2·5 (Continued)

CHROMOSOMAL DISORDER	CHARACTERISTIC SYMPTOMS
Superman syndrome (XYY)	Tall, muscular build Aggressiveness Acne persisting into adulthood Thought to be associated with criminal behavior

SOURCE: Adapted from Ian Porter, *Heredity and Disease,* McGraw-Hill Book Company, New York, 1968.

out symptoms of illness, they lead normal lives. Only if two carriers marry is there a problem. Then, statistically, the probabilities are one in four that their child will have the disorder, two in four that he will be a carrier like his parents, and only one in four that he will be normal. This does not mean that always one of each four children will be affected. It only means that the average chance or probability is one in four that the child will have the disease.

Inborn Errors of Metabolism PKU, galactosemia, Tay-Sachs disease, and cystic fibrosis are but a few of the disorders inherited by autosomal recessive transmission. Many of the inborn errors of metabolism, such as PKU, can be detected during the newborn period. The alert nursery nurse is usually first to note changes of differences in the infant affected with an inborn error of metabolism. Typical symptoms, no matter which disorder is involved, include vomiting, poor weight gain, failure to thrive, tremor, seizures, and strange-smelling urine or feces. Unfortunately, there is not room in this chapter to go into detail about all or any of the inborn errors. We can only talk about them in general. Porter (7), Stanbury and Wyngaarden (17), and Nyhan (18) have written about them in detail. Nelson's *Textbook of Pediatrics* (19) is another excellent resource. The important thing to remember is that many of the inborn errors, if detected early, are treatable, so that gross defects such as the mental retardation produced in untreated PKU can be prevented.

Careful observation in the nursery and in the pediatrician's office, pediatric clinic, or home is of primary importance in discovering an inborn entity which might otherwise go undiagnosed.

PHENYLKETONURIA An inborn error of metabolism is never cured. In some cases, treatment properly instituted can compensate for the missing elements and keep the condition well under control. Early detection and dietary treatment of PKU provide an example. The child who has PKU is missing the enzyme *phenylalanine hydroxylase*, which converts the amino acid phenylalanine to tyrosine. Because this conversion cannot take place, excess phenylalanine accumulates in the blood. In an attempt to get rid of this excess, the body converts it to phenyl pyruvic and phenyl acetic acid, which are excreted in the urine. These can be tested in the urine with Phenistix or by the ferric chloride test. Treatment involves reducing phenylalanine intake by using Lofenalac formula, never giving regular milk or protein foods, and carefully measuring all fruits and vegetables, since almost no food is free of phenylalanine. Without proper treatment, the probability is extremely great that the child will become severely retarded (20). In late childhood, it is possible to allow more freedom in the diet, but the girl who has PKU should again be careful to control her phenylalanine intake if she becomes pregnant.

TAY-SACHS DISEASE Until very recently, nothing could be done to assist families of children born with metabolic disorders of lipid metabolism. Recently this situation has begun to change, as witnessed by advancements concerning Tay-Sachs disease. This inborn error of metabolism, most common among European Jews, results in total loss of central nervous system function and finally in death. Infants appear normal at birth. At about a year of age, failure to thrive begins. Inability to sit or do any of the previously developed activities, seizures, blindness, and mental retardation follow, leading to death within a few years. There is no treatment. In 1971, tests for carriers and detection of affected fetuses through amniocentesis became possible (21).

Since most people do not know if they are carriers of hereditary disorders, the danger of having a child with the inborn error is not usually known until one is already born. The probabilities of two carriers marrying is not too great (about 1 in 12,000) for the general population. However, since people tend to marry those like themselves as far as family background, religion, and nationality are concerned, the chances are higher among some groups for some conditions. For example, the incidence of PKU is extremely high among the Pennsylvania Amish and fair-skinned northern Europeans, as is that of Tay-Sachs disease among Eastern European Jews.

Sex-linked Genetic Disorders Another group of inherited disorders comprises those which are *sex-linked*. Sex-linked conditions are transmitted by mothers to sons. The woman is a heterozygote in the sex-linked conditions. The genes for these disorders are located on the X chromosomes. Since women have two X chromosomes, if a gene on one of them is missing, one-half her sons will have the disorder. If a son inherits the X chromosome with the missing gene, he will have the disorder because the male karyotype is XY. If he inherits the normal chromosome, he will be normal. Naturally, half the daughters of a woman heterozygous for sex-linked disorders will be carriers. No daughters will have the disorder, since the father will have contributed a normal X chromosome. Sex-linked conditions include classical hemophilia, Duchenne's muscular dystrophy, and Lesch-Nyhan syndrome.

environmental factors influencing genetic change and altering fetal development

We now know that many factors in the environment produce mutation through a change in the genes themselves, as dictated by a "mistake" or change in the DNA itself. A genetic change, i.e., a change in the genetic material itself, in turn alters body chemistry and metabolism. It is conceivable that a mutation could in some instances be positive, i.e., helpful. In human beings at least, such changes are difficult to detect. The mutations that are noticed and are of concern are the harmful ones. As stated previously, they may result in inborn errors of metabolism which could be passed on to offspring.

A defect in body structure and form that is due to environmental problems which alter the growth of the fetus after fertilization is termed a *congenital defect* or *anomaly*. Those chemicals or viruses which cause damage are called *teratogenic* agents. The same kinds of agents which produce damage to an egg or a sperm prior to fertilization (resulting in genetic defects) can also produce damage to somatic cells of the developing baby after fertilization (resulting in congenital defects). Let us look at some of the agents which produce genetic change and congenital abnormalities.

RADIATION

Radiation of all types presents a potential hazard. The risk is proportional to the amount of radiation and the length of exposure, as well as to the nature of the particular tissue involved. Rapidly growing and immature cells are particularly vulnerable to radiation. Thus ova, sperm, fetal cells, and blood cells are most susceptible to radiation damage. This was demonstrated unfortunately by the hundreds of survivors of two atomic bomb attacks, who show more chromosomal breaks and have a higher incidence of leukemia than the general population (22). X-rays in the early weeks of pregnancy can damage the developing fetus: thus x-rays for diagnostic purposes should be avoided if at all possible and should be considered only with careful precaution (23). Prior to pregnancy, a person (either male or female) should avoid overexposure to x-rays. Lead aprons should be worn by nurses and technicians who are frequently exposed to radiation in the x-ray department when they assist patients during the taking of x-rays.

Emissions from microwave ovens, cosmic radiation, ultraviolet radiation, and perhaps even radar and sonar may pose potential hazard. Often cells damaged by such agents repair themselves before producing offspring, but under some circumstances mutations can be induced by the types of radiation mentioned, and then the mutant cell will produce abnormal offspring. Much of this radiation is present in our natural environment from solar and other astronomic sources independent of man. We are more concerned with man-made radiation hazards and other dangerous sources of genetic change in the environment as a result of poor control of industrial and other wastes.

INDUSTRIAL POLLUTION

In the long run, atomic power may be less of a potential hazard than some forms of chemical and industrial pollution. Hydrocarbons, plastics, insecticides, and metals such as lead, copper, and mercury are known to be as-sociated with birth defects. Birth defects among children born to parents who work in lead mines have been reported in Germany and elsewhere. Styrene and other chemicals used in the making of plastics have been known to induce leukemia in fetuses and in adults.

NUTRITIONAL DEFICIENCY

Nutritional deficiency during pregnancy may be the cause of some birth defects. Spina bifida, meningomyelocele, and cleft palate with harelip have been produced in laboratory animals lacking vitamin C in their diet. On the other hand, Cooke (25) reports that excessive vitamin A and also lack of vitamin B may produce similar results in rats and mice. McKibbin and Porter (26) report vitamin C deficiency in human children with myelomeningiocele which seems to be related not to poor diet but to failure to use vitamin C in the body once it is ingested. What relationship the faulty vitamin C metabolism may have in terms of cause or effect remains unclear.

DRUGS

Any drug given during pregnancy, especially in the early weeks, could endanger the fetus. LSD, barbiturates, caffeine, and cyclamates have been known to cause chromosomal breakage, which could result in severe birth defects of the skeletal, nervous, and cardiovascular systems. Thalidomide, used as a mild tranquilizer by pregnant women in Europe, is known to have been responsible for the production of hundreds of children without arms or legs (Fig. 2·14). It is ironic to think that the very drug that was intended to help their mothers maintain better equilibrium during pregnancy results in a lifetime of misfortune for them. Steroids rank high among the problem drugs. A single dose of testosterone given to a mother who is spotting early in

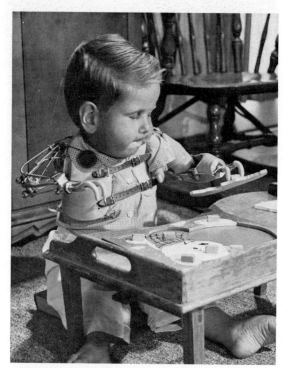

fig. 2·14 Phocomelia. (*Courtesy of The National Foundation–March of Dimes.*)

pregnancy may produce ambiguous genitalia and adrenal cortical hyperplasia in the female fetus. Additional examples of how drugs may affect the fetus are given in Chap. 19, where drug implications for the newborn are discussed.

VIRUSES

Viruses are great inducers of genetic change. Since a virus is either RNA or DNA enclosed in a protein coat and contains no ribosomes or mitochondria, it injects its genetic material into the living cell it invades, then takes over the cell to reproduce itself. In doing so, it alters the normal arrangement of the cellular DNA. If the cell lives, it grows and reproduces abnormal cells altered by the virus. Mutant cells may be involved in some malignant disorders and may contribute to the uncon-

trolled carcinogenic process. Viral infections may well prove to be a contributing factor in some forms of leukemia. Rubella virus and herpes virus are especially detrimental to the human fetus (see Chap. 20).

genetics, the nurse, and the future

Prenatal care and family health care can contribute much to the prevention of congenital and genetic defects. If one knows a person's whole family and understands something about the family background and history, it is possible to make some speculations about the kinds of health (and especially gene-associated) disorders most likely to develop. Communication skills and a basic nurse-patient relationship which involves trust are essential for gathering much of the data required about a family in order to give appropriate genetic counseling of a more involved nature. Current techniques in amniocentesis and cytology have contributed methods for detecting problems during early fetal life with little risk to mother or fetus. During these procedures the nurse must give support and understanding to help alleviate fear.

As knowledge about enzyme structure and activity increases, it may become possible in the future to make artificial enzymes, just as insulin is given as a substitute in the diabetic. These enzymes may then be used to treat individuals with inborn errors of metabolism, just as diabetics are currently being given medical treatment and nursing guidance. Genetic engineering may come about in the future, though man probably will never control intelligence or make a "super race" in test tubes as the science fiction writers would have us expect. Psychologic characteristics are either multigenetic (meaning that they involve complex interaction of many genes which man cannot duplicate) or they are influenced greatly by environment. Future treatment of a number of diseases (hemophilia, cystic fibrosis, sickle-cell anemia, and possibly even Tay-Sachs disease, leukemia, and other malignancies induced by interactions of heredity and environment) does fall within the potential reality of genetics in the near future. What role the nurse will have in this exciting future depends upon her own willingness to become involved.

references

1. Julian Huxley and H. B. Kettelwell, *Charles Darwin and His World*, Random House, Inc., New York, 1965.
2. J. M. Barry, *Molecular Biology and Chemical Control of Living Cells*, Prentice Hall, Inc., Englewood Cliffs, N.J., 1964, pp. 44–56.
3. George Beadle, *The Language of Life*, Doubleday & Company, Inc., Garden City, N.Y., 1966.
4. Victor McKusick, *Human Genetics*, Prentice-Hall, Inc., Englewood Cliffs, N.J., 1965, p. 10.
5. Alex Fraser, *Computer Genetics*, McGraw-Hill Book Company, New York, 1970.
6. Victor McKusick, op. cit., p. 5.
7. Ian Porter, *Heredity and Disease*, McGraw-Hill Book Company, New York, 1968, pp. 42–50.
8. Kay Corman Kintzel and Delores Lake, "Medical Genetics and the Nurse," in Kay Corman Kintzel et al., *Advanced Concepts in Clinical Nursing*, J. B. Lippincott Company, Philadelphia, 1972, pp. 80–105.
9. *Chromosome 21 and Its Association with Down's Syndrome*, The National Foundation—March of Dimes, New York, N.Y.
10. Ian Porter, op. cit., pp. 42–43.
11. Ibid., p. 244.
12. Ibid., p. 53.
13. Ibid., pp. 54–55.
14. Lytt Gardner, *Endocrine and Genetic Diseases of Childhood*, W. B. Saunders Company, Philadelphia, 1969, pp. 632–635.
15. F. Sergovich, et al., "Chromosomal Aberrations in 2,159 Consecutive Births," *New England Journal of Medicine*, Apr. 17, 1969, pp. 851–855.
16. Ibid., pp. 569–574.
17. J. B. Stanbury and J. B. Wyngaarden, *The Metabolic Basis of Inherited Disease*, McGraw-Hill Book Company, New York, 1969.
18. William L. Nyhan, *Amino Acid Metabolism and Genetic Variation*, McGraw-Hill Book Company, New York, 1967.
19. Waldo Nelson, *Textbook of Pediatrics*, W. B. Saunders Company, Philadelphia, 1969.
20. Delores Lake, "Nursing Implications from an Investigation of Diet, Development and Mothering in Two Groups of Children with Phenylketonuria," in *ANA Clinical Sessions, 1968*, Appleton-Century-Crofts, Inc., New York, 1968.
21. Albert Gerbie et al., "Amniocentesis in Genetic Counseling," *American Journal of Obstetrics and Gynecology*, **109**(5): 765–768, 1971.
22. Henry L. Nadler, "Intrauterine Detection of Genetic Disorders," in J. P. Greenhill (ed.), *Yearbook of Obstetrics and Gynecology*, Yearbook Medical Publishers, Inc., Chicago, 1972.
23. Ian Porter, op. cit., p. 418.
24. Joseph Sternberg, "Irradiation and Radio Contamination during Pregnancy," *American Journal of Obstetrics and Gynecology*, **108**(3):490–495, 1970.
25. Cooke, Robert, *The Biologic Basis of Pediatric Practice*, McGraw-Hill Book Company, New York, 1968.
26. B. McKibbin, and R. Porter, "The Incidence of Vitamin C Deficiency in Meningomyelocele," *Developmental Medi-*

cine and Child Neurology, **9**:338–344, 1967.

bibliography

Asimov, Isaac: *The Genetic Code,* Signet Books, New American Library, Inc., New York, 1962.

Becker, Kenneth: "Successful Use of Therapeutic Androgenization in Klinefelter's Syndrome," *Modern Medicine,* Nov. 13, 1972, p. 57.

Brady, Rosco: "Hereditary Fat Metabolism Diseases," *Scientific American,* August 1973, pp. 88–97.

Brown, Donald: "The Isolation of Genes," *Scientific American,* August 1973, pp. 20–30.

Carr, D. H.: "Chromosomal Errors and Development," *American Journal of Obstetrics and Gynecology,* **104**:327, 1969.

Douglas, Gordon: "Rubella in Pregnancy," *American Journal of Nursing,* December 1966.

Ferreira, Antonio J.: *Prenatal Environment,* Charles C Thomas, Publisher, Springfield, Ill., 1969.

Forbes, Nancy: "The Nurse and Genetic Counseling," *Nursing Clinics of North America,* **1**(4):679, 1966.

Gooder, Jennifer: "The XXY Male," *Nursing Mirror,* **130**(15):20–22, 1970.

Hecht, F.: "Genetic Diagnosis in the Newborn," *Pediatric Clinics of North America,* **17**:1039, 1970.

Marlow, Dorothy: *Textbook of Pediatric Nursing,* W. B. Saunders, Philadelphia, 1973, pp. 578–581.

Nitowsky, H. M.: "Prenatal Diagnosis of Genetic Abnormality," *American Journal of Nursing,* **71**:1551, 1971.

Reisman, L. E.: "Chromosomal Abnormalities and Intrauterine Growth Retardation," *Pediatric Clinics of North America,* **17**:101, 1970.

Rothberg, L.: "A New Sound in Obstetrics," *R.N.,* **34**:38, 1971.

Schiff, Gilbert, and Joseph Rauh: "Rubella Control," *American Journal of Diseases of Children,* **122**(2):112–116, 1971.

Sparkles, Robert S., and Barbara F. Crandall: "Genetic Disorders Affecting Growth and Development," chap. 4 in Nicholas Assali (ed.), *Pathophysiology of Gestation: Fetal-Placental Disorders,* vol. 2, Academic Press, Inc., New York, 1972, pp. 208–64.

Stone, David, et al.: "Do Artificial Sweeteners Ingested in Pregnancy Affect the Offspring?" *Nature,* **231**(5297):53, 1971.

Stutz, S. D.: "The Nursing Challenge of OB: When the Baby Isn't Normal," *R.N.,* **34**:40, 1971.

Taussig, Helen: "The Thalidomide Syndrome," in *Scientific American Resource Library Readings in Life Sciences,* vol. 7 (Offspring, No. 1100), W. H. Freeman and Company, San Francisco.

Tjio, J. H., et al.: "LSD and Chromosomes," *Journal of the American Medical Association,* **210**:849, 1969.

Watson, James: *The Double Helix,* Signet Books, New American Library, Inc., New York, 1969.

Wilson, James G.: "Environmental Effects on Development and Teratology," chap. 5 in Nicholas Assali (ed.), *Pathophysiology of Gestation: Fetal-Placental Disorders,* vol. 2, Academic Press, Inc., New York, 1972, pp. 270–314.

OTHER RESOURCES

National Foundation—March of Dimes
P. O. Box 2000, White Plains, N.Y. 10602

Ross Laboratories
Columbus, Ohio 43216

Mead Johnson Company
Evansville, Ind. 47721

Victor McKusick, M.D.
Department of Genetics

Johns Hopkins University
Baltimore, Md.

John Bartram, M.D.
Handicapped Children's Unit
St. Christopher's Hospital for Children
2603 North 5th St.
Philadelphia, Pa.

Mental Retardation Abstracts
Department of Health, Education and Welfare
300 Independence Avenue, S.W.
Washington, D.C.

National Institutes of Health
Bethesda, Md.

National Society for Crippled Children
and Adults
2023 West Ogden Ave.
Chicago, Ill. 60612

National Association for Retarded Children
420 Lexington Ave.
New York, N.Y. 10017

National Cystic Fibrosis Research Foundation
3379 Peachtree Road N.E.
Atlanta, Ga. 30326

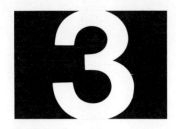

conception and fetal growth and development

Roberts Rugh

origin of primordial germ cells

All higher animals have reproductive organs
—ovaries and testes—within which the germ
cells mature. Even before any woman is
aware of her pregnancy, her embryo sets
aside about 100 cells for the specific purpose
of reproduction, the most far-sighted example
of a savings account for the future that occurs
in biology! These 100 cells arise apart from
the embryo, within its attached yolk sac, and
then pass through its junction to the embryo.
They begin the journey about 3 to 4 weeks
after conception, before any other organs are
formed, even the gonads within which they
will gather and reside. The cells continue to
divide and multiply, so that by the time they
reach the *gonad primordia,* which are simultaneously developing within the body of the
embryo, they constitute millions of similar
descendant cells which are to populate the
gonads, whether ovaries or testes. In both
sexes, the primitive germ cells cannot be
distinguished from one another in the embryo
until they begin to go through a process
known as *maturation* which is typical of germ
cells and is found exclusively in them.

maturation of germ cells

The maturing process occurs after the cells
have reached the gonad. Beginning usually
at about puberty, it involves meiotic cell
divisions, resulting in haploid daughter cells,
unlike the parent cell in that they contain only
half the normal number of chromosomes. The
reduction of the chromosomes to half is an
obvious necessity because, when the sperm
and ovum are joined in fertilization, there
would otherwise be a doubling of the number
of chromosomes with each generation. So,
while every cell of the human embryo or fetus
contains 23 *pairs* of chromosomes, the matured sperm or ovum of the postpubertal adult
contains only *23 chromosomes,* representing
one member of each of the original pairs.
Since each of the chromosomes may carry as
many as 20,000 hereditary units (*genes*) and
the genes on any chromosome may differ in
many instances from those on any member
pair, one can readily see that no two ova or
two sperm could be identical with respect to
hereditary potential. The twenty-third pair in
the embryonic or fetal cells determines the
sex of the individual; its members are identified as the XX or XY chromosomes. If the
twenty-third pair is XX, the individual is female, if XY, it is male. But since the XY
situation occurs only in the male, and by
division in the process of maturation the
members of pairs are separated, each mature
sperm as a haploid cell will carry either (but
not both) the X or the Y chromosome, while
every ovum carries only an X chromosome.
One can thus understand that sex of the
offspring is determined by the father rather
than the mother, in the sense that it depends
upon whether the X or Y carrying sperm first
reaches the mature ovum and fertilizes it.

Since the ratio of male to female babies
born in the general population is about
106:100, one can speculate that since the X-
and the Y-carrying sperm are produced in

exactly equal numbers, the production of a few more males than females may be related to the possibility that the Y-carrying sperm (male-producing) is infinitesimally lighter and hence faster moving than the X-carrying sperm, and hence gets to the ovum more quickly. There is some experimental evidence to support this theory.

MITOSIS

The potential sperm divide equally, as in simple *mitosis*, so that if there are at first 100 cells in the yolk sac beginning their migration to the site of the testes, these become 200, 400, 800, etc., dividing and thus multiplying until vast numbers are produced. The potential ova divide equally many times, giving rise to 7 million oocytes by the time the fetus is five months old. By the time of birth, the number is reduced to about 2 million; it is further reduced to about 300,000 by age seven, and to about 30,000 by age twenty-one. This drastic decrease in numbers may suggest that nature has overproduced in order to ensure ultimate propagation. One can readily understand that even during ovulatory cycles, from about the ages of twelve to fifty in the female, only about 400 of these oocytes become ova, maturing at the rate of about one each month, and fewer than 40 could possibly produce the offspring of a single woman! What happens is that the vast majority of these cells become *nurse cells*, known as follicle cells, assisting the 400 potential ova in becoming mature and acquiring some nutritive reserve (Fig. 3·1).

MEIOSIS

The first division of the final maturation of the primordial germ cell, which is meiotic, has resulted in what is called the *primary* oocyte, plus one discarded nucleus. The primary

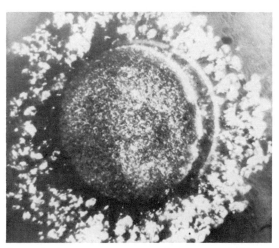

fig. 3·1 Mature human ovum entirely surrounded by follicle cells. (*Courtesy of Landrum B. Shettles; from R. Rugh, and L. B. Shettles,* From Conception to Birth: The Drama of Life's Beginnings, *Harper & Row, Publishers, Incorporated, New York,* 1971.)

oocyte nucleus then prepares for the second division by reaching the metaphase state in chromosome reduction and remains thus until the stimulation of fertilization by a mature spermatozoon. This stimulation causes the secondary oocyte to complete the second meiotic division; it discards its extra nucleus (second polar body), and its remaining haploid nucleus combines with the sperm nucleus (all within the ovum) to form the *diploid zygote nucleus,* which is ready to proceed in the developmental process. The original discarded nucleus from the immature ovum has undergone independent division to give rise to two small nuclei, and these three nuclei are known as *polar bodies*; they are functionless. Thus, the preferred ovum arises at the expense of the cytoplasm originally associated with all four nuclei (Fig. 3·2).

These two meiotic divisions not only reduce the number of chromosomes from 46 to 23 but eliminate three-fourths of the nuclear material in favor of the fourth nucleus, which

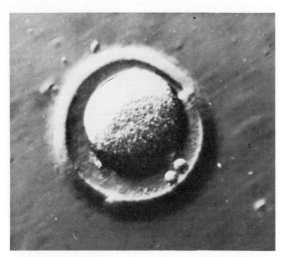

fig. 3·2 Fertilized egg with two polar bodies. Photographed through a phase microscope 12 h after being fertilized by a human sperm. The surrounding follicle cells and extra spermatozoa have been dispersed, and the two polar bodies (discarded nuclei) are seen in the perivitelline space. There is no external evidence of the dynamic changes that are occurring within the egg for the first division into two cells. (*From R. Rugh and L. B. Shettles,* From Conception to Birth: The Drama of Life's Beginnings, *Harper & Row, Publishers, Incorporated, New York,* 1971.)

is surrounded by cytoplasm and some yolk, and is now ready for fertilization. No one yet knows how the selection of a particular oocyte is made, nor why certain primordial oocytes give rise to mature ova, others become nurse cells, and still others simply die and are absorbed (Fig. 3·3).

In the male, Sertoli cells arise in the testes, and in the cytoplasm of these cells will lodge the heads of maturing spermatozoa, deriving therefrom such nutrition as is required to mature and survive until they are needed for fertilization. The sperm is little more than an encased nucleus (Fig. 3·4), with a middle piece and a tail for propulsion; there is no accumulation of nutrient reserve. Presumably each primordial sperm cell, *spermatogonia,*

gives rise to at least four equivalent, but not genetically identical, haploid sperm cells. This is one reason why a male can produce trillions of mature spermatozoa from puberty to advanced old age. Though this seems like a great waste, it tends to ensure propagation of the species, especially since most sperm are destroyed in the reproductive tract of the female as they progress upward toward the mature ovum (Fig. 3·5).

Basically the changes known as maturation (meiosis) are the same for sperm and ova, since the ultimate result is a haploid cell capable of joining a complementary cell and initiating the development process. Following maturation, the sperm and the ovum can indeed be distinguished, even though they are both of microscopic dimensions. The mature ovum measures about $1/125$ in in diameter, and the sperm measures about $1/500$ in in length, including its long tail. These two types of cells are developed for the specific purpose of together producing another generation by bringing together their two complementary nuclei and thus reestablishing the diploid or paired chromosome state neces-

fig. 3·3 Summary of ovum development. (*From A. J. Vander, J. H. Sherman, and D. Luciano,* Human Physiology, *McGraw-Hill Book Company, New York,* 1970.)

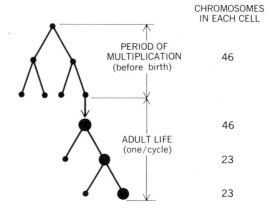

CHROMOSOMES IN EACH CELL

PERIOD OF MULTIPLICATION (before birth) — 46

46

ADULT LIFE (one/cycle)

23

23

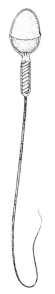

fig. 3·4 A mature human sperm. (*From A. J. Vander, J. H. Sherman, and D. Luciano,* Human Physiology, *McGraw-Hill Book Company, New York, 1970.*)

sary for the initiation, production, and survival of an embryo, fetus, and, after 266 days, a newborn human being.

general structure of mature gonads

THE MATURE MALE TESTES

Paired, oval organs measuring an average of $1^1/_2$ to 2 in in length and 1 in in thickness develop within the peritoneal cavity until the third month of gestation, when they begin their slow descent through the inguinal canal toward the external sac, the scrotum, located directly behind the penis. The scrotum is filled with loose connective tissue and is divided vertically by a partition (septum) so that each testis comes to lodge in a separate compartment (Fig. 3·6).

The mature testis is an organ closely packed with miles of seminiferous tubules, each of which has layers of maturing cells in its walls. Clusters of tubules are separated from one another by connective tissue septa, within which are formed testosterone-secreting, or *Leydig,* cells; it is *testosterone* which induces the secondary sexual characteristics of typically male muscle texture, skeletal size, deeper voice, and hirsutism. All tubules converge into the rete testis, leading thence to the efferent ductules and the epididymis, which are numerous tiny tubules within which mature sperm collect, awaiting propulsion through the vas deferens. Since millions of sperm mature daily, after puberty, the cross section of any tubule will reveal all the maturational steps from primary spermatocyte to mature spermatozoon.

Spermatogenesis At puberty a boy's anterior pituitary gland sends out hormones (FSH) which reactivate his testes. The original cords of the testes become seminiferous tubules, with spermatogonia and Sertoli cells lying against the basement membrane of the tubule epithelium. These cells begin to enlarge without mitosis, through the accumulation of nutri-

fig. 3·5 Summary of spermatogenesis. (*From A. J. Vander, J. H. Sherman, and D. Luciano,* Human Physiology, *McGraw-Hill Book Company, New York, 1970.*)

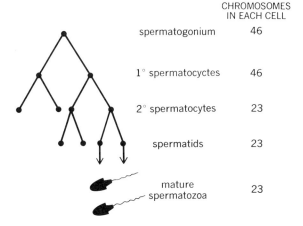

	CHROMOSOMES IN EACH CELL
spermatogonium	46
1° spermatocyctes	46
2° spermatocytes	23
spermatids	23
mature spermatozoa	23

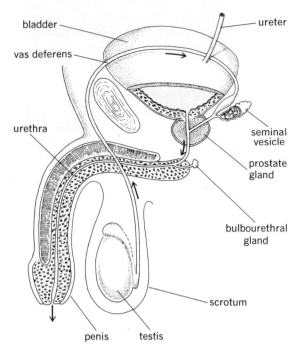

fig. 3·6 Anatomic organization of the male reproductive tract. (*From A. J. Vander, J. H. Sherman, and D. Luciano*, Human Physiology, *McGraw-Hill Book Company, New York*, 1970.)

tional reserve, and after about 26 days, become a relatively large, spherical cell known as the primary spermatocyte. At this stage, the primary spermatocyte still has its original 23 pairs of chromosomes (i.e., 46, one set from the mother and one set from the father), but there follows immediately a division giving rise to secondary spermatocytes, which are haploid. It is at this division of the nucleus that the X and Y chromosomes are separated, but each is associated with 22 separate chromosomes known as the *autosomes,* or nonsex chromosomes. However, just before this division, the pairs of chromosomes often exchange parts (called crossing-over), so that some genes originally contributed by the mother get onto chromosomes originally contributed by the father, and vice versa. Thus, we must not think of these chromosome pack-

ages as totally unchanging. Then follows another division, with the resulting cells, called *spermatids,* identical to that cell from which each is derived. It is now estimated that this entire process takes about 64 days in the human male, but it is a process which goes on continually and gives rise during the lifetime of a male to literally trillions of sperm cells (Fig. 3·7).

The mature sperm have very little nutritional reserve and hence cannot survive long apart from their nurselike Sertoli cells, or in the female genital tract. But each contains in the chromosomes in its nuclear head the DNA

fig. 3·7 Summary of male hormonal control. The negative signs indicate that testosterone inhibits both the hypothalamus and the anterior pituitary. Testosterone reaches the seminiferous tubules to stimulate spermatogenesis both by local diffusion and by release into the blood and recirculation to the testes. (*From A. J. Vander, J. H. Sherman, and D. Luciano*, Human Physiology, *McGraw-Hill Book Company, New York*, 1970.)

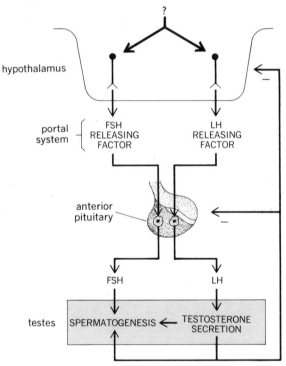

concentrate which is the carrier of its hereditary potential. After development in the epithelium of the seminiferous tubules, the mature sperm are liberated into the central lumen of the tubules, passing into the rete testis, the efferent ductules, and the epididymis, where they generally are retained until ejaculation. The volume of free, motile sperm builds up in the epididymis, and the sperm move through the vas deferens into a chamber (the ampulla) where they are mixed with a thick, glycogen-rich secretion (semen) and pass through the prostate (which contributes a serous alkaline secretion) to the ejaculatory duct. This trip takes about 12 days. The ejaculatory duct receives fluid from the seminal vesicle, the prostate, and Cowper's glands. This *seminal fluid* supports the mature and activated sperm. The ejaculatory duct from each testis opens into the urethra, which then becomes truly a urogenital duct.

THE MATURE FEMALE OVARIES

The ovaries are paired, almond-shaped organs about 1 in long and half as thick, each suspended between the broad ligament and the ovarian ligament, and intimately surrounded by the fimbriae of the *ostium*, or opening, into each fallopian tube. The ovary is thus actually suspended within the peritoneal cavity, but the ostium is so endowed with vibrating cilia, all beating toward the tube, that, as the ovum is liberated from an ovary, it is quickly scooped up by these vibrating cilia and propelled toward and into the 4-in-long tube (Fig. 3·8).

In contrast with the testes, the ova develop toward the periphery of the ovary, in the cortex, and as they mature they descend from the surface until they begin enlarging in a *graafian follicle*, whence they move toward the surface again in anticipation of ultimate rupture (ovulation) into the body cavity, at the rate of about one each 28 days.

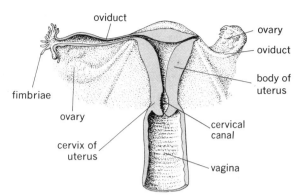

fig. 3·8 Uterus, fallopian tubes, and ovaries. (*From A. J. Vander, J. H. Sherman, and D. Luciano*, Human Physiology, *McGraw-Hill Book Company, New York, 1970.*)

THE UTERUS AND THE BIRTH CANAL

The uterus is pear-shaped and very muscular, with its smooth muscles capable of expansion to at least 60 times their resting length. It is about 3 in long in the resting state, located between the bladder and the rectum, so that it is easily palpated via the rectum during an obstetric examination. It consists of a *body,* with uterine cavity, and a tapering *isthmus* leading to a narrow internal *cervical os* and finally to the external cervical os, which is a very small opening into the vagina. The most anterior (upper) part of the uterus is the dome-shaped *fundus,* which measures at least 2 in from side to side. A woman's resting, or virginal, uterus may be estimated to be about the size of her closed fist. The recesses around the uterus, anterior to the cervix, are the *fornices.* The vagina is about 4 in in length, enclosing the lower end of the uterus; it has a single opening, the *introitus,* to the outside, laterally flanked by the small and large *labia* (Fig. 3·9).

hormonal control of reproduction

The growth of the graafian follicle is stimulated by FSH, the follicle-stimulating

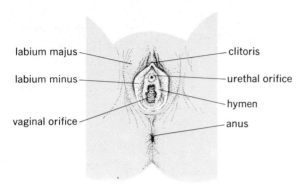

fig. 3·9 External view of perineal structures. (*From A. J. Vander, J. H. Sherman, and D. Luciano,* Human Physiology, *McGraw-Hill Book Company, New York, 1970.*)

that cooperates with prolactin and estrogen to thicken the cervical mucus, causes a brief rise in basal body temperature, and increases the elaboration of iron and glycogen in the endometrium of the uterus and vaginal mucosa. Estrogen prepares the uterus for the reception of the ovum, and progesterone aids in the implantation and maintenance of the implanted embryo (Figs. 3·11 and 3·12).

fertilization

For fertilization to occur, the germ cells not only must be at the proper stage for conjoin-

hormone. The graafian follicle produces estrogen, which enters the bloodstream in increasing amounts to influence the development of secondary female sexual characteristics, i.e., development of female contours (involving shoulders, hips, and breasts), the growth of pubic and axillary hair, and, more significantly, the beginning of the menstrual cycle at about age twelve. It is believed that oxidation products of estrogen in the bloodstream, arising from stimulation or activity of FSH, in turn stimulate the pituitary to secrete another hormone, luteinizing hormone (LH), which, in collaboration with FSH, causes the follicle to enlarge, ripen, and ultimately to rupture and release the maturing ovum. As ovulation occurs (Fig. 3·10), LH stimulates the ruptured follicle to secrete both *estrogen* and *progesterone,* the latter known as the pregnancy hormone. Continuation of secretion of these hormones is dependent upon release into the blood of a third pituitary hormone known as *prolactin* (LTH). It is the estrogen of the ovary that causes changes in the breasts, uterus, fallopian tubes, and vagina, particularly in their lining glands, which begin to proliferate in preparation for reproductive function. It is progesterone, after ovulation,

fig. 3·10 Summary of hormonal control of follicle and ovum development. Compare with Fig. 3·7. (*From A. J. Vander, J. H. Sherman, and D. Luciano,* Human Physiology, *McGraw-Hill Book Company, New York, 1970.*)

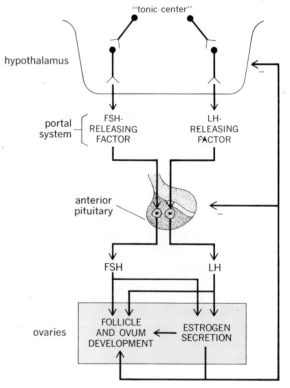

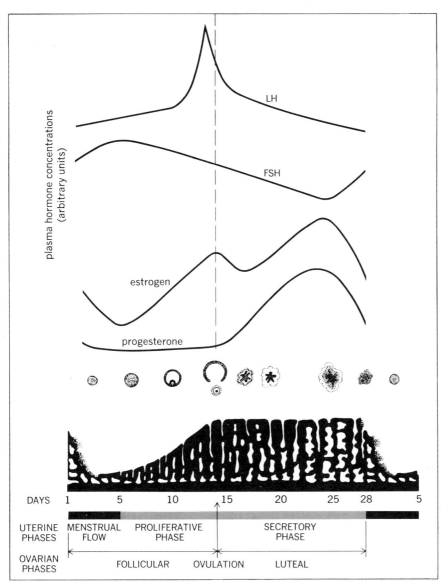

fig. 3·11 Plasma hormone concentration. Note LH peak before ovulation. (*From A. J. Vander, J. H. Sherman, and D. Luciano,* Human Physiology, *McGraw-Hill Book Company, New York,* 1970.)

ing but must come together deep within the female genital tract, usually high in the fallopian tube or near the ovary, just after ovulation has occurred. Ejaculation of hundreds of millions of motile sperm occurs at the height of the sexual act, during coitus, when the penis is inserted deep within the vagina and the semen is expelled from the male urethra into the vagina to cover the cervical os, or opening into the uterus. The volume of the

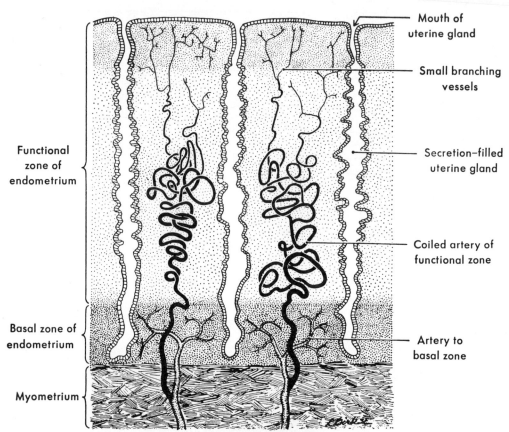

Functional zone of endometrium

Basal zone of endometrium

Myometrium

Mouth of uterine gland

Small branching vessels

Secretion–filled uterine gland

Coiled artery of functional zone

Artery to basal zone

fig. 3·12 Uterine mucosa during the secretory phase of the menstrual cycle. (*From B. M. Patten, Human Embryology, 3d ed., McGraw-Hill Book Company, New York, 1968.*)

ejaculate may be from 2 to 10 ml, and the concentration of sperm, 60 to 120 million per milliliter in fertile males. Some 80 percent of the sperm are active 2 h after ejaculation, and most of these are likely to be structurally normal. They are still not functional until they go through a chemical maturing process known as *capacitation,* which is believed to take 8 h.

The process of ejaculation by the male is the second part of the involuntary reflex-type act beginning with the delivery of semen into the prostatic urethra. Urethral and bulbourethral fluid acts as a lubricant for the insertion

of the penis; this is followed by rapid pulsations, overlapping one another, which ejaculate the cumulated semen with its sperm through the penis into the vagina, where the sperm become very active in the neutral and bacteria-free semen and where they swim in every possible direction. With appropriate psychologic and physical reactions, the female, too, may have pulsations (in the clitoris and vagina, and known as the *orgasm*), which are usually pleasant but are not necessary for the propelling of sperm into the uterus, where the more alkaline cervical secretions are favorable to survival and motility of the spermatozoa. The invasion of the uterus by millions of active cells calls forth the scavenging *phagocytes*, which arrive to attack and devour many of the sperm. Since so many sperm are provided, some survive and reach the mature ovum. Only the first spermatozoon to make contact with the surface of the ovum will function in fertilization, all others being immediately repelled. Those that are not successful, even though they could function in fertilization, lose that power within about 36 to 72 h, die, and are absorbed within 6 to 7 days, with no deleterious effect on the female genital tract or the developing ovum.

conception

Conception occurs at the precise moment when a motile, mature sperm encounters an immobile, mature ovum, stimulates it to begin a long process of complicated development, and, at the same time, causes the ovum to establish an instantaneous block to the invasion of any more sperm.

Usually the encounter occurs in the outer third of the fallopian tube (oviduct) as about 2000 sperm, having successfully overcome the hurdles en route from the cervix, converge upon the mature ovum. It is believed that the ovum does not actually attract the sperm, and that the sperm swim randomly about until one—entirely by chance—encounters the surface of the ovum.

The invading male nucleus is only the head of the sperm plus the small middle piece, and is, therefore, very small. It tends to swell as it moves through the egg cytoplasm toward the egg pronucleus to attain fusion, known as *syngamy*. The tail of the sperm is usually left at the surface, but the head is important because it contains all the hereditary potentials from the father, and the middle piece contains the granule (centriole) which regulates the spindle formation and subsequent

division of the fused nuclei. The centriole rotates 180° with the head, so that it precedes the head inward. It divides into two centrosomes, which soon will separate and take up positions on opposite sides of the congregating chromosomes from the two germ cells in order to form the first division or cleavage spindle. The membranes around the two pronuclei disappear, chromosomes form, and many vesicular nucleoli appear. All the chromosomes then line up on the spindle and split lengthwise; the pairs separate and then begin to migrate toward one or another of the poles, each marked by a centrosome. The entire process takes about 12 h to achieve pairing of the chromosomes from the sperm and the ovum, and another 12 h before there is evidence that the nucleoli have disappeared and the first mitotic division of the fertilized ovum, known now as the *zygote*, begins. The ovum is no longer dormant but is a dynamic, rapidly changing complete cell which would show, under ultramicroscopic magnification, almost violent activity.

The molecular material in the new cell, consisting of RNA-coded ribosomal precursor, directs the synthesis of the materials necessary for the early growth of the embryo before a placenta can be formed or the hereditary influences can play a part.

cleavage

Cleavage is simply the division of the fertilized ovum into equal and equivalent daughter cells, each possessing exactly what the other does with respect to hereditary potential (genes). But when one realizes that the single cell measures only about $1/125$ in in diameter and gives rise by proliferation to trillions of daughter cells which compose the newborn infant, the potency of this microscopic unit is beyond calculation. This first cleavage is attained by about 22 h, so that if

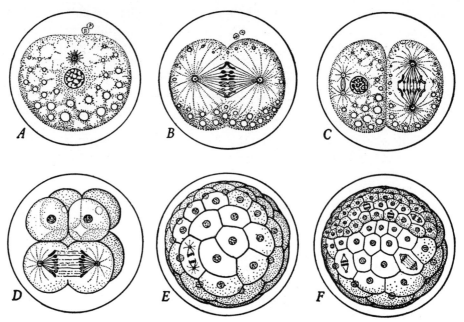

fig. 3·13 Sequence of events in cleavage. (*From B. M. Patten,* Human Embryology, *3d ed., McGraw-Hill Book Company, New York,* 1968.)

identical twins are to result, this is probably when the separation of the equipotential cells occurs. As early cleavage occurs, the embryo is slowly propelled downward through the fallopian tube toward its very small entrance into the uterus, where it arrives about 3½ to 5 days later to start implantation (Fig. 3·13). Before it begins to implant, it has reached the blastocyst stage, which may comprise as many as 128 or more cells in a rather spherical ball.

blastulation

The blastocyst begins to form on postconception day *4* and (Fig. 3·14) persists for about 1½ days until there are up to as many as 200 cells. As in almost all vertebrates, these cells do not remain in a solid sphere (morula) but acquire an eccentrically placed blastocyst cavity (blastocoel), probably as a result of imbibition from the surrounding fluids of the

fallopian tube and uterus as well as some secretions from its constituent cells. With the inner cavity eccentrically placed, the opposite pole of cells is thicker and is called the *inner cell mass,* within which the embryo will develop. The remainder of the sphere, a somewhat thinner layer of cells, will be the trophoblast, which is destined to give rise to the membranous chorion and the placenta, plus other extraembryonic structures. Later some of the *inner mass* cells will help to form the *amnion* and the *yolk sac.*

With the increasing size of the inner blastocoelic cavity and no significant change in the total mass of cells as yet, the whole blastocyst increases in volume until its diameter may be twice that of the fertilized egg, or about 300 μm. With this expansion, the zona pellucida is stretched and eventually torn and discarded. It must be presumed that all the nutrition for this early embryo is derived from the sparse yolk granules found in the mature human ovum.

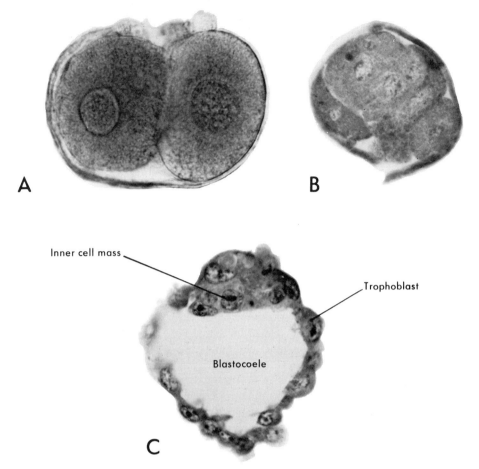

fig. 3.14 Human embryo in cleavage and blastodermic vesicle stages. (*From B. M. Patten, Human Embryology, 3d ed., McGraw-Hill, Book Company, New York,* 1968.)

implantation

Every embryo goes through certain crises, and it is estimated that about half the embryos started do not survive even the first crisis, e.g., implantation. Though the embryo must be at the morula-blastula stage of development, and the maternal hormones must be activated in order for implantation to occur, it is believed that the embryo itself determines whether implantation will succeed and that the state and function of the endometrium of the uterus play a lesser role in determining success. In any case, the embryo must establish a new and very intimate association with the lining of the uterus in order to derive the necessary nutrition, have access to oxygen, eliminate wastes, and be provided with physical protection. Implantation precedes the formation of the placenta, but these two processes will be considered together as continuous.

Usually the fertilized ovum reaches the uterus between 3½ and 5 days after conception as an enlarged blastocyst or trophoblast. The nonliving zona pellucida ruptures at about day *6 or 7* so that the surface of the trophoblast can make intimate contact with the inner surface of the uterus. Invasion of the highly vascular and secreting endometrium begins by day 7 or 8, as if the embryo were a parasite boring its way into the very lining of the uterus. As this occurs, a second inner, amniotic cavity appears within the trophoblast and separates the embryonic from the trophoblastic areas. This new cavity is entirely surrounded by mesoderm, the third of the three primary germ layers of the embryo (the others being ectoderm and endoderm). It is by proliferation of cells from the nonembryonic outer trophoblast that tissues of the placental villi will be derived. These cells become a *syncytium* (cells without clear boundaries), which forms the thousands of fingerlike functional villi, each with its core of stroma and capillaries. It is the syncytial portion of the trophoblast that is actively invasive and destructive, and which makes implantation possible. The embryo with its forming membranes constitutes an aggressive organism at this stage, destroying, digesting, and eliminating uterine tissues in its path, but, as a result, becoming surrounded itself in a blood lake. As the embryo burrows inwardly, it reaches the thicker, muscular *stratum compactum* of the wall of the uterus, and even some of these cells are destroyed by the enzymes from the chorion, but before dying they give off quantities of nutrient glycogen, which bathes and nourishes the embryonic tissue. The entire embryo is covered by regenerating maternal epithelium by *8* to *9* days.

development and functions of the placenta

The embryo is derived from the inner cell mass of the blastocyst, and its membranes and placenta arise from the opposite wall of the blastocyst. The placenta is not fully formed until after the first trimester, but it begins from the time of implantation, at *7¹/₂*

days. Lacunar spaces appear within the syncytium at 9 days, and villi by 11 to 12 days. These villi are wholly of embryonic origin; they become vascular, fingerlike processes of the *cytotrophoblast* which invade the lacunar spaces, now filled with maternal blood. By 16 days, the ever-increasing numbers of villi become branched and emerge from around the chorion of the entire embryonic mass. It is these villi that later comprise most of the placenta, the multiservice transmission organ for the embryo and fetus, a substitute for the undeveloped structures of the organism until it can develop its own digestive system, kidneys, liver, lungs, and endocrine glands and become independent of its mother. The placenta could be called the most perfect and efficient of exchange devices. By 3 weeks it covers 20 percent of the uterus; by 5 months, 50 percent. At 6 months, it weighs about 8 oz; at birth it weighs 1¹/₂ lb and will make up the *afterbirth*. It is always connected to the embryo by the umbilical cord, which will measure an average of 20 to 40 in at birth (Fig. 3·15).

Within the villi, now appearing as *cotyledons,* or little trees, blood vessels develop and form a continuous network to communicate between the emerging vascular system of the embryo and the placenta via a body stalk which becomes the umbilical cord. Since the heart starts to beat irregularly at day 24, a closed circulatory system between embryo and placenta must be established by then to bring diffusible materials to the embryo from the mother's blood, and to remove soluble and diffusible wastes. There is *no direct connection* between fetal and maternal circulatory systems. Intervillous maternal blood returns to the maternal circulation via the endometrial capillaries and venous sinusoids, carrying with it the collected fetal wastes for excretion through the kidneys, lungs, and skin of the mother.

The flow of blood from the uterus to the placenta increases from about 50 ml/min at

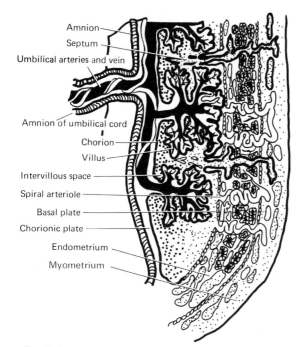

fig. 3·15 Placental formation.

10 weeks to about 500 ml/min at term. Just before birth, the placenta carries 30 l of blood per hour between the mother and fetus at the rate of about 4 miles/h. Each single round trip takes about 30 s. The blood in the intervillous spaces is somewhat independent of blood pressure changes, so that the fetus is protected against variables in the maternal supply which might cause asphyxia in the fetus. Estrogens from the ovaries cause dilatation of the uteroplacental vessels to meet the increasing nutritional needs of the growing fetus.

The human placenta does not reach its maximum size until about a month before delivery. Its growth seems to slow after the thirtieth week, and there is actual regression as the time for delivery approaches.

The umbilical cord carries two arteries and a single vein, none of which has valves. The blood flow through the cord is believed to be about 100 ml/kg/min, and arteries are sup-plied with abundant smooth-muscle fibers which contract at birth so as to reduce the lumina and cause hemostasis in the umbilical circulation. This is one reason why the cord is not clamped after an emergency delivery unless sterile equipment is at hand.

PLACENTAL HORMONES

The placenta is primarily an organ for the diffusion of substances between the fetal and maternal circulations, but it also has endocrine functions. In addition to the anterior pituitary, it is another source of *human chorionic gonadotropin* (HCG), production of which peaks at 2 months, falling to a low level by 5 months (see Fig. 4·3). HCG helps to prolong the life of the corpus luteum during implantation and is believed to provide the progesterone precursor substances and ensure the maintenance of ovarian steroid hormones. When detected between days 40 and 100 of a suspected pregnancy it is a sure sign of pregnancy, and when its assay is below normal in two consecutive tests at 10-day intervals, this may be a sign of a missed abortion or trophoblastic failure.

Lactogen, prolactin, and *somatotropin* also are provided by the placenta; the first two have to do with milk production, and the latter is concerned with breast growth. Lactogen has been demonstrated as early as 3 months after conception. The placental lactogen may be similar to the pituitary-derived prolactin, both promoting breast growth in anticipation of lactation, as well as suppressing the pituitary gonadotropic hormones to prevent ovulation during pregnancy.

The *estrogens* were the first hormones to be detected in the human placenta; they can be reduced from the placenta by ovariectomy prior to the sixth week, but not thereafter. From the seventh week on, there is increased urinary secretion of the metabolites of estrogen (*estradiol* and *estrone*) in normal pregnancies (see Fig. 3·11).

Maternal urinary estrogens may be found very early in pregnancy, but their increase is only gradual until the seventh week. They help to maintain uterine growth and development of the endometrium, and after the eighteenth week, their presence in normal concentrations is regarded as certain indication of the normalcy of the fetus.

Progesterone is also produced by the placenta and not by the ovaries, the adrenals, or the fetus. Its function is to maintain the vascular bed of the endometrium, as well as to prepare the implantation site for the zygote. Secreted throughout gestation, it is believed to supplement the corpus luteum in maintaining the pregnancy. It tends to keep the uterine musculature under control through the electrolyte potassium, a function which increases in importance with development of the fetus. Placental competence is indicated by the secretion of its metabolic product, *pregnanediol.*

The placenta also produces some enzymes which help both to synthesize and to break down carbohydrates, lipids, proteins, and their nucleic acids.

The products of placental metabolism designed for the fetus must get to it by intrauterine exchange across the placenta. The transfer mechanism is based largely upon the free diffusion of dissolved substances (i.e., breakdown constituents of the nutriments) from mother to fetus across semipermeable membranes, and the passage of excretory elements in the reverse direction. The flow may be nondirective except in the sense that it is usually from high to low concentration. Water and soluble items such as respiratory gases, acids and bases, electrolytes, vitamins, steroids, and the products of digestive metabolism move primarily by diffusion.

AMNIOTIC FLUID

By the eighth month there is at least a quart of amniotic fluid within the "bag of waters," the amniotic sac. The amount of fluid increases steadily in proportion to fetal growth (1), but the exact number of milliliters varies widely. At 4 weeks there is about 5 to 8 ml of fluid; at 8 weeks, about 20 ml; at 12 weeks, about 30 to 40 ml; at 16 weeks, about 175 ml; at 20 weeks, about 400 ml. In rare cases there may be little amniotic fluid. Amniotic fluid is secreted and reabsorbed in various ways, the major route being the cells of the amnion itself. At term, about 350 ml is absorbed and replaced each hour. The fetus swallows some fluid, which is reabsorbed through the intestinal tract into fetal circulation and then passed to the mother for excretion. The fetus adds a small amount to the fluid by voiding into it at intervals, a good reason for the rapid turnover of fluid! The fluid is mildly alkaline and has an electrolyte concentration somewhat similar to that of the mother's plasma. Amniotic fluid cushions the movements of the fetus and maintains a uniform pressure and temperature for it.

fetal development

THE FIRST 5 WEEKS

We have already described the development of the embryo from conception to implantation, which occurs not more than 10 days later. At this stage the embryo of a human being cannot be distinguished from that of any other mammal at a comparable stage. It has an enclosing amniotic membrane, which is becoming filled with an amniotic fluid that will cushion the fragile embryo against injury and keep it well separated from the maternal uterine tissues. It is the outermost, or chorionic, membrane that actually makes contact with the uterine lining and ultimately forms the placenta. Opposite the area of intimate contact with maternal tissues, there develops a yolk sac, so named because a similar structure is found in all vertebrate embryos and in the lower forms, becomes a source of fatlike nutritiment. The human yolk sac is connected with the embryo (Fig. 3·16) but contains no yolk. It does give rise at a very early stage to the precursors of all the germ cells which move to the internal gonads of the fetus at a later stage. It also produces the first blood cell precursors, prior to the functioning of the embryonic liver, spleen, and bone marrow, where blood will later develop. By the end of the second month, there is no trace of this yolk sac, and all its formative cells have migrated from it into the body of the embryo.

By 7 days after fertilization, the embryo has become a triple-layered organism (consisting of ecto-, endo-, and mesoderm) with a large cavity between the membranes of the amnion and chorion, and by 11 to 13 days, the outermost layer (ectoderm) shows signs of becoming the primitive streak, or major axis, of the future embryo, establishing its right and left sides, its anterior and posterior ends. From 18 to 28 days, this embryo is called a neurula, because this is when the major plan of the central nervous system is revealed. However, before this becomes very apparent other very significant organs begin to form, particularly the mesodermal heart, which is at first (at about 18 to 20 days) a mere tube. This tube will bend on itself and ultimately form a four-chambered heart, all the while pulsating, with the pulses beginning feebly and irregularly at 24 days after conception, smoothing out to a regular but rather rapid pulse in a few weeks, in preparation for the time when it will beat 100,000 times each day—never to stop for the rest of the life of the individual.

In the meantime, the beginnings of the endodermally lined digestive system appear, also as a single tube forming from anterior toward posterior and at first almost exterior to the mass of the embryo itself. But the all-important nervous system continues to develop by issuing primitive cells known as *neuroblasts,* all coming from the outermost

ectoderm (called *neurectoderm*) and migrating inward and away from, but always in communication with, the neural axis seen at 18 days. It is the nervous system that will integrate the functions of all the other systems later to develop and to coordinate the embryo, fetus, and baby to function as an efficient unit. Thus, the nervous system continues to develop throughout gestation, forming a network of communicating lines to and *from* every part of the body. By 6 weeks, this developing nervous system will be so hooked up to and in control of the developing musculature that it can direct the fetus to its first movements, although these could not be detected by the mother. By 28 days, there are 40 pairs of blocks of tissue which will give rise to all the major voluntary muscles of the body. Sense organs, such as the eyes, begin to form on day 19; they form in a manner similar to the building of a tunnel from two sides of the Hudson River so as to meet exactly beneath it. Parts of the eyes coming from the outermost layer of tissue (known as ectoderm) and growing inward, and parts from the innermost, endoderm tissue of the brain, growing outward, come together in perfect relationship to function for perfect vision.

By 22 days, the embryo begins to form its kidney system, long before it needs such a system, since the mother takes away all its waste products. Thus, before the mother knows that she is pregnant, her embryo has begun to form all its major systems. Though the human embryo cannot be distinguished from other mammalian embryos (all developing along the same general pattern), its basic organization has been revealed, and it is well on its way to becoming a human being.

THE FIRST TRIMESTER

This comprises the first 3 months of gestation and is probably the most sensitive, crucial, and important of the trimesters for the embryo, which will be called a fetus at about

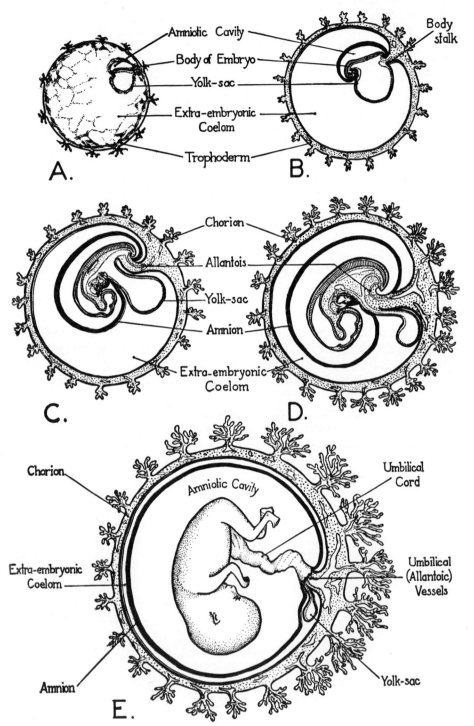

fig. 3·16 Early changes and interrelations of embryo and extraembryonic membranes. (*From B. M. Patten,* Human Embryology, 3d ed., *McGraw-Hill Book Company, New York,* 1968.)

5 weeks, when it first shows some organ formations. With each successive month, its security is greater and the probability of its reaching the delivery stage is enhanced (Fig. 3·17).

At 1 month, the human embryo is about $1/4$ in in length, yet within this tiny mass of protoplasm the mosaic of organ formation is well started. One can conjecture that the brain, heart, and digestive organs begin in that sequence because of their relative importance to the developing organism. The primary brain has three major parts which, since it develops early, may be the reason for the excessive growth of the anterior end, so that the head constitutes about one-third of the entire body and is bent forward onto the abdomen, almost meeting the tip of the tail. The sense organ systems—eyes, ears, and nose—begin to form. The early elements of the backbone appear, following the back bend, and can sometimes be seen through the skin. From the inner tube, representing the alimentary canal, grows the liver (day 21), and the gallbladder, thyroid gland, stomach, intestines, and pancreas are all defined. The lungs, offshoots of the digestive tract, appear (day 27) before the trachea develops. Paired buds appear on the sides of the body, forerunners of the arms and legs (day 31).

One usually thinks of the brain as a solid mass of nervous tissue, but on day 33 the three primary divisions of the brain acquire inner cavities as the first and third divisions further divide, giving rise to a five-sectioned brain with cavities in all, and all cavities connected. This transformation of relatively compact brain tissue to a cavernous structure is the very beginning of the outer cortex or cortical layer which has to do with all voluntary motor activity and where the learning processes reside. By 35 days, the hand plates are flat, serrated paddles, while the foot plates are mere bulges, lingering a little behind the forelimbs in development (Figs. 3·18, 3·19). At the same time, the primitive

germ cells are arriving in prolific numbers along the embryonic kidney ridge, where the gonads are beginning to form. By this time, the embryo has grown $1/3$ in and weighs about $1/1000$ oz. The face begins to look more human, and the umbilical cord is the lifeline from embryo to placenta. Even the pituitary gland, so important in the mother for the initial stages of human development, begins to form in this early embryo. By day 36, all 40 pairs of muscle blocks have formed and establish nerve associations which will incite them soon to function. As early as day 40, the pigment of the eyes forms, so that these sense organs can be detected through the skin. By day 42, the earliest reflexes begin; the embryo is only $1/2$ in in total length. Milk lines and rudimentary mammary glands appear in both sexes. The intermediate or mesonephric kidney displaces the nonfunctioning pronephros, and it too fails to function because the final step in kidney formation begins, namely the metanephros. By day 44, the sensory retinal cells of the eye form, which suggests that serious trauma of the embryo at this time could conceivably affect its vision for life. By day 46, the ovaries and testes are microscopically different, and the male external genitals begin to form.

By 7 weeks, the embryo is $4/5$ in in length and, having all its major organ systems in their earliest stages, begins to look more like the embryo of a human being than of any other mammal. By day 50, the female external genitals begin to form (Fig. 3·20), and both the ovaries and testes begin to move away from their site of origin toward the position in which they are found in the adult. Bone begins to replace cartilage and to give more rigidity to the body; though the head still constitutes about one-third of the body, it is more erect as the bones form. The hands and arms, feet and legs move laterally, and the digits begin to show. So many things are happening in these last few days that it is no wonder that the embryonic organs are hyper-

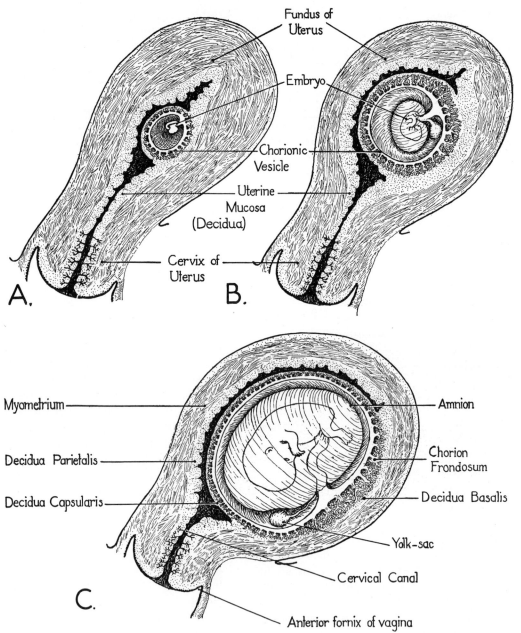

fig. 3·17 The uterus of a primipara in the third, fifth, and eighth week of pregnancy. (Drawn to actual size.) (*From B. M. Patten,* Human Embryology, 3*d ed.,* McGraw-Hill Book Company, New York, 1968.)

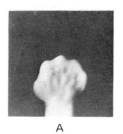 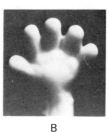 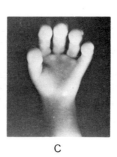 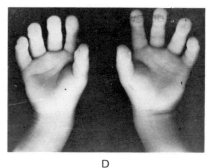

A   B   C   D

fig. 3·18 Development of human hands. A Hand plate, 5 weeks; B finger ridges, 6 weeks; C definite thumb and fingers with pads, 7 weeks; D regression of finger pads; 12 weeks. (*From R. Rugh and L. B. Shettles, From Conception to Birth: The Drama of Life's Beginnings, Harper & Row, Publishers, Incorporated, New York, 1971. Courtesy of Carnegie Institute, Washington.*)

sensitive to any environmentally imposed trauma such as smoking, disease, infections, drugs, or radiation. At 8 weeks the embryo is $1\frac{1}{4}$ in in sitting height (top of head to buttocks) and weighs about $\frac{1}{30}$ oz. An electrocardiogram taken at this time reveals all the typical phases of a normal adult heartbeat, but the pulse ranges only from 40 to 80 beats per minute. The heart is very small but structurally very similar to that of the adult, and it is functioning regularly and constantly.

The third and last month of the first trimester sees the fetus becoming active, indicating a newly acquired coordination of the neuromuscular junctions and controls, so that the mother may well feel the movements. Facial grimaces first form; the head turns a bit; and even the lungs and diaphragm simulate inhalation movements, causing the fetus to take in amniotic fluid through its mouth. The initial reflexes arc total in that they involve the whole body, not merely the area of stimulation. By the end of this third month, stroking of the lips causes a sucking reaction, while previously it would have stimulated involvement of almost the whole fetus.

This is also the month of further refinement of the differences between the sexes, but the genital tubercle could still become either the penis or the clitoris. The simultaneous development and proximity of origin of the genital and urinary systems of both sexes is emphasized, as the metanephric kidneys form and become separated from the gonads, which move further away from their original sites of origin near the kidneys. These kidneys soon begin to secrete urine, which is conveyed to the bladder and passes via the urethra into the amniotic fluid. Though certain parts of the urinary system remain always as functional parts of the genital system, separation of functions begins during this third month.

At 9 weeks, the fetus measures $1\frac{1}{2}$ in in sitting height (Fig. 3·21) and weighs about $\frac{1}{7}$ oz. Its posture is more erect, its abdomen less prominent. Finger- and toenails are forming, as well as hair in patches on the body. The eyes have iris diaphragms and lids, which seal the eyes closed for the next 3 months. Dentine organs appear in relation to the early-forming teeth. The heartbeat can now be heard easily via the stethoscope through the abdomen, uterine muscles, membranes, and

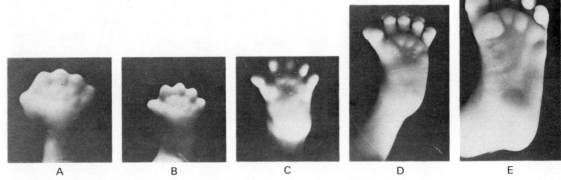

fig. 3·19 Development of human feet. A Foot plate, 6 weeks; B toe ridges, 2 days later; C heel development, 7 weeks; D walking pads, 8 weeks; E regression of toe pads, 12 weeks. (*From R. Rugh and L. B. Shettles*, From Conception to Birth: The Drama of Life's Beginnings, *Harper & Row, Publishers, Incorporated, New York*, 1971. *Courtesy of Carnegie Institute, Washington.*)

fluid surrounding the embryo. The potential male can now be distinguished by its enlarging penis, while the female external genitalia are less prominent but nevertheless forming.

At 10 weeks, the fetus measures $2\frac{1}{8}$ in in sitting position and weighs about $\frac{1}{4}$ oz. The head appears now to have slowed in its growth and, because of more rapid growth of the torso and related organs, no longer appears to make up such a large part of the whole body. Facial features (mouth, eyes, ears, and nostrils) appear more human, and nerve-muscle relations have increased enormously. Skeleton is displacing cartilage almost everywhere, even to the tips of the digits. Bone marrow forms for the first time, in which blood appears, thus taking over this function to some extent from the blood islands—the spleen and liver. The blood vessels are far more extensive and firm, propelling more and more blood to the many new tissue areas of the fetus.

During the eleventh week, the fetus measures $2\frac{1}{2}$ in in sitting height and may weigh $\frac{1}{3}$ oz. Tooth buds of all of the 20 temporary milk teeth appear, in proper relation to the ossifying jaws. It is important at this time that

the mother's diet contain adequate calcium both for the development of the fetal dentition and for protection of her own. These teeth will not normally erupt through the gums until the baby is six to twenty-four months of age, although there are known cases of exposed milk teeth at birth. The derivatives of the digestive tract (thyroid, thymus, larynx, trachea, lungs, liver, stomach, pancreas, and intestines) are all advancing very rapidly in their independent development. The liver, still forming blood, also pours bile into the intestines, although there is no fat to digest. The intestines begin to lengthen, ultimately to be about 30 ft in the adult. The mother still digests her food, breaks it down into such molecular size that it can diffuse through the various membranes into the blood vessels of the fetus, whence it is again resynthesized into protoplasm appropriate to the fetus. Before the fetus can do this for itself, it must produce over 20 million glands in its digestive tract.

By the twelfth week, the fetus measures 3 in and weighs about $\frac{1}{2}$ oz. It can oppose its thumb and forefinger, an accomplishment which is characteristic of all primates. Fe-

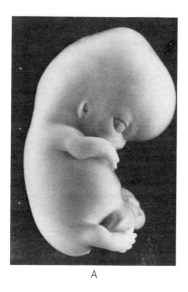 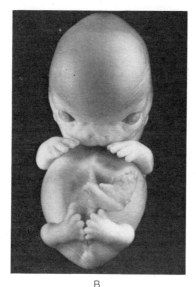 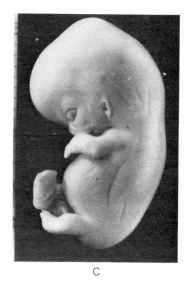

fig. 3·20 Human fetus, 54 days (22.5 mm or $7/8$ in). A right side; B front; C left side. (*From R. Rugh and L. B. Shettles,* From Conception to Birth: The Drama of Life's Beginnings, *Harper & Row, Publishers Incorporated New York, 1971. Photo by E. Ludwig.*)

tuses have been known to suck their thumbs and use their swallowing reflex. Milk glands of both sexes are able to secrete a milk substance and may even react to the same lactogenic hormones that are stimulating the mother's mammary glands to secrete.

Superficially, the fetus at the end of the first trimester appears to be a miniature human being, but this is deceptive because it is totally incapable of an independent existence. True, most of its organ systems have formed and are rather well developed and no really new organ systems appear in the next trimester, but such systems are unable to function properly, and no fetus of this age has ever been known to survive apart from its mother. The next trimester is, therefore, one of further development of these basic organ systems, with some attaining a degree of refinement that gives them better survival values. But it is not until the third trimester, particularly the seventh month, that the fetus

can survive outside the uterus with the skilled aid of the obstetrician and his coworkers in intensive care units for premature infants.

THE SECOND TRIMESTER

The intermediary second trimester in human intrauterine development lasts from about the thirteenth to the twenty-seventh week and is to be compared with the shakedown voyage of a boat just launched. The fetus has all or most of its organs, many of them functioning in a simple manner, but few have been tested. This is a period of rapid growth from about $3^1/_2$ in in sitting height (crown to rump) and 1 oz in weight to about 12 in and 2 to 3 lb.

The uterine invasion by the fetal chorionic villi is essentially completed, and the expansion of their absorbing surfaces has thinned them out so that diffusion between mother and fetus is more rapid, more extensive, and more efficient within the placenta. Fetal

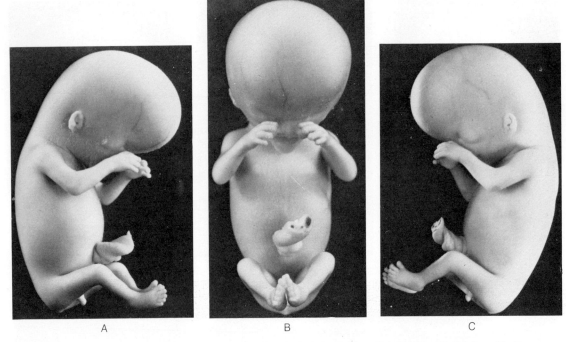

fig. 3·21 Male human fetus at 68 days (47 mm or 1⁷/₈ in). A right; B front; C left. (*From R. Rugh and L. B. Shettles,* From Conception to Birth: The Drama of Life's Beginnings, *Harper & Row, Publishers, Incorporated, New York, 1971. Photo by E. Ludwig.*)

growth is so rapid (an average of about 1.5 mm/day) that if this rate were continued to after birth the child could look over a two-story house before it was ten years of age! Growth is predominant in this trimester.

The skin of the fetus is thin and shiny; it tends to be reddish, with no underlying accumulated fat, so that even its face is wrinkled.

Most of the growth of the fetus relates to the elongation of its body; it begins to lose the disproportion that favored the head over the torso. At 3 months, the head is about one-third the total body length; by birth this is reduced to 25 percent; and in the mature adult, to about 10 percent. The nervous system, the first system to begin development in the embryo, retains its control over the entire

organism. The legs become relatively longer with growth of the fetus, from 25 percent of the total length to about 50 percent at birth. As the skeleton forms, the fetus becomes more and more erect and capable of supporting the enlarging visceral mass, with enlarging and more functional muscular masses.

The facial contours begin to fill out a bit and appear to be more human; the thin skin is pinkish because of the underlying capillaries; and the finger- and toe prints have formed for the life of the individual, being peculiarly different from those of every other fetus. The fetus exhibits more reflex responses which appear to be more purposeful, rather than all-inclusive, and exerts spontaneous stretching and other movements on its own. It is during this period that the mother can begin to become acquainted with her child—its habits and movements, and, to a certain extent, may train it to coordinate its activities with hers. If this is realized and an effort is made, the mother can avoid the disturbances that come from wanting to sleep undisturbed at a time when the fetus feels like galloping!

Oocytes are forming in large numbers in the newly formed ovaries, and female secondary sexual development begins, probably under hormonal influence. Late-starting female organogenesis begins to catch up on the earlier-starting male. The fetal heart pumps about 25 qt of blood through its circuit each day and grows steadily in its vigor and regularity of contractions (120 to 160 per minute) as it develops toward the adult stage, when it will pump 72,000 qt of blood through its miles of blood vessels each day. The lungs are structurally quite complete (except for alveoli) but are collapsed, filled with fluid, and inactive. The brain shows the beginnings of convolutions, with the forebrain (cerebrum) enlarging and overlapping the rest of the brain. Neuromuscular pathways are already established; electrical stimulation of the fetal brain would cause muscular responses even in distant parts of the fetus.

The general appearance of the fetus at 5 months suggests that it is a miniature human being, but it is still far from functionally independent of its mother. It cannot live alone, and it still has to acquire a thermostatic control mechanism.

It is well known that in the adult there is a constant loss of cells and replacement of such losses; it is said that even in an adult every 7 years a new person emerges in the image of the prior one. This anabolic vs. catabolic exchange begins during the fifth month, this trimester, even though the fetus is almost entirely made up of newly formed cells. Some of the discarded and dead cells accumulate on the surface of the skin and give it a cheeselike covering, *vernix*. Sweat

glands form close to the hair follicles, both of which will later help to control body temperature. When the hair on the body first appears, it is very fine and known as *lanugo*. Whitish eyelashes make the 5-month fetus look like an old man (Fig. 3·22).

The mother, and sometimes also the father, can identify some of the parts of the fetus as an arm, leg, or foot presses outwardly against the mother's abdomen. Hiccoughing and even crying of the fetus have been detected, but, of course, they do not involve air and, aside from frightening the mother when they first occur, are meaningless.

The hair on the head of the fetus now becomes considerable; if it continued to grow at the same rate, it would have to be cut shortly after birth. The cheeselike coating of dead cells covering the skin, which protects the tender skin against abrasions, begins to be sloughed off with the activity of the fetus, so that little is left at birth. A concentration of dead, greenish cells (meconium) accumulates in the unused intestines of the fetus, remaining there until passed out as feces shortly after birth.

The eyes, which begin to form about 4 weeks after conception, by this time are structurally complete. It is in this sixth month that the eyelids, which formed and sealed off the eyes, begin to part and open so that even by the seventh month, the eyes would respond to light, but not to specific objects. Bone-forming cells (osteoblasts) are very active in this month, utilizing what calcium the fetus can get from its mother's circulation, while at the same time bone-destroying cells (osteoclasts) are destroying some of the first bone to form. Thus, there is a constant forming and destroying of bone which favors the osteoblasts during this and succeeding months as the skeleton enlarges and becomes the very substantial, rigid structure it must be to support all the organs of the fetus in its late stages. The spine, for instance, is

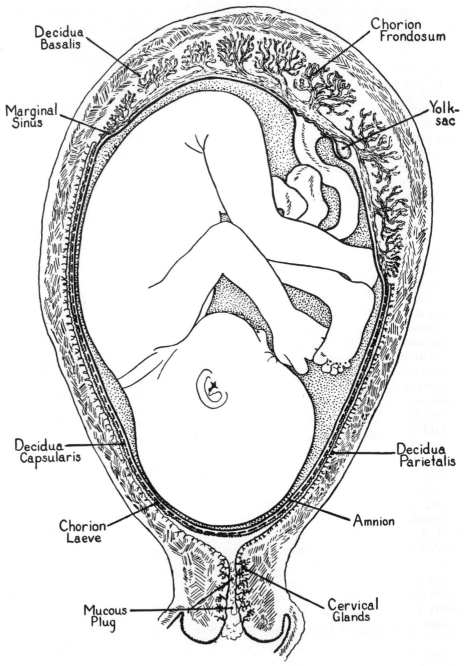

fig. 3·22 Relations to the uterus of a 5 month-old fetus and its membranes. (*From B. M. Patten, Human Embryology, 3d ed., McGraw-Hill Book Company, New York, 1968.*)

made up of 33 bony rings, 150 joints, and over 1000 ligaments, all coordinating in support of the fetus. A total of 222 bones are formed, but the muscles, ligaments, and tendons used in support are not all adequately attuned to use by the time of birth, and the newborn must strengthen and learn to coordinate these supportive structures. (Note: Though an x-ray of the mother's abdomen at this time would reveal the extent of the skeletal growth of the fetus, taking such an x-ray is not advised because of the possible hazard of ionizing radiations to the mother and her ovaries, and to the fetal organs still in the process of completing their development.)

THE THIRD TRIMESTER

The third trimester is the period during which both mother and fetus make final and essential preparations for the advent of the child. The placenta, so essential to every development of the fetus, begins to decrease in activity late in the seventh month, when chorionic villi are gradually inactivated and obstruct, rather than facilitate, diffusion between mother and fetus. Atrophy sets in, infarcts appear, blood vessel walls thicken, calcifications develop, and the placenta slowly becomes avascular and anemic so that the fetus is forced to fare for itself more and more. The volume of amniotic fluid is reduced by about 50 percent as the baby, by its continued growth, crowds the uterus.

At the beginning of this trimester, the fetus resembles a shriveled-up old man, with red, wrinkled skin and overhanging whitish eyebrows. It could probably survive if removed by cesarean section, but would still require intensive care by specially trained nurses, because though its organs are structurally almost completed, they are functionally unable to carry out their tasks. This applies particularly to the lungs, so that many babies delivered prematurely suffer respiratory difficulties. During this trimester, fat is deposited beneath the skin and the wrinkles begin to disappear. Certain chemical elements are so essential in this period that the mother's diet is more important than ever. About 80 percent of all the calcium the fetus needs will be accumulated, 40 percent in the last month before birth. This is also true of iron, much of which is stored in the fetal liver to supplement the mother's milk. About 70 percent of all the nitrogen required by the fetus, obtained from the mother's intake of protein, is accumulated now, and a serious deprivation on the part of the mother is now believed to hamper the proper development of the central nervous system and basic intelligence.

Even a 7-month baby sometimes has calluses on its thumb, indicating prebirth attempts at suckling. It is known to be responsive to taste variables such as sweet or sour, for it has more taste buds than it will retain for later use. It is active and responds to stimuli, but such responses are not yet purposeful. The human brain at birth is not completely developed, particularly with regard to the cerebellum, wherein resides much of the motor control and the sense of balance. It is probably 3 to 4 weeks before all these nervous connections are fully functioning.

Several reflex responses become evident during the *seventh month*, such as the sucking reflex, rooting reflex, Moro reflex, grasping reflex, and step reflex, but they are not normally demonstrated until after birth. We know that the seventh-month fetus can feel pain, and that it sometimes reacts vigorously when blood is being transferred into it in Rh-incompatibility operations.

The probability of survival of the *8-month* fetus, if delivered prematurely is about 70 percent; the average fetus of this age weighs 4 to 5 lb and is 13 in in sitting height. Artificial aid for respiration may still be necessary, even though the respiratory center in the brain is functional, because the alveoli are not yet fully prepared to transmit oxygen to the capillaries of the lungs. Temperature control is most important, and oxygen supply follows, with nutrition last as supporting supplements at this time (see Chap. 30).

During the *ninth month,* the apparent reduced activity of the baby sometimes tends to frighten the mother, but it is generally due to the greatly increased congestion of the enlarging child in the confined spaces available in the mother. Delivery at any time during this ninth month is usually safe for the child and easier for the mother; yet it is ill-advised to try to hasten the event. The child should be allowed to achieve full development while in its close relation with the mother unless extenuating circumstances involving the mother's health indicate the wisdom of inducing labor and delivery or resorting to cesarean section. It is during this month that the child acquires from its mother most of the antibodies, those disease-resisting proteins which she has developed as a result of bouts with infections; the child is thus fortified for at least six crucial months of its early life against many childhood ailments.

preparation for delivery

The birth of every one of 3.7 million babies born in the United States in a recent year is a major event in its life, but neither the beginning nor the end. It is major because it involves permanent adjustments on the part of both mother and baby to sustain a life that began its development some 266 days before as a living ovum and living sperm, conjoining in a truly symbiotic relationship. During at least 6 months of this development, it is a parasite in the mother's body, taking to itself all that it needs to grow and develop, even at the expense of the mother. But beginning at about 7 months, the fetus gives notice of impending maturity and self-reliance, while the mother gives evidence of impending eviction. Not until this time can the fetus be considered a viable baby, even with intensive aid from experienced doctors and nurses.

SIGNS OF IMPENDING DELIVERY

Several weeks before delivery, the uterus is lowered into the pelvis, the descent called "lightening" because it gives the mother a sense of decreased abdominal pressure and distension as the uterus moves away from the diaphragm, allowing deeper breaths. The fetal head enters the true pelvis toward the cervix and birth canal (Fig. 3·23). This adjustment is believed to be aided by a relaxation of the sacroiliac and symphysis pubis joints, but possibly also by aggressive movements of the fetus. The average uterus has a capacity of 4 l, but since it consists of smooth muscles, it is highly elastic and its volume and capacity can be adjusted to babies up to twice the average size. The mother-fetal relations become continuously more tense and strenuous, and if the mother gains more than 10 lb in this trimester she may have some difficulty at delivery. The baby grows to an average of 7 lb and a total length of 20 in—so that the mother becomes very anxious to have it delivered!

CHANGES IN FETAL CIRCULATION

From the protective environment of the uterus, the baby must get ready for the shock of cold air on its skin and within its lungs, must be ready and able to inflate those lungs for the first time, and must be prepared to use its own digestive system (the longer it delays in utilizing the latter, the more weight it will

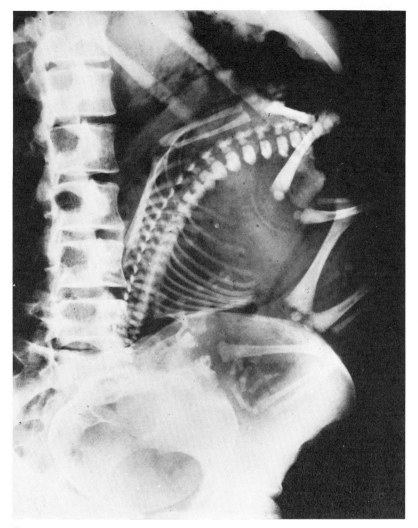

fig. 3·23 X-ray of the human fetus at term (in position for delivery). (*From F. Rugh and L. B. Shettles,* From Conception to Birth: The Drama of Life's Beginnings, *Harper & Row, Publishers, Incorporated, New York,* 1971. *Photo by T. R. Harlan.*)

gain). The extraembryonic blood supply with its oxygen and nutrition from the mother, via the placenta, is suddenly cut off, carbon dioxide accumulates in the baby's own blood, and, as a result, the respiratory center of its brain is stimulated to cause it to use its diaphragm, expand its lungs, and inhale the cold air of the environment. This is such a shock that the baby cries, starting the four main changes in the fetal circulation: shutting off the right and left umbilical arteries; closing off the ductus arteriosus which had connected the pulmonary artery with the dorsal aorta; forcing the fetal blood into the pulmonary artery, which had not previously reached full capacity; and closing off the foramina ovale between the two auricles (Fig. 12·1).

The fact that almost 100 percent of infants survive the crisis of birth is indication that the developmental process, if not interfered with by drugs, infections, radiation, etc., is quite consistently "normal" in the vast majority of pregnancies. The percentage of "normally healthy" babies that issue from mothers who have never before had the birth experience, who may not know the rudiments of diet and health, who may even have maltreated their own bodies, emphasizes the fact that the human embryo and fetus is truly a parasite, looking after its own survival and interests first, and surviving often in spite of the lack of rather than because of prenatal care. Within the range of normalcy, however, there is room for improvement of the fetal environment and prospects, and it is in the hope of contributing to such improvement that this chapter has been written.

reference

1. Delbert L. Smith, "Amniotic Fluid Volume," *American Journal of Obstetrics and Gynecology,* **110**:2, 1971.

bibliography

Davies, Jack: *Human Developmental Anatomy,* The Ronald Press Company, New York, 1963.

Goldman, A. S.: "The Influence of Hormones on Sex Differentiation," *Contemporary OB/GYN,* **3**(1):69, 1974.

Hamilton, William J., J. D. Boyd, and H. W. Mossman: *Human Embryology,* 4th ed., The William & Wilkins Company, Baltimore, 1973.

Patten, Bradley M.: *Human Embryology,* 3d ed., McGraw-Hill Book Company, New York, 1968.

Rugh, Roberts, and Landrum B. Shettles: *From Conception to Birth: The Drama of Life's Beginnings,* Harper & Row, Publishers, Incorporated, New York, 1971.

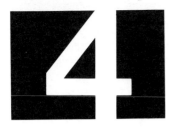

maternal development

Beatrice Lau Kee
Martha Olsen Schult

From the very beginning of its life, the new human embryo, while traveling through the fallopian tube, is going through rapid cell division on its way to nidate in the uterine lining. It is only in the first week of its life that the embryo is virtually unaffected by outside influences such as drugs, viruses, and pollutants, except for radiation. Only during that week is it free-moving.

Between the second and twelfth weeks of life the embryo is especially susceptible to substances inhaled or ingested by the mother, substances which will travel through her circulation and may affect the fetal environment. Many of the drugs and substances that might be taken in by the mother are harmless to the developing embryo, but others may be very harmful. Tragic experience with Thalidomide and the results of rubella virus are only two examples of the *teratogenic* effects of certain substances, organisms, or factors, i.e., of their ability to cause congenital malformations in the embryo.

The first 12 weeks of life of the fetus are the weeks of *organogenesis,* when the organs of the body are being formed and when there is the greatest chance of their malformation. Therefore it is most important that a woman seek prenatal care and guidance as soon as she suspects that she is pregnant.

Early prenatal care is one of our most potent ways to help prevent congenital anomalies, preterm birth, and maternal, neonatal, and infant mortality or morbidity.

Prenatal care can best be termed preventive, i.e., protective care of the mother and the growing fetus during its development. Everything done for the mother is based on the physiologic and psychologic changes that take place in these most important 9 months.

Perhaps the most dominant theme during pregnancy is that of growth and development. The experience of pregnancy is unique for every woman because the process is experienced differently in every case. And yet the experience is universal, in that the same basic physiologic process is happening in every pregnant woman.

Some women experience pregnancy as an exhilarating, exciting, welcomed occurrence, whether planned or "accidental." For some women it may be their *raison d'être*, the way to verify their feminine role. But for others, when pregnancy was unplanned, unexpected, or definitely unwanted, it may be a frightening time, a nuisance, or, at least, an interruption in their career plans. For all women, it is definitely a fact of life. Once conception has occurred no amount of emotional acceptance or rejection will cause the growth process to stop.

Approximately 95 percent of all pregnancies are normal in every respect; the others are called high-risk, complicated pregnancies. Prenatal care is directed toward preventing complications, toward modifying those that occur, and toward supporting the mother during this period in order to allow her to carry the fetus to the full term of growth.

Full development of the fetus takes about 266 days, or 38 weeks, after conception. When calculated from the last menstrual period (LMP), the duration is 14 days longer, i.e., 40 weeks or 280 days. Understood in calculating gestation from the first day of the LMP are the facts that women's menstrual cycles are somewhat irregular and that ovulation occurs approximately halfway through the cycle, 14 days ± 2 before the next menses (Fig. 4·1). An infant born before 37 full weeks of gestation will be incompletely developed in one or more of its body functions. A chart of the terminology related to the weeks of development is shown in Fig. 4·2. Before the end of the nineteenth week of gestation the fetus is not sufficiently matured to be able to survive out of the uterine environment. If labor begins before this time, the fetus cannot live and therefore is called *nonviable*; its birth is called an *abortion*. After the twentieth week some infants, weighing as little as 500 Gm, have been able to survive; therefore this period is termed the *viable* period. Between 20 and 28 weeks is a period of extreme fetal immaturity when the chances of survival are low. With each week after that and with each gram of weight added, the risks improve. *Preterm* birth is that which occurs between 20 and 37 weeks of gestation. The period of *term* birth, or *maturity*, is 38 to 42 weeks. After 42 weeks in the uterus, problems again develop, as *postmaturity* carries with it other complications.

physiologic changes caused by pregnancy

The hormones of pregnancy have a generalized body effect far beyond their effect on the reproductive system. Many of these alterations are the basis for the signs and symptoms of pregnancy and also underlie many of the discomforts the pregnant woman experiences. Other hormone-secreting glands in the body increase their function, particularly the adrenals, the thyroid, and the pancreas. With the variations in hormone levels, body systems are profoundly affected in ways that would be considered pathologic if the woman were not pregnant. These adjustments are *totally normal* during the gestation. Knowing the reasons for each change makes it possible for the nurse to explain to the woman the interrelatedness and meaning of the symptoms she is experiencing.

HORMONAL CHANGES DURING PREGNANCY

Estrogen and Progesterone After the woman conceives, the corpus luteum of the ovary begins to secrete increasing amounts of progesterone. Called the pregnancy-maintaining hormone, progesterone (for gestation) is necessary for nidation of the fertilized ovum and for the maintenance of the enriched endometrium, the *decidua*. The corpus luteum gradually diminishes in size as the placenta grows and takes over the production of progesterone.

In combination with estrogen, progesterone causes changes in the breast tissue, particularly influencing the development of the alveolar system of ducts and lobes in preparation for lactation. Montgomery's tubercles, the sebaceous glands in the areola surrounding the nipple, become more prominent and pigmented, as does the entire nipple tissue. In conjunction with the adrenal glands, progesterone and estrogen also cause other pigmentation changes in the skin.

Estrogen and progesterone together cause relaxation of smooth-muscle tissue in the body. Primarily this serves to keep the pregnancy intact by relaxing and reducing muscle tone of the uterus, but it also affects the gastrointestinal tract and, to some degree, arteriovenous elasticity and bladder function. Normal body water retention during the later part of pregnancy, *leukocytosis* (increased leukocyte formation), and increases in respiratory function are all responses to estrogen and progesterone.

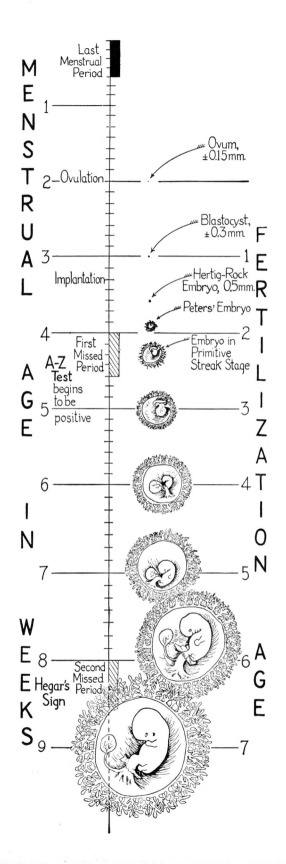

Estrogen is secreted by the ovary, the adrenal cortex, and during pregnancy, by the placenta as well. According to Hytten (1) some 27 estrogens have been identified, all of them chemically similar to progesterone and testosterone. The main work of estrogen is to control the growth and function of the uterus, but of course it interacts with the other hormones in their functions.

Relaxin Relaxin is an interesting hormone with a special effect during pregnancy. It functions in several ways, by increasing relaxation of pelvic ligaments in pregnancy and, synergistically with estrogen and progesterone, by stimulating breast growth and softening the cervix (2).

Human Chorionic Gonadotropin Although other gonadotropins are formed by the pituitary gland, human chorionic gonadotropin (HCG) is exclusively produced by the trophoblast of the chorion. Thus HCG is present only during pregnancy, or in a very rare chorionic growth called a *molar pregnancy* (see Chap. 22). It is this hormone which gives the positive results in urine-based pregnancy tests. HCG has been found in measurable amounts in the urine within 14 days of fertilization, in the early period of very active trophoblast growth. The amount of HCG peaks at about 60 days and then drops off sharply by 100 days to remain at a low level for the remainder of the pregnancy (Fig. 4·3).

Thyroid Hormones During pregnancy the thyroid gland enlarges and in many instances can be palpated in the neck. The thyroid produces increased amounts of hormone, which causes the basal metabolic rate (BMR) to rise gradually throughout pregnancy to

fig. 4·1 Actual size of embryos in relation to mother's menstrual history (left) and fertilization age of embryo (right). Based on 28-day cycle. (*From B. M. Patten, Human Embryology, 3d ed., McGraw-Hill Book Company, New York, 1968.*)

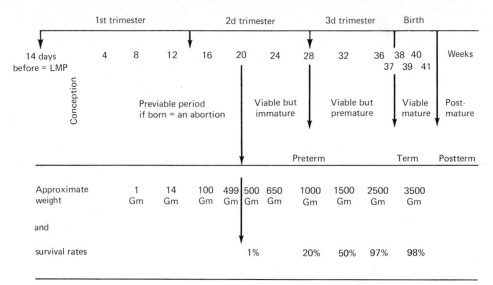

fig. 4·2 Terminology related to fetal maturity.

about 20 percent above the nonpregnant rate (see Chap. 24).

CARDIOVASCULAR SYSTEM

By the tenth week of pregnancy the maternal blood volume has increased by as much as 30 to 40 percent to provide for the needs of the enlarging uterus, breasts, and placenta. Most of the blood is concentrated in the pelvic region and does not unduly change the arterial blood pressure. Blood pressure, in fact, drops slightly during the first two trimesters, returning to the normal level or slightly above during the last trimester. A combination of the vasodilatation action of estrogen and the presence of an arteriovenous shunt in the placental circulation reduces pressure, much as a delta region does for a river. To accommodate the increased blood volume, however, the cardiac output increases and the pulse rises about 15 beats over the nonpregnant rate. Venous pressure in the lower extremities is affected, with an increase in femoral venous pressure from less than 10 mmHg to a level of 18 mmHg or more (3).

Hemoglobin and Hematocrit The increase in blood volume is primarily due to an increase in plasma. The result is a slight reduction in hematocrit but usually no significant change in hemoglobin levels. Hematocrit, normally 35 to 45 percent, may drop to as low as 30 to 33 percent (see Chap. 21). But hemoglobin levels, normally 12 to 14 Gm/100 ml, should fall to no lower than 11.5 Gm during pregnancy. Any change below these levels is considered iron-deficiency anemia, whereas a lowered hematocrit alone is called *hemodilution* of pregnancy.

The red cell count should remain above 3,750,000 per 100 ml of blood. Toward the end of pregnancy, the white cell count may be elevated normally, continuing into the postdelivery period. (See Chap. 21 for a detailed discussion of hematologic changes during pregnancy.)

Increased Blood Volume The increase in blood volume has several related effects causing minor discomforts during pregnancy. The first of these is a sensation of light-headedness or fainting (*syncope*). The literature on this subject indicates two causes—

postural hypotension and hypoglycemia. With the increase in volume of maternal blood in the pelvic region, pooling of blood can occur when the mother stands up suddenly, or for instance, moves from a horizontal position to jump up and answer the phone. A word of caution will usually prevent an episode of syncope from this cause. If the cause turns out to be hypoglycemia, the physician will advise frequent small meals during the day, with intake of quickly absorbed carbohydrate if the mother should feel faint.

Increased circulation may cause some women to have recurrent headaches as they become adjusted to the changes in volume. Emotional tension may contribute to headaches as well. Any persistent headache should be reported to the physician, as it may be a symptom of a more severe underlying problem.

Increased blood volume contributes toward the development of varicose veins in those women so disposed, and especially in those who have had preexisting varicosities. Varicose veins of the saphenous system and of the vulva and rectum (hemorrhoids) are primarily affected by the rising venous pressure in the lower extremities, induced by the enlarging uterus impinging on the venous flow. Varicosities are usually more common and pronounced in the multigravida. Besides being unsightly, they may be painful and throbbing, especially those in the vulva and rectum. Positional change to facilitate venous return—elevation of the legs above the level of the heart or placing legs and feet on a footstool whenever sitting, to avoid pressure of the chair on the lower part of the thigh—will be helpful measures. A woman with a tendency to have varicosities should wear support hose or elastic ace bandages to give support and counterpressure to the walls of the distended veins. (See Chap. 23 for further discussion of treatment.)

Edema of the lower extremities is also related to venous return. Standing for long periods of time and pressure of the uterus on the large veins returning from the legs tend to hinder the flow of venous blood, against gravity, to the right side of the heart. Positional change to one facilitating venous return will quickly reduce this dependent, *gravity-based* edema. The side-lying position during sleep or rest is the best position for efficient kidney function. The normal woman with dependent edema should find that it has disappeared by morning after a good night's rest. Edema that persists is a warning signal to be reported to the physician.

MUSCULOSKELETAL SYSTEM

Many women experience low-back strain and discomfort during later pregnancy because the muscles and ligaments in the pelvic joints become somewhat relaxed, causing discomfort and pulling. It is suspected that the

fig. 4·3 Urinary excretion of estrogen, progesterone, and chorionic gonadotropin during pregnance. (*From A. J. Vander, J. H. Sherman, and D. Luciano,* Human Physiology, *McGraw-Hill Book Company, New York, 1970.*)

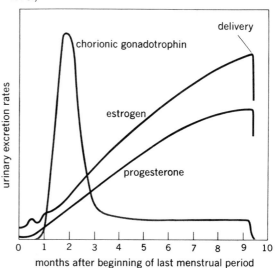

underlying hormone is *relaxin*, which, in conjunction with estrogen and progesterone, is preparing the body for the stretching of delivery.

Another factor contributing to back discomfort is the added weight and increasing abdominal girth that cause the pregnant woman to have the typical pregnant stance or walk. She leans backward to counterbalance the heavy uterus. The change in posture, unless noted and compensated for, will cause a strain on the lower-back and pelvic muscles. Improper shoes may aggravate the imbalance. The mother can be taught back exercises, such as the pelvic tilt (see Chap. 7), to strengthen her lower abdominal and back muscles. A bed board under the mattress will help to align her back. Occasionally a physician advises a maternity girdle for those women whose natural abdominal "muscle girdle" is not toned well enough to support the uterus. If analgesics are needed, they should be prescribed by the physician.

One of the most annoying problems of pregnancy, muscle cramps or spasms in the legs and feet, occurs during the second and third trimesters. Some of the causes are thought to be fatigue and decreased calcium when there is an increased phosphorus level. Pressure on the nerves caused by the enlarging uterus may also contribute to muscle cramping. Exercise, particularly walking, elevation of legs when sitting, and sufficient rest should help to relieve leg cramps. Standing on a cold floor and kneading the knotted muscle may relieve the cramp. Pointing the toes upward and exerting pressure downward on the kneecap helps to relieve the pain. Increasing the amount of calcium in the diet while reducing the amount of phosphorus may help to reduce cramping. To do this the physician prescribes calcium tablets and a reduced milk intake, for milk has a high content of phosphorus as well as calcium.

INTEGUMENTARY SYSTEM

The hormones from adrenal and placental steroids produce changes that are characteristic of pregnancy. The nipple and areola darken and become more prominent. A line between the symphysis and the umbilicus, called the *linea alba*, darkens and is then called the *linea nigra*. Some pregnant women develop a pigmented area on cheeks and forehead, known as *chloasma*, or the "mask of pregnancy." Stretch marks, or *striae*, on the abdomen, buttocks, and breasts are not due just to stretching (tiny tears in the lower skin layer), but are the effect of hormones from the adrenal cortex. Striae are purple-blue during pregnancy, changing to silver or brown scar tissue after pregnancy. They will never completely disappear, although they are usually scarcely noticeable between pregnancies.

The increased circulation of blood causes a variety of changes in the skin and hair. Fingernails grow faster. Many women notice the *erythema*, or redness, of the palms of the hands and soles of the feet. Nosebleeds and nasal congestions are the complaint of many women. On the positive side, many who were usually uncomfortable in cold weather find themselves tolerating cold more easily during pregnancy because of the increased circulation to the extremities.

According to Hytten (4), instead of the usual 85 percent hair growth there is a 95 percent hair growth during pregnancy. Since more follicles are active, fewer are falling out. Then with the sudden change in circulation and hormonal levels after birth, it appears that hair is coming out "in handfuls," probably because fewer follicles are active.

Sebaceous glands and sweat glands may be more active because of increased circulation. Oily skin, sometimes acne, may reoccur in the woman who struggled with this problem during puberty.

GASTROINTESTINAL SYSTEM

The circulating estrogens and progesterone exert a relaxing effect on the smooth muscles of the entire gastrointestinal tract. The primary purpose appears to be to increase the absorption of nutrients from the intestinal tract. The motility of the stomach is slowed, gastric secretions are reduced, and stomach emptying takes place more slowly. The cardiac sphincter is not as efficient as it was, and *regurgitation* with resulting heartburn becomes a problem for some. Toward the end of pregnancy the enlarged uterus may hinder the ingestion of large meals; in this case the woman should avoid fried foods and take smaller, more frequent meals to remain comfortable.

Morning Sickness Nausea is one of the most common complaints of the first trimester. For some women even the sight and smell of food bring on nausea or vomiting. Although psychologic factors, such as ambivalence toward the pregnancy, may be involved, there is a physiologic basis for nausea in the marked gastrointestinal changes. Fortunately, by the thirteenth week most women are free of morning sickness.

Women often are advised to eat a few dry crackers before arising from bed in the morning. Dry, easily digestible carbohydrate food in the stomach may prevent symptoms. Dry, low-fat meals ensure a smaller volume of food in the stomach. Since fat slows down peristalsis, low-fat meals would not aggravate the already slowed motility that underlies these symptoms. Liquids should be consumed between meals in order to prevent dehydration. If vomiting is severe or persists at other times of day, the patient should be advised to consult the physician for treatment. Medication to stop nausea must be by prescription, not an "over-the-counter" purchase (see Chap. 18 for a discussion of antiemetics).

Heartburn The cardiac sphincter between the stomach and the esophagus becomes slightly relaxed and may be opened by the pressure of the enlarging uterus, resulting in slight regurgitation of acids from the stomach. The acids irritate the mucosa, causing a burning sensation. Adding to the problems of heartburn, the increased movement of the diaphragm and the flaring of the rib cage may create a temporary, minor *hiatus hernia*, or an enlargement of the opening in the diaphragm where the esophagus enters the stomach. Surgical intervention is not necessary, as the problem will disappear after the baby's birth. Remedies may include drinking milk between meals and taking small, frequent meals. Any antacid should be prescribed by the physician. Early in pregnancy, when gastric acidity is already reduced, an antacid would not be advisable. Later in pregnancy the prescription may be given for an aluminum hydroxide gel. Patients should be especially advised not to take medications containing sodium bicarbonate to relieve heartburn.

Constipation With the slowing of peristalsis, the body is able to extract more vitamins, minerals, and other nutrients from the food that is eaten, but, in the process, the body also extracts more water from the food bulk as it passes through the large intestine. Slower motility and a drier stool contribute to constipation. If the symptoms persist, hemorrhoids soon develop (see Chap. 23 for treatment). Adequate exercise, increased fluid intake, and ingestion of foods containing roughage usually will alleviate constipation. Mineral oil is not to be taken because it interferes with the absorption of fat-soluble nutrients in the small intestine. Again, any cathartic should be advised by the physician, who often prescribes a stoolsoftener, such as Colace, instead of a laxative. For a summary of gastrointestinal changes, see Fig. 4·4.

THE RENAL SYSTEM

With the 30 percent increase in the amount of circulating blood, there is a corresponding increase in the amount that circulates through the kidneys. However, because of increased reabsorption by the tubules of sodium and electrolytes and hence of water, there is no appreciable increase in the volume of urine produced for excretion. Toward the end of pregnancy there is even a reduction of urine formation, as the woman retains more body water (5).

The renal threshold for glucose may drop slightly. A small amount of glucose may be found in the urine without being considered indicative of a problem. Later in pregnancy, *lactose*, part of the content of *colostrum* being produced by the breasts, may be found in the urine. (Diagnosis of diabetic changes in pregnancy is discussed in Chap. 24.)

The ureters and bladder are composed of smooth muscle and are therefore affected by progesterone and estrogen. The ureters dilate and relax, leading to some *stasis,* or pooling of urine. The bladder may not completely empty for the same reason; therefore infection, or *bacteriuria,* is more common during pregnancy (see Chap. 20.).

Nocturia is a common complaint among pregnant women. The basis for this problem is that fluid, affected by gravity, tends to accumulate in the lower extremities during the day. The horizontal position at night favors kidney function, and the fluid drains from the lower extremities and is excreted.

Positional changes affect kidney function because of the enlarging uterus. In the supine position the uterus presses upon the renal veins and arteries, reducing effective flow to the kidneys. Therefore, it is important for the pregnant woman, especially in the advanced stages, to lie on her side whenever resting.

Frequency is caused by the enlarging uter-us rising out of the pelvic cavity. The uterus compresses the bladder against the pelvic bones and reduces its capacity. The woman feels an urgent sensation to void even though there may be only $1/4$ to $1/2$ cup of formed urine. Then, again in the last weeks before delivery, after lightening has occurred, the uterus compresses the bladder to cause the same effect.

RESPIRATORY SYSTEM

During pregnancy the volume of tidal air increases with the increased movement of the diaphragm and the expansion of the lower ribs laterally to allow for a larger intake of air. An increased volume of CO_2 is expelled with expiration, allowing the CO_2 from the fetus to be transferred more easily to the maternal circulation because of the decreased P_{CO_2} of her blood. Likewise more O_2 is inspired.

Late in pregnancy, with the increase in the size of the uterus, many women, in spite of the flaring of the ribs, experience *dyspnea*. The uterus presses against the diaphragm, compressing the lungs, and the woman may become *orthopneic*. Once she experiences *lightening,* or tilting of the uterus forward, some of the pressure from the weight of the uterus is shifted away from the lungs and diaphragm and she can breathe more deeply again.

The increased circulation may cause swelling of the vocal cords and larynx, bringing about hoarseness or deepening of the voice.

signs and symptoms of pregnancy

It may be several weeks after conception before a woman suspects that she is pregnant. As changes are occurring within her body, she begins to notice symptoms, one of the first of which is *amenorrhea,* or the ab-

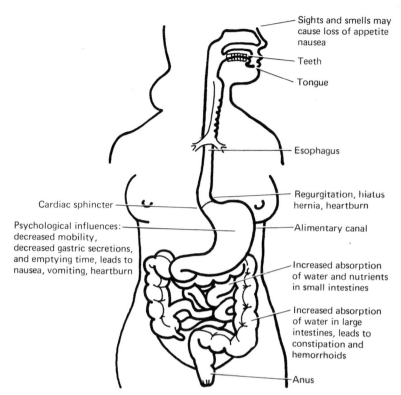

Sights and smells may
cause loss of appetite
nausea

Teeth

Tongue

Esophagus

Regurgitation, hiatus
hernia, heartburn

Cardiac sphincter

Psychological influences:
decreased mobility,
decreased gastric secretions,
and emptying time, leads to
nausea, vomiting, heartburn

Alimentary canal

Increased absorption
of water and nutrients
in small intestines

Increased absorption
of water in large
intestines, leads to
constipation and
hemorrhoids

Anus

fig. 4·4 Gastrointestinal tract showing minor discomforts during pregnancy.

sence of her menstrual flow. Her breasts may become tender and feel full. She may experience morning nausea. Fatigue is another early symptom. Many women, when asked how they knew conception had taken place, stated that they "just knew something was different."

Noticing that something is different about her body and then putting the symptoms together, the woman may decide to go to a clinic or private physician for confirmation of the pregnancy. (How early she goes depends a great deal on her understanding of what will take place there and how she will be received.)

The woman has experienced one or more early subjective *symptoms.* The physician will then look for *signs*, objective verification to confirm or disprove the beginning of a pregnancy. The signs and symptoms of pregnancy can be divided into two main groups: possible and positive.

Possible	*Positive*
Amenorrhea	Auscultation of the fetal heart
Breast changes	
Morning sickness	Fetal electrocardiogram
Frequency of urination	Palpation of fetal parts by examiner
Fatigue	
Abdominal enlargement	Visualization of the fetus by means of x-ray
Uterocervical changes	Ultrasound visualization of the fetus
Vaginal changes	
Positive pregnancy tests	
Quickening	

POSSIBLE SIGNS OF PREGNANCY

Possible signs of pregnancy are those which indicate a growing embryo but at the same time could occur with another condition of medical or psychologic origin. However, three or more of the possible signs taken together are a fairly good indication of the presence of a growing embryo. Positive signs are those which establish without doubt the presence of a fetus in the uterus; they usually may be confirmed after 16 to 20 weeks.

Amenorrhea Amenorrhea may be one of the earliest clues to pregnancy. In considering it as one of the signs, the physician and nurse must be aware of the possibility that other factors, such as low hormone levels, stress, anemia, and illness, can alter the menstrual cycle. The patient may suspect that she is pregnant, may worry about it, only to discover that her period is delayed for other reasons. Conversely, some women have a diminished flow at the regular period interval for 1 or 2 months after conception and for that reason do not recognize pregnancy or seek care.

Breast Changes The breasts become sensitive, full, and tender because of the increased blood supply and hormone effect. The nipple and areola darken. The tubercles of Montgomery become more prominent. For many women increased sensitivity and a tingling sensation in the breasts provide one of their first clues to the possibility of pregnancy. By 14 weeks *colostrum,* the precursor of milk, is being produced.

Morning Sickness Because it occurs on an empty stomach in the morning, the nausea of pregnancy is particularly easy to identify. Psychic factors plus hormone changes contribute to morning sickness. About 50 percent of pregnant women experience this bothersome nausea and vomiting. If the vomiting becomes excessive, so that it endangers the baby or the mother, the condition is referred to as *hyperemesis gravidarum* (see Chap. 24).

Frequency of Urination Frequency is caused by the pressure of the enlarging uterus as it rises out of the pelvic area. The bladder, compressed by the uterus, sends a message of urgency to void even though, as already mentioned, it may contain only $1/4$ to $1/2$ cup of urine. Frequency is also present when there is a bladder infection, but frequency during early pregnancy does not have the other symptoms of infection—burning and pain on urination.

Fatigue All the metabolic changes that are under way seem to cause an unusual amount of fatigue and sleepiness for a woman in early pregnancy. During later pregnancy, fatigue comes from the changes in body posture and the extra weight that must be carried everywhere.

Abdominal Enlargement Most primigravidas do not notice marked changes in abdominal size until the second trimester. By the sixteenth week the woman usually finds that she can no longer button her skirt or slacks. However, some multigravidas notice tightening of their clothes almost immediately after one missed menstrual period.

The rising of the uterus into the abdominal cavity is gradual and has completely occurred at about the twelfth week. From that time, the height of the fundus above the symphysis is a guide to the duration of the pregnancy because the uterus rises about 1 cm a week (Fig. 4·5). MacDonald's rule for calculating the duration of pregnancy is as follows: *measurement of height of fundus above symphysis (in cm) $\times$ $8/7$ = duration of pregnancy (in weeks)* (Fig. 4·6). The measurement is thrown off by obesity, multiple pregnancy, and an abnormally small or large amount of amniotic fluid.

Abdominal enlargement may occur in

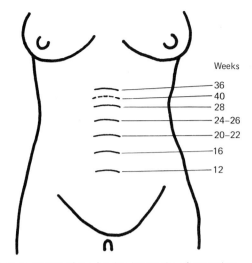

fig. 4·5 Height of the fundus by weeks of gestation.

Weeks
- 36
- 40
- 28
- 24-26
- 20-22
- 16
- 12

cases of *pseudopregnancy,* when the woman, believing that she is pregnant, goes through many of the preliminary signs. The physiologic basis for pseudopregnancy has been documented by Brown and Barglow (6), who showed that the corpus luteum can remain active under influence of stress-induced hormones, even though conception has not occurred.

Uterocervical Changes With increased circulation and hormonal activity the uterus and the cervix become increasingly soft. The softness is noted first as a spot on the anterior side of the uterus just above the uterocervical junction. This softening is known as *Ladin's* sign and may occur as early as the fifth week of pregnancy. The softening of the cervix itself is called *Goodell's* sign. In addition to these two signs, the lower uterine segment becomes very compressible. On bimanual examination of the junction, the fingers of the examiner seem to touch, apparently compressing the area to paper thinness. This is *Hegar's* sign and can be demonstrated as early as the sixth week. Before the use of isoimmunologic tests for pregnancy, Hegar's

sign was a very valuable indication of pregnancy.

Cervical Changes The tight, long, smooth muscle that guards the entry to the uterus changes by softening and by forming a large number of mucus-secreting glands near the external *os* (opening). These glands effectively close off the os during pregnancy. When labor begins and the cervix begins to open, these glands are shed in the form of a *plug* of mucus (Fig. 3·22).

Vaginal Changes Because of the increased blood supply to the pelvic region the vaginal mucosa and the cervix take on a bluish-purple coloration known as *Chadwick's* sign, or *Jacquimeier's* sign, demonstrable by the eighth week of pregnancy.

There is an increased supply of glucose to the cells of the vagina, as well as a general hypertrophy of the vaginal folds. The cervical secretions increase throughout pregnancy and may constitute a hygiene problem for the woman. *Leukorrhea,* or the increased secretion of cervical mucus, is thin, watery, milky white, and may be profuse enough to necessitate the wearing of a vaginal pad in later pregnancy. The secretions should not cause itching or irritation to the tissues unless there

fig. 4·6 Measurement of fundal height.

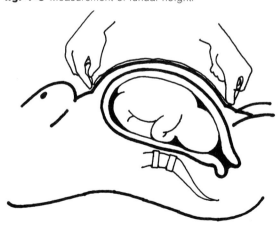

is an infection present. For hygienic reasons the pregnant woman is advised to cleanse the entire perineal area and keep it dry to prevent chafing. A mild vinegar and water solution is an effective external cleansing agent, but douches should not be used unless prescribed by the physician.

If the discharge becomes yellowish or thick and white, causes pruritus, or has an odor, it is no longer normal but is probably caused by one of the normally present organisms in the vaginal tract. The most common of these are *Trichomonas vaginalis* and *Candida albicans* (see Chap. 20). Medications are prescribed in the form of vaginal suppositories, gels, or solutions applied to the mucosa. The husband or sexual partner should also be treated, because of the possibility of reinfection.

Positive Pregnancy Tests There are two basic types of laboratory tests for pregnancy: biologic and isoimmunologic. Both types are based on the presence or absence of HCG in the urine (Fig. 4·3).

In biologic tests, the urine of the possibly pregnant woman is injected into an animal; resultant changes in its gonads are caused by HCG. In the *Friedman* test, the urine is injected into a rabbit; in the *Aschheim-Zondek* (A-Z) test, a mouse is used; and in the *Hogben* test, a frog or toad is used. If the woman is pregnant, the HCG will stimulate ovulation or the development of spermatozoa in the animal within a few days. These tests are all approximately 97 percent accurate. Urine can yield positive results 4 weeks after conception has occurred. Unfortunately, these tests require the breeding and sacrifice of test animals and thus are expensive.

The second method of testing for pregnancy, the *isoimmunologic* test, has virtually eliminated the cumbersome, time-consuming biologic tests because urine testing can be done in the clinic and takes from 2 min to 2 h, with a 95 percent accuracy rate.

One of the commonly used agents is the Pregnosticon test.[1] Instructions for use require that the patient void to give a fresh specimen; only a few drops of urine are necessary. The test is based on an antigen-antibody reaction; HCG is the antigen, and the serum from rabbits immunized against HCG is the antiserum. If no clumping of the HCG-coated latex particles occurs when mixed with the urine and antiserum, the test is considered positive for pregnancy. If clumping or agglutination occurs, the test is negative. A positive test can be found 12 days after the first missed menstrual period, or about 26 days after conception.

Quickening By the sixteenth to eighteenth week a primigravida will begin to feel the baby move within her uterus. Known as quickening or "feeling life," it is for many women a most significant point in their pregnancy. Even the woman who is anxiously waiting for the sign may mistake it for flatulence, for the flutter of fetal movement is so slight. A multigravida, being more experienced, may feel movements by the fourteenth to sixteenth week (7).

POSITIVE SIGNS OF PREGNANCY

There are *three types* of positive indication of a growing fetus: hearing or recording the fetal heart, feeling the fetal parts or movements, and visualizing the outline of the fetus by x-ray or ultrasound.

Auscultation Auscultation of the fetal heart rate (FHR) is possible at about the twentieth week after the LMP with a fetal stethoscope. An electronically amplified sound can sometimes be heard by the fourteenth to sixteenth

[1]Pregnosticon Dri-Dot, trademark, Diagnostic Products, Organon, Inc., West Orange, N.J. 07052.

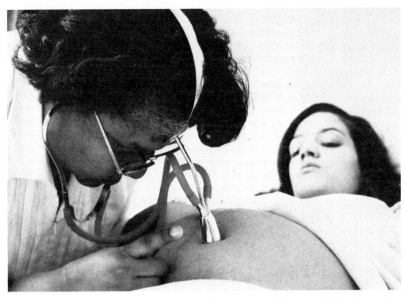

fig. 4·7 Placing stethoscope to hear fetal heart tones. (*Photo by Ruth Helmich. Courtesy of The Jamaica Hospital, Jamaica, N.Y.*)

week. The fetal heart rate is most clearly audible through the back of the fetus. Therefore, the stethoscope is placed over that site after the abdomen has been palpated (Fig. 4·7). It is important that the examiner differentiate between the mother's pulse and the fetal heart sound. The usual fetal heart rate varies from 120 to 160 beats per minute. The maternal pulse would range from 70 to 90, with the "average" pulse rate at 75 to 85 beats per minute. Both heart rates should have a regular rhythm. When listening to the heart the nurse may hear a slurring or blowing sound known as a *souffle*. The sound of the blood as it surges through the umbilical cord is called the *funicular souffle*; as it passes through the uterine vessels on the maternal side, it is called the *uterine souffle*. The funicular souffle is at the same rate as the fetal heart, since the baby's heart propels the blood through the umbilical cord. The uterine souffle sounds at the same rate as the mother's heart rate (Fig. 4·9).

Fetal Electrocardiogram A fetal electrocardiogram can be included as a positive sign of pregnancy, for electrodes applied to the mother's abdomen by 14 to 16 weeks can pick up the almost doubled rate of the fetal heart. This method is very useful in diagnosing the presence of a multiple pregnancy or in confirming fetal death.

Palpation of Fetal Parts Palpation of the fetal shape or body movement by the examiner is the second type of positive indication of pregnancy. By the twentieth week the examiner can usually differentiate between fetal kicking and what the mother may have described. By the twenty-sixth week the baby can be felt through the abdominal wall, and various parts identified. However, this sign can never be used as a sole indication of pregnancy, for some women have muscle tumors (myomas) in the uterine wall that could be misleading.

Visualization of the Fetus Visualization of the fetal outline or skeleton is possible by

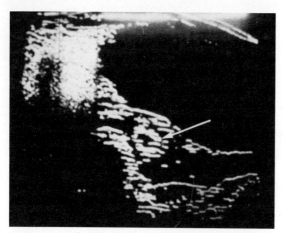

fig. 4·8 Ultrasonography indicating an embryo of 6 weeks gestation. Gestational sac at 6 weeks. (Fetal heart tones can be confirmed by Doppler effect after the 9th week.) (*Photo courtesy of Horace E. Thompson, M. D., University of Colorado Medical Center, Denver, Col.*)

these might have an influence on the course of the pregnancy. For example, it would influence the mother's care markedly if she were a diabetic or had a heart condition from a childhood bout with rheumatic fever. The following diseases are important in a medical history:

Past Illnesses	pelvic
syphilis, gonorrhea	perineal
heart disease	spinal
diabetes	lower-back
tuberculosis	*Family History*
measles	*of Illness*
rickets	any genetic
hypertension	diseases
anemia	hypertension
sickle-cell disease	diabetes
kidney infection	heart disease
Past Surgery	cancer
abdominal	tuberculosis

Included in the history would be the family history, for any disease that might be genetically carried would alert the examiner to possible disorders that could influence the health of the mother or fetus.

Social history, marital status, age, next-of-kin, insurance information, and occupation of patient and husband (if she is married) are recorded on the chart. Social habits, such as customary amount of drinking or smoking, may be included in this part of the record. (The patient should be assured of the privacy of her record.)

means of x-ray and ultrasound. Calcification of the bones takes place after the first trimester, so that the fetal skeleton shows more clearly after this time. X-ray merely to identify pregnancy is never done during the early part of pregnancy (Fig. 3·23).

Ultrasound On the other hand, ultrasound has not been proved to be harmful and can pick up very early the outlines of the fetal head in the enlarged uterus (see Chap. 27 for further discussion). Ultrasound is not available everywhere but is becoming an increasingly useful tool in obstetrics (Fig. 4·8).

the first prenatal visit

MEDICAL AND SOCIAL HISTORY

A complete medical/social history is taken at the first visit, with the interview often conducted by the nurse. The physician should know of previous operations and illnesses, as

OBSTETRIC HISTORY

At the clinic or office the woman's menstrual history is ascertained to determine the time of menarche, and the onset, duration, and regularity of her menses. Her past obstetric history is obtained, including the number of pregnancies, or her *gravidity,* and the number of deliveries of infants of more than 20 weeks'

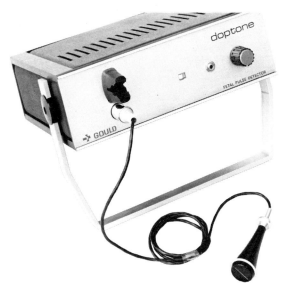

fig. 4·9 Doptone for auscultation of fetal heart beat. Amplified heart sounds can be heard early in the second trimester. (*Courtesy of Gould, Inc.*)

gestation, or her *parity*. Since many women have experienced spontaneous abortions during their reproductive period, the physician may closely question the woman about "miscarriages" (see Chap. 22) Miscarriages are recorded as part of her gravidity. The terms in Table 4·1 are special to obstetrics and are used as a shorthand way of referring to a woman's obstetric situation. As you learn more about pregnancy these terms will take on meaning. For example, if a patient has a *gravida IV, para 0* listing, it implies that she has never been able to carry an infant to term. She may have some underlying medical problem and may be tremendously anxious about the current pregnancy when she is seen in the clinic.

Gravidity and parity are described in two different ways. The first system explains only the number of times the woman has conceived (gravid) and the numbers of times she has delivered an infant of more than 20 weeks' gestation (para). The second system describes only her parity, but in more detail. The parity is listed in four categories, term pregnancies, preterm deliveries, abortions, and offspring now living. Shortened, these terms equal *T-P-A-L*. To determine gravidity from parity, add T, P, and A, always remembering to include the current undelivered pregnancy, should the woman be coming into the clinic or the labor room. Whether the viable (age in weeks) infant survived or not does not alter the parity; it is merely reflected in L (now living). Multiple births count only as one para but show in the column of living children (if they survived). Some institutions add a fifth category, multiple births, to make parity more accurately reflect what happens. Parity, like gravidity, is a shorthand reference system.

Transfer between the systems can be made as in the following examples, which take into account the current pregnancy.

table 4·1
GRAVIDA AND PARA TERMINOLOGY

Gravid = pregnant, the state of being pregnant

Gravida = a pregnant woman

Primigravida = a woman who is pregnant for the first time

Multigravida = a woman who has been pregnant more than once (usually used for one who has delivered more than once, also)

Para = a woman who has delivered a *viable* infant (over the age of 20 weeks), whether alive or stillborn

Parity = the *number* of *times* a woman has delivered a viable infant*

Nullipara = one who *never* has borne a viable child (para 0)

Primipara = a woman who has had *one delivery* of a viable infant or infants (para I)

Multipara = a woman who has had *two or more* deliveries of viable infants (para II, III, IV, etc.)

*The birth of twins, triplets, etc., counts as one delivery.

table 4.3

	System 1			System 2		
	GRAVIDA	PARA	TERM	PRETERM	ABORTION	LIVING
Case A	II	I	1	0	0	1
Case B	III	I	1	0	1	1
Case C	VII	V	3	1	2	4
Case D	II	I	0	1	0	2 (twins)

To make a complete history, there must be recorded the quality of past pregnancies, labors, and deliveries, and whether they were normal or complicated and whether postpartum complications occurred. It is desirable, of course, for the woman to go to the same doctor for every delivery, but the mobility of our society precludes this in many cases.

All these facts may be gathered by interview with several staff members in the clinic, but the purpose is the same—to assist in determining the direction of care for the individual patient. The physician needs to "know" the patient's idiosyncrasies in order to individualize care, and the nurse must always counsel and teach each patient according to her peculiar life circumstances, without generalizing information.

Duration of Pregnancy The usual length of time from conception to birth is 266 days, but some races have a shorter gestation period. For instance, in some areas black women have a period of pregnancy of about 8 days less than Caucasian women. (This difference may merely reflect socioeconomic factors such as poverty, nutrition, etc.) Some women, particularly primigravidas, go beyond the average period by 1 or 2 weeks without difficulty. Since the exact day of conception is rarely known, calculation is done from the first day of the last menstrual period. If the length of pregnancy is estimated from the first day of the last menstrual period, the duration becomes 14 days longer, or 272 to 280 days. (All calculations are based on a 28-day cycle in which ovulation occurs 14 days ± 2 after the period starts, even though 50 percent of all women have a shorter or longer interval between menses.) Using *Nagele's rule,* the estimated time for delivery, or the EDC (estimated day of confinement), is figured as follows:

LMP + 7 days − 3 months + 1 year = EDC

For example:

LMP = Nov. 15, 1975
Add 1 week (7 days) = Nov. 22, 1975
Back 3 months = Aug. 22, 1975
Add 1 year = Aug. 22, 1976

It should be kept in mind that only a very small percentage of women actually deliver on their EDC. It is merely an estimation, an actual delivery date 2 weeks either way is not unusual.

In the event that the woman cannot remember her LMP or when her menstrual cycle is so irregular as to make the date of conception unknown, other means can be used to determine when the infant will be born. The height of the fundus can be measured and MacDonald's rule used. If the mother is sure of her quickening date, Rawlings and Moore suggest a method of calculation (8):

Date of quickening + 20 weeks and 2 days = EDC for a primigravida
Date of quickening + 21 weeks and 4 days = EDC for a multigravida

This method is more exact and requires the use of a calendar for accuracy. For example:

Primigravida's date of quickening =
        Mar. 20, 1975
        + 20 weeks and 2 days
        ─────────────────────
        = Aug. 9, 1975
Multigravida's date of quickening =
        Nov. 26, 1974
        + 21 weeks and 4 days
        ─────────────────────
        = Apr. 27, 1975

A combined calculation using both methods probably would give a more accurate EDC than either one used alone.

PHYSICAL EXAMINATION

At the first visit, a complete physical examination will be made. For many healthy women, this may be the first time they have ever been examined; certainly it will be the first time for several of the tests they will have. Therefore, explanations of each procedure will greatly ease anxiety.

General Examination Ears, eyes, nose, and throat (EENT) are examined to determine any infections, abnormalities, dental caries, or gum problems. The condition of blood vessels can be seen when the fundus of the eye is examined with a fundoscope.

Skin and hair often give clues to the overall health of the woman. A skilled examiner can gain a general impression fairly rapidly by observing the color, turgor, and condition of the skin.

Neck and chest yield information about the thyroid gland, the lymph nodes of the axillary area, and the breasts. Every woman can and should be taught about breast self-examination during her pregnancy examinations.

Heart and lungs are auscultated for irregularities in function. The findings, coupled with a medical history, may permit diagnosis of a borderline cardiac condition during this first examination.

Extremities are examined for varicose veins and edema. The physician notes any signs of infection or restriction of movement.

Abdominal examination is done to determine the size and shape of the uterus. The fundus usually is measured at each visit, to permit recording of the rate of fetal growth. Patients often are very tense about abdominal palpation and need help in relaxing enough to allow the examiner to complete the task.

Pelvic Examination A vaginal speculum is inserted to provide a clear view of the cervix. The color, condition, and amount of leukorrhea from the cervix are observed. At this time most physicians take a Papanicolaou smear for screening of cervical cancer cells, and a smear for detection of gonorrhea. The speculum is removed, and a bimanual examination is performed to determine Hegar's sign. A few pelvic measurements are made at this time: the *biischial diameter* is the distance between the ischial tuberosities (normally 8 cm or more), and the *diagonal conjugate* is the distance between the lower margin of the pubic bone to the promontory of the sacrum (normally 11.5 cm or more). (Measurements are discussed in detail in Chap. 8.)

Vital Signs At every visit the vital signs will be taken and recorded. Of these signs, the blood pressure is the most significant and diagnostic indication of potential problems. An early base-line reading is important to have for comparison with later changes. A slight drop in pressure is expected in the first 24 weeks, with a return to normal or slightly above base line in the last trimester. Any elevation over base line of 30 points systolic and 15 points diastolic may be an indication of hypertension or preeclampsia (see Chap. 23). Older women often have preexisting high blood pressure. Early documentation during the prenatal clinic visits helps to diagnose and treat this type of hypertension.

The Warning Signals Sometime in the early prenatal visits each woman should be instructed about when to notify the physician of problems. Warning signals of problems other than the normal minor discomforts should be clearly taught. Unknowingly, a woman may endure a pathologic change in her condition, assuming that it is "just one of those things that happen." Warning signals can be divided into groups as below:

Bleeding. Any bleeding during pregnancy is abnormal. It may warn of impending abortion, a poorly implanted placenta, or a sudden separation of the placenta. And a few women have vaginal bleeding from cervical erosion due to chronic infection.

Infection. Signs of infection in any part of the body are warning signals, but during pregnancy, those conditions that might affect the fetal condition are especially serious. Fever, chills, and signs of kidney, bladder, or vaginal infection are all reportable.

Pain. Pain during the course of pregnancy is abnormal. (The abdominal aching and perineal pressure of prelabor or the "catching," brief pain in the side due to a pulling sensation of the round ligament as it supports the uterus are the only exceptions.)

Preeclampsia. A group of signs and symptoms related to developing preeclampsia may demonstrate as (1) severe continuous headache, (2) edema in face, hands, or legs upon arising in the morning, (3) scanty, concentrated urine, (4) visual disturbances. Any of these must be reported at once as the preeclampsia syndrome can develop very rapidly.

Laboratory Tests *Urine* tests can detect hormonal, cellular, and chemical products in the urine. The first visit includes the most thorough testing for glucose, protein, and cells. If there is a question about an early pregnancy, HCG in the urine will be indicative. At every later visit a dip-stick test is made for glucose and protein levels. The nurse directs the patient to obtain the urine specimen collected free of vaginal secretions which, being protein, would falsely affect the results of the albumin test. Most clinics ask for a clean voided midstream urine sample: easily used kits are available or can be constructed with cotton balls and warm water. If an antiseptic is included, the woman must rinse well, as the remnants of the hexachlorophene or aqueous Zephiran would disturb the test results. If a culture and sensitivity test of urine are ordered, a clean voided specimen is preferable over a catheterized one.

Blood tests are done as part of the initial examination of the pregnant woman's status. Complete blood count, hemoglobin, and hematocrit will indicate the normality of her hematologic system. Blood usually is typed as to group—A, B, AB, or O—and for the presence or absence of the Rh factor. In the event that the mother is Rh-negative, the father should be typed. A test for *antibody titer* is done for all women who potentially could have an antibody buildup in their own blood against the fetal Rh-positive erythrocytes or the A or B blood type inherited from an Rh-positive father or one with A or B blood type. The Hemantigen test can be done on each of these women as a general screening for antibodies. Hemantigen is a serum containing pooled antigens which, when mixed with the mother's blood, will show agglutination if any maternal antibodies are present. Specific tests for the type present can be performed subsequently (see Chap. 29).

Screening for some genetically carried diseases is possible, and specific screening for thalassemia and sickle-cell trait will be done on patients of Mediterranean or African heritage. (The effect of these problems is discussed in detail in Chap. 21.)

By state law, every pregnant woman in the United States must be screened for syphilis. The serology test usually is done at the first visit and may be repeated before labor begins.

Many clinics require that the patient have a

routine chest x-ray. The early chest x-ray shows heart size and can be used as a base-line view if later cardiac symptoms develop. X-rays are also done to screen high-risk populations for tuberculosis. Many private obstetricians do not perform this type of x-rays on their patients in the middle and upper income groups who are less exposed and thus less likely to have contracted tuberculosis. When a pregnant woman has a chest x-ray, her abdomen and perineal area should be shielded by a lead apron to prevent scatter. Although the amount of radiation for a chest x-ray is very small, precautions of this sort should never be ignored.

Many clinics are now screening for the presence of the *rubella antibody.* Any woman with a low antibody titer (see Chap. 20) is a candidate for rubella immunization immediately after delivery.

The pregnant woman may need a great deal of interpretation about what is happening to her. Chapter 5 details the nurse's role in teaching and supporting the patient throughout the period of her pregnancy.

nutritional needs during pregnancy

PREPARATION FOR PREGNANCY

Nutritional preparation for pregnancy does not begin just prior to conception. Nor does it begin in adolescence. It should be a lifetime process for the mother-to-be. It is a known fact that the nutritional health of the newborn depends upon the nutritional status of the mother at the time of conception as well as upon her nutritional practices during pregnancy. It is important for her to have adequate stores of nutrients in her body tissues to provide for all the nutrient needs of the fetus. The adequacy of nutrient stores is a result of a lifetime of good eating practices rather than a quick transformation from poor to good nutrition when pregnancy occurs.

Dietary studies of various age groups in the United States show that adolescent girls tend to have the worst food habits. Infants and young children, still under parental influence, usually are well fed. They continue good eating habits in their school years until they reach adolescence. Adolescent boys usually have ravenous appetites that go along with their linear growth and activity. By eating large quantities of food to meet the demands of their appetites, their nutrient needs usually are met. Girls do not fare as well.

Adolescent girls usually are not as active as boys, nor do they grow as tall; therefore their caloric needs are not as great. Usually concerned about maintaining slim figures, they may cut down their caloric intake or omit meals and follow bizarre weight-losing schemes at the expense of good nutrition.

Dietary studies have shown that the most prevalent nutrition problem among adolescent girls today is iron-deficiency anemia, shown by low hemoglobin and hematocrit levels and by diets with low iron levels. The problem may be magnified among adolescent girls from lower socioeconomic backgrounds.

In order to be in good nutritional health, the daily food plan shown in Table 4·3 is suggested for the adolescent girl and adult woman prior to pregnancy.

This plan represents approximately 1500 and 1800 kcal for the adult and adolescent, respectively. If skim milk is used instead of whole milk, the caloric content is reduced by approximately 80 kcal for each cup of milk. Additional calories are obtained from accompanying free-choice foods. The Recommended Dietary Allowance for adolescent and adult women is available in Table 4·4.

ADAPTATION OF DIET DURING PREGNANCY

According to an old Chinese tradition, a baby is a year old when he is born. Actually, at birth

table 4·3

DAILY FOOD GUIDE—BASIC FOUR FOOD GROUPS

FOOD GROUP	IMPORTANT NUTRIENTS	RECOMMENDED DAILY AMOUNTS

Milk	Calcium
	Proteins
	Riboflavin
		Adolescents: 4 cups
		Adults: 2 cups
		Equivalents:
		  8 oz fluid milk or
		  1 oz cheddar cheese = 1 cup milk
		  1/2 cup cottage cheese = 1/3 cup milk
		  1/2 cup ice cream = 1/4 cup milk

Meat	Protein
	Iron
	B vitamins
		Two servings.
		One serving is equivalent to:
		  2 oz lean, cooked meat, poultry,
		  or fish
		  2 eggs
		  1/4 cup cooked dry peas, beans, or lentils
		  4 tablespoons peanut butter

Fruit/
vegetable
	B vitamins
	Iron
		Four or more servings.
		One serving is equivalent to:
		  1/2 cup vegetable
		  1/2 cup fruit

	Vitamin C	One serving of citrus fruit or other fruit or vegetable rich in vitamin C daily; and
	Vitamin A	One serving of a dark green or deep yellow vegetable or fruit *every other* day

Breads/
cereals
(whole grain
or enriched)
	B vitamins
	Iron
		Four or more servings.
		One serving is equivalent to:
		  1 oz dry ready-to-eat cereal or
		  1/2 cup cooked cereal, rice,
		  spaghetti, macaroni, or noodles

the newborn is nutritionally 9 months old. The mother's nutrient reserves at the time of conception and her nutritional intake during pregnancy are essential factors in the nutritional health of the infant. If a woman begins in poor nutritional health, it is absolutely essential for her to have first-rate food intake during her pregnancy.

It is known that during the first part of pregnancy, gastrointestinal motility is slowed to enable the nutrients to be absorbed more efficiently in the small intestines. Better absorption of nutrients helps meet the nutrient demands of the first trimester before the women realizes that she is pregnant. When she does recognize the pregnancy, she should evaluate her dietary pattern (often with nursing or nutritionist help) to make sure that she is receiving all the foods necessary to provide the balance needed by the fetus.

Maternal Needs during Pregnancy If during the entire gestation the mother adds 300 kcal over and above her base-line, nonpregnant intake, she will supply the caloric needs for the estimated average 12.5-kg (27.5-lb) weight gain. The figures are calcu-

table 4.4

RECOMMENDED DIETARY ALLOWANCES (REVISED, 1973)

AGE, yr	FEMALES, 11–14	FEMALES, 15–18	FEMALES, 19–22	FEMALES, 23–50	PREGNANT FEMALES	LACTATING FEMALES
Weight, kg, lb	44–97	54–119	58–128	58–128		
Height, cm, in	155–62	162–65	162–65	162–65		
Energy, kcal*	2400	2100	2100	2000	+300	+500
Protein, Gm	44	48	46	46	+ 30	+ 20
Fat-soluble vitamins:						
Vitamin A activity, RE†	800	800	800	800	1000	1200
IU	4000	4000	4000	4000	5000	6000
Vitamin D, IU	400	400	400		400	400
Vitamin E activity, IU	10	11	12	12	15	15
Water-soluble vitamins:						
Ascorbic acid, mg	45	45	45	45	60	60
Folacin, μg	400	400	400	400	800	600
Niacin, mg	16	14	14	13	+2	+4
Riboflavin, mg	1.3	1.4	1.4	1.2	+0.3	+0.5
Thiamine, mg	1.2	1.1	1.1	1.0	+0.3	+0.3
Vitmain B_6, mg	1.6	2.0	2.0	2.0	2.5	2.5
Vitamin B_{12}, μg	3.0	3.0	3.0	3.0	4.0	4.0
Minerals:						
Calcium, mg	1200	1200	800	800	1200	1200
Phosphorus, mg	1200	1200	800	800	1200	1200
Iodine, μg	115	115	100	100	125	150
Iron, mg	18	18	18	18	18+‡	18
Magnesium, mg	300	300	300	300	450	450
Zinc, mg	15	15	15	15	20	25

*kcal = kilo calories.

†RE = retinol equivalents.

‡This increased requirement cannot be met by ordinary diets; therefore, the use of supplemental iron is recommended.

Source: *Recommended Dietary Allowances*, revised, 1973, Food and Nutrition Board, National Academy of Sciences–National Research Council.

lated by taking into account the reduced energy expenditure during the last trimester. The nutrient needs as indicated by the Recommended Dietary allowances (1973) are now increased for the entire pregnancy (Table 4.4), rather than for the last half of pregnancy, as was recommended in 1968.

Realistically speaking, it is neither practical nor desirable for anyone to count a daily caloric intake. Therefore, the best way to evaluate intake during pregnancy is for the mother to record and observe her *rate* of weight gain. If she is gaining too rapidly or not gaining enough, her diet can be further evaluated.

Weight Gain The "energy cost" of making a baby is about 80,000 kcal for the normally active housewife in the United States. Of course, the working mother, or one more active than usual, may need to take in proportionately more calories. Barring excessive fluid retention, her caloric intake, then, can be measured by periodic weighing. Many sets of figures are given for normal sequence of

table 4·5

PROTEIN CONTENT OF MAJOR FOODS

FOOD	APPROXIMATE PROTEIN CONTENT
Lean meat, fish, or poultry (cooked)	1 oz (7 Gm)
Egg	one (7 Gm)
Milk	8 oz (8 Gm)
Split peas (cooked)	¹/₂ cup (10 Gm)
Pasta (cooked)	¹/₂ cup (3 Gm)
Beans, dry (black-eye, navy, kidney, Great Northern), cooked, drained	¹/₂ cup (7 Gm)

weight gain, all of which are averages. The growth and development sequence of the infant would indicate that the least weight is gained in the first trimester and the most toward the end of pregnancy. The first trimester may include a loss of weight, or a gain of up to about 3 lb, or 1.5 kg. Each week after the twelfth, about 0.8 to 1 lb, or 400 to 500 Gm, is gained in a normal pattern. Hytten (9) gives the following rates of weight gain:

By 10 weeks 650 Gm (about 1.5 lb)
By 20 weeks 4000 Gm (about 9 lb)
By 30 weeks 8500 Gm (about 19 lb)
By 40 weeks 12,500 Gm (27.5 lb)

Heavier patients tend to gain less than thinner women, and young women tend to gain a little more than older women. Each woman is individual in her response to her pregnancy, and dietary counseling must be flexible. A large increase (2 lb/week or more) or a decrease in weight should be evaluated as to its cause. For this reason, the woman is weighed during every prenatal visit, with the weight recorded on the chart and compared with the previous weight.

In the past, many physicians advised their patients to limit their weight gain during pregnancy to avoid a difficult and prolonged labor and delivery. Women were anxious to follow this advice so that they would return more quickly to their normal size after delivery. However, inadequate food intake sometimes has resulted in undernourished, low-birth-weight infants and some birth defects—thus the new recommendations of the Committee on Maternal Nutrition of the National Research Council that the healthy woman should gain *at least* 25 lb. Nurses can interpret these facts to the mother who is anxious about regaining her figure and who may be skimping on her food intake.

Careful study of the components of weight gain in a normal pregnancy has detailed the elements of the average 12.5-kg increase.

	No. of grams
Fetus	3300
Placenta	650
Amniotic fluid	800
Uterus	900
Breasts	450
Maternal blood	1250
Maternal fat stores	5200
	12,500 (12.5 kg, 27.5 lb)

The maternal stores once thought to be protein were found to be fat. The increase of fatty tissue is gained in proportion to the total

table 4·6

CALCIUM IN MILK FOOD GROUP

FOOD	AMOUNT	CALCIUM CONTENT, mg
Whole milk	8 oz	288
Skim milk	8 oz	296
Modified skim	8 oz	352
Cheddar cheese	1 oz	213
Cottage cheese	1/2 cup	115

weight gain and cannot be considered as excessive weight, for this fat probably is stored in preparation for lactation.

If weight gain is excessive and there appears to be no abnormal retention of fluid, a moderate calorie restriction may be advised. The mother is instructed to limit intake of sugar, butter, margarine, oil, fried foods, gravies, and rich desserts. Skim milk may be substituted for whole milk. The nurse should never advise her patients to omit bread and potato from the diet. These foods provide valuable nutrients and are necessary for her health. Any reduction from the recommended diet should be by prescription from the obstetrician and be under his supervision.

CHANGES IN NUTRIENTS

Protein Needs To meet the nutrient needs for the growth and health of the fetus, and for the growth of the maternal accessory tissues, an additional *daily intake* of 30 Gm protein is recommended. The base-line recommendation for women of childbearing age is 46 Gm daily; thus, in pregnancy 76 Gm daily is recommended.

Protein is needed for the growth of the fetus, uterus, mammary glands, and placenta, and for formation of amniotic fluid and plasma. These additional needs are over and above the normal anabolic needs of the woman.

Foods providing high-value, complete proteins are meat, fish, poultry, eggs, and milk. Plant sources supply useful but incomplete proteins to the diet. Vegetables, cereals, nuts, dried peas, beans, and lentils are sources of about one-third of the protein in North American diets. In some cultural groups the proportion of protein from plant sources increases (Table 4·5).

Calcium Even though calcium absorption is more efficient during pregnancy, additional intake of calcium is needed, especially during the period of bone formation and growth of the fetus. The recommended daily amount during pregnancy is 1200 mg (see Table 4·6).

Calcium is unevenly distributed in foods. The highest amount is found in milk and milk products. A small quantity is found in dark green leafy vegetables. An intake of approximately 4 cups of milk daily will meet the calcium needs during pregnancy.

Iron Before pregnancy the average woman absorbs about 10 percent of the iron in her diet. The additional needs for the increased maternal blood volume and fetal stores are partially compensated for by the lack of menstruation and by the increased iron absorption by the body. During the third trimester, almost three times the usual amount of iron can be absorbed by the body. At the same time, the fetus is demanding iron from the mother to form red cells and to accumulate stores that should last from 3 to 6 months after birth. The fetus will take the iron it needs from the mother; therefore she needs at least the recommended amount. Since it is very difficult to get the needed 18 mg iron daily in the diet, many physicians recommend an iron supplement (see Table 4·7).

table 4·7
IRON CONTENT OF FOODS

FOOD	AMOUNT	IRON, μg
Meats group:		
Pork liver, fried	3 oz	24.9
Calf liver, fried	3 oz	12.2
Beef liver, fried	3 oz	7.5
Heart, beef, braised	3 oz	5.0
Beef, lean, broiled	3 oz	3.0
Pork, roast	3 oz	2.7
Egg, cooked	1 large	1.1
Haddock, breaded and fried	3 oz	1.0
Tuna, canned	2 oz	1.0
Frankfurter	1, 2 oz	0.8
Vegetable-fruit group:		
Baked beans in tomato sauce	½ cup	2.6
Red kidney beans, canned	½ cup	2.3
Prune juice	½ cup	0.9
Spinach, cooked, drained	½ cup	2.4
Raisins	½ cup	1.6
Peas, cooked	½ cup	1.5
Beet greens, cooked, drained	½ cup	1.4
Prunes, dried, uncooked	4	1.3
Broccoli, cooked, drained	1 cup	1.2
Apple juice	½ cup	0.3
Potato, baked	1 medium	0.7
Beets, cooked, drained	½ cup	0.5
Bread-cereal group:		
Bran flakes, 40%	¾ cup (1 oz)	1.2
White bread, enriched	1 slice	0.6
Whole wheat bread	1 slice	0.6
Corn flakes	½ cup	0.2
Farina, enriched, cooked	½ cup	5.0
Macaroni, enriched, cooked	½ cup	0.7
Noodles, enriched, cooked	½ cup	0.7
Rice, enriched, cooked	½ cup	0.7
Milk Group:		
Milk, whole	1 cup	0.2

Source: From B. K. Watt and A. L. Merill, "Composition of Foods, Raw, Processed, Prepared, Agriculture Handbook No. 8," U.S. Dept. of Agriculture, 1963.

Iron-deficiency anemia is common in those women who have diets deficient in proteins, leafy green vegetables, dried peas, beans, and enriched breads and cereals. Teenagers most commonly have iron-deficient diets and may need extensive counseling to correct their nutritional habits. Where a clinic population has a history of poor diet, iron (taken orally) is routinely prescribed (see Tables 4·7, and 4·8).

Vitamins The additional intake of B vitamins is obtained with the foods added for the calorie and protein intake. *Folacin* (folic acid) is found in proteins and leafy green vegetables. Many doctors now advise supplementation of 200 to 400 μg folic acid.

table 4·8

DAILY DIET PLAN IN PREGNANCY

FOOD	BASE-LINE DIET	DIET DURING PREGNANCY
Milk	Adult: 2 cups	4 cups
	Teen-ager: 4 cups	4 cups
Meat, fish, poultry, eggs, nuts, dried peas or beans	2 servings (2 oz each)	2 servings (3 oz each)
Vegetable/fruit: Include:	4 servings	4 servings
High–vitamin C fruit or vegetable	1 serving daily	1 serving daily
Dark green or deep yellow vegetable	1 serving every other day	1 serving every other day
Bread/cereal, enriched or whole grain	5 servings (4, if one serving is a breakfast cereal)	5 servings

Additional intake of 15 mg vitamin C is recommended during the latter part of pregnancy. Since the North American diet is likely to be low in vitamin C, special emphasis should be given to foods which provide this nutrient. Ascorbic acid is unevenly distributed in foods, but certain foods stand out as high vitamin C sources. To provide the recommended minimum daily requirement of 60 mg vitamin C, the woman should take one of the following foods daily:

Fruits

Orange juice	1/2 cup
Orange	1
Grapefruit	1/2
Grapefruit juice	1/2 cup
Tangerine juice	1/2 cup
Papaya	2/3 cup
Strawberries	3/4 cup

Vegetables

Broccoli, cooked	1/2 cup
Cauliflower, cooked	1 cup
Greens, cooked (kale, collards, mustard, turnip)	1 cup
Green pepper	1

The recommended intake of vitamin D, 400 IU, is supplied by 1 qt fortified milk. Cheese, which often is used as a milk substitute, is a good source of calcium but is not fortified with vitamin D. Vitamins A, D, E, and K are fat-soluble and are stored in some measure in the body. Therefore, excess intake is not recommended and may be harmful to the developing fetus. Counseling about self-medication with vitamins is important, since in this culture many women are accustomed to taking large doses of vitamins during dieting periods or because a neighbor has recommended vitamin ingestion for a variety of ills. Water-soluble vitamins are excreted by the body and overdose is not harmful, but fat-soluble vitamins are dangerous in high doses. Most obstetricians prescribe a low-dose multivitamin during pregnancy. Instructions to the mother will include cautioning her to take just what is prescribed.

One of the most important aspects of prenatal care is that of nutritional counseling for the mother. When the pregnant woman understands that what she eats has an influence on her unborn baby, she will usually try to cooperate with a diet plan. One way of stating this simply is found in a pamphlet from The

National Foundation—March of Dimes, "Nutrition and Birth Defects Prevention" (10): "Malnutrition comes from not eating enough of the right foods. Malnutrition is different from hunger: you can eat just about anything and hunger will go away. But you have to eat the right kinds of food for malnutrition to go away." Every woman seeks the highest level of health for her growing baby and can respond positively to diet counseling that begins "where she is," i.e., that takes into consideration her life style and the foods to which she is accustomed.

The nurse may have to work closely with the pregnant woman to determine her dietary habits, because different sources of essential nutrients are "favorite foods" in different cultural groups. The nurse who works in a prenatal-care setting should become informed of the cultural patterns of her area.

references

1. Frank E. Hytten, and Isabella Leitch, *The Physiology of Human Pregnancy,* 2d ed., Blackwell Scientific Publications, Ltd., Oxford, 1972, p. 197.
2. *Ibid.,* pp. 203–204, 214.
3. *Ibid.,* p. 84.
4. *Ibid.,* pp. 104–105.
5. *Ibid.,* p. 153.
6. E. Brown, and P. Barglow, "Pseudocyesis: A Paradigm for Psychophysiological Interaction," *Archives of General Psychiatry,* **24**:221, 1971.
7. R. C. Benson, *Handbook of Obstetrics and Gynecology,* 4th ed., Lange Medical Publications, Los Altos, Calif., 1971, p. 38.
8. E. E. Rawlings and B. A. Moore, "The Accuracy of Methods of Calculating the Expected Date of Delivery for Use in the Diagnosis of Postmaturity," *American Journal of Obstetrics and Gynecology,* Mar. 1, 1970, pp. 676–679.
9. Hytten and Leitch, *op. cit.,* p. 285.
10. "Nutrition and Birth Defects Prevention," The National Foundation—March of Dimes, White Plains, N.Y. 10602.

bibliography

Prenatal Care

Anderson, Edith H.: "Today's Parents and Maternity Nursing," in Betty S. Bergersen et al. (eds.), *Current Concepts in Clinical Nursing,* vol. 1, The C. V. Mosby Company, St. Louis, 1967, pp. 355–364.

Benson, Ralph C.: *Handbook of Obstetrics and Gynecology,* 4th ed., Lange Medical Publications, Los Altos, Calif., 1971.

Bruser, Michael: "Sporting Activities during Pregnancy," *Obstetrics & Gynecology,* **32**:721–725, 1968.

Falconer, Mary, et al.: *The Drug, the Nurse, the Patient,* 4th ed., W. B. Saunders Company, Philadelphia, 1970.

Fitzpatrick, Elsie, et al.: *Maternity Nursing,* 12th ed., J. B. Lippincott and Company, Philadelphia, 1971.

Hellman, Louis M., and Jack A. Pritchard: *Williams' Obstetrics,* 14th ed., Appleton-Century-Crofts, Inc., New York, 1971.

Hytten, Frank E., and Isabella Leitch: *The Physiology of Human Pregnancy,* 2d ed., Blackwell Scientific Publications, Ltd., Oxford, 1972.

Rugh, Roberts, and Landrum B. Shettles: *From Conception to Birth: The Drama of Life's Beginnings,* Harper & Row Publishers, Incorporated, New York, 1971.

Slatin, Marion: "Why Mothers Bypass Prenatal Care," *American Journal of Nursing,* **71**:1388–1389, 1971.

Steinberg, J.: "Radiation and Pregnancy," *Canadian Medical Association Journal,* **109**:51, 1973.

Tanner, Leonide M.: "Developmental Tasks of Pregnancy," in Betty S. Bergersen et al. (eds.), *Current Concepts in Clinical Nurs-*

ing, vol. 1, the C. V. Mosby Company, St. Louis, 1969, pp. 292–297.

Williams, Barbara: "Sleep Needs during the Maternity Cycle," *Nursing Outlook,* February, 1967, pp. 292–297.

Nutrition

Bradfield, Robert B., and Thierry Brun: "Nutritional Status of Mexican-American," *American Journal of Clinical Nutrition,* **23**(6):798, 1970.

Committee on Maternal Nutrition/Food and Nutrition Board, *Maternal Nutrition and the Course of Pregnancy,* National Research Council, National Academy of Sciences, Washington, 1970.

Cross, A. T., and H. E. Walsh: "Prenatal Diet Counseling," *Journal of Reproductive Medicine,* **7**:265–274, 1971.

Fernandez, Nelson A.: "Nutritional Status of the Puerto Rican Population: Master Sample Survey," *American Journal of Clinical Nutrition,* **24**(8):952, 1971.

Jerome, N. W.: "Northern Urbanization and Food Consumption Patterns of Southern-born Negroes," *American Journal of Clinical Nutrition,* **22**(12):1667, 1969.

"Nutrition in Pregnancy and Lactation, Report of a WHO Expert Committee," *World Health Organization Technical Report Series No. 302,* 1965.

Recommended Dietary Allowances, Eighth Revised Edition, 1973, National Research Council, National Academy of Sciences, Washington, 1974.

Rosso, Pedro: "Nutrition and Abnormal Fetal Growth," *Contemporary OB/GYN,* **2**(3):53, 1973.

Shanklin, D. R., et al.: "Nutrition and Pregnancy: An Invitational Symposium," *Journal of Reproductive Medicine,* **7**:199–219, 1971; and **8**:1–12, 1972.

Watt, B. K., and A. L. Merrill: *Composition of Foods, Raw, Processed, Prepared; Agriculture Handbook No. 8,* USDA, Washington, 1963.

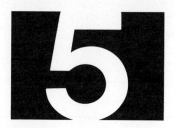

prenatal care

M. Christine Dobson
and
Dorothea M. Lang

The prenatal phase of the perinatal cycle is the most crucial period for the development of the baby and for its healthy outcome. Nursing care during this phase is totally concerned with the education and supportive care of the mother.

Observers who studied the needs expressed by pregnant women found that basic psychologic needs did not vary in relation to economic status or class but that parity of the mother and her educational level significantly influenced the frequency of her questions and the anxieties that she expressed. "Frequency of concerns related to childbirth, family, subsequent pregnancies and finances increased as education level decreased" (1).

Tanner has identified the basic developmental phases through which most women pass during pregnancy. During each trimester, questions and interests reflect the phase with which the woman is involved. As Tanner states:

> Pregnancy is a period of disequilibrium involving profound endocrine and general somatic as well as psychologic changes. This constitutes a significant turning point in the life of the individual, the resolution of which will affect future adjustments (2).

first trimester

Today the woman having a baby has generally *chosen* to become pregnant. Her feelings, then, toward the experience are usually predominantly positive. This is true at present because for many women there are the options of practicing family planning or of having an abortion.

First-trimester needs vary according to whether the pregnancy is a first one. A first pregnancy is like any other "first" experience. Curiosity and concern are felt about the unknown that lies ahead, the "somewhere I have not yet traveled."

Although the woman may have chosen to become pregnant, there will always be an ambivalence at first until the idea of being pregnant is fully accepted by her and an acceptance of the growing fetus, or *integration,* takes place (3).

Most pregnant women are concerned during the first trimester with the changes in their own bodies and how these changes will affect their lives. Some of the concerns expressed have to do with:

1. Normality of symptoms of pregnancy ("Should I worry?" "Am I normal?" "What shall I do?")
2. Changes in life-style that will result from the pregnancy ("I wonder how pregnancy will make me different?")
3. Changes in relationship with the woman's partner ("How will he accept this pregnancy?" "How will it change sexual responses?")
4. Medical care—the sequences and reasons for visits ("How can I get help between visits?")

The woman may appear to be very self-concerned and will reflect the ambivalence of the phase through which she is going. Because she probably will not be able to focus on instructions concerning future events such as labor, delivery, child care, or contraception, such topics are best discussed in later visits.

SEQUENCE DURING VISIT

Since most women choose clinics or private doctors on recommendations of other patients, they more or less know what to expect on the first visit. In the clinic setting, the sequence is planned to move patients efficiently through each aspect of care.

A nurse usually has the first contact with a patient following the registration procedure. Ideally, every clinic patient should be briefed by a nurse on what she can expect during the rest of her visit. (To do this effectively in large clinics, some nurses have made introductory films or videotapes.)

The patient should be assured of the confidentiality of her record and of the importance of having a complete history for background information that will be useful in assessing this particular pregnancy. This background information and family history are usually taken by the nurse, after which the patient's weight, height, and urine specimen results are noted on the chart. The physical examination, including a vaginal examination for signs of pregnancy and possible infection, is performed by the physician or midwife. Following this, blood tests are performed for screening. If a pregnancy test is needed, it is done at this time, and the result is made available before the woman leaves the office.

The interval for subsequent visits may vary; the usual pattern is one visit per month until the thirty-second week, after which the visits may be scheduled every 2 to 3 weeks because signs of beginning complications are more likely to occur as the patient nears term.

The patient needs to know that on subsequent visits, brevity will not mean poor care. The blood pressure, urine, and weight can be explained as important indices to the physician of a healthy progression of her pregnancy.

REFERRALS

Before the end of the first visit, the woman will receive a referral to the dental clinic, for three reasons: (1) since patients sometimes neglect their teeth when they are not pregnant, this provides one way to do dental screening of a large group of women; (2) if sufficient calcium is not ingested, decay may occur; (3) the doctor needs an assessment of the state of the patient's dental health from the beginning of pregnancy.

Other referrals may include one to the nutritionist for evident nutritional problems, or to the social worker when the mother is very young, is an emancipated minor, is involved with drugs, or has family problems needing social service assistance.

The clinic patient should be provided with information regarding the availability of help, if and when she needs it between visits. In contrast to the private doctor, the clinic is not available after hours. In order to provide assistance many hospitals have set up a telephone number, usually in the admitting labor area, by means of which a patient can reach professional counsel or help when trouble arises. During the day the patient can reach the conference or teaching nurse at her special number. Such reassurance is important to patients who perhaps in the past have found clinics to be somewhat inaccessible and impersonal.

EDUCATION OF PATIENTS

Every office or clinic waiting room should have available literature for perusal by the patient. Take-home pamphlets are most effective when they are carefully chosen on an individual basis, and even then frequently are helpful only if much of the material has been already discussed either on a one-to-one basis or in a group. Reading material serves as a reinforcement or a summary of subjects already discussed.

Nurses, more than doctors, do the counseling or hold conferences in clinics. The nurse is the one who may be deluged with questions on each visit if she is perceived by the patient as a person who will listen and answer questions. (Nurses can choose to take the role of educator or can avoid this role by spending all their time with technical tasks.)

In the clinic sequence, the patient, when seen by the conference nurse, is likely to be tired and hungry. It is therefore best to keep the initial nursing conference short and to the point; coffee or juice may be most welcome. The nurse elicits questions from the patient on any point she did not understand in the process she has just been through. She goes over the chart and the doctor's recommendations with the patient, and plans with her for the next visit.

Emphasis should be placed on giving the patient a sense of the availability of supportive services throughout the pregnancy, as well as the feeling that there is concern for her well-being. Some evaluation of the examiner's findings (shown on the patient's chart) is reassuring following the initial visit and examination.

Conferences are personal and sensitive for both the patient and the nurse. The setting should be chosen to ensure privacy, relaxation, comfort, and freedom from as many distractions as possible. Knowledge of interviewing techniques is helpful (4). Sensitivity to the length of the conference, the nature of information sought, and the response given is important. Patients who do not ask questions may be very inquisitive. Some who ask many questions may be anxious; others may simply need to socialize.

Individual conferences are an important part of each patient's visit. When the patient comes in for subsequent visits to the clinic, even though a different physician, resident, or intern may see her, she is given a sense of continuity by being able to talk with the conference nurse each time. Conferences can take place before the examination to ascertain what the patient has experienced and may be unable to articulate to the midwife or the doctor. The nurse should relay this information. Conferences afterwards may be used to clarify instructions further, to give anticipatory guidance about the changes of the next few weeks, and to explain referrals. The nurse should check up on referrals that were made at the last appointment.

second trimester

By the end of the first trimester, discomforts from physiologic changes have usually disappeared. The expectant mother is well on her way to settling down to exactly what she needs to do for herself and the growing baby. Her concerns begin to shift from her own bodily changes during the first trimester to the growing baby. It is during the second trimester that the baby takes on its own identity as a separate being. The psychologic task of perceiving the fetus as a growing baby, separate from herself (5), is normally completed by the end of the second trimester. If the nurse wants to test the mother's perception of the baby's individual identity she can ask how the mother responded to the feeling of quickening. Mothers who have successfully accepted the baby's presence usually respond in positive ways. In general, the mother is interested in protecting the health of the infant, and her concerns will now reflect her awareness of the infant's needs. The more general concerns are these:

1. Nutritional intake ("Am I gaining too much?" "Too little?")

2. Amount of exercise, travel ("What restrictions are necessary?")
3. Progression of fetal growth ("How big is the baby this month?")
4. Warning signs of problems
5. Changing body image (how reflected in clothes, hygiene, hair, skin)
6. Changes in sexual desires (concern about restrictions and misconceptions)

If the patient visited the clinic initially after missing two periods, by the second trimester she is returning for her second or third visit. By now she will be familiar with clinic personnel and will know where to get juice, fruit, or coffee and where the bathroom is located. The process she will be going through does not frighten her. She relaxes and socializes with other patients.

Individual conferences are continued, as suggested earlier. By this time, however, most patients have begun to participate in group discussions or the teaching program that the particular clinic may have set up. Most of the woman's waiting time in the clinic should be taken up in giving, sharing, and receiving information. Various approaches are used in clinics toward this end. One useful way is to schedule the group conference into the sequence of the visit, in 30-min segments, staggering the appointments, so that no one has to wait too long in boredom before seeing the doctor. The specific topic for discussion may be posted for sessions in a given morning or afternoon. Thus, if the patient missed a session she can elect to sit in on the discussion of the current topic. Perhaps the hardest type of conference to handle sucessfully is the ongoing group discussion in which patients come and go as their interest and time permit.

Several nurses may be assigned to conduct "bench conferences" on a selective basis with patients who, by appearance (bodily attitude) or other nonverbal signs, indicate a need for private discussion. Closed-circuit

TV, video-tape cassettes, and a variety of cartridge films may be utilized in small groups of patients for information purposes. By whatever means the staff may choose to disseminate information, the goal is usually to utilize the available time for patient-based concerns (Fig. 5·1).

With each recommendation for health maintenance, the nurse should give a reasonable explanation based on the physiology of pregnancy. There are few hard-and-fast rules today; recommendations are tailored to each woman's life-style, the aim being to bring her to an acceptable level of health, and to maintain her at that level, while preventing problems.

EXERCISE, REST, AND RELAXATION

Exercise and rest should be discussed in terms of relieving minor discomforts of pregnancy during the second and third trimesters. For most women, especially if they are working, the activities of the home provide enough activity and exercise. Physicians often recommend long walks as the best form of exercise when the woman is not employed outside the home. Rest intervals with feet elevated will help prevent edema and will improve lower-extremity circulation.

Muscle-toning exercises are taught as early as the need is indicated; e.g., if a patient lives in a walk-up apartment, discussion of the best way to climb stairs without strain may be helpful. Ways of stooping, bending, and lifting are often taught earlier than exercises for labor and delivery.

Relaxation is sought in individual ways and discussed whenever there are problems.

SEXUAL INTERCOURSE

Questions regarding intercourse usually come from women who are pregnant for the first time and are anxious to follow instructions to the letter. In the absence of complica-

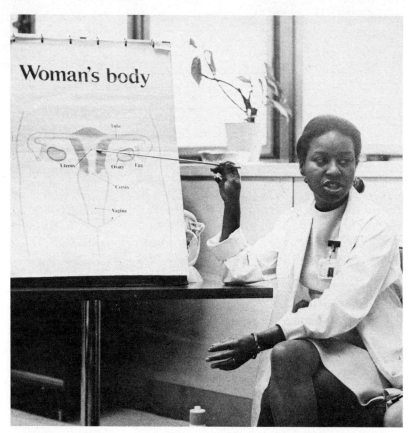

fig. 5·1 Teaching in the clinic. (*Photo by Nancy Goodman.*)

tions, however, there is no advice peculiar to pregnancy. Couples may continue their sexual relationship as usual. Some men have reported that there is a difference in the feeling of the vagina. This, of course, results from the physiologic changes which have taken place.

In the past, intercourse was restricted at intervals during the first 3 months, and again 6 weeks before delivery, because of fear of complications. Now, physicians merely advise the couple to use common sense about position and pressures (6). Chapter 6 discusses some of the sexual fears and fantasies women may experience.

EMPLOYMENT

Socioeconomic factors, cultural considerations, safety aspects, and the therapeutic value of work all help in determining whether to continue one's employment. A consultation with the physician or midwife gives direction to the expectant mother.

SMOKING

Excessive smoking is detrimental to the growing fetus.

There is a strong inverse relationship between maternal smoking and mean birth-weight of offspring. The mean birthweight decreases over 400 grams in Whites and over 250 grams in Negroes and the low birthweight rate more than doubles between babies of nonsmokers and those smoking over 30 cigarettes a day (7).

Should a woman be unable to reduce her smoking habit, she should be encouraged to smoke only one-fourth a cigarette, thus cutting down on nicotine intake.

TRAVEL

After midpregnancy, trips of over 2 to 3 h by car, train, or plane are unwise, because of the prolonged sitting time. If a trip has to be made, the woman should change positions frequently and, if driving, stop to walk around at least every 2 h.

Prolonged sitting or standing still is associated with a marked increase in sodium retention, a change caused by the postural effect on the dynamics of blood flow through the kidneys. Sodium retention leads to water retention (see Chap. 23) and consequently to edema, first in the lower extremities and then, when severe, throughout the body (8).

Seat belts According to the 1967 American Medical Association Committee on Medical Aspects of Auto Safety, seat belts continue to be an important safety factor for pregnant women. Lap and shoulder belts provide the best protection, with the lap belt fastened, of course, below the bulge of the uterus.

HYGIENE DURING PREGNANCY

Most women practice good daily hygiene. Sensitivity can be exercised in the case of a mother who has special needs. A reminder can be given to women about safety during bathing, the most important point to make since baths, both tub and shower, can be taken right up until the time of delivery.

Increased vaginal secretions may be bothersome during pregnancy. Discussion will help women to recognize leukorrhea as normal (Chap. 4); they should be taught to report to the physician if it becomes excessive enough to necessitate the wearing of a pad, if it is odorous or discolored, or if it causes itching. Douching is not advised, and tampons, feminine hygiene suppositories, creams and jellies are usually prohibited, unless ordered by the physician. Perineal care several times a day should relieve any discomfort that might occur.

the third trimester

No matter what the background of the mother, her needs in the third trimester will be expressed in approximately the same ways. She focuses on the outcome of the baby, the process of labor, her own changing physical condition and emotions, and her figure during this last trimester. Even multiparas have questions about the differences in labor and delivery with each baby. If a program has been designed for education in childbirth for the last trimester, it usually begins around the thirtieth week of gestation. By this time the mother has been working through her emotional task of separation from the fetus in preparation for its delivery. She is getting ready to take up the care of the infant (9). Concerns expressed in this trimester tend to be about:

1. The baby's well-being (questions on birth defects, signs of fetal well-being, how birth affects the infant, effect of medication and anesthesia)
2. The costs of having a baby (fees, having to stop work, expenses for equipment)
3. The process of labor and delivery (pain, fears, misconceptions, when to come to the hospital)

4. Family (how other children will accept the infant, how to plan for them during hospitalization, how father will respond to the infant)

The changing contours of the woman's body become more prominent, backaches, leg aches, lower abdominal pressure, ligament pain, fatigue, extra weight, concern about normal dependent edema, and anxiety over the warning signals of preeclampsia all cause her to be impatient for labor to begin.

Thus the woman is eager to learn any methods and techniques to relieve discomforts and those which will be of assistance to her during the later part of pregnancy and during the labor process. She will use exercises and practice breathing in these weeks when she would not have done so before. If this is a first pregnancy, she will need instruction to reduce the fear of the unknown in labor. If it is a second or third pregnancy, a review is usually welcome. The approach to childbirth education will vary according to the method used in each hospital. The one commonality is to reduce the fear-tension-pain cycle by information and discussion of sources of anxiety (see Chap. 7). Usually, after discussion, an informational brochure is given to each woman to reinforce the material.

Counseling continues on an individual basis and may now include preparation for the baby. Many women still cannot focus on baby care. The outcome of the pregnancy is as yet unreal. Therefore, postdelivery classes should be held on the unit for those who become aware that they do not really know what to do for the new infant.

Many women are superstitious about buying anything for the infant before its birth; to do so might risk death or injury to the child, they have been told. The nurse may acknowledge that this is a belief that some do hold, and can skillfully turn the conversation to a discussion of the equipment that will be needed by the new baby, even though layette purchasing can begin any time the mother wishes. The father or grandparents may have this task during her hospitalization, but the mother will want to know how to plan. The only important fact to emphasize is that planning should be in advance of taking the infant home. Mothers who have limited apartment space and/or income will usually welcome suggestions on how to economize.

When Light and Fenster questioned women after delivery, they found that concerns took a different order of priority than before delivery (10). High on the list at that time was the concern about how to prevent subsequent pregnancies; indications are that the woman after delivery is highly motivated to learn about contraception.

Of course, not every woman follows the "average pattern." Nurses can become skilled in individualizing the teaching and support of patients during prenatal care. In the sections to follow we will discuss the adaptations necessary for the care of the adolescent who becomes pregnant before marriage, and the care of the drug-addicted woman who becomes pregnant, both particularly difficult problems to deal with.

The role of the nurse-midwife in prenatal care will be discussed in relationship to the role of the maternity nurse. The new relationship between the certified nurse-midwife (C.N.M.) and the registered nurse (R.N.) provides avenues to be innovative and to change areas of inadequate care for the mother and infant in our society.

One family's viewpoint about receiving care from nurse-midwives is included at the end of the chapter.

adolescent pregnancy

EARLY ADOLESCENT PREGNANCY

If we view the adolescent age span as that from eleven to eighteen, developmental tasks during this period will divide adolescence into two groups, early and late. Assuming that the level of maturity differs with experiences, exposure to challenges, and rate of body maturation, we will first consider the adolescent who might become pregnant between eleven and fourteen, the early adolescent.

Sexual involvement at this young age is naturally experimental, most often without much previous education or without assimilation of the education that has been received. Sometimes the young adolescent, beset by turbulent emotions, seeks love outside the family circle. In this case, she is often rebellious and is seldom directed toward parenthood but toward proving that she is lovable (11). The father of the unborn child is often four or more years older or may be an adult.

For a variety of reasons, pregnancy may not be discovered in very young girls until the second and sometimes even the third trimester. The young girl's knowledge of menstruation and hormonal activity is limited; periods are often irregular for the first year or two, so that she herself may not suspect that she has become pregnant. Weight gain is natural during this period. Overweight girls often do not seem much larger until the fifth or sixth month of pregnancy. The girl may be frightened by the prospect of parental, teacher, or peer disapproval and may hide her symptoms by wearing a tight brassiere and girdle. Elaborate measures may be taken to conceal the pregnancy, and there are known cases of a girl's coming to term without parental knowledge of the pregnancy.

Once it becomes evident that the pregnancy is a fact, the girl and her mother are usually counseled. The issue may be approached by assessing the parent-teen relationship, the counselor having talks with the girl and her mother, first on an individual basis and then together, and trying to reconcile any differences in their feelings as to the solution of the situation. If the pregnancy has been discovered early enough, interruption is often recommended, for obvious reasons. The child is not mature enough to assume the role of parent, nor can she assume economic support of a child of her own. Medically, she is at risk for more complications than an older teen-ager. However, cultural, ethnic, religious, and socioeconomic constituents of the decision must be balanced against the girl's own attitudes and reactions. To force interruption may be more detrimental to her than to carry the infant to term. It is not a lightly reached conclusion and needs careful counseling and support from social worker, physician, psychiatrist, and nurse (12).

If the girl goes on with the pregnancy, hospitals routinely provide concomitant psychiatric support in the child psychiatry department, or through social service. Some girls may be placed in foster care or in a home for girls with premarital pregnancies, especially if the parents are unable to be supportive during the pregnancy (13).

The young adolescent experiences the pregnancy with detachment. For example, it is very difficult for her to be responsible in adjusting eating patterns. If she has the "quickie" snack habit, she may be used to consuming candy bars, potato chips, peanuts, sodas, etc. When the emphasis is on nutrition, the girl's mother needs to be brought into the conference for necessary health support. In fact, the mother will be needed at every step in health care during pregnancy, to ensure the keeping of appointments at the clinic and the carrying out of referrals.

Pregnancy may be viewed by the girl as a transient childhood disease, unpleasant, but soon over and "cured." During the last trimester, much support and preparation should be afforded for the process of labor and delivery. Growth of the girl is still in progress, so that cesarean section may have to be done in cases of a small pelvis. When this is the case, needless to say, the experience is even more unreal and similar to a disease for which surgery is necessary.

The medical approach to the delivery of young girls is made with very special humane, sympathetic care. To minimize the trauma during labor and delivery, medication will be used to keep the girl as comfortable as possible through the entire process. This is in keeping with the thought that future pregnancies will be experienced with less fear and fantasy and with more maturity if this one is not frightening. One teen-ager expressed the panic she experienced during an unmedicated, unprepared-for delivery in this way: "I thought I was going to turn inside out. How could the big baby push out my rectum, and how ever would they push my insides back in again?"

LATE ADOLESCENT PREGNANCY

Older teen-agers (fifteen to eighteen) are naturally viewed and counseled in a different light. Barring immaturity, it is highly unusual that pregnancy within this age group is accidental because of ignorance. With more information available on family life, sex, and child-spacing methods, and with the growing availability of abortion services, the late adolescent may be fairly sophisticated about her options. Some of the reasons given by girls for not protecting themselves against pregnancy remain romantic—not wanting to plan ahead or to seem aggressive or to "spoil the mood." Rebellion and the desire to have a "baby of my own to love me" may lead desperately unhappy girls to seek pregnancy. Many documented studies attest to the unconscious wish for pregnancy (14).

The nurse can expect to see this adolescent earlier in pregnancy, usually not for confirmation of the pregnancy but for medical care and counseling, either with the parent or with the father of the unborn child. As with the young adolescent, counseling, once the older girl reaches the clinic, is directed first toward assessing the family relationship and then toward attempting to reconcile any differences that may exist between parent and daughter on the plan of care.

Emancipated minors Hofmann states that the traditional definition of emancipated minors is "adolescents who are married, in the armed forces or who with parental consent are self-supporting or living away from home under such circumstances that (they) make most of (their) own decisions" (15).

There are, however, many cases of minors over fifteen who have been treated by physicians without parental consent. An informed judgment must be made as to the adolescent's need, maturity, and life situation. Problems of consent apply to contraceptives, pregnancy testing, venereal disease treatment, and all other adolescent health services. As yet, few states have realistic statutes reflecting adolescent needs for health care.[1]

In many urban areas, special facilities for adolescent health services are available for pregnancy and venereal disease (VD) testing. Some schools are using peer-group counseling by older prepared students to handle the common concerns of adolescents and to provide free referral for pregnancy and VD testing without parental consent. These school services, always backed up by medical personnel and clinics, are an attempt to teach teen-agers, who are a high-risk group for VD and early pregnancy (16).

Continuing Education Some schools have provided special programs for the pregnant teen-ager. These facilities are being phased out as public attitudes toward premarital pregnancy have become less stringent (17). Girls are encouraged to stay in school. Finishing education is the practical solution to the situation, since if the girl keeps

[1]Information about laws in each state can be found in *Contraception, Family Planning and Voluntary Sterilization: Laws and Policies of the United States, Each State and Jurisdiction*, U.S. Department of Health, Education, and Welfare, January, 1973.

the child she will have to assume its economic support if the father of the child does not. In most programs it has been discovered that these girls benefit from personal attention and may bloom in confidence and ability to cope with their new situation. Therefore, even if education is provided in the same school, special supportive discussion groups and personal interest of a sympathetic counselor are important ways of assisting the girl to gain confidence.

Depending on the ethnic makeup of the school, the girl returning to school may have some difficulty with social pressures and adjustments. In black communities, the baby is usually assimilated into the family as another child, with the grandparents taking ultimate parental responsibility. The usual option in the white culture has been to require marriage or to give the child up for adoption. Adoption is traumatic for the mother, and teen-age marriages have led to a much higher divorce rate, since both partners are immature. The recognition of these facts and the more permissive trend in society are making more options available. No matter what the situation, the emphasis with teenagers should be on the importance of finishing basic education and on becoming economically able to support a family, and psychologically mature enough to assume the role of parent. Thus, the need for more widespread education for parenting is reemphasized each time a premarital pregnancy occurs.

drug addiction in pregnancy

Drug addicts are the outcasts of our society. Recent trends reflect less sympathetic understanding than was accorded them in the past, largely because of the intensity with which public health agencies have worked to inform the population about addiction. Commonly existing feelings, both of medical personnel and of laymen, are that one who becomes addicted now does so by choice. In addition, there are feelings that already addicted persons are antisocial because of the existence of varied agencies with enough approaches to provide detoxification, regardless of the drug classification. It is still admitted, however, that widespread devastating socioeconomic conditions continue to ravish the poor, affecting ego strength and mental hygiene. Such conditions may have a forceful impact on the individual who is ill prepared to cope with life. The alternatives, however, continue to remain philosophic.

Drugs used most commonly vary with locale, e.g., the use of LSD is more widespread on the West Coast, while 50 percent of heroin users in the United States are in New York (18). Varying degrees of drug usage and habituation are common as well. Because heroin addiction is by far the most common drug problem in large inner-city hospital clinics, our discussion will focus on the female heroin addict who becomes pregnant.

The female drug addict who appears in the clinic because of pregnancy is perhaps the most pathetic of all drug addicts. Our treatment of her surely tests our humanity, our degree of civilization, and our medical knowledge.

To begin with, pregnancy and the birth of the baby represent to her the last claim to a worthwhile purpose for her entire feminine being. The pregnancy represents a new lease on life—another beginning. Sometimes it means a release of old guilt feelings. Often, at the time, the woman makes a sincerely felt resolution to reform and be different.

The woman may or may not be aware that heroin addiction has contributed to irregularities in her menstrual cycle. Thus, pregnancy may be several months advanced before she realizes that she is pregnant. She may conceal the fact then, for her own ego gratification and to prevent being forced into a decision, or she may come at once to the clinic for confirmation to ensure the health of the baby.

PRENATAL CARE

On first visits to the clinic, most addicts are defensive and paranoic. They expect that the initial counseling will include pressure and suggestions to interrupt the pregnancy. They have usually been involved with prostitution, for themselves and often for their male counterparts; and often they have been jailed for shoplifting and other misdemeanors. Statistics show that the majority of drug-addicted women have had two to four pregnancies (19). Thus some women may have children placed in foster care, or, as they perceive it, "taken away from them." In abortive attempts to reclaim other children or to gain credentials in an effort to reestablish in some measure their claim to be responsible, they may have gone into institutions for treatment.

In spite of all the expressed and unexpressed goals of a drug addict, general traits of the addicted personality need to be kept in mind. Some of the more common characteristics are that they will attempt to be manipulative by trying to please the counselor, while seldom being truthful. They may falsify the amount of daily drug intake because a large amount reinforces a feeling of being "bad." They may make unsolicited promises, that they are in the process of becoming involved in rehabilitation or are already involved.

The nurse must have an understanding approach regardless of personal feelings, keeping in mind the addictive profile. This means adopting a firm, consistent, direct manner in seeking information for medical purposes and in counseling for the possible prevention of deterioration during the pregnancy.

If the nurse sees the patient early, she can assume that the mother has made the choice to come of her own accord for the sake of the baby. Because the mother usually feels a sense of worthlessness and uselessness, the pregnancy then represents her one act of decency, a way to feel human again. In the light of this situation, to suggest interruption of pregnancy would be a catastrophe. Nonsympathetic personnel who may not be acquainted with the psychology of the addicted female might be inclined to force their solutions on her through manipulative, threatening persuasion. Such an approach would eradicate any cooperation the patient might give and would most likely result in complete loss of rapport or possibly in loss of contact with the woman until the time of delivery.

On the other hand, counseling toward traditional health maintenance is a waste of time with the addict in early pregnancy. She is likely to continue in her same destructive patterns until late in pregnancy. Recognizing this, the nurse should not become frustrated in attempts to counsel or place restrictions on her regarding nutrition, hygiene, and rest.

Usually toward the end of the second trimester, the nurse counselor has the best chance of helping the expectant mother safeguard the outcome of the baby because the woman begins to worry about the infant's health. It is at this point that the counselor can encourage the mother to adhere to some of the most important aspects of prenatal care.

Nutrition is critical. In every possible way the nurse can encourage the mother to increase her protein intake. For example, sweets probably constitute the major part of her usual diet. To be useful and realistic, diet substitutions should be in keeping with what she *will* eat—milk shakes with an egg added, hamburgers and cheeseburgers, french fries, ice cream, oatmeal cakes or cookies, "Orange-Julius," and fruit. Her diet is particularly deficient in vegetables, because most of them require some kind of preparation.

Substitutions, such as diet soda for regular soda, can be encouraged. Juice, chocolate drink, tea, and coffee are means of getting the needed fluid intake. Vitamins, folic acid, and iron will be prescribed and should be stressed as supplements necessary for the baby's health.

Negative counseling is often necessary to impress the addict with the importance of having an adequate intake of certain food constituents. One may have to say, for example, "Your baby's brain is developing more rapidly during the last 3 months than at any time during your pregnancy. Too little protein (meat, cheese, milk, eggs, etc.) will result in your having a baby who will be less intelligent than it could be." This method of counseling is not ordinarily the best approach. Purposely to inspire fear, however, may elicit better health practices and avoid a higher percentage of complications.

Personal hygiene and sexual habits are serious considerations for counseling. Prostitution often continues to term, so that it is not unusual for the patient to contract venereal disease very late in the pregnancy after routine screening.

The addict's irregular life pattern with regard to rest, food, and hygiene contributes to the detrimental environment experienced by the growing fetus. Medical complications in patients who do not seek care or follow prenatal care guidelines include problems related to drug dependency. Infections, especially venereal disease and hepatitis, and thrombophlebitis and iron-deficiency anemia may occur.

Obstetric complications include preterm labor with low-birth-weight babies (50 percent), preeclampsia, and precipitate labor (20).

When a woman participates in prenatal care and in a rehabilitation program, the incidence of complications drops sharply.

In areas where drug addiction is common, urine testing should be routine on clinic visits and on admission to labor. The presence of heroin, methadone, codiene, barbiturates,

amphetamines, phenothiazines, and quinine can be detected by these urine tests.

DETOXIFICATION

Referral for detoxification and rehabilitation is routine in most hospitals. The pregnant addict is inclined to feign interest in such a program or to go through it just to reduce her daily dosage needs. A woman may even go through detoxification several times during the pregnancy. She may participate (reluctantly) because she realizes that the baby will not be released in her custody at the time of discharge if she is still on heroin.

Detoxification of heroin addicts is now accomplished almost universally in the United States with methadone. The detoxification with methadone for the person willing to enter rehabilitation follows a decreasing dosage schedule for a period of a week. To remain drug-free after this period a woman must be in a strong supportive program. The alternative is to place her on a methadone maintenance program. Use of methadone, however, is simply a new addiction. In every possible case, therefore, patients should be supported and encouraged to become drug-free. Nurses should make themselves knowledgeable about all the implications of the use of methadone as an agent for detoxification.

Withdrawal of the patient without some kind of drug therapy is contraindicated during pregnancy because of the possible dangers to the baby. For instance, smooth-muscle spasms affect the circulation through the placenta. In severe cases of maternal withdrawal, the baby may die.

Toward the latter part of pregnancy, the patient's concern as to whether the baby will be addicted is most pronounced. The nurse needs to give the patient as much information as possible about the drug's effect on the baby. The patient should know that the baby will become addicted through her habit and the degree of difficulty during the baby's withdrawal will depend upon the size of her habit. She can be reassured that in the absence of psychologic dependency, medical treatment of the baby usually alleviates withdrawal symptoms. The baby's recovery may be affected by its poor intrauterine environment, most commonly causing *intrauterine growth retardation*, a complex result of many factors—among them poor nutritional supply and intrauterine stress.

DELIVERY

Deliveries, often premature either by weight or by date, are complicated by inability of the doctor to use traditional medication or anesthesia during labor or delivery. Stone states that in the study from Metropolitan City Hospital in 1969 80 percent of the drug-addicted mothers admitted to, or gave evidence of, drug use on the day of admission to labor (21). Because of inability to determine how much drug a mother has in her system, dosages particularly of narcotics and anesthetics, are prescribed with extreme care.

Remembering that this patient usually has not attended the clinic regularly or participated in classes in preparation for childbirth, the nurse must be especially alert and watchful for untoward responses during labor.

POSTPARTUM CARE

Following delivery, the patient's first concern is usually to satisfy her need for drugs. Old habits become apparent again. If the patient is not on a methadone regimen or receiving tranquilizers, she will make attempts to acquire drugs from the outside through visitors to avoid withdrawal symptoms (nausea, tremors, sweating, abdominal pain, cramps, and yawning), which will appear in 2 or 3 h after delivery.

The nurse must be alert to the possibility of stealing from other patients, must notice the length of time the patient spends in the bathroom, and must not leave medication rooms or carts unguarded. Some way must be planned for unobstrusive surveillance of visitors to drug-addicted patients when they are not separated from other patients. Withdrawal is not attempted without drug therapy (tranquilizers), because of the complex changes in the woman's body during this recovery period.

Fears of separation from the baby may be intensified following delivery because the addicted mother cannot feed or hold it; in most instances, the infant is placed in an intensive care unit for observation and treatment.

The social worker has usually been involved in discussing placement of the baby in foster care until the mother is either completely drug-free or involved in an approved program for rehabilitation. Guidelines for approved programs are set up by the bureau of child welfare in most cities or states when policies are regulated by a governmental agency.

Care of the addicted pregnant patient is one of the most difficult aspects of maternal and infant nursing. The outcome is often negative and sad. Nurses in this area find themselves wanting to become more and more involved in prevention of drug addiction. Certainly the high infant morbidity and mortality rates and the tragedy in the mother's life appear to justify aggressive programs to this end.

modern midwifery[2]

A phone rings in the midwifery office, and a concerned voice asks for the midwife. What might be her concern? It is a young pregnant mother asking a seemingly simple question

[2]By Dorothea M. Lang.

about a "little ache" in her side. For the next 18 min the midwife's friendly yet detailed questions regarding other possibly related symptoms which might, or might not, point to the simplest muscle strain or to the warning signs of a developing complication of pregnancy, finally result in a reassuring answer. This young mother was at the end of her eighth month of pregnancy. The midwife and her colleagues have managed her prenatal care since the day of her positive pregnancy test. Last Wednesday she had her prenatal checkup, and the midwife will see her again the day after tomorrow, and when she arrives at the hospital in early labor, and throughout the delivery, and then with the baby at feeding time, and for her first month's postpartum visit, and for interim counseling.

This is a modern midwife, a *certified nurse-midwife* (C.N.M.), who functions as a part of the professional obstetric team. She might be employed by the hospital, by a medical center–affiliated, community-based maternal and child health service, or by an obstetrician-midwife group practice. She manages the complete maternity care for mothers with an essentially normal course of pregnancy. She always functions with readily available medical direction, should any sudden medical complications arise (1). Today's modern midwife is prepared to function in all areas of woman's health maintenance concerned with reproductive processes, including family planning and childbirth. Perinatal care and newborn health management are integral parts of midwifery practice.

Although midwifery management of labor and birth in most countries takes place in the patient's home (over 80 percent of the world's babies are delivered by nonphysicians, most of whom deliver at home), the American midwife, the C.N.M., performs the delivery functions in a hospital setting. Being aware that familiar homelike surroundings and close family support can have a relaxing influence

on the laboring mother, the midwife attempts to integrate these family-centered supportive measures into today's hospital setting, where, in case of sudden complications, the mother or baby can benefit from the most modern emergency facilities.

Midwifery practice endorses the philosophy that each woman has the right to personalized health care, and the right to acquire family health education which will help her to understand her own psychophysiologic functions as a woman, wife, and mother. Therefore, a midwife is committed to provide each woman with quality health care. This means that along with quality physical care there must be educational opportunities provided which will guide the family to the security they desire through personalized family planning; that individualized education will enable them to have quality in the childbirth experience itself and have satisfaction in the nuturing of the newborn; and to help them acquire the ability to form rewarding family relationships within the cultural setting of their choosing.

Although a C.N.M.'s functions may vary slightly from setting to setting, she will function in any or all of the described typical patient-care activities.

TYPICAL ACTIVITIES IN THE CARE OF PATIENTS

Traditionally the obstetrician follows his patients from office to hospital; similarly, today's certified nurse-midwife is the consistent and continuing link between the community-based ambulatory care center, office, or clinic and the in-patient services of the affiliating hospital. She acts as a liaison between the community hospital health care teams and serves as a "patient advocate" throughout all units of the hospital (2).

In the ambulatory care center the midwife may care for approximately 8 to 10 prenatal revisit patients and one or two new prenatal patients during a 2-h prenatal session. The same number of patients can usually be cared for in the postpartum or family planning session.

At all times, whether in the hospital or in the community, in areas pertaining to obstetric management, the C.N.M. works with the readily available consultation and supervision of a physician.

A typical day for a nurse-midwife may start out in a prenatal care center in the community. After a new maternity patient has been admitted to the center, attended a public health nurse's "new-patient orientation conference," and had her laboratory work completed, she is introduced to the midwife by a public health worker whose responsibilities may include the guidance of patients to the examining room.

The midwife evaluates the laboratory findings and, through a friendly interchange of feelings and concerns, obtains a complete medical and obstetric history, adding any other pertinent information to the family history which may have been previously taken by the public health nurse. The patient then is ushered onto the examining table, and the midwife performs the total physical examination, including breast examination, abdominal palpation, complete pelvic examination and evaluation, and the taking of a Papanicolaou smear (Fig. 5·2).

Throughout her clinical work-up, the midwife encourages questions from the patient, thus providing information on maternity care, family planning, and general health maintenance. This on-the-spot discussion of problems related to the mother's discomforts or facts regarding growth and development of the fetus is most reassuring to the mother.

After the patient's total physical and emotional findings have been evaluated, the appropriate midwifery management is implemented; this includes the initiation of appropriate referrals and the prescribing of appropriate

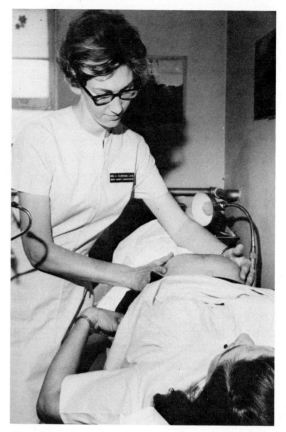

fig. 5·2 Nurse-midwife examines mother to determine fetal position. (*Photo by Ruth Helmich.*)

proved medications, vitamins, and treatments. Should findings reveal early signs of complications or obstetric problems, the physician is contacted directly or by telephone, and consultation is provided the midwife as necessary. If the patient is found to have a medically complicated condition, she is referred to the obstetrician for management.

During a revisit appointment, the prenatal patient is individually counseled by the midwife regarding her interim history. Each mother is encouraged to select the degree to which she (and her husband and family) wishes to participate in the birth process. Classes in preparation for childbirth and responsible parenthood are offered and encouraged, but are optional. Personalized information and support are provided by the midwife throughout the maternity cycle. Newborn health care is emphasized and family planning counseling is offered.

In the hospital, C.N.M.s manage the complete obstetric course of mothers with a normal or near-normal labor. Mothers with minor complications are comanaged with the resident and the attending medical staff. The physician manages the medical problems, and the midwife manages the course of labor and performs the spontaneous delivery.

That C.N.M.s can successfully manage the obstetric course of mothers who have no medical complications has been adequately demonstrated. A 5-year report of one of New York City's midwifery services demonstrated that certified nurse-midwives, as part of a medically directed obstetric-perinatal team, can also successfully manage the care of mothers with certain complications, such as mild preeclampsia, hypertension, premature ruptured membranes, prematurity, persistent posterior position, shoulder dystocia, anemia, severe varicosities, drug addiction, etc., and maintain a low perinatal mortality rate (3).

When a patient presents herself in labor the midwife will perform the admission physical examination, evaluate the status of labor, secure appropriate comfort measures, and provide reassurance as needed by the patient and her family members. The attending obstetrician or the resident in charge of the unit is notified of the admission and the physical findings. In preparation for emergencies or unforeseen complications, and depending upon the policies of the unit, a physician will evaluate the status of the patient's heart and lungs so that general anesthetics could be administered, if necessary.

Throughout labor, the midwifery management includes supportive care and continuity in implementing those childbirth concepts that the patient believes in and has learned during her preparation for labor sessions. This type of continuity of personalized care is of utmost importance in attempting to minimize the need for medication during labor and birth.

During the course of labor, the physician and obstetric nurse in charge of the unit are kept informed of the course of labor, and the midwife consults with the obstetrician or the maternal-fetal perinatologist whenever she or the supporting nursing team notices any deviation from the normal. Any necessary treatments, infusions, and medications, such as sedatives and analgesia, are prescribed by the midwife in accordance with the Approved Certified Nurse-Midwife Orders as described in each hospital's *Midwifery Policy Manual.*

Throughout labor and delivery, every possible comfort measure and relaxation technique is employed by many obstetric team members. As long as the course of labor and delivery is normal, the midwife will perform the delivery (Fig. 5·3). If required, the midwife provides local anesthesia or gives a pudendal block prior to performing an episiotomy. She manages the third stages of labor and prescribes oxytocics as needed. She repairs the episiotomy or any lacerations if indicated, and manages the fourth stage of labor.

The midwife provides immediate care of the newborn, and if necessary performs simple resuscitation. She confirms the official Apgar score and signs the birth certificate. Early mother-newborn interaction is also encouraged by the midwife, as nonmedicated or minimally medicated mothers are often ecstatic when given the opportunity to hold (and breast-feed) their newborn before they leave the delivery room. The father should be given the opportunity to hold his newborn, and as soon as possible family members or other significant persons are encouraged to share those early moments of joy.

At all times, the nurse-midwife works in close cooperation with the maternity nursing team. Management of the patient depends to

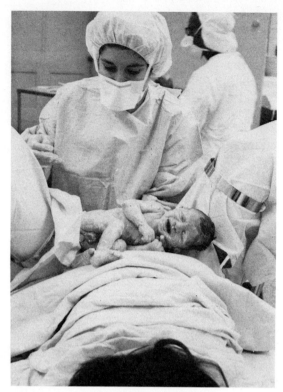

fig. 5. 3 Nurse-midwife shows newly delivered infant to its mother. (*Photo by Ruth Helmich.*)

course experiences in normal labor and delivery.

Postdelivery care includes individual visits by a midwife to each of her patients in the postpartum unit. As part of the perinatal team, the midwife checks each newborn during the daily newborn nursery visits and, if possible, visits mother and baby in the postpartum unit at feeding time, offering counseling as indicated.

To follow through with the education which every patient received during the prenatal period, the midwife continues to instruct the mother, emphasizing postpartum self-care, newborn care, and family adjustment. Instructions are also given regarding postpartum and pediatric health care appointments.

As desired by the patient, the midwife may prescribe contraceptives. Family planning counseling is an integral part of patient education. Midwives deal with a population of proved fertility and serve the patient at a point of highest motivation. As a patient entrusts herself to the midwife for delivery and newborn care, she is also inclined to accept family planning advice and services from the same individual.

The continuity of care which such arrangements can provide is self-evident. According to feelings that have been expressed by patients, it is most satisfying and comforting for them to see a familiar person in the hospital, one whom they have learned to trust during their prenatal period, and to know that they will see her again in the community clinic or office for the postpartum, family planning, and interconceptional care.

MIDWIFERY IN THE UNITED STATES

Midwifery as currently practiced in the United States must be understood through the richness of its heritage, which comprises the work of tireless pioneers in the midwifery profession and the sustaining support of friends outside the profession. This fine her-

a great degree on their findings and their observations of the patient. The midwife regularly reviews and compares the medical, midwifery, and nursing notations on the records and participates actively in the team conferences on care of the patient. Whenever the midwife provides maternity nursing care, she follows the nursing policies of the unit. Frequently she will provide consultation to student nurses and to the members of the maternity nursing team and participate in the development of new policies for care of patients and new tools for their education. The midwife is an expert in the management of normal labor and childbirth. As such, at many medical centers she is also involved with the education, demonstration, and supervision of midwifery and medical students during their itage enables the C.N.M. to function as a coequal with other professionals in today's health teams and health care programs.

Historically, the profession of midwifery precedes almost every other profession. The earliest Biblical writings mention midwifery as a personalized service that women offered to women (4). At that time, the profession was perpetuated mostly by the apprentice-tutorial pattern of education, the traditional form of education throughout early civilizations until the twentieth century.

Compared with the other women of their time, midwives were usually the most educated, and rightfully earned respect from the families in the communities which they served. These midwives were the only professionals who officially assisted at birth, cared for the newborns, and provided supportive services to the mother and family.

In American history, the earliest colonial records tell us that the midwife was a very important person in the newly settled territories. The services of a midwife were guaranteed by several charter companies as an inducement to women to travel to the new lands. In 1641, the General Court of Massachusetts showed its respect and esteem for midwives by ordering that they, along with "physicians and chirurgeons," should have transportation first on all ferry boats in the colony" (5).

In the early nineteenth century, a new vogue of employing physicians to assist in childbirth was brought from other countries. Soon the use of forceps was introduced, and the hospital was encouraged as the place for delivery and for the education of physicians in midwifery/obstetrics.

As the immigrants continued to flock to the New World, they brought with them their midwives, who often neither spoke English nor were familiar with the American customs and practices of hygiene. Vast misunderstandings between the medical hierarchies and the midwives developed and inevitably were magnified by the complex health problems that prevailed during these decades. Midwives were not invited to practice in hospitals; because of the lack of opportunities for progressive midwifery education, they had little chance to keep pace with new approaches to health care and could not become part of the American obstetric scene (5, 6).

At the turn of the century, worsening social and health conditions in the urban areas contributed to infant and maternal mortality. The low status of women at that time furthered the atmosphere in which all midwives were blamed for the deaths of infants born at home during those preantibiotic times. As a result the midwives were gradually discouraged from practicing in most urban areas.

In 1905 New York City became concerned about the fact that over 3000 practicing midwives were delivering 40 percent of all babies in New York City. Many tried to condemn the midwives; others suggested that the work of the midwife could and should be raised to higher planes by proper education and state licensure. Two years later the Board of Health started to license midwives (6, 7).

One early attempt to bring the midwife into the main stream of health care was initiated by the New York City Health Department when, in 1911, it opened the Bellevue School of Midwifery, the first American school of midwifery. In this educational program midwives and obstetricians worked as a team in providing maternity care. The school's midwifery students included women from New York City and surrounding states, some local lay-midwives, immigrant midwives and some nurses. However, the school closed in 1936 when less than 10 percent of New York City's births were attended by midwives (8, 9).

In 1925, the late Mary Breckinridge founded the Frontier Nursing Service to provide primary health care for the people in the mountain counties of Kentucky. Because of the maternity care needs of the area, Mrs. Breckinridge recruited midwives and nurse-midwives from England and founded the first organized nurse-midwifery service in America (10). The first recognized school of nurse-midwifery in the United States is the Maternity Center Association School of Nurse-Midwifery (9). It was organized in association with the Lobenstein Midwifery School and Clinic which accepted its first student group in 1931. Thereafter, most schools required nursing education and experience as a prerequisite to American midwifery education.

Acceptance of the full scope of the nurse-midwife's services by American hospitals seemed painfully slow. As a result many nurse-midwifery graduates became educators of maternal and child health in schools of nursing or actively encouraged the family-centered approach to childbirth by demonstration, graduate nurse education, and parent education (9, 11). Many midwifery graduates also chose challenging consultation assignments in maternal and child health programs with the United States Children's Bureau or state health departments which encouraged educational preparation in midwifery. Some graduates went overseas to travel and work under government auspices or to serve as missionaries providing leadership in international health (8, 9).

Pioneering endeavors of the Maternity Center School of Nurse-Midwifery and the Frontier School of Midwifery stimulated several demonstration programs in the 1940s to 1950s, and nurse-midwifery educational programs developed at Yale, Johns Hopkins, Columbia, and Catholic University-Catholic Maternity Institute (12). Gradually over the next 20 years additional educational programs developed at the State University of New York–Kings County, University of Utah, Mississippi, Illinois, Loma Linda, St. Louis, Meharry Medical College, New Jersey Medical College, and by the United States Air Force (13).

In 1964, the Roosevelt Hospital in Manhattan became the first voluntary hospital to employ nurse-midwives to function as part of the obstetric team to provide comprehensive maternity and family planning care (14). Midwifery service programs in many states were started in affiliation with health departments and medical centers. Acceptance of midwives by patients was overwhelmingly positive (15).

As obstetric nurses, midwives, obstetric residents, and obstetrician-gynecologists worked together in an increasing number of hospitals, mutual respect, trust, and colleague-team relationships developed. The team approach was exemplified in the "Joint Statement on Maternity Care," which was published in January 1971, by the American College of Obstetricians and Gynecologists (ACOG) and their Nurses Association (NAACOG) and the American College of Nurse-Midwives (ACNM). With this statement midwifery entered the mainstream of American health care, as it specifically provided that, as part of a medically directed health team, "qualified nurse-midwives may assume responsibility for the complete care and management of uncomplicated maternity patients" (16). In his Health Message of 1971, the President of the United States mentioned the allocation of funds for the education of nurse-midwives, and federal guidelines for the Maternal and Infant Care Projects across the country included recommendations that certified nurse-midwives be employed on the health care teams (17).

Public media started to carry information on the return of the "midwife in modern style" (18,19). Large numbers of nurses applying for entrance into the nurse-midwifery educational programs encouraged new programs to develop. An up-to-date listing of these educational programs may be obtained by writing to the American College of Nurse-Midwives, 1000 Vermont Avenue, N.W., Washington 20005.

In May, 1971, the American College of Nurse-Midwives initiated the National Certification Examination to standardize the basic competency level of the professional midwife practitioner.

International recognition was given the American midwife as early as 1956, when the American College of Nurse-Midwives (ACNM) became a member of the International Confederation of Midwives (ICM). The ICM selected the United States as the site for its Golden Anniversary International Congress. It had selected the President of the ACNM, Miss Lucille Woodville, C.N.M., as its international president to preside at the Congress. In 1972, the triennial Congress was held in Washington, D.C. The ACNM had the honor of hosting over 2000 midwives from over 100 countries (20).

Thus in the United States, professional midwifery has taken its rightful place among the health professions in today's modern health care system.

DEFINITIONS IN MIDWIFERY

Midwifery Midwifery is the art and practice of combining the scientific, philosophic, and human approach to the provision of health maintenance of women in their normal reproductive processes including childbirth, with involvement of the family and/or significant others. Midwives practice within a health team and a framework of an organized regional or local health service with qualified medical direction.

Certified Nurse-Midwife A certified nurse-midwife (C.N.M.) is a professional midwife who possesses evidence of being certified according to the requirements of the National Certifying Board of the American College of Nurse-Midwives. Such a person is entitled to use the initials C.N.M. after her(his) name. She(he) is educated in two disciplines: nursing and midwifery. A nurse-midwife may be further qualified by having a baccalaureate, master's, or doctoral degree in public health, nursing, or a health-related science.

International Definition of Midwife A Midwife is a person who, having been regularly admitted to a midwifery educational program fully recognized in the country in which it is located, has successfully completed the prescribed course of studies in midwifery and has acquired the requisite qualifications to be registered and/or legally licensed to practice midwifery.

The sphere of practice: She must be able to give the necessary supervision, care and advice to women during pregnancy, labor and postpartum period, to conduct deliveries on her own responsibility, and to care for the newborn and the infant. This care includes preventive measures, the detection of abnormal condition in mother and child, the procurement of medical assistance, and the execution of emergency measures in the absence of medical help.

She has an important task in counseling and education—not only for patients, but also within the family and community. The work should involve antenatal education and preparation for parenthood and extends to certain areas of gynecology, family planning, and child care.

She may practice in hospitals, clinics, health units, domiciliary conditions or any other service.[3]

American College of Nurse-Midwives The ACNM is the professional organization for certified nurse-midwives in the United States. It establishes the standards for the practice of midwifery, provides a national certification mechanism for the professional midwife, and offers guidelines and accreditation for midwifery educational programs in the United States. The ACNM collaborates with all other professional groups who share

[3]This international definition was accepted by the ICM Membership in 1972, as well as by the Joint Study Group on Maternity Care, FIGO, WHO (20, 21).

its primary concern for quality maternal-infant health care for all women and babies. The organization was formed in 1929 and incorporated in 1955.

International Confederation of Midwives The International Confederation of Midwives (ICM) is an international organization whose membership consists of national groups of midwives. It was established with the belief that the profession of midwifery will be advanced by greater international cooperation and that this will promote the health and well-being of the family throughout the world. This international organization was founded in 1922.

a family's viewpoint[4]

In modern society the hospital has become the center of medical care, increasingly geared to the needs of science. Professional and technical specialization has led to the fragmentation and depersonalization of the care of the patient. Too often the social and emotional needs of the patient and the family are overlooked. It is evident that maternity services have not escaped these trends.

Quality maternity care must be concerned not only with the physical well-being of mother and child (an area being handled with increasing effectiveness) but also with the emotional and social needs of the entire family, including father and siblings.

JENNIFER

Our first childbirth experience, in 1967, was a lonely, unprepared-for delivery in a traditional general hospital setting—alone for

[4]By Janice T. Kuhlmann and Edward G. Kuhlmann. Paper presented at the Sixteenth Triennial Congress of the International Confederation of Midwives, held in Washington, Oct. 28 to Nov. 3, 1972, and published in the report of the Congress proceedings, *New Horizons in Midwifery* (Waverly Press, Baltimore, 1973).

mother in the third-floor labor room with few nurses during the 11 P.M. to 7 A.M. shift, and alone for father in the waiting room on the second floor during the five tired, anxious hours before my 7:30 A.M. delivery. Demerol was the only resource offered me during labor, for husbands were considered "germs" from the outside world. I had not been aware of childbirth preparation courses which would have provided other tools in the form of breathing and relaxation techniques and increased knowledge of what was occurring in the birth process. Fortunately, the Demerol wore off as the expulsion contractions began, and the obstetrician offered the choice of an awake delivery. I had a pudendal block and came away from the event with the positive feeling that this was the hardest piece of work in my life, yet the most rewarding. However, it was *my* experience and my husband had the loneliest part in the whole process, excluded from helping me and from sharing the joyful reward of delivering.

JONATHAN

As we anticipated the arrival of our second child, in 1970, we met our first nurse-midwife, the instructor of our childbirth preparation course, sponsored by the Childbirth Education Association. She was jolly and sensitive and a medically knowledgeable person; however, to us her role as a professional participant in the birth process was very theoretic. We were well established with a team of two fine obstetricians and probably subconsciously relegated her practical skill to the needs of rural populations or perhaps to the urban poor who could not afford rising obstetric costs. For this delivery we used the same obstetric team and the same hospital that we had used for our first birth. Enlightenment, however, had begun to creep in. Husbands were permitted to be present during labor and delivery, and we pioneered as the first couple to have rooming-in. Still, we were an oddity at the hospital. We repeatedly taught the principles of our childbirth preparation courses to many of the doctors, nurses, and students who were observing the couple have a good time delivering their baby. As our rooming-in began, our oddity continued. Although our obstetrician was supportive, this was all so new to the rest of the staff that we had frequent battles with nurses who felt threatened by the fact that we were able and eager to care for our child ourselves.

On the first night of Jonathan's life, one nervous nursery nurse awakened me at 2 A.M. to say that it was not safe for him to be alone with his mother all night. As Jonathan lay sleeping peacefully beside me against a background chorus of crying babies in the central nursery, she explained that her babies were constantly watched and I could not possibly be doing that for mine.

Labor, delivery, and rooming-in were a tremendous improvement over our first experience. The three of us enjoyed our family times together instead of being separated by a glass wall. However, Jennifer, our two-and-one-half-year-old, was unable to see her mother and baby brother until their return from the hospital, and we found pioneering a strain.

DAVID

A relocation, combined with the expectation of our third child in 1972, necessitated a change of obstetricians. At that time we were presented the option of a new family-centered maternity program at Booth Maternity Center in Philadelphia. This program was conceived when a frustrated consumer, a nurse-midwife, and an obstetrician with vision, sharing a common concern for low-cost, personal, family-centered maternity care, found in an existing institution an ideal basis for activating this idea. Booth had historically been a home and hospital for unmarried mothers.

Because of the decline in number of clients, whom they continue to serve, the staff grew concerned to make better use of their facilities by providing a new service to the community—the option of progressive, flexible, personal, family-centered maternity care at lower cost to the consumer, with a total program of prenatal visits, delivery, and postpartum care provided by a team of nurse-midwives and obstetricians. This option seemed precisely what we desired, and this time there were many differences.

Our initial surprise came when the obstetrician met with us as a couple to discuss our ideas and desires for this childbirth experience, as well as his moderate fee, which he was willing to move downward in accordance with our budget. We were somewhat aware that nurse-midwives were involved in the Booth program, and a month later at my next prenatal visit a nurse-midwife examined me and arranged an appointment for the following month. I was surprised and disappointed that I had not seen the doctor, but I rationalized that he must have been busy delivering a baby. And it was nice that other medical people were around, so that we didn't have to wait. On my next visit, I was examined by another one of those "other medical people," and began to sense that I was not being neglected. The nurse-midwives seemed as competent as the obstetrician, and I was not receiving second-rate prenatal care. I felt more assurance about the team relationship of the midwives and doctor when at an early prenatal appointment, in response to a question, the midwife said she would check with the doctor. She quickly returned with confirmation of the opinion she had expressed. I have always respected a general practioner who is secure and wise enough to know when to refer a patient to a specialist. Thus, my estimation of this nurse-midwife soared as I observed her judgment in this situation.

I began to enjoy the rotation which allowed me to become acquainted with all the midwives on the staff. My understanding of nurse-midwifery and my confidence in midwives as skilled professionals increased gradually during the course of my prenatal visits.

D-Day was approaching. One midwife gave me a reminder of what to do if I delivered en route. Her casual attitude emphasized that delivering a baby is a natural experience rather than a catastrophic event. Three days after the anticipated date, contractions began at about 4:30 A.M., I arrived at the Maternity Center, and was relaxing in the labor room at 7 A.M., with my husband timing contractions and assisting me with my breathing pattern. As I approached transition, I reminded the nurse-midwife that I preferred to deliver in bed in the labor room. Twelve minutes after I had entered the intense transition period, expulsion contractions began. David was arriving faster than the doctor could make it to the hospital. I was not anxious, since the midwife was not a stranger to me, and by this time I felt complete confidence in her skill. Our philosophy of childbirth was that my husband, the baby, and I were the main actors, and the medical person was a skilled assistant for the technical part of the drama. As the expulsion progressed, the four of us chatted about progress between contractions. Without the walls created by drapes and stirrups, we felt marvelously closer and more actively involved in the birth process. Our 9-lb, 8½-oz, red-haired son arrived in a delightful, unmedicated, prepared-for delivery.

Although I had thought that the nurse-midwife worked with us on delivery only because the doctor had not yet arrived, I later learned that the nurse-midwives are active in most normal deliveries at the Maternity Center. The doctor is available in the hospital in the event of complications, but his confidence in the nurse-midwives is evidenced by his supporting them in this most signifi-cant role of working with couples in the normal birth process.

The role of the nurse-midwife did not end for us at delivery. During our two previous childbirth experiences we had carefully listed our concerns to discuss with the busy obstetrician when he paid his brief daily visit. It was often frustrating to realize after he left that some of our questions had been omitted and would have to wait at least 24 h until he returned. In contrast, we valued the availability of nurse-midwives on each shift to answer questions as they arose. We were further impressed when one of the midwives telephoned a few days after we returned home to inquire how mother and child were feeling and how nursing was progressing. This was a personal touch that we had not expected. Another highlight of this third experience was that during the hospital stay, Jennifer and Jonathan could visit with mother.

references

1. Harriet K. Light and Carol Fenster, "Maternal Concerns during Pregnancy," *American Journal of Obstetrics and Gynecology,* **118**(1):47, 1974.
2. Leonide M. Tanner, "Developmental Tasks of Pregnancy," chap. 28 in B. S. Bergersen, et al., *Current Concepts in Clinical Nursing,* The C. V. Mosby Company, St. Louis, 1969, p. 293.
3. Ibid., p. 292.
4. R. R. Wilson (ed.), *Problem Pregnancy and Abortion Counseling,* Family Life, Inc., Publications, Box 427, Saluda, N.C. 28773, 1972, p. 5.
5. Tanner, op. cit., p. 293.
6. Barbara Quirk and Ruth Hassanein, "The Nurse's Role in Advising Patients on Coitus during Pregnancy," *Nursing Clinics of North America,* **8**(3):501, 1973.
7. Kenneth R. Niswander and Myron Gordon

(eds.), *The Women and Their Pregnancies,* The collaborative perinatal study of the National Institute of Neurological Diseases and Strokes, W. B. Saunders Company, Philadelphia, 1972, p. 72.

8. J. Atkinson, "Salt, Water and Rest as a Preventative for Toxemia of Pregnancy," *Journal of Reproductive Medicine,* **9**(5):224, 1972.

9. Tanner, op. cit., p. 293.

10. Light and Fenster, op. cit., p. 50.

11. Francis L. Curtis, "The Pregnant Adolescent," *Nursing '74,* March, 1974, p. 77.

12. American Academy of Pediatrics, "Teenage Pregnancy and the Problem of Abortion," Report of the Committee on Youth, *Pediatrics,* **49**:303, 1972.

13. National Council of Illegitimacy, *Directory of Maternity Homes and Residential Facilities for Unmarried Mothers,* New York, 1966.

14. L. B. Johnson, "Problems with Contraception in Adolescents," *Clinical Pediatrics,* **10**:316, 1971.

15. A. D. Hofmann and H. F. Pipel, "The Legal Rights of Minors," *Pediatric Clinics of North America,* **20**(4):989, 1973.

16. S. L. Hammar, "The Approach to the Adolescent Patient," *Pediatric Clinics of North America,* **20**(4): 1973.

17. A. Foltz, L. V. Kleeman, and V. Jekel, "Pregnancy and Special Education: Who Stays in School?" *American Journal of Public Health,* **62**:1612, 1972.

18. American College of Obstetrics and Gynecology, "Addictive Drugs and Pregnancy," Technical Bulletin 21, April, 1973, p. 1.

19. Ibid., p. 3.

20. Ibid., p. 4.

21. Martin L. Stone et al., "Narcotic Addiction in Pregnancy," *American Journal of Obstetrics and Gynecology,* **109**(5):717, 1971.

Midwifery

1. "Qualifications, Standards and Functions," The American College of Nurse-Midwives, 1000 Vermont Avenue, N.W., Washington 20005, 1975.

2. Dorothea M. Lang, "Providing Maternity Care through a Nurse-Midwifery Service Program," *Nursing Clinics of North America,* **4**(3):1969.

3. "Progress Report, Maternity, Infant Care–Family Planning Projects," Department of Health, The City of New York, 1972.

4. *The Holy Bible,* Exodus, 1:16.

5. Claire Gilbride Fox, "Toward a Sound Historical Basis for Nurse-Midwifery," *Bulletin, American College of Nurse-Midwives,* **14**(3):1969.

6. David Harris, "The Development of Nurse-Midwifery in New York City," *Bulletin, American College of Nurse-Midwives,* **14**(1):1969.

7. David Harris, Edwin F. Daily, and Dorothea M. Lang, Nurse-Midwifery in New York City, *American Journal of Public Health,* **61**(1):1971.

8. M. Theophane Shoemaker, Sr., *History of Nurse-Midwifery in the United States,* The Catholic University of America Press, Washington, 1947.

9. Maternity Center Association, *Twenty Years of Nurse-Midwifery 1933–1953,* 48 East 92 St., New York, N.Y. 10028.

10. Mary Breckinridge, *Wide Neighborhoods,* A Story of the Frontier Nursing Service, Harper & Row, Publishers, Inc., 1952.

11. Hazel Corbin, "Historical Development of Nurse-Midwifery in this Country and Present Trends," *Bulletin of the American College of Nurse-Midwifery,* **4**(1):1959.

12. *Education for Nurse-Midwifery,* American College of Nurse-Midwifery, Washington, 1958.

13. American College of Nurse-Midwives,

What Is A Nurse-Midwife, American College of Nurse-Midwives, 1000 Vermont Ave., N.W., Washington 20005.

14. Johanna Borsellega, "The Role of Nurse-Midwife in a Voluntary Hospital," *Bulletin, American College of Nurse-Midwifery,* **7**(4):1967.

15. Ann Simon, "A Satisfied Patient Views Nurse-Midwifery," *Bulletin, American College of Nurse-Midwives,* **17**(2):1972.

16. "Joint Statement on Maternity Care," American College of Obstetricians and Gynecologists (ACOG), The Nurses Association of the American College of Obstetricians and Gynecologists (NAACOG), and The American College of Nurse-Midwives, *ACOG Newsletter,* February, 1971.

17. Health Message from the President of the United States, Relative to Building a National Health Strategy, 92d Congress, 1st Session, House Document 92-49, Feb. 18, 1971, p. 9.

18. Judy Klemensrud, "Midwives Carry New Image into Hospital Delivery Room," *The New York Times,* Sept. 20, 1972.

19. Dorothea M. Lang, "The Midwife Returns Modern Style," *Parents' Magazine,* October, 1972.

20. "New Horizons in Midwifery," The International Confederation of Midwives, 47 Victoria St., London, England, 1973, p. 220.

21. "The Midwife in Maternity Care," Report of a WHO Expert Committee, WHO Technical Report Series, no. 331, 1966.

bibliography

Anthony, E. J., and T. Benedek (eds.): *Parenthood, Its Psychology and Psychopathology,* Little, Brown and Company, Boston, 1970.

Bancroft, A. V.: "Pregnancy and the Counterculture," *Nursing Clinics of North America,* **8**(1):67, 1973.

Cobliner, W. G., H. Schulman, and S. L. Romney: "The Termination of Adolescent Out of Wedlock Pregnancy and the Prospects for Primary Prevention," *American Journal of Obstetrics and Gynecology,* **115**(3):212, Feb. 1, 1973.

Combs, A. W., D. L. Avila, and W. W. Purkey: *Helping Relationships: Basic Concepts for the Helping Professions,* Allyn and Bacon, Inc., Boston 1971.

Curtis, Francis L.: "The Pregnant Adolescent," *Nursing '74,* March, 1974, p. 77.

"Effective Services for Unmarried Parents and Their Children," National Council of Illegitimacy, New York, 1968.

Elliott, J. M.: "Pica and Pregnancy," *Nursing Clinics of North America,* **3**(2):277, 1968.

Fink, P. J.: "Dealing with the Sexual Pressures of the Unmarried," *Medical Aspects of Sexuality,* March, 1970, pp. 42–53.

Finnegan, L. P., and B. A. MacNew: "Care of the Addicted Infant," *American Journal of Nursing,* **74**(4):685, 1974.

Helfer, R. E., and C. H. Kempe: *The Battered Child,* The University of Chicago Press, Chicago, 1968.

Hilliard, M. E.: "The Changing Role of the Maternity Nurse," *Nursing Clinics of North America,* **3**(2):277, 1968.

"Illegitimacy—Today's Realities," National Council of Illegitimacy, New York, 1971.

Kramer, J. P.: The Adolescent Addict: The Progression of Youth throughout the Drug Culture, *Clinical Pediatrics,* **49**:303, 1972.

Krepick, D. S., and B. L. Lang: "Heroin Addiction: A Treatable Disease," *Nursing Clinics of North America,* **8**(1):41, 1973.

McBride, A. B.: *The Growth and Development of Mothers,* Harper & Row , Publishers, Incorporated, New York, 1973.

McKenzie, R. G.: "A Practical Approach to the Drug-using Adolescent and Young Adult," *Pediatric Clinics of North America,* **20**(4):1035, 1973.

Raugh, J. L., L. B. Johnson, and R. L. Burket: "The Reproductive Adolescent," *Pediatric Clinics of North America,* **20**(4):1021, 1973.

Richardson, S. A., and A. F. Guttmacher (eds.): *Childbearing—It's Social and Psychological Aspects,* The Williams & Wilkins Company, Baltimore, 1967.

Semmens, J. P., and W. M. Zlamers, Jr.: *Teenage Pregnancy,* Charles C Thomas, Publisher, Springfield, Ill., 1967.

Slatin, M.: "Why Mothers Bypass Prenatal Care," *American Journal of Nursing,* **71**:1388, 1971.

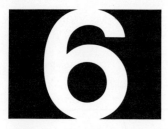

6

psychology of the pregnancy experience

Nancy Thoms Block

Pregnancy, climaxing in the birth of a new baby, opens for a time mysterious doorways to the main participants. Although no one knows exactly what the baby's feelings are at the time, parents' reactions have been studied and described in detail.

In all times and cultures, man has regarded the human reproductive process with special awe and reverence, giving it great religious significance, feeling that through the mysteries of conception, pregnancy, and birth there is participation somehow in the ongoing creative process at work in the universe. This spiritual dimension of human life, which sets it apart from lower animal nature, is perhaps man's most unique and precious possession. Unfortunately, our modern health care system in many ways tends to disregard, and even destroy, man's sense of pride, dignity, and spiritual power which normally finds its most poignant expression in ushering a new life into the world.

the role of the professional

It is the immense privilege of the obstetric team to witness and participate daily in the drama and miracle of human pregnancy and birth. At the same time, it is their respon-

sibility to be understanding, compassionate, and above all, humble in their ministrations. In the midst of crowded waiting rooms, noisy labor rooms, and harried delivery rooms, it is all too easy to lose sight of the unique meaning which each delivery, together with the preceding months of preparation, signifies for the particular human beings involved.

This chapter is intended to assist nurses to become aware of the tremendous importance of feelings and attitudes in achieving and maintaining good health during pregnancy. Mental and physical well-being are closely linked together. This means that a good obstetric nurse tunes in to the mother's state of mind as attentively as to the baby's heartbeat, and evaluates the position of the mother within her family as carefully as the position of the fetus within its mother.

Furthermore, medical personnel must understand that people are exquisitely sensitive to the attitudes of those on whom they must depend. In this case the prospective mother, looking to the obstetric team for assistance and support, may be greatly affected in the way she experiences pregnancy and motherhood by the way they respond to her. Therefore, it is important that nurses and doctors do not simply observe the progress of the pregnancy in a clinical way, merely noting problems as they arise. They must also provide understanding and encouragement to the patient and her family.

Is this asking too much of the busy professional? Actually, doctors and nurses who make the effort to know and relate to their patients find their work easier, more enjoyable, and far more successful.

An obstetric nurse, then, should know the answers to the following questions:

1. How is a healthy woman likely to feel and think throughout her pregnancy and delivery?
2. How can her husband and older children be expected to react?
3. What should be the roles of the medical

people involved, and how are they likely to feel?

4. Where may things go wrong emotionally?

Let us consider these questions in order.

reactions of the mother

As each woman's personality and background are different, so each woman's reaction to pregnancy is somewhat individualized. Furthermore, no two pregnancies are just alike for the same woman. After all, each time she is carrying a different child, under different circumstances. Fathers' reactions, of course, vary in a similar way from individual to individual and from pregnancy to pregnancy. However, investigators who have studied and worked closely with large numbers of "pregnant parents" find that certain patterns of feelings and reactions are fairly predictable at different stages of pregnancy, for both parents.

It is helpful for the obstetric team, from the beginning of pregnancy, to encourage the prospective parents to express these feelings, both to the medical personnel and to other prospective parents. Parents are by turns frustrated, amused, troubled, mystified or ecstatic, and bursting to talk to someone. They are usually anxious to be reassured that these changing moods constitute a normal human experience rather than a sign of mental imbalance.

We will begin, then, considering the changing feelings of the average pregnant woman, remembering that her reactions are closely tied to those of family, friends, and medical helpers.

THE FIRST TRIMESTER:
ACCEPTING PREGNANCY

Psychophysiologic Needs Life's earliest and most urgent needs are for food, sleep, warmth, and human closeness. Their fulfillment provides life's first experience of love,

which develops trust and provides a basis for future relationships and learning. The physical and psychologic stresses of pregnancy reawaken these needs. Sleeping, eating, and affection become major issues again in early pregnancy, just as they were in early childhood. It is often said—and not always sympathetically—that pregnant women want to be "babied." This is quite literally true, and for good reason.

The drastic shifts in her body hormones cause the pregnant woman to feel strange and often disturbing sensations. Her appetite is changed—she may actually be quite nauseous. She feels tired and sleepy much of the time. Her emotions are difficult to control; she may feel like laughing or crying without much explanation. She must depend on others for help. Outside activities may be restricted. All this interferes with her routines, focuses her attention inward on herself, and forces on her a change of pace. She becomes aware of a process taking over her body and mind, her present and her future, over which she has little control.

The symptoms which are thrust on a woman in early pregnancy seem to be nature's way of ensuring that she gets the extra rest and attention she needs for the tremendous new task she has undertaken in her body, mind, and emotions. Perhaps nature does her a favor in this way because she is forced to begin, right away, to think about and deal with the big change which is coming into her life, rather than put off facing it, which is the usual human tendency.

Perhaps this is the reason, also, why pregnancy is a time of increased emotional activity and openness. Nature, it seems, refuses to tolerate procrastination or indifference at that time. Husbands and children are drawn into the excitements and uncertainties. Indeed, prospective parents are surprised at the richness and unpredictability of their own feelings, scarcely recognizing themselves as the "commonsensical" beings which they were formerly and which they will become again once the pregnancy is over. All this fuss and turmoil may serve the same sort of purpose as the squirrel's frantic scramble for nuts in the fall—preparing for stressful times ahead.

Problems and Fantasies Pregnancy is an unmistakable sign of femininity. Most women who accept and take pride in their sexual identity welcome the discovery that they are pregnant.

Many women, however, are somehow dissatisfied with their sexual role. Some reject femininity in obvious outward ways, claiming that pregnancy and motherhood are unfair burdens thrust upon the female sex. Such a woman might feel very resentful or humiliated at becoming pregnant. She might, of course, seek an abortion—or she might refuse to face the fact of her pregnancy. She may suffer from fears of pregnancy relating to her mother's experience. If her mother died at her own or a sibling's birth, she may feel frightened, or even guilty. If her mother had difficulty in becoming pregnant or in carrying a pregnancy to term, or if she is past the menopause and therefore infertile, the pregnant daughter may feel that she is competing, thereby putting her mother down.

Some women who want a baby may demonstrate unrealistic attitudes. Becoming pregnant may satisfy a need to compete with men, as it is something no man can do. Unconsciously, women who feel that they have been deprived of a penis and who envy males their physical characteristics, may try to find compensation for being females in imagining that the fetus is a male organ. Pregnancy is therefore reassuring for the time being, but the woman's illusion that the new "appendage" is there to stay is bound to be shattered before long, leaving her more dissatisfied and depressed than ever.

Psychoanalysis has shown that, in many cases, a girl has a strong unconscious wish for a baby as evidence of the love of her own father—a little girl's first "boyfriend." Since she has learned very early that he actually belongs to another female, her mother, she shifts her hopes to a baby, as though it were a gift from her father which will be her very own and love her unconditionally in his place. This fantasy may live on well into adulthood.

Many unmarried teen-age girls, especially lonely ones who lack parental love and protection, allow themselves to become pregnant for this reason. Of course, they are bound to become disillusioned and to make poor mothers, because the baby, it soon turns out, demands far more love and attention than it can immediately repay, from the very girl who desperately wishes to be loved and protected herself. Such an immature, emotionally deprived mother may neglect or abuse her child after birth, or care for it mechanically and capriciously as if it were a doll. As the shocking occurrence of serious child abuse in our country rises, it is the increasing responsibility of the medical and allied professions to be alert to such potentially abusive mothers very early in pregnancy. Psychiatric help, or possibly even abortion, might be offered to them, though resistance to suggestions may be great.

In some unusual cases, a woman who desperately wants a child develops "pseudocyesis," or false pregnancy. Remarkably convincing physical changes may occur, as the woman herself steadfastly believes she is pregnant. Psychiatric help is obviously needed in persistent pseudocyesis.

There are a number of other fantasies which a woman may experience in early pregnancy. She may feel and imagine that she and the baby are one and interchangeable. This is not hard to understand. The tiny embryo is deep down and hidden inside her, like one of her own organs. It has given no sign yet of having a life of its own. The mother has felt no separate movement, heard no separate heartbeat. Her own body shape, especially in a primipara, remains deceptively normal for some time. Yet she knows there is a baby within. Sometimes she fancies that she is the baby.

A similar fantasy, one which is common to young children and may recur in pregnancy, connects conception with eating, as though the baby, like food in the mother's digestive tract, may be eliminated.

These fantasies make it easy to deny the real facts and implications of pregnancy, which many women tend to do at first. Some neglect for several months to seek confirmation of their pregnancy and prenatal care for this reason. One might say this is a sign of the babyishness a pregnant woman usually feels—failing to accept her new responsibility to herself and her anticipated child, and, instead, playing the child herself, depending upon others to bring her to the doctor or clinic for necessary medical attention.

THE SECOND TRIMESTER: DEVELOPING A NEW IDENTITY

By the end of the first trimester, the bulge of the growing uterus and the passage of time have helped convince nearly every pregnant woman that, beyond any doubt, she is to become a mother. Soon, the baby's movements will be proof positive. This brings her abruptly upon one of the most absorbing and important psychologic tasks of her life—pondering what it means to be a mother, and even more basically, a woman.

To be sure, she has done some thinking about this long before her pregnancy, and she will probably continue to consider and reconsider her role from time to time throughout the rest of her life. But there is a certain urgency—a deadline when she will suddenly have to *be* a mother—imposed by pregnancy.

Child vs. Mother Some consider pregnancy a woman's greatest time of personal testing. It is like a long mirror, a 9-month "moment of truth," in which she faces herself as a woman and takes inventory. She can neither avoid the confrontation nor speed it up, and during the wait she has plenty of time to explore her inner world, where the questions are written large, "Who am I?" and "Who am I to become?"

Deep within her, she recognizes that a transformation is about to take place. When pregnancy is terminated in delivery, she will have become, once and for all, a parent. This is a new role for her. At the same time, childhood is symbolically left behind, though many "child" longings remain within every adult. With mixed feelings, she prepares to step over the one-way threshold into parenthood.

What does she find as she takes stock? A prospective mother did not arrive at this point overnight. Even if she is still in her teens, she has years of infancy, childhood, and adolescence behind her. Bit by bit, during that time her personality was taking shape, her hopes and expectations were being formed, and her ideas of womanliness were developing. She considered many choices, tried out some, adopted a few. The whole process was gradual; changes were almost unnoticed as they occurred, and have been largely forgotten. Now, as if by magic, pregnancy opens up a window to her past. Her inner eyes are sharpened for a while, more than at any other period of her life. She relives childhood feelings, experiences, and relationships, trying to bring them into focus from her new point of view.

As she looks backward and inward, sensing herself a child again, the chief person she confronts is her own mother. She may become quite obsessed with thoughts of her and of their relationship. She may reexperience a confusing mixture of feelings—tender affection, frustrated anger, admiration and scorn, rebellion and dependency—which were present in years past. Her task is to sort out the good threads from the bad, weaving a garment for herself, and trying it on for size, so to speak. She must soon step out on the stage as a full-fledged mother herself, and wants very much to be a good one.

Conflicts about Motherhood Understandably, some women will have considerable difficulty accomplishing this. An extreme case may be a woman who had neither a real mother nor a good substitute and is bewildered for lack of any kind of model in her own experience. If she did have a mother, who is seen as a very bad example, it may still be difficult for her to construct a different pattern for her own motherhood. She will find it almost impossible to give to her child what she has not received herself. If she is fortunate, other "mothering" people in her life—relatives or friends—have filled this need. Even supportive doctors, nurses, and social workers can be of some help to her, for they not only care for *her*, but they can demonstrate to her some practical child-care techniques that will make her more competent and confident in actually handling her expected infant.

A pregnant woman, especially a primipara, who does not appear to be experiencing some struggles is a cause for concern. She may be mentally blocking out her pregnancy because of fear or resentment, or she may have the fantasy that her own mother is the baby's mother and will therefore take care of it, while she herself is only some sort of intermediary. In certain parts of society, where it is quite common for a young mother, married or not, to be living with her own mother, this does indeed happen. Such an arrangement may seem to work out satisfactorily, but the young mother may lose out sadly by not claiming this aspect of womanhood for herself.

The teen-age girl who becomes pregnant in competition with her mother, or in defiance of her, may have great psychologic difficulty in resolving her feelings. If her mother offers a poor example and little support, or if the girl rejects what her mother can indeed offer, she may be looking inappropriately to one or more boyfriends, siblings, or even her baby to take her mother's place.

Normally, the mother-preoccupation diminishes toward the end of the second trimester, to be replaced by a relatively calm, realistic concern for the coming baby and a busy, delighted interest in the practical concerns of preparation. Maternity clothes are purchased, financial matters are discussed, and space is provided for the baby.

Turning to the Father The expectant father now becomes more involved, in various ways. Practical and financial concerns require his attention. But beyond that, his wife may begin quite actively to draw him into the pregnancy experience. She insists that he must share in feeling the baby move, putting his hand on her enlarging abdomen. She may begin classes to prepare for childbirth, urging him to participate with her in the intimate physical concerns which are dealt with there. Her sexual appetite, which may have been very poor or unpredictable earlier in pregnancy, usually increases at this time. She may only want to be held and caressed, however, instead of seeking intercourse.

Does she require this attention of her husband simply because he is most available? Is he supposed to substitute for her own mother as comforter and protector? Perhaps. At any rate, the pregnant woman shifts her preoccupation from her mother to her husband, and begins to work out her mixed feelings toward him, much as she has already done toward her mother.

She feels in turn dependent or competitive, insecure or confident, tender or resentful, toward him. These feelings are frequently expressed as fears for his safety or as fluctuating moods. Needless to say, the husband, unless he is a flexible and confident man, may become confused and upset over all this. He may withdraw from her emotionally, or actually desert her, in which case she will feel very lost and helpless indeed.

THE THIRD TRIMESTER: PREPARATION FOR DELIVERY

By the third trimester, the pregnant woman has usually accepted her pregnancy and coming motherhood. She is the center of attention wherever she goes, practically popping with pride at her obvious accomplishment. Folklore has it that a woman is most radiantly beautiful when she is "great with child"—the "madonna mystique," one might call it. In her exalted, dreamy moments, she feels special, instrumental in the sacred rite of creation, destined to bring forth a new life. She is eager for the event.

Common Anxieties and Concerns Yet she must pause and recognize what will be required of her. This may be frightening. She cannot turn back the processes of nature, carrying her along like a great river. As though she were confronting an unknown stretch of rapids, she must now trust herself to the hands of others to aid her through labor and delivery to calmer waters beyond.

To relieve the anxiety, she becomes absorbed in various matters—the medical details of the coming delivery; clothing; equipment; a name for the baby; household preparations for her absence at the hospital; her own increasing awkwardness; and minor but annoying physical symptoms. Her legs and back may ache, her breath comes short, her bladder won't wait, and she can't reach down to put on shoes and stockings. Still, if she has a job outside the home, she may prefer to keep working until the last minute if allowed to, even though nature is giving her the message to slow down. A mother who already has one or more young children may not be able to slow down anyway. Indeed, older children, sensing that a new competitor is arriving soon, may become more demanding of her attention than usual.

Naturally, there are particular anxieties about whether something will go wrong with the delivery, and whether the baby will emerge normal and healthy. Such concerns frequently appear in dreams at this stage.

Sexual Intercourse Sexual relations become very awkward toward the end of pregnancy. Both husband and wife require some ingenuity, as well as mutual understanding, tenderness, and a sense of humor to work out their sexual adjustments. The pregnant belly is a real obstacle which comes between them. In addition, the wife's rapidly changing sexual feelings and physical shape may frighten or repel her husband, while she herself tends to be uncomfortable and self-conscious. Usually, in the course of a normal pregnancy, their obstetrician will impose few restrictions on sexual activity. There are a number of medical indications for doing so, including bleeding and a history of prenatal complications. Frequently the couple themselves will limit intercourse unnecessarily, out of fear or ignorance, at this time when intimacy and mutual support are especially vital to their relationship.

Because many couples are reluctant to discuss intercourse during pregnancy, some member of the medical team should routinely and explicitly deal with the issue early, and perhaps raise it again in the third trimester, to elicit questions, doubts, and fears. If coitus must be restricted for medical reasons, alternative avenues of reciprocal sexual gratification may be suggested, such as mutual masturbation by manual or oral means.

Anxiety about Labor If false labor occurs, it may be frustrating and bewildering to the pregnant woman, especially if she is ignorant or misinformed about what to expect. She will be offered all kinds of advice by relatives, friends, and neighbors who consider her pregnancy a community affair.

Finally, she is indeed in labor. The average woman then presents herself at some hospital. She may be accompanied by her husband, another relative, or a friend, or she may come alone. Ideally, she will have become familiar with the hospital during her pregnancy, in preparation for this event, though frequently it is totally strange to her. As she progresses through labor and delivery, she may be reassured by the familiar faces and voices of nurses and doctors whom she knows and has come to trust. More likely, if she is a clinic patient in a busy city hospital, she will find herself unable to recognize a single familiar person.

In most hospitals today, the final act of the pregnancy drama is curtained off from the everyday world of the main participants. The mother is snatched away from view, while the ritual of delivery is secretly performed in the inner sanctum of the delivery suite.

reactions of the father

Let us stop here for a bit to see how the expectant father has been faring for 9 months. He has his own predictable assortment of feelings. Some of them are due purely to his maleness or his own personality. Others are reactions to the particular way his wife rides out her pregnancy "trip."

TRADITIONAL ATTITUDES

As everyone knows, expectant fathers in this country are often pushed into the background. They are said to feel like "fifth wheels" throughout the pregnancies and deliveries of their wives. Actually, they may be "brainwashed" into accepting this state of affairs. The increasingly frequent man who tries to fight the system will very likely run into all sorts of obstacles, raised eyebrows, or ridicule. He finds himself in a kind of "lion's den" of jealous female relatives and sphinx-like doctors and nurses, all making him feel most unwelcome and uncomfortable. However, he is beginning, fortunately, to hold his head up now and then and stake out his claim to his rightful place as father of the child. After

all, it is his offspring which is creating all the fuss!

The news that his wife is pregnant is almost always a source of tremendous pride to a man, for he takes it as evidence of his masculinity and his power to create life. It is unfortunate when, as so often happens, a man feels that his involvement ends here (except, perhaps, to provide financial support to his family). Playing the part of emotional father to the expected baby, and husband to its mother, is a much more demanding role than that of becoming a biologic father through one act of intercourse.

TASKS, CONFLICTS, AND FANTASIES

Probably, every pregnant woman seems like a strange and unfamiliar creature to her husband at various stages of pregnancy, and he must adjust to her in some way. He frequently needs reassurance that he is not the cause of her emotional fluctuations. He also needs someone to whom to vent his own feelings (in case his wife is not in the mood to listen).

Furthermore, he has his own crucial inner tasks to perform which parallel those of his wife. He must also recognize and accept the fact of the new child who will soon intrude upon *his* life, making him a parent, too.

Our society makes this latter task especially perplexing for men because of the curiously irrational notion that men are not supposed to be tender, caring, patient human beings. A "real man" is portrayed in movies, comic books, and folklore as tough, domineering, and unemotional. Who is to tell the expectant father that love and concern for his wife and children are natural and thoroughly manly?

To be sure, a number of inner fears and conflicts crop up during pregnancy to plague the expectant father and handicap him in developing his new role.

Some men, harboring deep neurotic conflicts over their own sexual identity, with unconscious fears of being feminine or homosexual, cannot allow themselves to be "soft" in any way. Instead they are impelled to be tough, brusque, and defensive, and tend to make poor husbands and fathers unless they receive psychiatric help.

One of the natural feelings which a man often has to confront when his wife becomes pregnant is that of envy. As a little boy, he may have seen his mother pregnant and wished that he could perform an equally marvelous feat. If he said so, he was probably laughed at and told, "Only girls can have babies!" As he now watches his wife's abdomen enlarge and feels the movements of the fetus with his own hands, he is again reminded that *he* cannot bear a child. If he is otherwise insecure about his own abilities and worth, and his relationship with his wife is strained, he may at this time stay away from her as much as possible, keeping busy with his work, other hobbies, or associations which build up his sense of identity and achievement. He may seek out a girl friend at this time, for reassurance. He thus resorts to rejecting or competing with his wife, instead of supporting her in what is actually their joint production, the pregnancy.

Occasionally an expectant father will actually identify or compete with his pregnant wife strongly enough to produce the "Couvade syndrome." This term is derived from a French word meaning "to sit on" or "hatch," and refers to a psychosomatic condition mimicking pregnancy—the male version of pseudocyesis. This may include a variety of symptoms such as nausea, weight gain, abdominal distension, or pain, but is rarely severe enough to require psychiatric intervention.

The immature man who married in order to acquire the permanent, undivided attention of a "mother" for himself will, of course, begin to feel uneasiness and jealousy over the approach of a serious rival for his wife's attention. These feelings only tend to increase after the birth of the child unless he can discuss them and discover creative ways of handling them. The more actively and positively he can begin assuming supporting and caring roles as husband and father, the more readily he can give up competing with his own child. Parental preparation courses during the pregnancy, which include some practical instruction in child care for both parents, can be extremely useful to such fathers.

Besides competing with his own wife and child, the American husband very frequently feels that he has to compete with the obstetrician in importance to his wife and to the whole production. If he feels totally overshadowed and displaced, he may withdraw his interest and support altogether. It is an alarming fact that some fathers, especially of the lower socioeconomic classes in our urban areas, tend to desert their families, or at least fail to take on appropriate responsibilities in child support and upbringing. Yet they can hardly be blamed, it seems, when they are constantly given the message by the experts that babies are none of their business!

PROFESSIONAL SUPPORT OF THE FATHER

It is the opinion of this writer that one of the most urgent tasks of the obstetric team ought to be the proper care of the fathers of the babies who are being born daily in our nation's hospitals, both private and public. Alert and sympathetic professionals who support the father's self-esteem may help keep him in the picture at this crucial time, to the enormous benefit of the family and society. It might be an excellent innovation to pay as much attention to the fathers, if possible, as to the mothers of unborn babies. Their presence ought perhaps to be required, as a matter of course, at key office visits, instructive activities, labor room, and delivery suite (where they might be given the option to wait in a closely adjoining room if they prefer not to witness the actual delivery, or if there are complications necessitating surgical intervention) to signify their full participation in the pregnancy and birth processes of their children (Fig. 6·1). As things now stand, unfortunately, the obstetrician and other hospital personnel, for various reasons which we will discuss toward the end of this chapter, are often the greatest opponents of the father's active involvement.

the delivery experience

Having weathered the 9 months of pregnancy, the couple come—hopefully, together—to the final act of labor and delivery, the culmination of the whole experience. Some couples with a strong determination to share this experience firsthand, avoid going to a hospital altogether for fear of being separated, and arrange for home delivery.

Some hospitals allow the husband in the labor and delivery rooms if he is properly prepared and motivated. Actually, many couples still prefer to leave the delivery itself entirely in the hands of the medical team, with minimal participation themselves—she well sedated and he waiting somewhere outside; but all expectant parents ought to feel that they have the right to some choice in the matter.

The well-prepared couple will have discussed certain matters with the doctor and made certain decisions in advance, such as the place and expected method of delivery. They should know, as far as possible, what to expect and how to assist in the physiologic process of birth by proper breathing and relaxation.

Nevertheless, there are the inevitable pain, anxiety, and uncertainties which tax both the

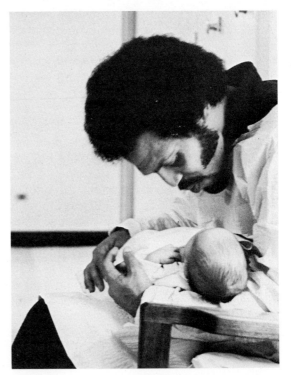

fig. 6·1 A father needs time with his new baby. (*Photo by Andrew McGowan.*)

medical and psychologic expertise of the medical team. When proper preparation is lacking, or the hospital regulations are cumbersome and its personnel insensitive, the laboring mother's anxiety can easily escalate into panic—especially if she finds herself alone among strangers. Her inability to relax and cooperate may in turn cause unnecessary complications in the delivery.

Some women panic even under ideal conditions, and need sedation. Medical complications may indicate further analgesia or anesthesia. In view of this, it is vitally important to prepare every expectant mother, especially the "natural childbirth" enthusiast, for the possibility that a need for medication might develop after all. She should be relieved of the fear, in advance, that she would be a "failure" in any way because of that. Among the most urgent questions in a laboring mother's mind are, "Can I do it?" and "Can I trust those who have to help me in this inescapable ordeal?" Being forced to depend on others, if her relationship with them is not good, may cause her to feel angry and helpless. Frank discussions with the medical team before the stresses of delivery arise will vastly increase rapport.

The most upsetting and bewildering time for the patient, according to Drs. Arthur and Libby Colman, is that of "transition" between the first and second stages of labor. There is a momentary pause after dilation of the cervix is complete, before the baby continues its descent. As her uterine muscles reorganize their efforts, the patient is uneasy and uncertain about what is happening to her. An otherwise cooperative, rational woman may become briefly irritable and unreasonable toward all those around her. This is likely to occur just as she is being transferred to the delivery room, thus increasing the turmoil of the moment.

If all goes well, however, the completion of the delivery, with the first sight and feel of the new baby, is for the parents an experience of incomparable fulfillment, and for the attending staff a moment of deep satisfaction. All share the elated feeling of having successfully completed an ambitious but rewarding family project.

ATTITUDES OF THE STAFF

The doctors and nurses have a legitimate place here emotionally as "parent figures" to the new parents. The actual relative ages of the participants is unimportant. Medical personnel, who are in the dominant position with their expertise and authority, can be either "bad" parents—judgmental, belittling, and domineering—or "good" parents—supportive and encouraging the couple to feel that *they themselves* have actually done a good job. The parturient mother has never worked harder in her life, and the father, perhaps, never agonized so much. They are entitled to enjoy a sense of accomplishment. Furthermore, they will be needing all the confidence and self-assurance they can muster for the difficult early period after they bring the new baby home from the hospital.

IMPACT OF HOSPITAL POLICIES

The hospital delivery and postnatal routines are significant in confirming the parents' central importance to their child. The mother needs to be reasonably well awake during and immediately after the delivery, though as free of pain as possible, to appreciate what she has done. Both parents should be allowed to see and hold their child at the earliest practical moment. True, there may be no father in the picture at delivery. Or the mother herself may have strong negative feelings about her baby, in which case it should not be thrust at her. Nevertheless, the message she receives from the medical team ought to be, "This is *your* baby—your accomplishment, and your responsibility."

The opposite message may be conveyed by certain hospital practices. In some hospitals, for instance, babies who are technically undersized (though otherwise normal) are kept in the nursery at feeding times, to be bottle-fed by the staff. Yet they are not released at any other times to the mothers because of inconvenience to the staff, or the fear of germs. The luckless parents may scarcely be allowed a peep at their child, who is kept "safely" at the back of the newborn nursery or even in the premature nursery, away from the windows. Hour by hour, their anxieties mount while their confidence wanes, until the moment of discharge from the hospital when they are abruptly handed a

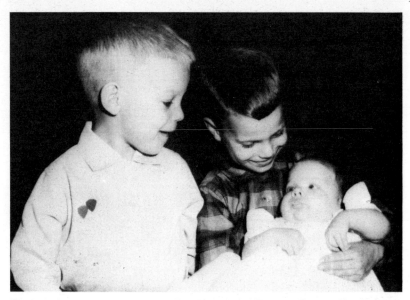

fig. 6·2 A new baby changes the family pattern. (*Photo by Russell Block.*)

mysterious, fragile bundle to deal with. Small wonder if they want just to drop it and run!

SIBLINGS' NEEDS

Where there are older children in a family, their needs must be considered in addition to those of the parents and the newborn. They tend to feel left out of the pregnancy and birth, and therefore become more demanding or babyish themselves. Their unhappy behavior, in turn, increases difficulties for both parents. Older children's competitive needs to feel important can be turned to very good use at this time by involving them in discussions of what is happening and enlisting their willing participation. Assignment of small but significant tasks within the household (elevating their status to competent helpers), along with some extra attention in their own right, can transform a very threatening experience into a happy and creative one for the newborn's siblings (Fig. 6·2). Some pioneering obstetric centers, recognizing this concern, allow older children to visit their mother and the new baby in a special area (see "Viewpoint," in Chap. 5).

postpartum emotional difficulties

A few words must be said here about postpartum emotional disturbances, which are relatively common and seem to stem from a number of causes, some of which may be preventable.

The grieving of a mother who has given up a baby for adoption, or whose baby was born dead or deformed, is normal. She must be allowed to undergo the mourning process, and may benefit from some help in working through the burdens of self-blame, guilt, and anger which she will experience (Fig. 6·3).

A woman who is subject to psychotic breakdowns of one sort or another is likely to suffer a relapse in the postpartum period. She should be carefully followed for at least 2 months after delivery, and given prompt psy-

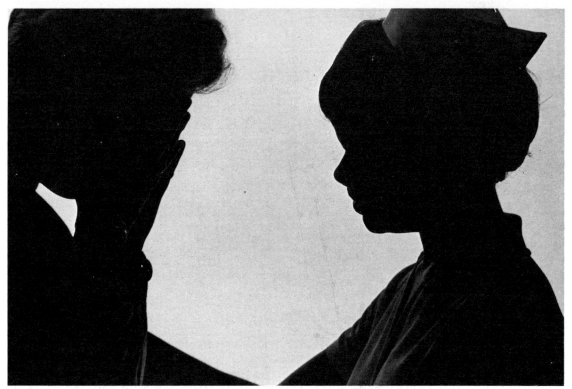

fig. 6·3 Nursing intervention as depression begins may avert more complex problems. (*Photo by Larry Mulve-hill.*)

chiatric attention if any signs of psychosis develop.

In addition, many apparently healthy women, following normal deliveries, experience a prolongation or exaggeration of the normal, brief, "after-baby blues," which seem to be hormonally related. Such depressions can also reach psychotic proportions, endangering the well-being and even the life of the mother, the baby, or other children, through violence or neglect. Again, psychiatric attention is urgent.

In some cases, alertness of the medical staff to psychologic problems during pregnancy may forestall a postpartum crisis. A pregnant woman who seems to have an unrealistic concept of the demands and dependency of a newborn baby on its mother, or who appears unduly immature herself, de-

pending heavily on the obstetrician, nurses, and relatives for constant attention, is a prime target for trouble. She can be helped somewhat by the obstetric staff even during her brief prenatal contacts. She should be seen regularly by the same doctor, nurse, or counselor, who would recognize and acknowledge her feelings but give her positive support, so that "growing up" internally to her new role is not so difficult.

Many women never truly accept their babies' separateness, even after birth. Feeling somehow incomplete or unfulfilled without the child—as though it were indeed a vital organ or appendage —they tend to keep at least one of their children bound to themselves emotionally throughout life, to satisfy their own unconscious need. They may suffer depressions, not only postpartum but whenever the child leaves the home in later years. Such women generally require extended psychotherapy for improvement.

So much for women's postpartum difficulties. It stands to reason that men must have their share as well, but adequate studies in that field are lacking—a further indication, perhaps, of the tendency to underplay fathers in our society.

psychologic problems of the medical staff

Most of this chapter, up to this point, has been aimed at helping obstetric teams to understand their patients. In order to be truly effective in helping their patients, however, doctors and nurses need a special degree of self-understanding. Being human, just as their patients are, they are subject to needs and attitudes of their own which may interfere seriously with their competence. Recognizing and dealing with these personal feelings may be the most difficult professional task which they need to face.

THE NEED TO CONTROL

A major psychologic issue for health care professionals is that of *control*. People, as a rule, try to control things they are afraid of. A doctor's or nurse's determination to control disease and eliminate death is commendable, but it is bound to fail at times. Death, disease, and unforeseen complications continue to occur in spite of the greatest human skill and dedication. If a person is actually frightened and angered by these forces, feeling helpless or guilty because he cannot forestall them, he may take out his feelings on his fellow workers, or even on the patient who is already the victim of circumstances.

Obstetricians may exercise their needs to control upon their women patients in inappropriate ways, such as failing to allow them to express their feelings or to participate in decisions. An authoritarian attitude may extend beyond medical to personal matters, such as how many babies to have and when, or what birth control methods to use. Or it may dictate the conditions of delivery, without consideration for the patient's feelings and convenience. Nurses have their own ways of overcontrolling patients, particularly through setting up inflexible or insensitive hospital routines.

FEELINGS OF ENVY

A somewhat different problem tends to apply mostly to male obstetricians it seems, but may be of concern also to female professionals; that is, some sort of *envy* of the pregnant woman's accomplishment in bearing children. A young nurse or female doctor who has never been pregnant herself, especially if she is having difficulty conceiving, may feel that she is being outdone, and thus may unconsciously resent the patients committed to her care. An older single or postmenopausal female may have similar feelings toward expectant mothers, even becoming depressed as a result. If she happens to work in the newborn nursery, she may tend to become openly possessive toward the babies and punitive toward their mothers, depriving them of contact with their infants or belittling their competence. When the time comes for mother and child to leave the hospital, such a nurse has been heard to exclaim reproachfully, "Are you taking *my* baby home?"

The obstetrician has available a different, though no better, avenue of expressing envious feelings without directly competing. He or she is in a position to take over the whole process by controlling the expectant mother. Such a physician tends to "baby" the mother, dismissing her role with such words as, "Don't worry, little mother, I'll have this baby for you!"

As noted earlier, some "mothering" is

needed by the pregnant patient. She may appropriately look to her doctors and nurses, as well as to her own parents and husband, for support and concern. Too often, however, medical people become patronizing, excluding the patient's family from involvement, thereby keeping her almost wholly dependent on themselves. This may be one of the reasons for the reluctance of personnel to make expectant fathers feel welcome and important.

AIDS TO THE STAFF

It is to be hoped that medical people will have the wisdom and courage to confront and correct their own unhelpful attitudes, for the benefit of their patients as well as themselves. It might prove highly useful for an entire obstetric service to initiate frank discussions of cases or situations which have aroused emotional problems for the staff. Regular airings of tensions, anxieties, and feelings of guilt or anger among the professional staff, if properly conducted, can be both instructional and therapeutic. Equally helpful are informal reading seminars based on such pertinent writings as Kübler-Ross's works on the subject of death and dying, Jacobson's studies of depression, Klaus's studies on maternal needs, and Brian Bird's book, *Talking with Patients.*

Finally, a special word to nurses—of whatever age, sex, or background. Although the modern approach to patient care is via the *medical team,* and although the nurse is the key person on the team with regard to regular, direct contact with the patient, he or she may hesitate to contribute openly some valuable observations, insights, and skills. As the team approach to medicine grows in acceptance, so the special role of the nurse increases in recognition and respect, as it rightly should. Timidity and false modesty generate only resentment and distrust. Team members, to be truly effective, must feel free to share and contribute as equals, though their particular responsibilities differ, in their common effort to serve people who seek their help.

bibliography

Benedek, Therese: "The Psychobiologic Approach to Parenthood," in E. J. Anthony and T. Benedek (eds.), part II *Parenthood, Its Psychology and Psychopathology,* Little, Brown and Company, Boston, 1970, pp. 109–206.

Bibring, Edward: "The Mechanism of Depression," in P. Greenacre (ed.), *Affective Disorders: Psychoanalytic Contribution to Their Study,* International Universities Press, Inc., New York 1961, pp. 13–47.

Bird, Brian: *Talking with Patients,* J. B. Lippincott Company, Philadelphia, 1955.

Chappel, John N., and Robert S. Daniels: "Puerperal Psychosis," *Hospital Medicine,* June, 1969, pp. 115–122.

Colman, Arthur D., and Libby Lee: *Pregnancy: The Psychological Experience,* Herder and Herder, Inc., New York, 1971.

Deutsch, Helene: *The Psychology of Women,* vols. I and II, Bantam Books, Inc., New York, 1973 (paperback ed.).

Erikson, Erik H.: "Eight Ages of Man," chap. 7 in *Childhood and Society,* W. W. Norton & Company, Inc., New York, 1963.

Heiman, Marcel: "A Psychoanalytic View of Pregnancy," in J. Rovinsky & A. Guttmacher (eds.) *Medical, Surgical, and Gynecologic Complications of Pregnancy,* 2d ed., The Williams & Wilkins Company, Baltimore, 1965, pp. 473–511.

Howells, John G.: "Childbirth Is a Family Experience," chap. 7 in J. G. Howells (cd.), *Modern Perspectives in Psycho-obstetrics,* Brunner-Mazel, New York, 1972, pp. 127–149.

Jessner, Lucie, et al.: "The Development of Parental Attitudes during Pregnancy," chap. 9 in E. J. Anthony and T. Benedek (eds.), *Parenthood, Its Psychology and Psychopathology,* Little, Brown and Company, Boston, 1970, pp. 209–244.

Kübler-Ross, Elisabeth: *On Death and Dying,* The Macmillan Company, New York, 1969.

Masters, W. H., and V. E. Johnson: *Human Sexual Response,* Little, Brown and Company, Boston, 1966.

Nadelson, Carol: "'Normal' and 'Special' Aspects of Pregnancy," *Obstetrics and Gynecology,* **41**(4):611–620, 1973.

Richardson, A. Cullen, and Lynn D. Webber: "The Noetic Dimension of Human Reproduction," *American Journal of Obstetrics and Gynecology,* July 15, 1971, pp. 808–822.

Wagner, Nathaniel N., and Don A. Solberg: "Pregnancy and Sexuality," *Medical Aspects of Human Sexuality,* March 1974, pp. 44–66.

"Women's Liberation and the Practice of Medicine," *Medical World News,* June 22, 1973, pp. 33–38.

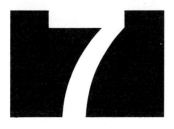

education for childbirth

Constance R. Castor

Girls and boys are informally educated for the childbirth experience from their own birth. Depending on their culture, this education varies in its positive and negative qualities. The availability of formal programs of prenatal education is a rather modern phenomenon. The change to the nuclear family in our society reduced the natural education source of mothers, aunts, and cousins in the extended family. Now, with the general movement toward self-awareness and responsibility for becoming pregnant, parents in unprecedented numbers are seeking to prepare themselves for the childbirth experience.

In preparation classes, by organized learning programs, parents can acquire information and specialized skills which will permit the woman to remain relatively comfortable and in control of herself during labor and delivery. She can participate actively in the process with no sacrifice of safety to either herself or the fetus.

methods of preparation

There are currently two major approaches to preparation for childbirth in the United States: psychophysical methods and psychoprophylactic methods.

PSYCHOPHYSICAL METHOD

This method evolved out of the natural childbirth movement of the forties and fifties, which was founded on the writings and work of Dick-Read, Thomas, and Goodrich. The program of education and exercise is directed toward breaking the fear-tension-pain cycle. Fathers are welcomed to class and are prepared for labor as well. The psychophysical method is the oldest approach to prepared childbirth in this country. Such courses frequently incorporate general prenatal education with specific labor techniques which the woman can apply as she chooses. With the changes in contemporary society and with the continued refinement in the education of parents, the differences between psychophysical and psychoprophylactic methods are rapidly diminishing. (More specific details on the psychophysical method are available from the Maternity Center Association, 48 East 92 St., New York, N.Y. 10028.)

PSYCHOPROPHYLACTIC METHOD

This method of childbirth preparation was introduced in the early sixties through the efforts of Marjorie Karmel and her book, *Thank You, Dr. Lamaze.* The method evolved out of the application by the Russians of Pavlovian classical conditioning to childbirth. Although differences in technique can be observed as it is practiced throughout the world, the central thrust of psychoprophylaxis remains a highly structured system based on conditioning, discipline, and concentration. On the surface, many of its techniques are similar to those of the psychophysical approach. Indeed, it can be said that the methods have mutually influenced one another. A closer evaluation of the actual teachings reveals a greater intensity in psychoprophylaxis, with a central emphasis on the role of conditioning. It is believed that the woman must undergo a period of highly disciplined training which teaches her to substitute new responses to the stimulus of labor contractions. The necessity for sound prenatal education and reduction of psychic tension is recognized as well. The support of a knowledgeable labor coach is inherent to the technique. In most Western countries, including the United States, the coach is the father. Within this and subsequent chapters, "husband" may be interchangeable with the person who will assist, coach, and encourage the woman—perhaps a parent, boyfriend, close friend, or other close relative.

The psychoprophylactic method is sometimes referred to as a nonpharmacologic analgesia, but it recognizes that the various obstetric modalities can be added to the prepared woman's efforts as circumstances warrant.

HYPNOSIS

Hypnosis is an effective approach to the alleviation of pain in childbirth, but is impractical as it depends on a sufficient supply of trained physicians. Through hypnosis, the woman learns to enter a trancelike state, focusing intently on the hypnotist or on prearranged self-hypnotic suggestions, which significantly reduce attention to outside stimuli. Some observers feel that there may be elements of self-hypnosis in the other methods discussed, but this has not been adequately demonstrated.

GENERAL CLASSES

Many physicians teach childbirth classes in their offices. General information is given on the pregnancy and labor process. Most physicians who take the time to educate their patients find a reduction in numbers of questions and a heightened sense of cooperation on the part of the couple.

SUMMARY

It should be understood that preparation for childbirth provides the modern couple with the means to cope effectively with the stress of pregnancy, birth, and the early postpartum period. The psychophysical and psychoprophylactic methods are similarly based on (1) accurate information to reduce anxieties and fears which are recognized to facilitate pain; (2) the acquisition of specific techniques of relaxation, muscular control, and respiratory activity to reduce or eliminate the pain of labor; and (3) the creation and maintenance of a calm, supportive environment.

THE MECHANISM FOR CHILDBIRTH PREPARATION

In the past, much of the effectiveness of preparation for childbirth was attributed by some to good education, dedication, courage, distraction, and luck. Grantly Dick-Read believed reeducation and antepartal and intrapartal support were essential in helping a woman achieve control during labor. Concentration and distraction played a part as well, as the woman practiced mental disassociation and performed relaxation and breathing activities. Lamaze and other proponents of psychoprophylactic preparation for childbirth believed that classical Pavlovian conditioning was the element responsible for the management of labor. This explanation was based on the principle of cortical excitation-inhibition. Women were deconditioned from harmful attitudes by an educational process and conditioned to perform various motor and neuromuscular skills during labor. These conditioned responses were thought to take precedence in the stimulus-response cycle and were registered in the cortex as an area of excitation which subsequently inhibited or interfered with the registering of painful stimuli in the brain.

More recent investigations on pain by Livingston, Melzack, and Wall suggest a fuller explanation for the effectiveness of psychoprophylactic childbirth preparation. According to this theory, referred to as the gate-control theory, the central nervous system is capable of effectively blocking or reducing pain under certain conditions. It is suggested that local physical stimulation, such as the stroking activity done in labor, can balance the pain stimuli by closing down a gate type of mechanism thought to exist in the cord. Activity within the cord itself, such as is created when the woman performs various neuromuscular and motor skills, further modifies the transmission of pain. Finally, selective and directed cortical activity, such as the various cognitive activities related to analyzing and directing one's behavior and concentrating on breathing and relaxation skills, is proposed to activate and close the gating mechanism as well. This theory points out the need for the creation and maintenance of a supportive environment and the development of trusting relationships as essential to the structuring of an atmosphere in which the various higher mental activities can be successfully implemented. The woman learns to respond to labor in an active and directed manner. As she concentrates on controlling and directing her behavior and activities, and as she performs these skills in a supportive situation, modification in the transmission of pain signals is thought to occur in the relays to and from the brain.

Perhaps other elements of behavior and learning, such as behavioral modification, also operate to create this highly structured system of preparation. Further exploration of these related areas is necessary before definitive explanations can be made.

preparation for childbirth

Family-centered maternity care was an academically accepted concept for decades, it was applied at first to the postpartum period, with rooming-in and flexible visiting for new fathers. At this level, husbands were included in prenatal classes but were permitted limited actual participation during labor. Their involvement was generally confined to the hours of waiting, at home or in the waiting room. If the husband was admitted to the labor room, it was under closely regulated conditions.

NEED FOR A COACH

For a long time in this country, the husband's presence during the actual birth was limited to a handful of men in unique circumstances. More recently, this situation has dramatically changed.

Informed couples sought to share this experience; prepared husbands began to be included as part of the supporting group throughout labor and delivery. Only then did family-centered maternity care become a practical experience as well as an academic idea.

The practitioners of the psychoprophylactic method of prepared childbirth, in particular, have strongly advocated the active participation of the husband or of a labor coach. It has been recognized that not only does the laboring woman desperately want to help herself (which preparation provides), but that the presence of a caring person, knowledgeable in what should be done for support, has a discernibly calming effect during this time of physical and emotional stress. Although proponents of psychoprophylaxis suggest that the husband may be best suited for this role, room must be made for the many situations where the father is not part of the woman's current environment. The father needs to be an involved participant in the preparation period so that he understands his role as coach as well as the mechanics of labor, his wife's responses, and appropriate techniques.

In studies of husband-coached childbirth, the couple's relationship, both as husband and wife and as parents, was found to be affected. Each spoke of the other in new appreciation; the bond seemed to be strengthened; couples had new perspectives on their marital and parental roles. These subjective findings are now gaining the attention of behavioral scientists, who are verifying in objective studies the validity of such observations.

EFFECTS OF PREPARATION

The effects of preparation for childbirth are seen during the prenatal period as both men and women acquire information, gain appreciation for each other's role, and evaluate and develop realistic goals. The anxieties of pregnancy are not limited to the woman, but extend to her husband or mate, creating the *pregnant couple.* Parent education in preparation for childbirth must deal with these anxieties as well. Such preparation seeks not only to present the husband with the same factual information as his wife, but to give him a sense of importance and relevance during the birth experience. He gains an appreciation of the physical effort of birth as well as the assurance that he, too, will be prepared to function in specific and definite ways as part of the childbirth preparation team.

In the psychoprophylactic method of prepared childbirth, the woman learns how to integrate the physical, emotional, and intellectual aspects of her personality so that she can work as a harmonious and focused unit throughout the complex demands of labor. This response is in contrast to that of the unprepared woman who remains out of focus as labor approaches and who finds the physi-

cal and emotional responses in labor dominating and opposing rational thought processes.

Through disciplined learning and through the concentrated application of technique and information during labor, the prepared woman is better able to cope with the strenuous demands of labor. She controls her body and checks the inclination of "flight"; she works cooperatively *with* the process of labor, enhancing the work effort during all stages. She has learned to minimize fatigue by reducing unnecessary and distracting activity, both during contractions and in the contraction intervals. By sophisticated and conscious control of her body, she effects a significant reduction of psychic tension and its components of anxiety, fearful anticipation, and heightened perception of pain. (The need for analgesics, anesthetics, and obstetric intervention is dramatically reduced, with benefit to both mother and baby.)

During birth, the prepared woman works more efficiently and is able to cooperate. Because she has been intellectually prepared to understand the mechanism of the second stage, she can use her body more effectively, again with benefit to herself and the baby (Figure 7·1).

Immediately after birth, the woman will be characteristically excited and pleased with her efforts. With the absence of analgesics or anesthetics, or a reduction in their use, potential aftereffects, such as alterations in vital signs, mental confusion, anxiety regarding the baby, headaches, are eliminated.

The cooperative efforts of the mother to enhance the work of labor and reduce or eliminate the use of medication and anesthetics produce important benefits to the newborn. Apgar scores are consistently good in normal infants; in low-birthweight and defective babies, such lack of depression and improvement of oxygenation may have an important impact on their survival.

Summary The total result of preparation

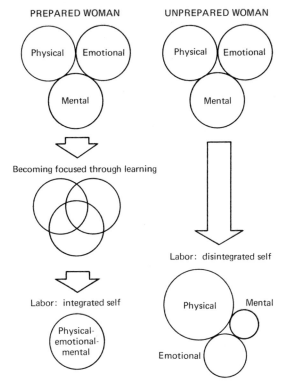

PREPARED WOMAN

Physical   Emotional

Mental

Becoming focused through learning

Labor: integrated self

Physical-
emotional-
mental

UNPREPARED WOMAN

Physical   Emotional

Mental

Labor: disintegrated self

Physical   Mental

Emotional

fig. 7·1 Diagram of results of childbirth preparation. Through preparation for childbirth, the woman learns to integrate herself, physically, emotionally, and intellectually, so that she remains focused and in control throughout labor. The conditioning process allows her to meet each contraction with an appropriate technique; she substitutes new, learned responses to the stimuli (contractions), which significantly reduce or eliminate pain. By contrast, the unprepared woman remains out of focus, so that her reactions disintegrate under the stress of labor. Anticipatory anxiety and the contraction itself signal "pain"; she responds with diverse and inappropriate reactions, breath holding, muscular tension, psychic tension, unnecessary activity, crying out, loss of control.
(*From Constance R. Castor,* Participating in Childbirth: A Parents' Guide, *2d ed., Council of Childbirth Education Specialists, New York, 1973. By permission of the author.)*

for childbirth extends beyond the specific performance of technique during labor into an improved physical and emotional readiness for parenthood for both husband and wife and discernible benefits to the newborn.

SELECTION OF PHYSICIAN, CLINIC, AND HOSPITAL

Parents-to-be should select their doctor, clinic, and hospital on the basis of their decision to be a prepared couple in the birth experience. Couples will be concerned with hospital facilities and policies. Most prepared women desire the atmosphere and milieu of a family-centered maternity care unit as a continuation of their prenatal education and labor participation. The medical community is responding with significant changes directly related to consumer demands.

Until recently the outlook for the clinic patient was bleak. The impersonal nature of many clinics, the staffing procedures, and other clinic policies made it difficult for the woman to be assured of a supportive situation or a sympathetic acceptance of the idea of prepared childbirth. As effective teaching practices are being perfected for the clinic situation, as clinic personnel are being educated regarding the benefits of preparation for childbirth, and as cultural differences are receiving more respect, effective classes are being formed in many clinic settings. It remains with the woman or couple to seek that clinic which provides the opportunity for sharing this experience. Word-of-mouth communication and public relations efforts will acquaint the community with the availability of these programs.

Participation in programs of preparation should not be limited to parent-initiated requests. As physicians, nurses, and hospitals become more familiar with its concepts and more comfortable with its practical implementation, all pregnant women when first entering prenatal care should be introduced to the availability of preparation and education for birth. The interview skills of the maternity nurse specialist will be able to make this a fact of information and not an expectation.

The couple needs to understand that physicians and health care facilities may not be enthusiastic proponents of husband-coached childbirth, but rather, will reflect a more modest acceptance and willingness to help the woman help herself within the bounds of good obstetric practice. With increased experience and information, however, the medical community must measurably progress toward the establishment of that ideal calm and supportive environment, sharing a mutual commitment and enthusiasm for education and preparation for childbirth.

SOURCES OF CLASSES FOR PREPARATION FOR CHILDBIRTH

The growing interest in prepared childbirth and the concurrent trend in obstetrics toward minimal use of pharmacologic agents have created an ever-increasing demand for classes in prepared childbirth. This need is being met by expanded parent education programs of hospitals, health agencies, specialized interest groups, and private practitioners.

Parent education courses offered by health agencies and institutions have commonly been general in approach and content. The classes vary in length from three to eight sessions and may be taken at any point in pregnancy. Informal group discussions led by a resource person focus on various aspects of pregnancy (hygiene, nutrition, exercise) and a general introduction to labor, delivery, postnatal recovery, and the newborn (care, feeding). The aim has been to help parents gain an understanding of the pregnancy-birth continuum, and to understand and cope with anxiety, rather than to teach specific techniques of prepared childbirth. More of these institutional programs are now incorporating techniques for labor, often in addition to the general prenatal series. The curriculum is then expanded to include some or all of the content discussed below. Many agencies prefer to continue the general courses, which they feel meet the total community's needs, and to refer interested parents to the childbirth educator in private or group practice.

The Red Cross offers prenatal classes and baby care classes without charge. Taught by a registered nurse, these classes usually are attended by women during the day. Visiting nurse services may offer classes to groups of pregnant women, especially to young teenagers in community agencies. In fact, the interest level is high enough so that classes could be started in many noninstitutional sites.

Concern for quality has emerged with the sudden upsurge of interest. Several groups now prepare childbirth education specialists. (Information about further preparation can be obtained from the Maternity Center Association and Council of Childbirth Education Specialists.)

THE CHILDBIRTH EDUCATOR

One of the most important sources for classes in specific techniques of prepared childbirth is the nurse engaged in private or group practice as a childbirth educator. As a private practitioner, the childbirth educator provides a program which incorporates current trends in technique and philosophy, whereas institutions must be responsive to more general community needs and more fixed hospital policies.

The course is more structured in format and extends for five or six weekly sessions near the end of pregnancy. The focus is on specifically preparing a couple for the work of giving birth. The program includes a presentation of the philosophy and goals of prepared childbirth, emotional and physical changes of pregnancy, detailed analysis of the stages of labor, and expectations for the immediate postpartum period. Central to the program is the learning of specific techniques and physical conditioning exercises. Parents are usually referred for baby care classes and hospital tours.

It is hoped that in future developments, complete childbirth preparation will be provided within the context of the woman's total prenatal and postnatal care, as an integral part of her physician's, hospital's, or clinic's program.

barriers to preparation for childbirth

We must consider the woman's culture, education, attitude, family, and economic status when seeking the barriers to preparation for childbirth.

In certain cultural groups, the lack of interest by the woman's husband or family, or their overt opposition to and degrading of her interest, is a sufficiently strong factor to deter her consideration of these programs *unless* such preparation is an integral part of her prenatal care, as suggested earlier. If she views her husband's active participation as essential, even though he might not oppose her interest, she is likely not to choose the course.

Other cultural, social, temperamental, or maturational factors influence the woman and her involvement. Such preparation for childbirth may violate sexual taboos, cultural expectations, or family structure. If the woman has unresolved conflicts about her sexuality, this pregnancy, and/or motherhood, the probability of her participation will be reduced.

Lack of participation may logically arise out of lack of information or misinterpretation. Although somewhat interested in the idea of learning to help herself, the woman may be unaware of the availability of classes in her community and, lacking strong motivation, fail to seek out such information.

She may be uninformed as to the basic concepts of childbirth preparation, especially if she is a member of a lower socioeconomic or a culturally deprived group. With a smattering of information, she may misinterpret the purpose and goals of these programs. These particular deterrents can be significantly modified by the accurate presentation of the purpose and availability of classes to the whole community.

Fatigue and other physical factors may seriously affect her attitude toward and her motivation in seeking out and attending classes. Intrinsic to her attitude is her self-image and her concept of the uniqueness of her role in the childbirth experience. If she lacks positive feelings about herself as a worthwhile person, as a mature individual able to cope with her life situation, she is apt not to consider this preparation. In addition, whether or not she and her husband see preparation for childbirth as a worthwhile expenditure of effort and money will influence consideration and choice of prenatal education.

Other factors are influential in excluding participation. Classes must be made available at convenient times and locations for the couple, and the cost must be reasonable for all socioeconomic groups. Childbirth educators in private or group practice must make known their willingness to accept reduced fees if low-cost programs are not otherwise available.

The attitude of the various authority figures responsible for her prenatal care cannot be overlooked. Unless a woman is highly motivated, rejection of the concepts of childbirth preparation and participation by doctor or nurse will block her from participating in a program.

In many instances, several factors are present simultaneously which effectively block preparation.

SUMMARY

We can say that classes in preparation for childbirth are becoming more widely available throughout the country. Programs are being broadened to include women and couples from low economic groups as well as the middle class.

Couples interested in active participation in the birth experience can be expected to investigate and select prenatal care and hospital on the basis of interest in and support of family-centered preparation for labor and postpartum care.

At the present time, many women and couples do not enter prenatal preparation or are excluded from participation despite its acknowledged benefits; for example, the teen-ager, the unmarried, those from minority groups, the immature, the very frightened, are seldom seen in class unless a special attempt is made to include them. Accurate information and an inclusion of preparation as an intrinsic part of prenatal care may act to eliminate many of these barriers.

nursing approach in childbirth education

The goals of parent education will determine the content of classes. The central goal should be the reduction of anxiety and fear through the dissemination of accurate information. The direction and depth of this information will be determined by the needs and interests of the participants. Keeping in mind the need to reduce anxiety, reinforce the normalcy of childbirth, and enhance each couple's self-esteem, the childbirth educator evaluates class objectives, content, and approach.

In presenting factual information pertaining to pregnancy, labor, and the postpartum period, the teacher directs the discussion to the needs, awareness, and intellectual capacities of the group. The content must be appropriate, relevant, and readily understood. There must be sufficient detail to give the couple an accurate and realistic picture of labor, presented in a positive manner which

will enhance self-esteem and not heighten preexisting anxieties. Effective learning can then take place. Since the classes take place in the third trimester, there must be an awareness of how the concerns and anxieties of the couple are focused. Concerns about the baby's normalcy, the woman's ability to give birth safely, and the ambivalence regarding parenthood are the major focus during this period.

The teacher works to create a pleasant, relaxed atmosphere so that the couples can verbalize questions and underlying anxieties without fear of rejection. The childbirth educator establishes herself as a concerned and knowledgeable resource person. Thoughtful and appropriate answers must be given, which reflect awareness of the meaning of the question. Does a husband simply want a piece of information, or is he expressing a particular anxiety? In asking about medication, is the woman reflecting on her goals, her fears for herself, or for her baby?

As an atmosphere of acceptance, knowledgeability, and self-awareness is established, the couple will begin to see themselves as unique and yet within the normal context of childbearing. The group experience itself assists in developing this attitude. The couple's reactions and feelings are no longer mysterious or capricious, but become more manageable and understandable. Independent and self-sufficient women in particular are helped to accept their new dependency needs and vacillating energy states.

As the couple perfects various neuromuscular and respiratory skills related to childbirth, the effective childbirth educator sees to it that important communication skills are also established. She gives opportunity for the exploration of feelings, continually involving the husbands in nonthreatening ways. As the classes progress, the nurse-teacher underscores the validity of the man's role both in class and during the childbirth. She directs comments and questions to the husbands, asking them to solve specific labor problems. Basic to all this is the introduction of the husband's role as chief supporter—or coach—from the very first session. His role is continually built as the important caring person needed by his wife during labor. In a more general way, the childbirth educator encourages a mutual respect for the specific roles of both husband and wife during the childbirth experience. She fosters the concept of birth as a family experience and of the couple as an informed and cooperating team.

Through this learning experience the couple becomes independent, knowledgeable, and cooperative, and learns that it can manage a stress situation. The skills and confidence thus developed will, it is hoped, encourage the growth of the couple as a family unit, able to deal with the ongoing stresses of family life.

SUMMARY OF BASIC GOALS OF CHILDBIRTH EDUCATION

1. Minimize anxieties, correct misconceptions, and reduce fear by providing factual information on pregnancy, labor, and the postpartum period in detail and terms suitable for pregnant couples.
2. Teach neuromuscular, motor, and respiratory skills, proficiency in which will enhance the woman's response to labor and her ability to deal with it intelligently and cooperatively.
3. Provide an accurate framework of reference for the pregnant couple in which they will see their responses, concerns, anxieties, and fears appropriately.
4. Create a setting in which cooperative, independent, and knowledgeable parents can effectively utilize both verbal and nonverbal communication skills.
5. Develop a relaxed and open atmosphere

conducive to learning and growing in self-awareness.

CONTENT OF CLASSES

Introductory Class The introductory class sets the tone of acceptance and credibility. The learning process by which the couple increases in self-awareness and ability to master the skills essential to control in labor begins. The childbirth educator excites the couple with the potential for control and comfort during labor when utilizing the techniques to be taught. The presentation is such that each couple determines its own needs and goals within the context of preparation for childbirth, and begins to learn how these needs and goals will be met during the classes. It is in this session that the couple can be helped to see themselves as a pregnant couple for which certain physical and emotional reactions are entirely normal.

The teacher facilitates group interaction by introducing herself and class participants by first and last names. (Couples should feel that they are all together as people about to become parents who share a mutual desire to learn how to help themselves.) Introductions should be limited to simple information: name, parity, due date, community, and hospital. Describing occupations might unnecessarily divide the group along socioeconomic lines.

General comments as to the purpose of the course are made. Realistic goals are presented and some basic concepts introduced. Parents need to understand that they will establish their own goals as the class evolves. Although couples are easily overwhelmed by a too complex explanation of theory and methodology, a discussion of the basic principles upon which the techniques operate is important.

Since the class is still a collection of persons and not as yet a group, couples respond more readily to concrete and factual details as opposed to theoretic concepts. Using visual aids, such as the Maternity Center's *Birth Atlas* (Fig. 7·2), the childbirth educator presents pertinent information on conception and the trimesters of pregnancy. By discussing this in a parallel outline of fetal development and maternal changes, the childbirth educator reinforces the reality of the baby and the understanding of self. Using words like, "Now your baby's heart can be heard," helps the couple to identify *their* baby, particularly if it is their first. Comments such as, "Many women feel very tired at this point," or, "You may have become very nervous about being home alone," not only establish the nurse's insight into pregnancy but again enhance self-awareness.

fig. 7·2 Using visual aids, the childbirth educator discusses the birth process with the parents.

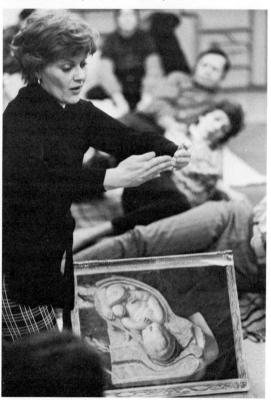

Physical conditioning exercises are appropriate to this first class (Fig. 7·3). Couples are anxious to *do* something. These exercises (described in Figs. 7·4 to 7·9) basically serve to increase the woman's sense of well-being and physical comfort during pregnancy. They are directed not toward the development of muscular strength, but toward improvement of circulation, ventilation, body awareness, and posture.

The couple also begins the mastery of neuromuscular control and the development of teamwork. Controlled relaxation is the foundation upon which all other techniques are applied. The woman begins to develop her body awareness. She learns how to be comfortable, to detect tension in her body, and to facilitate relaxation. Her husband begins to learn to detect tension in his wife by touch and observation. Together they concentrate on achieving the active (vs. passive) relaxation necessary for control during labor. The husband is encouraged to touch and stroke his wife in ways to enhance relaxation and rest. Stroking always accompanies the verbal cue, "Relax," so that stroking itself soon becomes a signal for relaxation.

Intermediate Classes Building on the information and rapport of the introductory class, the childbirth educator expands subsequent classes with a logical progression. Content is carefully structured to parallel the interest and awareness of the couple, their understanding of the mechanism of labor, and their emotional responses during labor, as well as the development of labor itself. Couples need a clear understanding of what happens, how the mother will feel and react, how she can cope with each particular phase, and how her husband can support and direct her efforts.

In teaching the second stage, for instance, the childbirth educator needs to be alert to the anxiety about and fear of giving birth. Attitudes of sexuality, fear of safety, misconceptions relating to the second stage, and

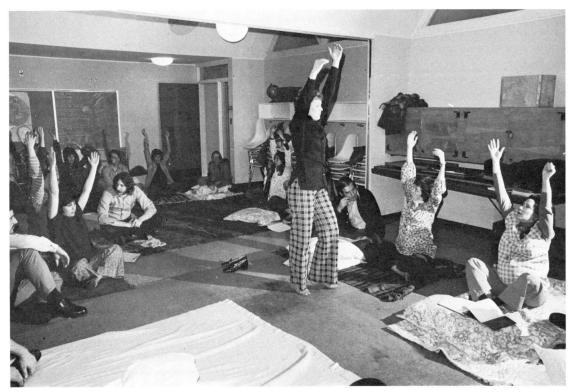

fig. 7·3 The childbirth educator starts the class with a warm-up exercise, which also helps to improve ventilation and increase the woman's sense of well-being.

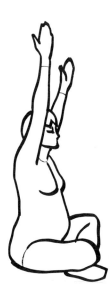

fig. 7·4 Tailor reach exercise. The woman alternately reaches (in a rhythmic pattern) with arms stretched toward the ceiling. This exercise tones both the upper part of the chest and the upper back muscles, and promotes good ventilation. (*From Constance R. Castor,* Participating in Childbirth: A Parents' Guide, *2d ed., Council of Childbirth Education Specialists, New York,* 1973. *By permission of the author.*)

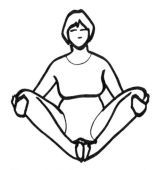

fig. 7·5 Tailor press exercise. Woman learns to use thigh muscles to press knees toward floor, using slight resistance with hands. This exercise helps to relieve hip tension and low backache. (*From Constance R. Castor,* Participating in Childbirth: A Parents' Guide, *2d ed., Council of Childbirth Education Specialists, New York,* 1973. *By permission of the author.*)

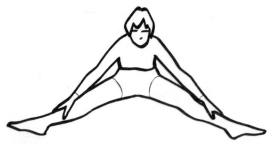

fig. 7·6 Tailor stretch exercise. Sitting on the floor and bending from the hips, the woman stretches forward, sliding her hands toward the ankles. This exercise also relieves hip tension and low-back distress. (*From Constance R. Castor*, Participating in Childbirth: A Parents' Guide, *2d ed., Council of Childbirth Education Specialists, New York*, 1973. *By permission of the author.*)

inaccurate information contribute to these fears of pain and injury held by both husband and wife. It is essential that the couple gain an accurate and positive understanding of the mechanism of birth and a realistic expectation about their ability to work with the birth process.

Concluding Class The couple's proficiency in technique and knowledge of labor must be reviewed and evaluated. One effective technique is the use of role playing in a variety of real-life situations. Their responses can be evaluated by the group to determine the most effective and appropriate approach.

The nurse can introduce material pertinent to the postpartum period. Couples need a

fig. 7·7 Childbirth educator demonstrates the back-roll exercise, used as a passive pelvic tilt for pregnancy and as a preparation for the expulsive technique to be learned later on.

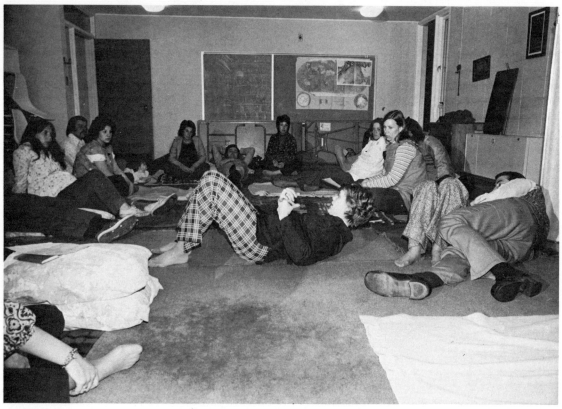

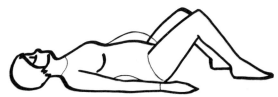

fig. 7·8 Pelvic tilt exercise. Using abdominal and buttocks muscles, the woman rotates the pelvis up, pressing the small of back against the floor. Knees are bent to stabilize the pelvis. This exercise relieves low backache and hip tension, as well as toning the abdominal muscles. (*From Constance R. Castor,* Participating in Childbirth: A Parents' Guide, *2d ed., Council for Childbirth Education Specialists, New York, 1973. By permission of the author.*)

basic awareness of the physical changes and emotional and social adjustments of the recovery period.

They also need to be prepared for the rather "unfinished" qualities of their newborn, as well as his demands and needs. The impact of the firstborn, both in terms of the mother's physical recovery and the parents' adjustments to being parents, must not be minimized.

First-time mothers need to be made aware that they will not suddenly be transformed into the romanticized image of motherhood but will grow into an ability to mother.

Many primigravidas are unprepared for the various aspects of physical recovery, such as lochial flow, involution, breast engorgement, fatigue, and emotional lability. A brief discussion of what to expect aids understanding of the physiology of the recovery period, as well as providing a few practical suggestions for dealing with this recuperative and restorative period.

SAMPLE CLASS OUTLINE: PSYCHOPROPHYLAXIS

I. Introductory class
    A. Introduce self and fellow class participants.

fig. 7·9 Bent leg lift exercise. The pelvis is stabilized by bending the knees and tilting the pelvis up. The woman alternately bends each knee over the abdomen, extends the leg toward the ceiling, lowers it, and slides it along the floor to the starting position. This exercise relieves low backache and hip tension, and tones the leg muscles. (*From Constance R. Castor,* Participating in Childbirth: A Parents' Guide, *2d ed., Council of Childbirth Education, Specialists, New York, 1973. By permission of the author.*)

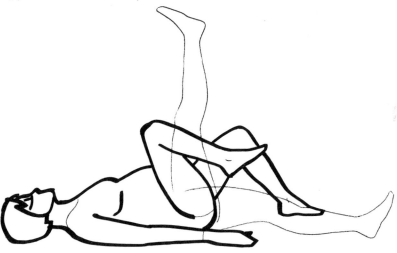

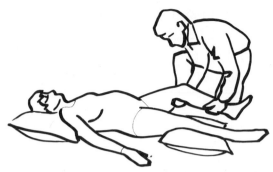

fig. 7·10 Controlled relaxation. In this neuromuscular technique, the woman learns to facilitate relaxation consciously while her husband learns how to enhance their teamwork through new verbal and nonverbal communication skills. (*From Constance R. Castor*, Participating in Childbirth: A Parents' Guide, *2d ed., Council of Childbirth Education Specialists, New York, 1973. By permission of the author.*)

B. Discuss basic purpose and goals of the course.

C. Present information pertaining to the basic concepts of psychoprophylaxis.

D. Discuss highlights of conception, fetal development, maternal reactions, and physical changes, using visual aids.

E. Teach physical conditioning exercises, discussing rationale and using demonstration and group participation.
   1. Tailor press
   2. Tailor stretch
   3. Tailor reach
   4. Pelvic tilt
   5. Bent-leg lift
   6. Perineal control (Kegal exercise)

F. Teach basics of controlled relaxation,

fig. 7·11 The nurse demonstrates how to encourage and facilitate relaxation.

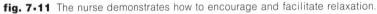

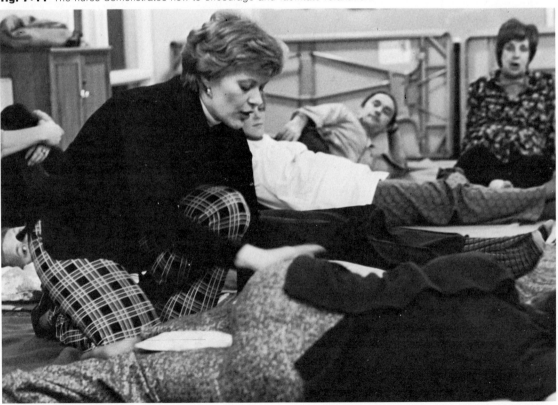

using demonstration and group participation: (Figs. 7·10, 7·11)

1. Achieving comfort
2. Facilitating relaxation
3. Self-detection of tension and relaxation
4. Husband/coach's detection of tension and relaxation
5. Role of touching and stroking to enhance relaxation
6. Use of precise verbal cues
7. Development of gross muscular control

II. Intermediate classes (three or four)

A. Perfect controlled relaxation technique
B. Introduce and develop the mechanism of labor, using visual aids.
C. Discuss related maternal reactions and emotional responses to the mechanism of labor.
D. Teach various labor techniques in which the couple needs to become proficient, using demonstration, visual aids, and group participation:
   1. Integration of controlled relaxation
   2. Rationale for respiratory techniques (Fig. 7·12)
   3. Rhythmic chest breathing

fig. 7·12 Practicing breathing technique for labor. The woman's coach is learning how to evaluate her breathing patterns and how to enhance relaxation under stress.

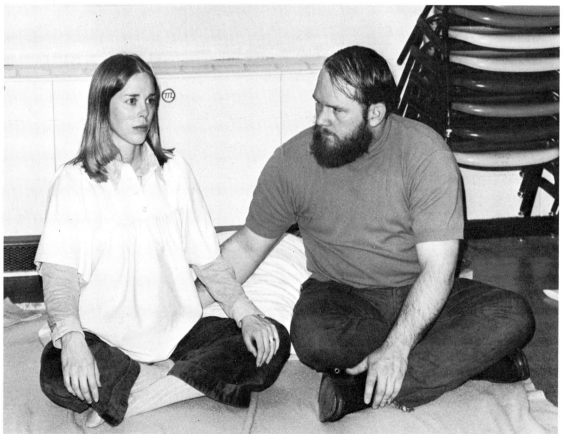

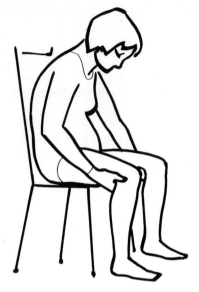

fig. 7·13 Expulsive technique. The woman must learn to master her body for effective and efficient work during the second stage. She learns how her position, respiratory rhythm, and voluntary muscular activity enhance the pushing effort. Her husband learns cue words to remind her of the correct technique. By first learning the expulsion techniques sitting in a hard chair, the woman becomes aware of how her body works while in a more comfortable position for advanced pregnancy. Once she has perfected this, she learns how to do these same actions in the more common labor position (Fig. 9·10). (*From Constance R. Castor,* Participating in Childbirth: A Parents' Guide, *2d ed., Council of Childbirth Education Specialists, New York, 1973. By permission of the author.*)

    a. Slow rate
    b. Modified rate
  4. Shallow chest breathing
    a. Combined with rhythmic chest breathing (modified rate)
    b. Rhythmic pattern of shallow breathing and short blows
  5. Recognizing, preventing, and dealing with hyperventilation
  6. Expulsion techniques
    a. Overcoming fear of pushing
    b. Integrating controlled relaxation (especially perineal)
    c. Effective use of abdominal muscles in directing pushing effort
    d. Correct position to enhance the work effort (Fig. 7·13)
    e. Respiratory patterns to enhance work effort
    f. Effective coaching in expulsion
    g. Control of pushing effort
  7. Managing back labor
 E. Develop the couple's confidence and self-awareness, through discussion.
 F. Introduce couples to various community resources, e.g., baby care classes, visiting nurse services, family planning services.
 G. Review class content through role playing, nonthreatening question periods, and class participation.
 H. Acquaint couples with local hospital facilities and policies, using tours, visual aids, and discussion.

III. Goals and content of concluding class
 A. Complete review of mechanism of labor, maternal reactions, labor techniques, and husband's role, through discussion, role playing, and visual aids.
 B. Discuss immediate postpartum period, using group discussion:
  1. Physical recuperation
  2. Emotional responses
  3. Emotional needs
  4. Hospital facilities: recovery area, postpartum unit, nursery
 C. Discuss newborn, using group discussion.
  1. Appearance at birth
  2. Care of infant in delivery room

3. Characteristics of newborn during first few days
4. Need for mother's physical contact
5. Feeding, if pertinent to class needs
D. Discuss postpartum period at home, using group discussion:
   1. Physical changes
   2. Emotional needs and responses
   3. Simple exercises to improve muscle tone and sense of well-being
   4. Husband's needs and role

bibliography

Chabon, Irwin: *Awake and Aware*, Dell Publishing Co., Inc., New York, 1969.

Chertok, L.: *Motherhood and Personality*, J. B. Lippincott Company, Philadelphia, 1969.

Goodrich, F. W., Jr.: *Preparing for Childbirth*, Prentice-Hall, Inc., Englewood Cliffs, N. J., 1966.

Lamaze, Ferdinand: *Painless Childbirth*, Simon & Schuster, Inc., New York, 1972.

Livingston, W. K.: "What Is Pain?" *Scientific American*, March, 1953, p. 3.

Melzack, R.: "The Perception of Pain," *Scientific American*, February, 1961, p. 3.

——— and K. Casey: "Neutral Mechanisms of Pain: A Conceptual Model," in *New Concepts of Pain and Its Management*, F. A. Davis Company, Philadelphia, 1967.

Richardson, S., and A. Guttmacher: *Childbearing—Its Social and Psychological Aspects*, The Williams & Wilkins Company, Baltimore, 1967.

Siegele, Dorothy: "The Gate Control Theory," *American Journal of Nursing*, **74**(4):498, 1974.

Tanzer, Deborah: *Why Natural Childbirth?* Doubleday & Company, Inc., Garden City, N.Y., 1972.

RESOURCES

Teacher Preparation Courses:

Council of Childbirth Education Specialists, 168 West 86th St., New York, N.Y. 10024 (psychoprophylaxis).

Maternity Center Association, 48 East 92 St., New York, N.Y.
(psychophysical).

Also: consult local childbirth preparation group.

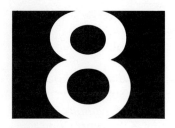

process
of labor

Jean C. Metzger

Birth is defined as "the act of being born or of bringing forth." During the period of time referred to as labor, the uterus must deliver the mature or nearly mature products of conception. To accomplish this the cervix of the uterus must open far enough to allow the baby's head, its largest part, to exit. Then the baby must be pushed down the birth canal and through the vulvar opening. As it descends, the fetus is maneuvered so as to aim its narrowest dimensions through the fixed dimensions of the mother's bony pelvis, thereby meeting with the least resistance possible.

Following expulsion of the fetus, the placenta separates from its site and is expelled, allowing the uterus to contract further to prevent excessive bleeding.

The human fetus customarily is adequately developed for survival outside the uterus at approximately 266 days of age, and labor normally occurs at about this time. Irregularities in the menstrual cycle make precise calculation of the date of conception difficult in some pregnancies. Beyond this, a variety of abnormal conditions in the mother and/or the fetus may cause labor to be initiated earlier or later. However, 2 weeks in either direction has generally been accepted as normal.

initiation of labor

Initiation of labor at the time of fetal readiness for survival, specific for each species including Homo sapiens, is a wonder which continues to be studied and debated in search of a cause. A combination of some or all of the theories put forth is most probable. The theories include:

1. A decrease in placental production of progesterone probably occurs as a result of placental aging. Progesterone is believed to prevent transmission of impulses which would cause contractions starting in one area to spread throughout the whole uterus. This has been difficult to demonstrate in human beings, but it has been demonstrated experimentally that a precursor of progesterone effected a decrease in frequency, though not in intensity, of contractions (1).
2. A limit to uterine volume or stretch may be reached. This theory is supported by the occurrence of premature labor in multiple pregnancies and hydramnios. (It is contradicted, however, by the occurrence of labor at what would be term when fetal growth has ceased several months earlier because of intrauterine death.)
3. A sudden decrease in uterine size often occurs just before labor starts. Also, labor often is stimulated by spontaneous or artificial rupture of membranes, perhaps as the result of sudden shortening of muscle fibers.
4. Endogenous hormonal stimulation of a "ready" uterus may be part of labor initiation. The uterus has been shown to be increasingly responsive to exogenous oxytocin as pregnancy moves toward term. Though increases in the circulating blood have not been observed before labor, there is an increase of endogenous oxytocin in venous blood during labor (2).

Prostaglandins, which also have a positive effect on uterine contractility, are being studied as to their relationship to labor. Though they have not been detected in the plasma prior to onset of labor, they are present in blood and amniotic fluid during labor (3).

5. Fetal adrenal activity has been demonstrated to affect the timing of onset of labor. Destroying the pituitary or hypothalamus in animal fetuses has been shown to prolong gestation, while premature labor was produced when the fetal adrenals were stimulated by injecting ACTH directly into the fetus. The former situation is paralleled in the extended gestation of a human anencephalic fetus in which the pituitary is missing and the adrenals, therefore, are very small (4).

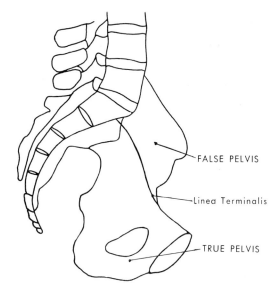

fig. 8·1 True pelvis and "false pelvis," divided by the linea terminalis. (*Courtesy of Ross Laboratories, Clinical Education Aid No. 18.*)

maternal pelvic dimensions

The pelvis is divided longitudinally at the linea terminalis into the false pelvis above and the true pelvis below (Fig. 8·1). The false pelvis, together with the abdominal muscles, provides for protection and support of the growing fetus after it rises out of the pelvic cavity, and directs it into the true pelvis at term.

The true pelvis provides the framework of the birth passageway. For a normal delivery, this passageway must be large enough to accommodate the baby. The pelvic cavity has ample room on the whole, but there are three narrow points which require evaluation.

1. The *pelvic inlet—(superior strait)* (Fig. 8·2). The boundaries (the pubis, the sacral promontory, and the linea terminalis of the ischium) form a slightly oval circle with a posterior indentation caused by the sacrum. The *gynecoid pelvis* (Fig. 26·3) has dimensions which are best suited to the shape and size of the baby's skull. The

dimensions can be approximated on vaginal examination by measuring from the sacral promontory to the lower edge of the symphysis pubis (the diagonal conjugate) (Fig. 8·3), and making adjustments for the dimensions of the conjugata vera and the obstetric conjugate. If the diagonal conjugate is more than 11.5 cm it is considered normal.

2. The *interspinous diameter* in the midpelvis. The distance between the ischial spines is the narrowest diameter in the canal and is therefore of great significance. It can be estimated digitally or measured with a special instrument, and is considered normal if at least 10 cm. The anteroposterior diameter parallel with the ischial spines from the sacrum to the lower surface of the pubis should measure 11.5 cm.

3. The *pelvic outlet (inferior strait)* (Fig. 8·4). This consists of two triangles with the transverse intertuberous diameter providing the base for both. This diameter can be

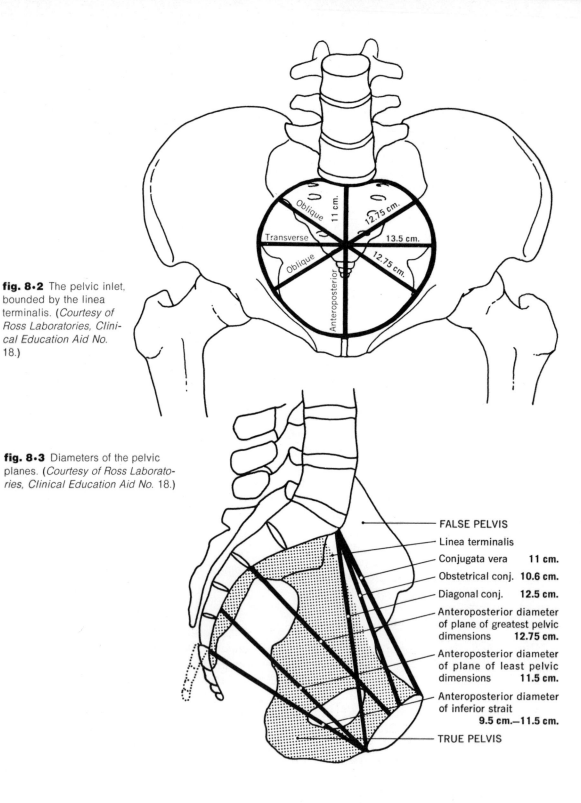

fig. 8·2 The pelvic inlet, bounded by the linea terminalis. (*Courtesy of Ross Laboratories, Clinical Education Aid No. 18.*)

fig. 8·3 Diameters of the pelvic planes. (*Courtesy of Ross Laboratories, Clinical Education Aid No. 18.*)

Oblique 11 cm.

12.75 cm.

Transverse 13.5 cm.

Oblique 12.75 cm.

Anteroposterior

FALSE PELVIS

Linea terminalis

Conjugata vera   **11 cm.**

Obstetrical conj.   **10.6 cm.**

Diagonal conj.   **12.5 cm.**

Anteroposterior diameter of plane of greatest pelvic dimensions   **12.75 cm.**

Anteroposterior diameter of plane of least pelvic dimensions   **11.5 cm.**

Anteroposterior diameter of inferior strait   **9.5 cm.—11.5 cm.**

TRUE PELVIS

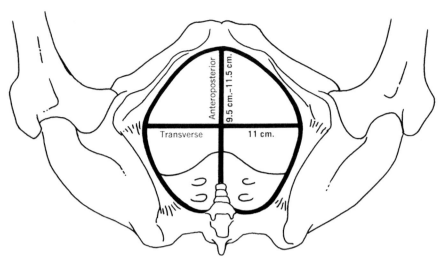

fig. 8·4 The pelvic outlet. Note pubic arch of at least 90°. (*Courtesy of Ross Laboratories, Clinical Education Aid No. 18.*)

estimated externally, using a fist, or measured with calipers; 8 cm or more is considered adequate. If the angle of the pubic arch is at least 90°, it will allow the baby's head to fit closely as it pivots around the pubis on exit. In measuring the anteroposterior diameter, the mobility of the coccyx is evaluated, as it may be able to move back as much as 2.5 cm when the baby's head pushes against it.

While doing the vaginal examination, the doctor will also evaluate the slope of the walls above and below the spines. If these are straight or almost straight, it is an indication of adequate space. The depth of the sacral curve is also noted, as indication both of space and of forward angulation of the canal toward the outlet (Fig. 8·5). The difference in length between the anterior and posterior surfaces of the canal can be noted, the former being approximately 4 to 5 cm (the height of the pubis), and the latter, 10 to 14 cm (the length of the sacrum).

Precise measurements are sometimes needed if there is suspicion of contraction in one of the areas or an unusually large fetal head. They can be obtained by x-ray or ultrasonography; the latter is preferred to avoid radiation of both the maternal and the fetal gonads. If an x-ray must be obtained, this is done at or near term so as to have the advantage of comparison with the fetal measurements, and care is exercised to keep radiation as low as possible.

fig. 8·5 The angle of the birth canal. A "stovepipe" curve must be negotiated by the fetus during the process of birth. (*Redrawn from E. A. Friedman and J. P. Greenhill,* Biological Principals and Modern Practice of Obstetrics, *W. B. Saunders Company, Philadelphia, 1974.*)

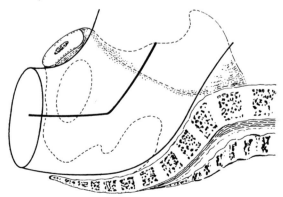

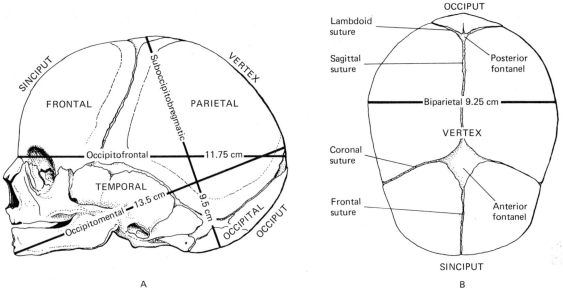

fig. 8·6A Side view of the fetal skull. B Vertex view of the skull. (*Courtesy of Ross Laboratories, from "Phenomena of Normal Labor."*)

dimensions and construction of the fetal skull

Since it is the size of the fetal head relative to that of the maternal pelvis which is of ultimate significance, average diameters of the normal neonatal skull are used for comparison. By noting the several diameters (Fig. 8·6A), it is readily seen that the *suboccipitobregmatic* is the smallest of the anteroposterior dimensions. This explains the desirability as well as frequency of the vertex presentation. Note also the *parietal* diameter, the broadest transverse dimension (Fig. 8·6B).

The baby's head is constructed in such a way that it can change shape as it passes through the birth canal. The bony plates which make up the skull are relatively soft and are loosely joined by membranes, allowing for space between. Not only can the angle of the head be adjusted to present the smallest diameters, but the head can be compressed by means of a narrowing or elimina-

tion of the spaces, or even by an overlapping of the plates. The elongation produced is called *molding*, and may persist for a period of days in the neonate. It is probably not harmful to the fetus if pressure is placed on *just one dimension* of the skull at a time, so that total intercranial space is not decreased. Care is taken to avoid compression over a long period of time, or sudden decompression.

fetal positions during descent

Well into the third trimester the fetus has ample room and may still be found in a variety of positions in the course of a week. During the last few weeks of gestation, as the fetus approaches maximum size and the amount of amniotic fluid decreases somewhat, the *lie* becomes relatively stabilized, although *position* may change in the course of labor.

Lie refers to the relationship of the long axis (or spine) of the fetus to that of the mother. In 99 percent of pregnancies at term, the fetus exhibits a longitudinal lie. Other types are transverse and oblique.

Attitude refers to the position of the parts of the infant's body in relation to itself. Most commonly, the infant assumes what has come to be called "fetal position," with back curved, head flexed so that the chin is close to the chest, knees flexed with thighs resting on the abdomen, and lower legs across the abdomen. Arms are at sides or flexed and crossing over the chest.

The *presenting part* is that part of the fetus closest to the cervix which will be delivered first. This is most commonly *cephalic*, or head first; it is thought that this is because of the pear shape of the uterus, the breech seeking the roomier fundus to allow for movement of the lower limbs.

Presentation refers to the leading area of the presenting part, determined by attitude of the part. In a cephalic presentation, the *vertex* leads in 85 to 90 percent of cases.

By *position* is meant the relationship between an arbitrary point of reference on the presenting part and the four quadrants of the maternal pelvis. The point of reference in a vertex presentation is the *occiput*; in a face presentation, the *chin* (mentum); and in a breech presentation, the *sacrum*. Most commonly at engagement the fetus is in the LOT position (left occiput transverse—see further on, under "Mechanism or Cardinal Movements of Labor") and changes to LOA (left occiput anterior) as it descends (Fig. 8·7). This means that the baby's occiput is directed toward the mother's left side and turns toward the abdominal surface as it descends the birth canal.

STATION

If the head is above the inlet and freely movable, it is said to be *floating*. When the broadest diameter is at or into the pelvic inlet it is said to be *engaged*. When the forward portion has reached the level of the ischial spines it is said to be at *station 0*, which

fig. 8·7 Positions assumed during internal rotation. (*Courtesy of Ross Laboratories, Clinical Education Aid No.* 18.)

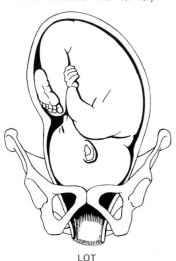

LOT

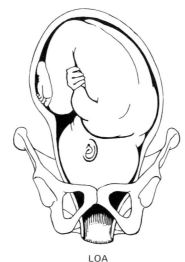

LOA

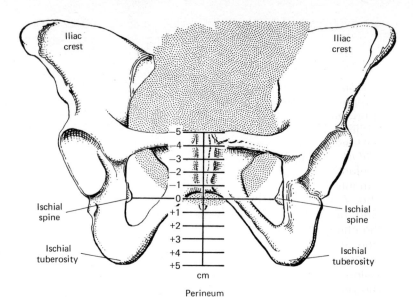

fig. 8·8 Station in relation to descent of the fetal head. (*Courtesy of Ross Laboratories, from "Phenomena of Normal Labor."*)

usually, but not always, indicates engagement. Station refers to the relationship of the presenting part to the ischial spines. Stations above the spines are designated in centimeter gradations as −1, −2, etc.; those below are designated +1, +2, etc., down to the pelvic floor (Fig. 8·8).

DETERMINATION OF FETAL POSITION

It is possible to determine lie, presentation, position, and degree of descent of the fetus by abdominal palpation using the "four maneuvers of Leopold" (Fig. 8·9A, B, C, D). After cervical dilation has begun, vaginal palpation of the fontanels and sutures of the skull, or of other landmarks of face or breech are helpful in determining position and attitude of the presenting part, as well as descent of the fetus in relation to the ischial spines. In certain instances where these methods would be unsuccessful, and it is considered necessary to have the information, x-ray and ultrasonagraphy are considered.

uterine contractions

DESCRIPTION AND MEASUREMENT

As the uterus has grown to fourteen times its prepregnant size, much elastic and fibrous tissue has been added, which strengthens its walls and enhances its contractility. Two different kinds of contraction have been identi-

fig. 8· 9A With thumb and forefingers, press into the lower part of the abdomen just above the symphysis. If the part is hard, round, and freely moveable, it is the head and is not engaged. If the part is firmly fixed, the head is probably engaged. B Press gently with the palms on each side of the abdomen. The general examination will reveal whether the oval shape of the fetus is parallel with the long axis of the mother. Press deeply to feel the smooth curve of the back as contrasted with the unevenness of the extremities. C Palpate the fundus with the fingers. The breech feels soft and irregular, the head hard, round, and freely moveable. D Using the first three fingers of each hand, press deeply into the pelvis, moving toward the inlet. If the fingers almost meet, it indicates that the part is high; if the part is difficult to distinguish, the head has probably become engaged. (*Photos by Ruth Helmich.*)

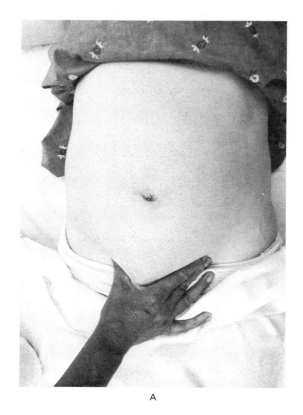

A

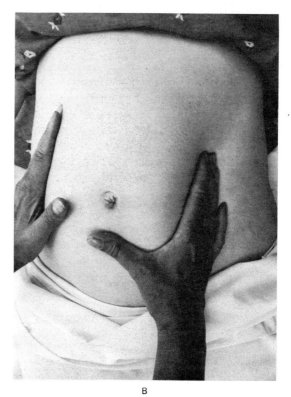

B

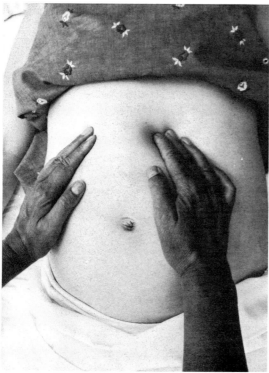

C

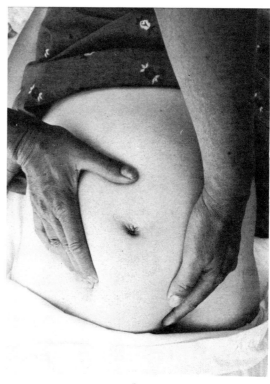

D

fied throughout pregnancy by electronic devices; one kind is regular but very faint, the other stronger and irregular.

In the last trimester, particularly in the last month, one type of contraction becomes stronger, longer-lasting, and more rhythmic. These are called *Hicks contractions*, or sometimes *false contractions*. They can be perceived by the mother and usually by an observer using abdominal palpation. Early ones may be uncomfortable or just detectable. Shortly before onset of active labor, some mothers experience them as quite uncomfortable, though rarely as painful. If measured electronically they rarely exceed 20 mmHg pressure, with a resting tone of 5 to 8 mm, whereas contractions of the first stage average 40 mmHg with a resting tone of about 10 mm.

Contractions are characterized by an *increment* (buildup), an *acme* (plateau), and a *decrement* (relaxing phase) (Fig. 8·10). Electronic equipment is sensitive to the total contraction, measuring and graphically recording the picture, including the rest periods before and after.

In the absence of monitoring equipment, contractions can be measured by palpating the abdomen near the fundus. Provided there is not too much adipose tissue, and the contraction increases in intensity by more than 10 mm over the resting tone, the frequency, duration, and intensity of contractions can be assessed with a reasonable degree of accuracy. The early part of the increment and the late part of the decrement will not be detectable, but *frequency* (from the beginning of one to the beginning of the next contraction), *duration* (from the beginning to end of one contraction), and *intensity* (degree of muscle contraction), can be assessed.

THE WORK

In labor the uterus becomes divided into two portions: the upper muscular portion, which contracts, and the lower uterine segment, which thins and dilates. The *physiologic retraction ring* becomes the dividing line. The contractions are strongest in the area of the fundus, and carry out their work from the top downward, the muscles running approximately vertically in this portion. The activity in the two portions is reciprocal. When the contracting muscles of the upper segment relax, they remain somewhat shortened rather than returning to their prior length. They are en-

fig. 8·10 Intensity, shape, duration, active pressure area, and area of pain sensation of uterine contractions. The contraction is a bell-shaped curve, with a steeper slope during increment. The relaxation phase (decrement) lasts two-thirds of a contraction. The resting tone (lowest intraamniotic pressure between contractions) amounts to 10 mmHg. The area above 10 mmHg is considered as the active pressure area. The pain threshold is that intrauterine pressure above which a contraction is painful—about 10 to 15 mmHg over resting tone. (*Redrawn from Helmuth Vorherr, chap. 3 in N. Assali and C. R. Brinkman, (eds.),* Pathophysiology of Gestation: Maternal Disorders, vol. I, *Academic Press, Inc.,* New York, 1972.)

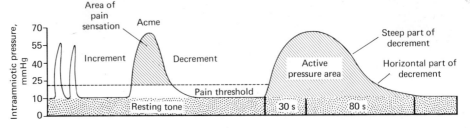

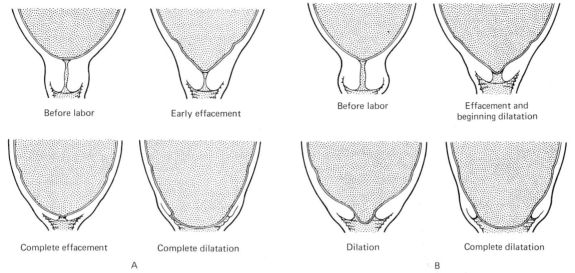

fig. 8·11 Degrees of effacement and dilation. A Primigravida. B Multigravida. (*Courtesy of Ross Laboratories, from "Phenomena of Normal Labor."*)

abled to do this only as the fibers in the lower uterine segment stretch and do not contract to their former length, but become progressively longer. The *work* thus involves the power of the contractions to overcome the resistance of the cervix.

The cervix is made up of only 10 percent smooth muscle, this portion circling the os in sphincter fashion. The connective tissue which makes up the major portion is rich in collagen fibers, which, having lost some of their binding substance, are enabled to stretch. Changes in the endocervix are such that much of the cellular substance is cast off with the mucus, leaving the area considerably thinned. Progressive contractions above produce progressive thinning until the cervix is no thicker than the rest of the lower segment. Before this process, known as *effacement*, is complete, the cervix begins to dilate, continuing until it is large enough for the passage of the fetal head (about 10 cm) (Fig. 8·11A and B).

Perhaps helpful to the above process are the equalized pressure exerted at first by the enclosed membranes and later the more di-rect pressure on the cervix by a bulge of fluid-filled membranes and the presenting part itself.

the pain of labor

The pain threshold level is considered to be between 15 and 20 mmHg though many persons do not experience pain until pressure has risen at least 15 mm above the current resting tone. Pain of labor is believed to have a number of causes:

1. Uterine ischemia, with resulting lack of oxygen and buildup of waste products in the cells
2. Pressure of the presenting part on nerves in the cervix and lower uterine segment
3. Stretching of the cervix and peritoneum
4. Radiation along the pathways of the sacral and lumbar plexuses causing pain in the back and sometimes down the legs.
5. Stretching of the vagina, ligaments, and vulva during the second stage.

Many other factors enter into the amount of

physical stress placed on the body during labor. In addition, pain threshold and response are tempered by individual physical and emotional differences, as well as the kind and amount of preparation for labor and current emotional support being given. This is discussed more fully in Chap. 9.

The use of analgesia and anesthesia in labor is discussed in Chap. 18. Decisions regarding drugs, their dosage and time of administration, require great care so that they will not delay the progress of labor or compromise the safety of the baby. Seeing these as an adjunct to supportive measures, rather than as a replacement, will help in overall management of the delivery.

onset of labor

The onset of labor is usually equated with onset of regular contractions as experienced by the mother. Many doctors are of the opinion that some effacement and dilation of the cervix must have taken place before labor can be said to have begun in a particular patient. Some patients, unaware of contractile activity, may report for a routine appointment and be found to have an almost fully effaced and dilated cervix.

When patients are examined throughout the month prior to delivery, in most of them the cervix is found to be effacing and dilating progressively. One study showed the average dilation of nulliparas to be 1.8 cm and of multiparas 2.2 cm when they were examined within 3 days of delivery. Nulliparas came into labor with an average effacement of 70 percent, multiparas with 61 percent. Because of the extra degree of effacement, the presenting part is often engaged at term for the nullipara. Very few patients come into labor without some dilation; those who have not dilated adequately are considered to have a potential labor problem.

Readiness for labor is the key factor in how long the body will take to accomplish the work of the first stage. This readiness, as discussed above, is what is looked for when induction of labor is being considered. What controls the intricate timetable coordinating these factors with those initiating labor is not fully understood (see Chap. 25).

Some of the work of getting ready for labor evidences itself with characteristic symptoms.

SIGNS OF APPROACHING LABOR

1. Strong *Hicks contractions* may persist for several hours at a time with a fair degree of regularity. They are sometimes called "false" labor, but it is often impossible to know this until it is seen that dilation has not been accomplished and the contractions have ceased. The contractions may sometimes be recognized in that they tend to be low in the pelvis or groin rather than in the back or over the fundus, and they may be relieved, rather than aggravated, by walking.
2. *Lightening* usually occurs in the nullipara approximately 10 to 14 days before onset of active labor. This settling of the fetus into the pelvic cavity is characterized by relief from pressure in the upper part of the abdomen, but by renewed pressure on the pelvic organs, with increased urinary frequency as one symptom. This usually does not occur in the multipara until after the onset of active labor.
3. Discharge from the vagina of clear tenacious mucus (the mucous plug from the cervix). This is called *show* when it becomes mixed with the blood from breaks in small cervical capillaries as a result of dilating activity. Show usually occurs in the preliminary phase of labor.

stages of labor

Classically, labor has been divided into three (or four) stages.

First stage—from onset of labor to full effacement and dilatation of the cervix

Second stage—from full dilatation through descent and birth of the baby

Third stage—from birth of the baby through delivery of the placenta

A fourth stage is sometimes defined as the period of recovery—1 to 2 h following delivery of the placenta.

The first stage is divided into latent and active phases. The latent phase technically extends from the beginning of effacement (long before labor becomes evident) to approximately 4-cm dilatation of the cervix. Various terms are used to describe divisions of the latent phase—*preliminary* and *early* are used in this text. The *active phase* describes active dilation of the cervix from 4 to 10 cm. This phase is divided into either the active and advanced active (transitional) phases by one method, or the acceleration phase and phase of maximum slope by another method. Friedman has redefined the phases of labor by functional divisions to describe the dilating and descent processes (9) (see Fig. 26·1).

Preparatory division = latent and acceleration

Dilatational division = phase of maximum slope

Descent division = rim of cervix (9 cm) through birth

Progress of effacement, dilation, and descent can be determined only by internal vaginal examination. (Rectal examinations can be done, but are less accurate and are more likely to cause infection.) These determinations should be made as often as needed to keep aware of progress, but not *more* often than needed. It is most important to maintain strict asepsis to avoid introduction of bacteria into the birth canal. Sterile gloves are used, and pouring antiseptic solution, such as Zephiran Chloride, over the glove for lubrication is routine procedure. With the patient in the dorsal recumbent position in the labor bed, the examiner separates the labia widely before introducing the first two fingers, in order to avoid contaminating the gloves. Some labor room policies require the wearing of a mask by the examiner, and cleansing of the whole perineum prior to examination.

In assessing the progress of dilation, use of *centimeters per hour*, rather than total number of hours, makes possible early recognition of a labor problem. Friedman (9) gives the time for the latent phase (preliminary and early) for the nullipara as an average of 8.6 h, but not more than 20, and for the multipara an average of 5.3 h, but not more than 14. During active dilation the pattern for the nullipara averages 3 cm/h and at least 1.2 cm, while that for the multipara averages 5.7 cm/h, rarely less than 1.5 cm. This pattern is for the dilation beyond that which was accomplished prior to active labor. In a study by Hendricks et al., 90 percent of patients attained full dilatation in from 1 to 8 h (5).

When the cervix is almost completely dilated, the patient may experience an increase in pain and frustration. There may be an increase in bloody show, the cervical rim developing small fissures as it completes dilation and retracts around the presenting part. Shortly, the characteristic grunt is heard as pressure on the pelvic muscles and rectum stimulates a reflex expulsive response. Strong abdominal and diaphragmatic muscles are brought involuntarily into action to move the fetus through the remainder of the birth canal.

The contractions are now forcing the fetus out of the uterus, which gradually decreases in length, becoming thicker in the upper segment. (This could roughly be compared to squeezing meat out of a sausage skin by squeezing the far end and rolling up the excess skin.) As the uterus contracts, the supporting round and uterosacral ligaments pull the fundus forward and the cervix back, so that the fetus is directed behind the pubis and into the sacral curve.

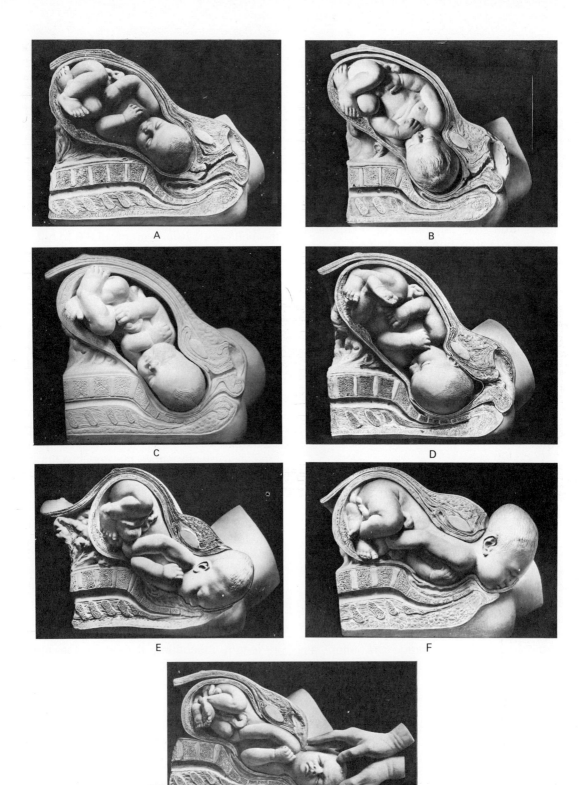

A

B

C

D

E

F

G

It is important to remember that descent does not *begin* at this time—the fetus has been descending since it became engaged, as allowed by the effacing and dilating cervix.

Throughout the period of labor, as the fetus descends and conforms to the shape of the birth passage, it makes certain movements or turns which have been called the *mechanism of labor*.

MECHANISM OR CARDINAL MOVEMENTS OF LABOR

Descent of the fetus is essential to and concurrent with the movements. Only in the theoretic sense can they be isolated.

Engagement is the first landmark for the fetus as it descends from floating in the false pelvis, usually in the left or right occiput transverse (LOT or ROT) position, somewhat less frequently in the LOA (left occiput anterior) (Fig. 8·12A).

Flexion. As the head approaches the spines, if not before, it tends to flex acutely, probably as a result of resistance. The chin rests on the sternum, so that the smaller suboccipitobregmatic dimension, instead of the occipitofrontal, is now presented to this narrowest part of the canal (Fig. 8·12B).

Internal rotation. As the occiput passes the midpelvic plane, if not before, the head begins to rotate so that the occiput moves toward an anterior position (OA) (Fig. 8·12C, D). Completion of this movement may not occur, especially in nulliparas, until the occiput reaches the pelvic floor; several strong contractions may be required to effect it. The head is getting into position to take advantage of the greater anteroposterior diameter of the outlet (Fig. 8·12E).

If the sacral curve is deep, the occiput may turn toward the mother's back on passing the spines to an OP (occiput posterior) or, more commonly, ROP (right occiput posterior) position. In this case rotation to the anterior position involves a 135 to 180° rotation instead of the 45 to 90° rotation from an LOA or OT position.

Occasionally the head stops when it reaches the transverse position, or remains in the posterior position. These are complications of labor and are discussed in Chap. 26.

Extension. As the occiput passes the symphysis, it maintains contact with it, so that the nape of the neck comes to pivot around it. The occiput is directed anteriorly, and the head extends (Fig. 8·12F).

Restitution and external rotation. As soon as the head is free, it rotates or untwists in order to realign itself with the shoulders. These will have turned with the head during internal rotation, but they often stop in the oblique position rather than rotating fully to the transverse. In that case, the head rotates to LOA or ROA. Shortly, the shoulders rotate internally to the anteroposterior position. External rotation describes the head turning the rest of the way to transverse as it follows the shoulders (Fig. 8·12G).

Expulsion describes the birth of the shoulders and the remainder of the body, which follows easily.

RUPTURE OF MEMBRANES

Membranes will usually rupture toward the end of the first stage if they have not done so previously. If the break is high, there may be only a trickle of fluid, and this only during a contraction. If there is uncertainty as to

fig. 8·12 Mechanisms of labor in the vertex position (LOT). A Head at the entrance to the true pelvis. B Engagement and flexion completed. C and D Internal rotation in progress. E Crowning. F Extension completed G External rotation and beginning delivery of shoulders. (*Reproduced with permission, from* A Baby Is Born, *Maternity Center Association, New York, 1964.*)

whether or not membranes have ruptured prior to or after admission, *nitrazine paper* will give a neutral or alkaline reaction in the presence of amniotic fluid in a usually acid vagina. A microscopic test can be performed if this is not conclusive.

Whenever the membranes rupture, it is important to check the fetal heart beat. Particularly if the rupture is accompanied by a gush of fluid, the umbilical cord may be washed downward, so that it could be compressed between the presenting part and the cervix. If membranes are ruptured artifically by the physician, the FHT (fetal heart tone) should be checked before and after the procedure.

FETAL RESPONSE TO LABOR

The fetus is passive in the birth process, and is wholly dependent on its environment for survival. The stresses of the labor and delivery, in themselves, may leave the infant poorly equipped for the major adjustments which must be made in the first few minutes following birth if it is to survive extrauterine existence. If the labor process is overlong, if the contractions are long and intense, and particularly if intervals between contractions do not allow for full circulatory recovery, problems may be expected. Particularly crucial is the period of time between crowning and expulsion of the infant, as evidenced by fetal bradycardia (6).

Prolonged bradycardia is associated with acidosis, which decreases responsiveness to resuscitative measures. Infants who are depressed from analgesic or anesthetic drugs which have crossed the placental barrier, tend to have lower cord blood oxygen levels, to be more acidotic, and to respond more slowly, either independently or with recusitation (7). Choice of drugs, as well as timing and dosage of these agents, is therefore of extreme importance.

It has been possible to observe the fetal response to the labor process both electronically and by auscultation; the former process is more accurate and reliable. Such observation is usually coordinated with the measurement of contractions previously discussed, so that the relationship can be readily seen (see Chap. 27 for details).

If electronic recording equipment is not available, auscultation of the fetal heart must be carried out to evaluate the status of the fetus. The frequency for taking the FHT is determined by the findings, but should not be less than every 10 to 15 min in the active phase of the first stage, nor less than every 5 min in the second stage.

Indications in the mother for immediate readings and close follow-up would include:

1. Rupture of membranes
2. Anything which might reduce maternal blood pressure and therefore diminish blood supply to the fetus via placental circulation. The latter might include a drug reaction, reaction to conduction anesthesia, and occasionally, supine hypotension.

While the specific underlying problem is being remedied, oxygen administered to the mother as a supportive measure will help to prevent oxygen deprivation to the fetus.

The fetal heart is best heard through the upper part of the back of the fetus, so the position of the fetus should first be ascertained. If the fetus is in the LOA position, the FHT will be heard best to the left and slightly below the level of the umbilicus early in the first stage, and correspondingly lower as the baby descends.

Auscultation can be done with an ordinary stethoscope but is greatly facilitated by specialized equipment which amplifies the heart sounds. Gentle pressure must be put on the area, sufficient to overcome the distance created by adipose and other intervening maternal tissue. The fetoscope adds bone conduction vibrations to those heard (Fig. 4·7). The Leffscope both amplifies the sound

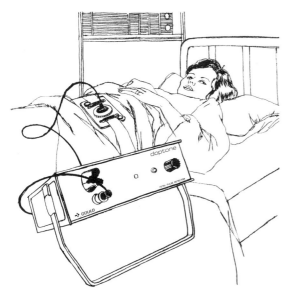

fig. 8·13 Doptone for fetal heart monitoring. (*Courtesy of Gould, Inc.*)

and provides its own weight, so that pressure need not be maintained. The Doptone and other similar devices magnify and broadcast the sounds (Fig. 8·13).

It is difficult, if not impossible, to hear the FHT during a strong contraction, but it is important to get a 30-s reading during the decrement, and another 1 min later for comparison.

Patterns are more meaningful than an isolated reading. Using graph paper to record would help in seeing both patterns and their relationship to contractions.

When describing the FHT, the base-line level of the heart rate should be termed as follows:

	Beats/min
Marked tachycardia	Above 180
Moderate tachycardia	161–180
Normal range	120–160
Moderate bradycardia	100–119
Marked bradycardia	100 and below (8)

Many normal labors are not being monitored routinely at the present time; however, the trend is toward increasing use of monitoring equipment. It is considered advantageous, at least for evaluation purposes, especially during active dilation and descent. It would be of great benefit to have accurate knowledge of fetal condition during that crucial period just before birth.

SECOND STAGE

The major function of the second stage of labor is descent. To accomplish this, the resistance of the vaginal canal, the muscles and fascia of the pelvic floor, plus the superficial muscles, fascia, and connective tissue of the vulva and perineum, must be overcome. Coaching and encouraging the patient will enable her to maximize the energy expended, adding her voluntary expulsive efforts during contractions.

With these forces functioning adequately, the advancement of the fetus should be constant and continuous, the rate of progress dependent upon the resistance met. Friedman has defined normal limits of descent as a guide to aid in recognizing problems early. The guide is for normal presentations, uncomplicated by any malposition or other known problems. For the nullipara whose birth canal has not been previously distended, the fetus can be expected to descend at least 1.5 cm/h, descending in most cases at 3 cm/h. In the multipara the fetus can be expected to progress faster than 2.1 cm/h, most often at about 5 cm. The upper limits of normal descent are stated as 6.4 and 14 cm, respectively (9).

The pelvic floor, made up chiefly of the levator ani muscles and their fasciae, must be displaced downward and outward by the fetal head. The resistance is variable and can be evaluated on internal manual examination.

The folds of the vagina are obliterated as it stretches to form a lining membrane for the canal. The fascial layers are thinned as they stretch, making them and the vagina susceptible to tears.

During contractions the perineum will be seen to bulge progressively. Fecal particles may be passed because of pressure on the rectum. The anus opens, and hemorrhoids, if present, swell. Gradually the labia separate, the slit becoming progressively larger until the fetal scalp is seen. Between contractions the head is forced back by the elasticity of the muscles of the pelvic floor. After a few contractions the labia have flattened with distension, and the head maintains the perineal opening during the relaxation phase. This is called *crowning* (see Fig. 8-12E).[1]

The skin over the perineum glistens as it is stretched to its limit. If there is adequate elasticity, the occiput will progress, with the head in flexion, until the largest area is encircled. The occiput emerges and then the face and chin slip out over the perineum by extension of the head.

The delivery of the head should not be hurried. If progress seems too fast, either for adequate stretching of the perineum, or to avoid rapid decompression of the head, the mother can be coached to pant rather than push during the contractions. The doctor may then ask her to exert some pressure between contractions so as to ease the head out under better control. *Forcible* pressure must never be put on the head to restrain its progress. If there is question that the perineum may tear, or if the pressure and time required for adequate perineal stretching are causing fetal distress, the physician will perform an *episiotomy* (see Chap. 26). Following this the head slips out easily.

As soon as the head is born, the nose and mouth are cleared of mucus and amniotic fluid to prevent their aspiration when the infant first breathes. The physician feels for the cord. If it is wrapped around the neck, he attempts to slip it over the head. If the length is inadequate, the cord is clamped and cut.

[1]Another definition of *crowning* will also be found—that of the largest circumference of the presenting part being encircled by the vulva.

Usually the anterior shoulder advances to the pubic arch, which acts as a pivot. The posterior shoulder is forced forward over the perineum, allowing the anterior shoulder to follow. Sometimes the anterior shoulder is delivered first. The rest of the body slips out easily.

There are differences of opinion regarding whether the cord should be cut before or after draining the residual volume of placental blood to the fetus. The prevailing opinion is that this extra blood increases the likelihood of *hyperbilirubinemia* in the neonatal period.

THIRD STAGE

Immediately after the birth of the infant, there may be a slight flow of blood until the uterus contracts firmly around the placenta. Close observation is maintained to see that it remains well contracted. With the contraction, the site of placental attachment becomes smaller than the placenta itself, severing the villi and thin-walled blood vessels by which it is attached. If the central portion separates first, bleeding from the sinuses may aid further in the separation process. In most instances, by 1 to 5 min several indications that the placenta has separated and moved into the lower segment and vagina will be noted:

1. The uterus becomes smaller and spherical.
2. There is a slight gush of blood from the vagina.
3. The umbilical cord lengthens by several inches.
4. The uterus may rise in the abdomen because the separated placenta displaces it upward.

If the patient is awake, the physician will probably ask her to bear down to deliver the placenta (Fig. 8-14). If she is anesthetized, fundal pressure may be exerted after ascertaining firm uterine contraction, but this

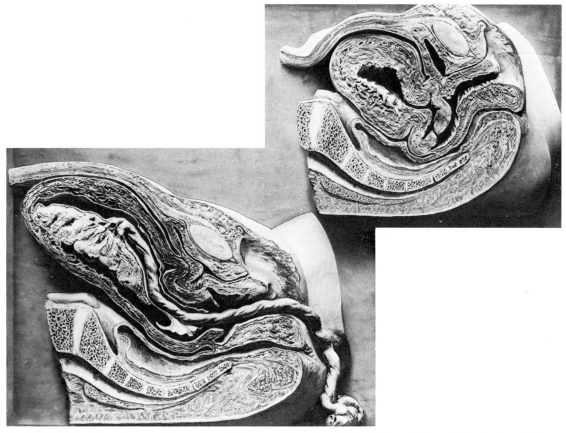

fig. 8·14 Birth of the placenta. (*Reproduced with permission, from* A Baby Is Born, *Maternity Center Association, New York,* 1964.)

must be done with great care. The placenta must be inspected to be certain that it is complete, i.e., that no parts have been left in the mother.

In some instances, separation may take somewhat longer. At no time may traction be put on the cord or membranes when still attached, as they may tear, leaving fragments attached to the uterus, or worse, traction could cause inversion of the uterus.

If there is delay in separation of the entire placenta, resulting in considerable bleeding, or if the placenta is found to be incomplete, the placenta or what is left of it must be removed manually. Many physicians are doing this procedure relatively routinely to

shorten the third stage and therefore minimize bleeding. Obviously this must be done with care and with meticulous asepsis. The patient must be anesthetized; then the cervix and vagina must be carefully inspected so that they can be repaired if necessary and blood loss prevented.

The first hour following delivery is a critical period for the mother. The blood vessels and myometrium are intertwined in such a way that natural ligatures are created when the uterus is contracted. Careful and frequent observations must be made to see that firm contraction is maintained until clotting can take place.

Nursing care of the laboring mother is

discussed in Chap. 9. Complications of labor and delivery are discussed in Chap. 26.

references

1. A. Scommegna, "The Effect of Pregnenolone Sulfate in Uterine Contractibility," *American Journal of Obstetrics and Gynecology*, **108**:102, 1970.
2. Edward J. Quilligan, "The Initiation of Labor," *Hospital Practice*, **1**(11):47, 1968.
3. Emanuel Friedman and J. P. Greenhill, *Biological Principles and Modern Practice of Obstetrics*, W. B. Saunders Company, Philadelphia, 1974, p. 187.
4. Louis Hellman, Jack Pritchard, and Ralph Wynn, *William's Obstetrics*, 14th ed., Appleton-Century-Crofts, Inc., New York, 1971, p. 351.
5. Charles Hendricks, William Brenner, and Gary Kraus, "Normal Cervical Dilatation Pattern in Late Pregnancy and Labor," *American Journal of Obstetrics and Gynecology*, **106**:1076, 1970.
6. Mario Zilanti, Carlos Segura, et al., "Studies in Fetal Bradycardia during the Birth Process, II," *Obstetrics and Gynecology*, **42**:842, 1973.
7. Ibid., p. 843.
8. Hon, Edward H., *An Introduction to Fetal Heart Monitoring*, Corometrics Medical Systems, Inc., Wallingford, Conn., 1973, p. 52.
9. Emanuel Friedman and Marlene Sachtleben, "Station of the Fetal Presenting Part, IV: Slope of Descent," *American Journal of Obstetrics and Gynecology*, **107**(15):1032, 1970.

bibliography

Friedman, Emanuel A.: "The Functional Divisions of Labor," *American Journal of Obstetrics and Gynecology*, **109**:274–280, 1971.

———, and J. P. Greenhill: *Biological Principals and Modern Practice of Obstetrics*, W. B. Saunders Company, Philadelphia, 1974.

———, and Marlene R. Sachtleben: "Station of the Fetal Presenting Part, IV: Slope of Descent," *American Journal of Obstetrics and Gynecology*, **107**(15):1031–1034, 1970.

Hellman, Louis M., Jack A. Pritchard, and Ralph Wynn: *Williams' Obstetrics*, 14th ed., Appleton-Century-Crofts, Inc., New York, 1971.

Lasater, C.: "Electronic Monitoring of Mother and Fetus," *American Journal of Nursing*, **72**:728–730, 1972.

Matousek, I.: Fetal Nursing during Labor, *Nursing Clinics of North America*, **3**:307, 1968.

Oxhorne, Harry, and William R. Foote: *Human Labor and Birth*, 2d ed., Appleton-Century-Crofts, Inc., New York, 1968.

Smith, B. A., R. M. Priore, and M. K. Stern: "The Transition Phase of Labor," *American Journal of Nursing*, **73**:448, 1973.

Williams, Barbara, and Sharon Richards: "Fetal Monitoring during Labor," *American Journal of Nursing*, **70**:2384, 1970.

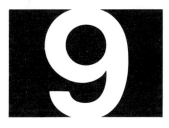

nursing during the birth process

Constance R. Castor

Labor is work and progress. It is the work of regular uterine contractions which results in progressive cervical changes and culminates in the birth of a baby and the expulsion of placenta and membranes. This work requires the integration of both physical and mental effort and total concentration if the woman desires to be an active participant during labor. The following discussion is oriented to the psychoprophylactic method of childbirth preparation.

the body prepares for labor

The preparation for this work is an ongoing process throughout pregnancy which accelerates during the final weeks. The uterus has accommodated the growing fetus by the elongation and hypertrophy of its muscle fibers as well as the formation of a few new fibers. There is simultaneous development of a network of *fibroelastic tissue*, permitting a significant increase in strength and elasticity, imperative to the accomplishment of labor.

CHANGE IN THE CERVIX

The softening of cervical consistency noted earlier in pregnancy becomes more pro-

nounced in the last few weeks of pregnancy, in response to hormonal influence. The cervix is said to *ripen*. The degree and timing of this softening may vary for each woman, but the cervix will be "ripe" within the week of delivery.

During the entire pregnancy the vagina has been prepared for the stretching process by forming extra blood vessels, increasing secretory action, and developing increased elasticity. There is a generalized relaxation of the tissue, and a deepening of the vaginal folds.

CHANGE IN FETAL POSITION

Primigravidas frequently experience the phenomenon known as *lightening* during the final 2 weeks of pregnancy as the fetal head descends into the pelvic cavity. With this descent, the uterus also descends and tilts slightly forward. The woman will feel off balance after this happens and may also sense increased perineal pressure. There will be less pressure on the diaphragm to ease breathing, but the increased pressure on the bladder will result in urinary frequency. For some primigravidas and most multigravidas, lightening does not occur until the onset of labor (Fig. 9·1).

CHANGE IN METABOLIC RATE

Metabolic changes characteristic of the latter part of pregnancy may produce varying energy states which alternately result in a sense of increased work capacity (energy spurt) and increased fatigue. The woman's metabolism increases to facilitate the work of labor. During antepartal education, women learn to recognize this possibility and pace their activities, trying not to deplete energy stores and resting as the body demands. It is not unusual for women to undertake ambitious projects, only to be frustrated by quickly fading energy. They might also experience a

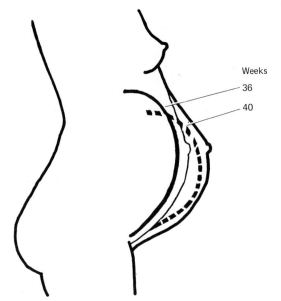

Weeks
36
40

fig. 9·1 Lightening causes a release of pressure on the diaphragm as the fetal head descends into the true pelvis to engage.

nesting impulse to get things in order for the baby. The urgency of this impulse is not always understood by husbands and families. These same metabolic changes may also result in a weight loss of several pounds in the final week or two of pregnancy.

signs of labor

Although the earliest indication of labor for a primigravida may be *lightening,* other women experience increasing pressure sensations throughout the pelvic area. Multiparas particularly complain of perineal or groin pressure.

Loss of weight and *varying energy levels* are particularly apparent just prior to labor.

The *mucous plug* (cervical secretions) which, during pregnancy, has acted as a safeguard against ascending infection, is usually expelled shortly before or at the time of labor. As this happens, cervical capillaries frequently rupture and mix with the mucus, making it pink-tinged. Referred to as the *show*, this is often the first indication of the beginning of labor. Though the show most frequently occurs within the 24 h immediately prior to labor, it may be observed several days before.

The amniotic membranes most often rupture during the active phase of labor. A few women experience a *premature rupture of membranes,* before the onset of labor. The amniotic fluid usually leaks in small amounts, as there are no contractions to exert force; however, labor usually begins within 36 h. Although a tear is present, and the fluid is leaking, the body continues to manufacture amniotic fluid; therefore, a *dry birth* is impossible. The physician should be notified when the membrane ruptures, since another protective barrier has been removed and infection may follow if labor does not begin within 24 h. At this time, the baby's position, presenting part, and condition should be checked by the physician.

Some women experience episodes of diarrhea, intermittent backache, or generalized abdominal cramping immediately before labor begins.

With or without any preliminary indicators, the woman will begin to feel uterine contractions, which become progressively longer, stronger, and closer together.

The mother may experience very early irregular contractions and be convinced that she is in labor. These misleading signs indicate *prodromal labor,* often called *false labor*. The contractions prove ineffective, irregular, and poorly defined (i.e., without much increment or decrement). During contractions, the abdomen remains relatively soft and can be indented with gentle finger pressure. Activity—showering, walking, busyness—generally causes the contractions to cease. On examination, no cervical dilatation is noted and

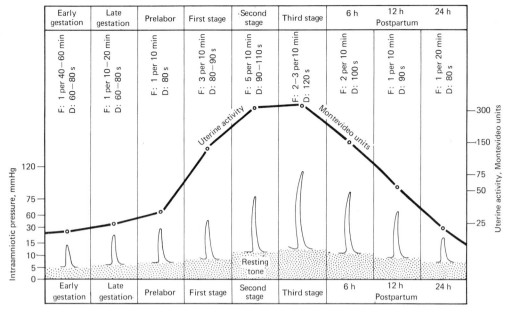

Early gestation	Late gestation	Prelabor	First stage	Second stage	Third stage	6 h	12 h Postpartum	24 h
F: 1 per 40—60 min D: 60—80 s	F: 1 per 10—20 min D: 60—80 s	F: 1 per 10 min D: 80 s	F: 3 per 10 min D: 80—90 s	F: 5 per 10 min D: 90—110 s	F: 2—3 per 10 min D: 120 s	F: 2 per 10 min D: 100 s	F: 1 per 10 min D: 90 s	F: 1 per 20 min D: 80 s

fig. 9·2 Contractions throughout pregnancy: frequency (*F*), duration (*D*), and intensity of uterine contractions in relation to uterine activity, as observed in different phases of gestation, labor, and postpartum. During gestation uterine activity is low, less than 25 Montevideo units. (Montevideo unit = product of frequency and intensity of uterine contractions in each 10-min period.) Prelabor begins a rapid increase in myometrial contractility. The highest pressures are during the second and third stages. Within 24 h the myometrial activity declines rapidly. The initially high pressures after delivery are required for uterine hemostasis. (*Redrawn from Helmuth Vorherr, chap.* 3 *in N. Assali and C. R. Brinkman (eds.),* Pathophysiology of Gestation: Maternal Disorders, *vol.* I, *Academic Press, Inc., New York,* 1972.)

the presenting part has not begun to descend.

The woman experiencing prodromal labor is often embarrassed, discouraged, and susceptible to fatigue. A skillful nurse can be a source of encouragment and renewed self-esteem in emphasizing the vague nature of early labor, even to the trained observer. Ready access to the physician or other attendant for labor evaluation in the office or clinic examining room also helps to diminish the woman's feelings of frustration. With antepartal education, women become more sophisticated in judging the quality of contractions, as false labor seldom requires special techniques (Fig. 9·2).

Advancing labor is characterized by:

1. Contractions of increasing frequency, increasing duration, and increasing intensity
2. Cervical effacement and dilatation
3. Descent of presenting part
4. Intensification with walking
5. Presence of a show

Prodromal labor is characterized by:

1. Contractions at irregular intervals, constant or irregular duration, and constant or irregular intensity
2. Lack of cervical effacement or dilatation
3. Failure of presenting part to descend

4. Absence of a show
5. Walking produces relief

Imprecise, sketchy, or unintelligible information to the pregnant woman regarding contractions and labor, both in clinics and in private practice, is a major factor in the repeated trips or phone calls to physician, clinic, or hospital which result from anxiety. The nurse can be a calming influence in this period of heightened stress by planning and implementing a realistic plan for the dissemination of accurate and appropriate information, in terms understood by the woman.

the preliminary phase of the first stage

The preliminary phase is characterized by irregularity and variability, but differs from prodromal labor in that cervical changes occur, the baby may begin to descend, and there is a progression in contractions, however erratic. The preliminary phase should be seen as a latent but essential period of intermittent contractions which are irregular in frequency, mild in intensity, and poorly defined.

This phase can be confusing to the woman until progress becomes evident. During antepartal instruction, the preparatory aspect of the preliminary phase is emphasized. This knowledge reduces the incidence of early hospitalizations during this period.

CONTRACTIONS

Contractions (1) are characteristically short —30 to 40 s in duration; (2) come at irregular intervals, from 20 to 5 min; and (3) may be interpreted as a recurring urge to defecate, as intestinal cramping, or as intermittent backaches. Diarrhea may occur (Fig. 9·3).

DURATION

In the primigravida, the duration of this phase is highly variable—from zero to many hours. If a multipara experiences this phase, its duration is usually under 6 h. Confident and well-prepared women frequently are unaware of this phase until the contractions are better defined.

WORK

As part of the continuum of labor, cervical changes occur in response to contractions. The descent of the presenting part and the effacement process continue slowly. Although the membranes are usually intact at this time, should they rupture, the clear, odorless fluid generally escapes in small spurts with each contraction.

WOMAN'S MOOD

Just as the physical characteristics of the preliminary phase are variable, so are the woman's reactions. She is comfortable; her mood may be described as excited, ambivalent, and/or anxious. With antepartal preparation, her most frequent reactions are a sense of excitement ("This may be it!") tempered by ambivalence ("Am I ready? Can I handle it?"), until a predictable pattern is established and she begins to use appropriate techniques. Her mood parallels the ambivalence of the first trimester.

COMFORT MEASURES/TECHNIQUES

The woman should be encouraged to keep occupied with activities which divert her attention but do not tire her. She should be encouraged to rest periodically when this phase occurs during the day.

She should urinate often to prevent bladder distension and interference with labor. Her

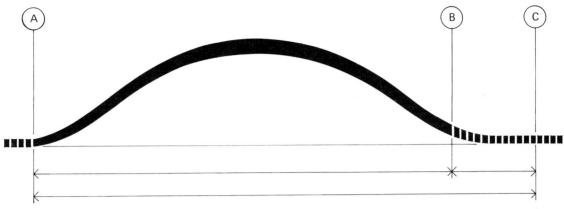

fig. 9-3 Contraction: preliminary phase. Contraction duration, 30 to 40 s (A to B); intervals, 20 to 5 min (A to C); strength, mild and irregular. (*From Constance R. Castor,* Participating in Childbirth: A Parents' Guide, *2d ed., Council of Childbirth Education Specialists, New York,* 1973. *By permission of the author.*)

diet is usually restricted to easily digested foods and liquids which will sustain her for the long work of labor but which will neither be a safety hazard if an anesthetic becomes necessary nor result in distracting nausea and vomiting. Many physicians now encourage the prepared woman to consume *small* amounts of sweetened tea, water, gelatin desserts, or toast with jelly. Women frequently lose their appetite and need encouragement to maintain fluid and energy balance.

If she awakens with mild contractions, the woman is encouraged to get up, take a warm shower and cup of tea, and then try to sleep. When she understands that the more pronounced contractions of active labor *will* awaken her, rest becomes possible.

If a woman is unduly apprehensive at this time, she may utilize the technique of *controlled relaxation.*

THE COACH

Circumstances may indicate that someone other than the father act as coach: friend, relative, or nurse. The role of the coach remains essentially the same. The mother primarily needs the coach to be available during the preliminary phase to indicate love and concern for her. Although it is not necessary for the father to return home at this point, if he is already there (e.g., during a weekend or evening) he should be alert to signs of tension in the mother. He then can coach her in relaxation techniques. He reminds her to empty her bladder and maintain fluid intake as permitted. The record of labor during this phase should simply include hourly comments on duration, interval, and strength of contractions.

NURSING APPROACH

If the childbirth educator can be available for consultation during the earlier phases of labor, her suggestions on technique, her aid in maintaining the self-confidence of the couple, and her validation of their appraisal of labor are very supportive.

The office or clinic nurse, who may be in contact with the couple during this phase, can give encouragment and interpret instructions from the physician in a manner which is positive and supportive. The nurse needs to be oriented to the emotional susceptibility of the laboring woman, realizing that positive remarks are understood by her as important, meaningful encouragement.

If they have come to the hospital or clinic too early, the couple should not be sent home with an abrupt dismissal. Here is a good opportunity for important reinforcement of learning, in which the nurse can underscore the need for rest and the maintenance of fluid balance and energy reserves, and remind them of the nature of the labor process. The couple at this point see themselves as amateurs and appreciate a few moments of specific directions relevant to their needs.

If a unique situation occurs in which the woman is hospitalized, the nurse's focus should be on the maintenance of a restful and relaxed environment. The husband also should be encouraged to rest. If he returns home to rest, both he and his wife need to be assured that he will be summoned promptly when labor becomes active. The nurse must take responsibility for carrying out this promise.

If the husband remains in the labor room with his wife, he should be encouraged to keep his wife occupied with diversional activity as he would do at home, and he can assume most of the responsibility for her comfort.

The nurse will monitor both the woman's and baby's conditions by observing vital signs, fetal heart tones, and contractions. Despite the fact that the woman is not yet in active labor, the nurse should make frequent visits to the woman so that she does not feel abandoned.

SUMMARY OF NURSING CARE DURING PRELIMINARY PHASE

If the nurse is in contact with the couple, she (1) creates a relaxed and supportive situation; (2) reinforces antepartal teaching; (3) interprets doctor's instructions; (4) encourages restful and diversional activities; and (5) observes vital signs, fetal heart tones, and contractions.

early phase

Progressive labor patterns become established during the early phase. The pace of labor is more consistent, with better-defined contractions at more predictable intervals. This is the longest, but easiest, phase of labor. The woman will be comfortable during most of the phase without any specific labor technique.

CONTRACTIONS

1. Most of the contractions have a duration of 30 to 45 s and are of moderate strength.
2. Increment, acme, and decrement of the contractions are better defined and more apparent.
3. Contraction intervals become more regular, from 10 to 5 min apart. Earlier in the phase they are closer to 10 min apart; as the phase concludes, intervals shorten to 5 min.

During classes, parents are reminded that some degree of irregularity will be present throughout labor, but that within a given period of time, most contractions will conform to a specific pattern.

DURATION

Duration of the early phase, also, is variable—from 2 to 6 h. Primigravidas average 4 to 6 h; multiparas, 2 to 4 h.

WORK

Cervical changes become more evident during this phase, as the contractions work to almost complete effacement and bring dilation to 4 cm. Usually the presenting part gradually moves deeper into the pelvis. The rupture of membranes does not profoundly influence labor in the early phase.

MOOD

During the earlier part of this phase, the woman is comfortable and in control. Her mood is confident. If she has not experienced the preliminary phase, she may feel the flush of excitement and anticipatory anxiety characteristic of the beginning of regular contractions.

As the phase progresses, she finds herself increasingly drawn into the experience of labor, in contrast to the peripheral attentiveness of the beginning of labor. The woman's confidence in herself, and in her coach, is reinforced as she begins to apply techniques appropriately.

COMFORT MEASURES AND TECHNIQUES

The prepared couple should be encouraged during classes to view the woman's work in labor as a close parallel to that of a long-distance runner or swimmer. The warm-up completed, the race is begun. The runner paces himself with controlled effort, coordinated muscular effort, and rhythmic breathing patterns. He resists the impulse to panic into premature speed in response to the efforts of other competitors. In this same way, the prepared couple relies upon the effectiveness of their training program and upon their ability to interpret labor correctly, to make appropriate responses.

At the beginning of the early phase, the woman continues diversional activity, interspersed with rest periods.

The woman is confronted with a sense of urgency to deal with the progressively stronger contractions as the phase continues. She finds she can no longer walk or talk through a contraction; she pauses as it be-

gins, perhaps takes a little gasp of air, or may perceptively tense. These are indications that she should begin the active use of learned techniques.

She utilizes the skill of *controlled relaxation,* by taking a deep breath as the contraction begins, relaxing her body completely as she exhales, letting it concentrate on the contraction. She may breathe normally as she permits the contraction to work. This ability to let the body work without interference by concentrating on the controlled relaxation skills may be sufficient to deal with tension. If not, she can begin controlled breathing activities.

BREATHING TECHNIQUES

The couple has learned a series of precise respiratory techniques so that in labor, the woman may effectively pace the intensity of her labor pattern with the appropriate respiratory pattern. Just as the runner finds that erratic breathing interferes with his ability to perform, whereas rhythmic breathing enhances his stride and effort, so the laboring woman has learned the necessity of rhythmic respirations, and her coach has learned the importance of monitoring her efficiency and technique.

The couple learns that certain aspects of the techniques remain constant and are in fact basic to all respiratory effort.

1. *Chest breathing,* which is said to diminish diaphragmatic interference on the uterine fundus, is employed throughout. The woman feels as though she is breathing higher and higher in the chest as she progresses with the techniques, using more of the intercostal muscles and an increasing shallowness of respiratory depth.
2. *A deep breath* initiates and concludes each contraction. This is an important sig-

nal for both the woman and her coach. The woman has learned to relax consciously as she exhales this breath, in preparation for the work of the contraction. The coach reminds her of this by stroking or saying "Relax." These beginning and ending breaths make each contraction into a single entity that terminates, as opposed to the sense of relentless contractions. The demarcation also facilitates the use of contraction intervals for rest.

3. A *focal point* increases the woman's concentration and diminishes distraction. It serves to direct her attention to dealing with the contraction constructively, rather than running from it.

4. *Verbal cues* are used in practice to indicate when the woman will use a breathing technique, e.g., "Contraction begins . . . contraction ends." The conditioning to such verbal cues is readily transferred to the actual contraction. At times, these may even be used by the coach during labor, if the woman has become drowsy, tired, or uncertain as to the actual onset of each contraction.

5. A *comfortable position* is important for effective relaxation and efficient respiration. It has been determined that the usual recumbent flat position not only may interfere with the progress of labor but may cause undesirable intraabdominal pressure on the large blood vessels. The woman may assume any safe position. She usually chooses a tailor-sitting, side-lying, or semi-Fowler's position.

The first respiratory pattern she will use is *rhythmic chest breathing,* at the slower rate of about eight breaths per minute. The inhalation is through the nose, and the exhalation through the mouth, stressed and slightly prolonged. In rhythm with the breathing, the woman can use a circular *stroke* over the abdominal area, using her fingertips. This type of stroking, known as *effleurage,* en-

hances her comfort and becomes another precise motor skill on which to concentrate. It may be done with one or both hands, or by her coach. This type of breathing is continued for as long as it is effective (Fig. 9·4).

With the advance of dilation as the phase progresses, the woman may need to progress in breathing activity as well. If so, she modifies the rhythmic chest breathing by increasing the rate to 16 or 20 breaths/min, continuing with the rhythmic stroking.

COACH

The need for active coaching usually coincides with the woman's use of specific breathing activities. The coach assists with the controlled relaxation technique, observes breathing technique for rhythmic quality and correct performance, and makes note of progress. He reminds the woman to empty her bladder, and to take sips of water if permitted. He helps her determine what position is most comfortable. He may initiate the use of technique, on the basis of observation of her responses, or suggest that she progress with techniques if he detects diminished effectiveness with the one she is using.

NURSING APPROACH

The need for positive encouragement and validation of the couple's own observations remains constant throughout labor. The couple needs to see the nurse as a caring resource person, to whom they can readily turn. The more knowledgeable the nurse is in technique and method, the more effective the assistance becomes. From admission to the labor unit through transfer to the postpartum unit, the nurse sets the tone of acceptance and encouragement.

The prepared couple is well informed in the mechanics of labor and has worked hard to develop teamwork and skills. The couple needs to be kept posted on the progress of

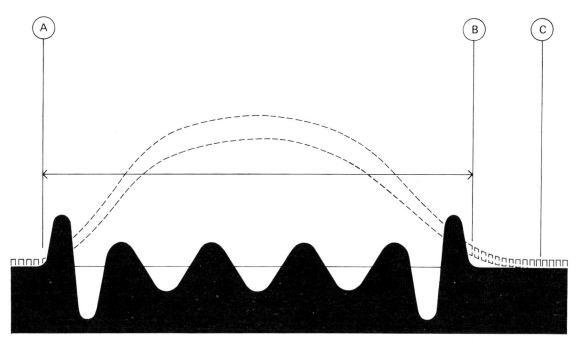

fig. 9·4 Early phase and rhythmic chest breathing. Contraction duration, 30 to 40 s; intervals, 10 to 5 min (A to C); strength, mild to moderate; regular. Rhythmic chest breathing at rate of eight breaths per minute. Deep breath begins and ends each contraction. (*From Constance R. Castor,* Participating in Childbirth: A Parents' Guide, *2d ed., Council of Childbirth Specialists, New York, 1973. By permission of the author.*)

labor. When such progress is slow, as it typically is with first babies, the nurse's wise choice of words means the difference between perseverance and discouragement; for example, contractions should be referred to as such, rather than as "pains."

The nurse should demonstrate respect for the bond which exists and grows between the members of the couple as they work together. If knowledge of technique permits, the nurse may make alternate suggestions, confirm the couple's choice of technique, or even take over while the coach has a coffee break. If the coach indicates that his suggestions on technique are different, the nurse should defer to him, understanding that the couple's confidence is based on a familiarity which has grown with weeks of practice; they are not rejecting the nurse personally.

During the admitting procedure and con-

tinuing throughout the monitoring of labor, the nurse should interfere as little as possible during a contraction.

SUMMARY OF NURSING CARE DURING EARLY PHASE

1. *Performing* required admitting procedures such as:
   a. Perineal shave (total or partial)
   b. Admitting enema (as ordered)
   c. Obtaining of urine specimen (clean-voided, especially if show is present)
   d. Care of personal belongings
   e. Accurate identification of the woman
   f. Complete record taking, including listing of allergies, last food-fluid intake
   g. Vaginal examination (depending on setting, these exams may become a nursing function)

h. Drawing blood for hematocrit, type, and cross matching (as ordered)
2. *Establishing* a comfortable, relaxed, and supportive environment by:
   a. Introduction and welcome to the couple
   b. Familiarizing the couple with facilities and equipment
   c. Using quiet, calm voice
   d. Assisting woman into a comfortable position
   e. Providing couple with comfort aids: extra pillows, blanket, washcloths, emesis basin, drinking cup, ice chips, comfortable chair, supply of clean bed pads
3. *Evaluating* the woman's condition and progress in labor by:
   a. Taking base-line vital signs—blood pressure, pulse and respirations, and temperature
   b. Ascertaining the quality of contractions, their duration and intervals
   c. Observing for show and rupture of membranes
   d. Determining progress made at home by questioning couple on contractions, appearance of show, and condition of membranes
4. *Evaluating* fetal condition by:
   a. Listening to fetal heart tones for quality and rate
   b. Palpating position, lie, and presentation
   c. Attaching external electronic equipment, if it is to be used

active phase

At the midpoint of cervical dilation, labor accelerates and the woman enters the active phase. Contractions become strong and consistent in quality, with shorter rest intervals. This phase demands the total concentration of the laboring woman and the encouragement of those attending her, if she is to remain in control.

CONTRACTIONS

1. The duration of contractions now consistently extends from 50 to 60 s; they are of moderate to strong intensity.
2. Contractions have a well-defined curve and a distinct peak (acme) lasting from 40 to 50 percent of each contraction (Fig. 9·5).

DURATION

The phase varies widely in length, but averages 2 to 3½ h. It is now calculated in terms of cm of dilation and descent per hour (see Chap. 8).

MOOD

The carefree, confident, talkative mood which often characterizes the early phase is quickly replaced by an intense, total absorption in the work of labor. As the phase continues and fatigue increases, the woman's confidence begins to waver; she requires active supportive measures.

COMFORT MEASURES AND TECHNIQUES

Her familiarity and skill with respiratory techniques will enable the woman to direct her conscious efforts to *controlled relaxation.* She becomes more and more aware of the critical importance of this concentration to her ability to deal with the contractions. Her performance of the breathing activities becomes almost automatic.

In order to deal with the more intense contractions of the active phase, the woman progresses to a *combined pattern* of the modified rhythmic chest breathing and shallow breathing. She matches the increment

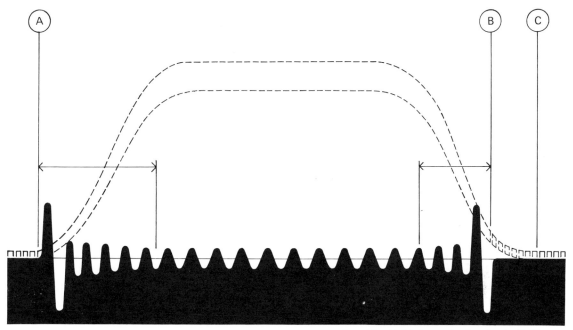

fig. 9·5 Active phase and shallow breathing. Contraction duration, 50 to 60 s (A-B); intervals, 5 to 3 min (A-C); strength, strong; well-defined peaks. Shallow breathing is coordinated to the intensity of each contraction. Rhythmic chest breathing, at the increased rate of 16 to 20 breaths per minute, is used during this increment and decrement; shallow breathing is used for the acme. (*From Constance R. Castor,* Participating in Childbirth: A Parents' Guide, *2d ed., Council of Childbirth Specialists, New York, 1973. By permission of the author.*)

and decrement with the rhythmic chest breathing pattern; she utilizes the lighter, faster shallow breathing for the acme. The rhythmic *stroking* is continued if the woman finds it soothing. As the contractions demand, she may use the *shallow breathing* for the entire contraction, permitting greater flexibility in rate and depth. When employing this technique, the woman breathes lightly and evenly, both inhaling and exhaling through her slightly opened mouth. The rate is just fast enough to ensure respiratory exchange (as opposed to simply moving tidal air) with minimal effort and depth of respirations (Fig. 9·6).

"Back Labor" Should the woman experience so-called *back labor,* because of either a posterior position of the fetus or a focus of tension, she and her attendants must or-

fig. 9·6 In active labor, this mother is concentrating on relaxing and the shallow chest breathing. Her husband is checking the contraction to help her coordinate the breathing to the contraction.

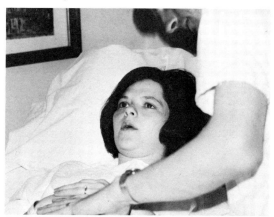

ganize response and action for effective control. While using appropriate breathing techniques, the woman directs her total concentration on releasing tension both generally and specifically in the sacrum, perineum, buttocks, and thighs. She avoids lying on her back; her coach applies firm counterpressure to the sacral area. Some women find relief by the application of cold or warm compresses, or by doing the pelvic rock exercise, rounding the back and tilting the pelvis forward.

Ice chips, if allowed, and cool-water mouth rinses are refreshing (mouthwash is nauseating). Some women prefer to suck on sour lollipops between contractions. Talcum powder will make stroking of either abdomen or back easier.

Hyperventilation If, despite good teaching, adequate practice, and good coaching, a woman begins to *hyperventilate,* a respiratory imbalance of decreased CO_2 levels will develop. She must rebreathe her exhaled air from a small paper bag or her cupped hands. This usually quickly corrects the imbalance and relieves the symptoms of dizziness, lightheadedness, and tingling.

COACH

The need for active coaching coincides with the active phase. As the contractions heighten and occur more frequently, the woman's perspective becomes distorted. She needs to be reminded to take one contraction at a time. Her coach helps her accurately focus on the contractions by counting off each 15-s interval within the contraction. During the contraction, her degree of relaxation is observed; specific instructions are given to facilitate relaxation, especially during the peaks.

NURSING APPROACH

Though the couple has learned and perfected various skills, this does not mean the total abolition of discomfort or the elimination of all sensations of labor. The couple understands that medication, anesthetics, and other obstetric techniques may be indicated for the accomplishment of the stated goal.

In observing labor and the woman's reactions, the nurse relies on the woman's judgment of her comfort. She may appear to be in distress when actually she is concentrating and working hard. Comments such as, "You're working very hard," "Having a baby is hard work. You're doing a good job," or "That contraction was not easy, but you managed it," underscore the nurse's appreciation of the work of labor and the effectiveness of the woman's efforts.

Should intervention become necessary, the skill with which the nurse presents it will strongly influence the couple's acceptance of help in the accomplishment of their goals. The nurse needs to convey the idea that such measures are used to help the woman's efforts, not to take over for her.

Even with expert teaching, an occasional couple enters labor with unrealistic goals and exaggerated reactions. In dealing with this kind of couple, the nurse continually directs them toward realistic and attainable goals, reinforcing what is known to be stressed in prenatal preparation. "As you learned in class . . . ," is a helpful emphasis.

SUMMARY OF NURSING CARE DURING THE ACTIVE PHASE

1. *Completing* admitting procedures as described earlier. Most multiparas and some primigravidas will enter the hospital during this phase.
2. *Evaluating* the woman's condition, tolerance of labor, and progress by:
   a. Checking vital signs
   b. Observing contractions by palpation or monitoring
   c. Noting show and condition of membranes
3. *Evaluating* fetal condition by:

a. Palpation of position
b. Checking fetal heart tones (quality and rate) by fetoscope or monitoring
c. Observing activity
d. Observing amniotic fluid for color

4. *Maintaining* a comfortable, relaxed, and supportive environment by:
   a. Courteous attitude when entering and leaving room
   b. Introduction of new personnel
   c. Supporting the efforts of the couple
   d. Interpreting appropriate information in a positive manner
   e. Enhancing physical comfort for both father and mother
   f. Being aware of techniques being utilized by the couple

5. *Assisting* the physician and performing tasks as directed by him. These might include:
   a. Preparing for artificial rupturing of membrane. In explaining this to the couple, emphasis should be on the painlessness of the procedure, the need for sterility, and how this will affect the progress in labor. Following this procedure, the nurse is expected to monitor closely both contractions and the fetal heart tones.
   b. Administration of sedatives or analgesics, if required. Dosages usually will be significantly reduced for the prepared woman. The father is reminded that the mother's responses are dulled and that she will require active coaching.
   c. Assist with the administration of regional anesthetics as necessary.

advanced active phase (transition)

As cervical dilation nears completion, the woman enters the most intensive and demanding part of the first stage. Fatigue, the inconsistency and discomfort of the contractions, and the intensity of labor make control difficult.

CONTRACTIONS

The pattern of contractions intensifies as the uterine muscles work to complete dilation.

1. The duration of these contractions can be palpated at 60 to 90 s.
2. Intervals shorten to 3 to 2 min.
3. Contractions build rapidly into very strong peaks, which last about two-thirds of the contraction. The contraction also subsides quickly, but the woman often feels as though it never totally disappears as the uterine tonus rises (Fig. 9·7). Some multiparas experience multiple peaks.

DURATION

In a woman having her first baby, this final phase usually lasts up to 1 h; the advanced phase is completed in 20 to 45 min for multiparas.

WORK

The cervix now dilates fully, from about 8 to 10 cm, with the baby pushed deep into the pelvis and against the cervix. This produces a heavy show as more cervical capillaries rupture. The presenting part may cause strong sensations of pressure in the rectum, back, groin, or perineum. Many women feel as if they must have a bowel movement and will call for a bedpan.

MOOD AND PHYSICAL REACTIONS

The woman becomes agitated and intense during the advanced phase. The physiologic changes of labor and fatigue make her irritable, restless, and discouraged. She finds it difficult to cope with contractions; relaxation during the brief rest intervals is almost

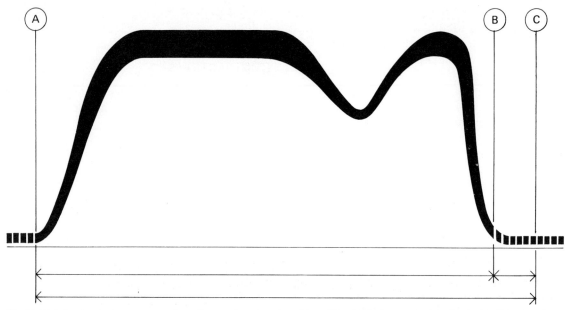

fig. 9·7 Advanced phase contraction. Contraction duration, 60 to 90 s (A-B); intervals, 3 to 2 min (A-C); strength, intense. Contraction may have multiple peaks. The increment and decrement are brief; the contraction does not seem to subside entirely. (*From Constance R. Castor*, Participating in Childbirth: A Parents' Guide, *2d ed., Council of Childbirth Specialists, New York,* 1973. *By permission of the author.*)

impossible. She may sweat profusely, become chilled, or alternate between these reactions. Her legs may tremble and cramp. She may complain of nausea or a backache. She may feel overwhelmed and discouraged; she wants to give up. Her perspective is severely distorted.

COMFORT MEASURES and TECHNIQUE

To handle this tough period, the woman must deal with each contraction with a rhythmic pattern of *shallow breathing and short puff-blows*. The sequence is usually three or four shallow breaths and one puff-blow, which can be altered to meet the contraction's intensity. A sequence of one shallow breath and one puff-blow is particularly effective for strong peaks or sensations of pressure. If she experiences the urge to push before dilation is complete, she uses a repeated blow-blow-

blow until given permission to bear down (Fig. 9·8).

To assist in her efforts to relax between contractions, restore respiratory balance, and foster a sense of well-being, the woman uses the *rhythmic chest breathing* at its slowest rate, eight breaths/min, during the brief intervals.

Stroking (effleurage) is irritating and distracting during the advanced phase, but the woman may find relief in supporting the lower abdominal area with her hands.

COACH

Coaching must be specific and direct. The woman's reactions frequently require active and continual direction. The coach must insist that she take one contraction at a time, because she anticipates them all and panics. She must be reminded to use the *rhythmic*

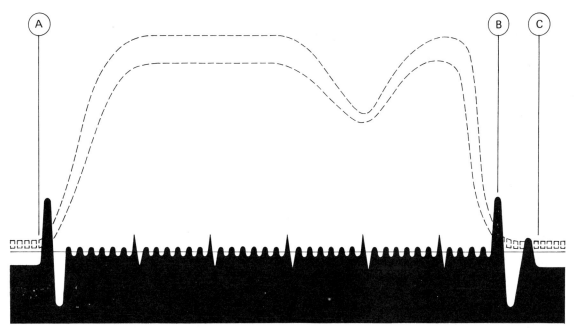

fig. 9·8 A rhythmic pattern of shallow breathing and short puff-blows is used to control the intense contractions of the advanced phase. Rhythmic chest breathing is used between contractions to aid relaxation and restore respiratory balance. (*From Constance R. Castor*, Participating in Childbirth: A Parents' Guide, *2d ed., Council of Childbirth Specialists, New York, 1973. By permission of the author.*)

chest breathing between contractions. The coach may have to touch the abdominal area lightly to help her discern the absence of a contraction. Communication, both verbal and nonverbal, is very important to her ability to remain in control. The coach cannot allow her to waste the rest periods, no matter how brief, in purposeless activity or tenseness.

NURSING APPROACH

The woman's need for the reassurance of the nurse intensifies. The nurse's continued interpretation of the physician's findings and her support and encouragement of the couple's efforts increase their tolerance and enhance their effectiveness. A woman at this point in progress must not be left alone. The nurse, therefore, plans the various preparatory activities—seeing to the coach's gowning, check-

ing on delivery-room setup and required equipment, arranging for one person to remain with her at all times. During this phase, the nurse is expected to monitor the fetal condition more frequently. This needs to be done skillfully, so as not to interrupt the woman's activities. The nurse is alert to any sudden changes in the position of the fetal head, particularly with multiparas, in whom dilation may dramatically progress from 8 to 10 cm in a few minutes, with concurrent descent of the baby.

SUMMARY OF NURSING CARE DURING THE ADVANCED PHASE

This care remains focused on points previously discussed:

1. Evaluating the woman's condition and progress

2. Evaluating the fetal condition
3. Maintaining a calm, relaxing environment
4. Assisting the physician
5. Readying the delivery-room facilities

second stage

With full dilatation, the forces of labor focus on descent. The baby must pass through the dilated cervix, maneuver down through the pelvis, then distend the vagina, pass through the perineal muscles, and emerge. Controlled and efficient voluntary bearing down by the woman contributes to an effective and safe delivery. Bearing-down efforts add about 40 lb of pressure to the uterine contraction work. Fortunately, the expulsive action of the uterus, the woman's sense of renewal, and prior instruction will enable her to be an effective and active assistant.

CONTRACTIONS

The tumultuous quality of the advanced phase subsides. Once again the contractions become regular and predictable.

1. Duration of contractions remains at 60 to 90 s.
2. Intervals change to 5 to 3 min, with a well-defined rest period.
3. Increment, acme, and decrement are well defined and consistent. Contractions are strong. The uterus can be seen rising up within the abdomen during each contraction; the fundus perceptibly lowers (Fig. 9.9).

DURATION

With the cooperative efforts of the prepared woman, it takes 20 to 90 min to accomplish the second stage for a primigravida, with an

fig. 9.9 Second stage contraction. Contraction duration, 90 s; intervals, 5 to 3 min; strength, intense but defined. Increment and decrement lengthen, helping to make contractions more manageable. (*From Constance R. Castor, Participating in Childbirth: A Parents' Guide, 2d ed., Council of Childbirth Specialists, New York, 1973. By permission of the author.*)

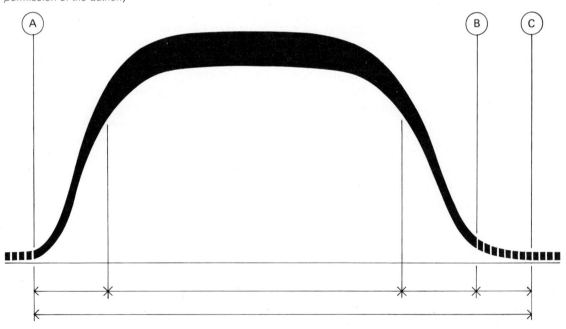

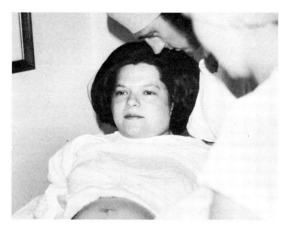

fig. 9·10 The mother is in the pushing position. Her husband gives her the necessary cues as she bears down with the contraction. It is obvious that she is concentrating and working hard.

average duration of 40 to 60 min (and 20 pushes). Lack of muscle resistance in a multipara usually reduces the second stage to 10 to 40 min (and 10 pushes).

WORK

The mechanical work of labor involves the *flexion, descent,* and *rotation* of the baby's head through the pelvis and vaginal canal. Indeed, birth is impossible without these maneuvers (see Fig. 8·12).

MOOD

The irritability, discouragement, and agitation which marked the final hour of the first stage, rapidly disappear at full dilatation and the beginning of the woman's cooperative efforts. As she senses active progression with each push, and as the contractions resume a more manageable pattern, the woman gets the feeling of a second wind, a renewal of energy and stamina. Modesty is replaced by a greater work sense; position and bodily covering are unimportant to her.

The father's encouragement to sustain the

immense pushing effort is very important to her, and she focuses intently on him. Although she becomes oblivious to peripheral activity, she is susceptible to confusion if conflicting directions are given or several people attempt to direct her. The woman's pushing effort may be timid and inefficient at first. As she senses that the harder she pushes the better it feels, and as she is specifically directed by her coach, her efforts become rhythmic and efficient (Fig. 9·10).

It is important that the woman be prepared for the sensations which accompany expulsion so that they can be put in proper perspective: the distension of the vaginal tissue; the increasing pressure on the perineum; rectal pressure; the absence of perception of the contraction itself with the pushing effort. As the baby exerts greater and greater pressure on the perineal musculature, her pushing effort may temporarily diminish. She may also feel the full weight of the responsibility of getting this baby out, which can be overwhelming to her unless her efforts are continually encouraged and unless her progress is continually noted. Some women require detailed direction; others need only occasional reminders (Fig. 9·11).

A tremendous sense of relief accompanies the birth of the head. Though some women report that it feels good to push, most women will be absorbed in a great work effort and the overriding urge to get that baby out.

COMFORT MEASURES and TECHNIQUE

Technique focuses on controlled relaxation, correct positioning to influence favorably the axis of the birth canal, effective use of the abdominal muscles and diaphragm, and the direction of pushing effort toward the vagina. The woman learns to push during the peak of each contraction, permitting the contraction to build by taking a series of deep breaths. She learns to push several times during the peak, which, for many women,

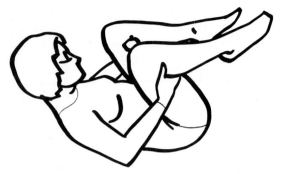

fig. 9·11 The woman concentrates on pushing at the peak of each contraction. To do this, she takes a series of deep breaths during the increment, then holds her breath, bearing down with the abdominal muscles while consciously relaxing the perineum to enhance pushing efficiency. She quickly exhales, inhales, and holds her breath several times during each peak. During the decrement, she takes several deep breaths. (*From Constance R. Castor,* Participating in Childbirth: A Parents' Guide, *2d ed., Council of Childbirth Specialists, New York, 1973. By permission of the author.*)

seems to maintain pushing efficiency better than one sustained push. She restores respiratory balance by taking several deep breaths as the contraction declines. Pushing effort must come from the abdominal muscles, and not consist simply of straining in the throat. Between contractions she must rest, utilizing controlled relaxation once again. She learns to cooperate with the physician's instructions during the delivery of the head, controlling her pushing effort by utilizing the shallow breath and blow sequence to control the strong urges to expel the baby at once (Fig. 9·12).

The woman is also prepared for the *episiotomy* and understands its place in normal delivery. Since this is often feared out of ignorance and misinformation, the episiotomy is carefully explained as being a painless procedure, even without local anesthesia, when done at the peak of a contraction, as pressure from the baby's head causes a natural anesthesia to the perineum. As the physician enlarges the vaginal outlet with surgical scissors, the woman experiences a sensation not unlike being unzipped. She now pushes the baby out with decreased resistance. (Local anesthesia is, of course, used in most instances.) (Figs. 9·13, 9·14.)

COACH

The implications of the coach's continued involvement through delivery are now being more completely understood. The former banishment of the father at this time, after hours of active involvement, caused an acutely felt emotional wrenching. He felt left out, and his wife felt isolated.

In contrast, the father's presence at the birth of their child can be a profound experience for the new parents, and orients them in a beautiful way to parenthood as a mutual and shared effort.

The father remains at the mother's side, speaking directly into her ear, if need be. He also has learned the correct pushing technique so that he can encourage her efforts. Both in practice and in delivery he uses cue words:

(Breathe) *In, out; in, out; hold* (your breath) *Relax key areas* (jaw, mouth, perineum)

fig. 9·12 As the mother bears down with the contraction, the baby's head comes down onto the perineum, causing it to bulge. *Caput* is seen.

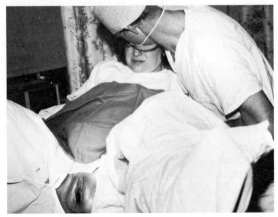

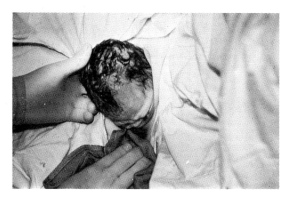 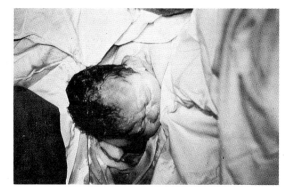

fig. 9·13 Birth of head in OA position (left), rotating to ROA (right).

Push out (use the abdominal muscles; push out through the vagina)
Release air

He repeats the sequence several times for each contraction and slowly counts to help her sustain pushing for each 20- to 30-s block.

He reminds her to maintain a correct position with her sacral area flat, so that the pelvis is in a slight tilt upward and knees are flexed.

Between contractions, he encourages her to relax by speaking in soothing tones, stroking, or using a cool cloth.

NURSING APPROACH

The nurse plays a dual role during the second stage, as she assists the physician in assuring the safe delivery of a healthy baby and as she undergirds the efforts of the couple.

Recognizing that a woman most often relates best to a single source of direction, the nurse defers to the father or the physician, except for general encouragement. However, if the woman's efforts falter, the nurse should recognize that she needs specific directions, not general statements such as "Push!" General directions are frustrating, because the woman feels she *is* pushing. The nurse can help the husband give specific, detailed help.

When the hospital prohibits the father's presence during the second stage, the nurse assumes the coaching role.

SUMMARY OF NURSING CARE DURING SECOND STAGE

1. *Continues* to maintain a supportive, comfortable environment by:
   a. Safe and comfortable positioning both in the labor bed and on the delivery table, including efficient *transfer between contractions* without interruption of the woman's efforts
   b. Adjusting lighting
   c. Explaining nursing activity: perineal scrub, draping, fetal monitoring, ad-

fig. 9·14 Birth of body.

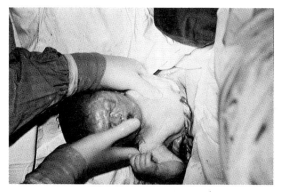

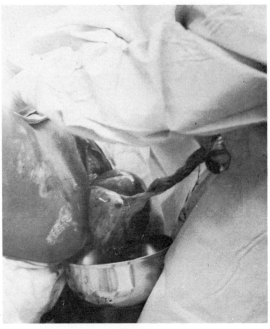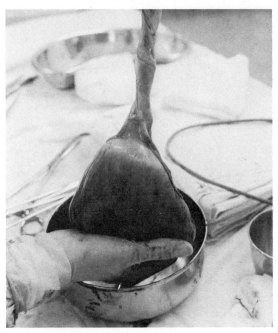

fig. 9·15 Explusion of placenta. (*Photos by Ruth Helmich.*)

ministration of intravenous solutions or medications

   d. General encouragement of the woman's efforts

2. *Assists* the physician to ensure a safe delivery of a healthy infant from a healthy mother by:

   a. Monitoring fetal heart—every 5 min as possible

   b. Monitoring woman's condition: contractions, vital signs, blood pressure as ordered

   c. Preparing necessary equipment for delivery and immediate care of the newborn

3. *Provides* immediate care of the newborn (discussed in detail in Chap. 13) by:

   a. Assuring clear air passage

   b. Evaluating the infant's condition by Apgar score

   c. Caring for the cord

   d. Providing prophylactic eye care, after parents have seen the baby

   e. Properly identifying the infant

   f. Keeping the baby warmly wrapped in incubator

   g. Providing necessary physical contact: gentle holding, allowing parents to hold the baby as soon as they are ready

third stage

The placenta, having completed its intricate life-sustaining function, now separates from the wall of the uterus as it once again contracts. The uterus, now considerably smaller, rises up and assumes a globular shape. The placenta is painlessly expelled as the mother pushes for the last time.

CONTRACTIONS AND DURATION

Mild contractions of approximately 1-min duration occur 5 to 30 min after the birth of the baby (see Fig. 9·2), and then continue at longer intervals through the recovery period. The uterine contractions exert pressure which causes the placenta to move into the lower uterine segment or upper part of the vagina, from which the woman can then push it out (Fig. 9·15).

MOOD

Following the birth of the baby, the mother usually is exhilarated and talkative, irrespective of the length or intensity of labor and/or delivery. She feels very close to the father; she reaches out physically and emotionally for her baby. Her prevailing reaction is one of elation, tempered with a sense of new responsibility: parenthood. The transition into parenthood can be facilitated by the continued support of the professional maternity care specialist, the provisions for contact with the infant, and the physical care of the new mother (Fig. 9·16).

The mother may express annoyance at having to exert herself to push out the placenta or at the repair of the episiotomy. She is highly perceptive at this time and will pick up any signals of anxiety or concern. If any variance from the norm occurs, she needs accurate information and positive reassurance.

COMFORT MEASURES AND TECHNIQUES

The mother appreciates anything which increases her comfort, such as wiping her face, giving her ice chips, or adjusting the delivery table.

COACH

This is a sharing time, as the couple waits for the completion of delivery.

NURSING CARE DURING THIRD STAGE

Once the newborn's condition is seen to be stable, the nurse assists the physician with the care of the new mother, still in a critical stage of labor. The nurse's responsibilities at this stage include:

a. *Observing* the mother's general condition in relation to the third stage.
  a. Watching vital signs as directed by the physician
  b. Observing for signs of placental separation: (1) rising up of uterus in globular shape as it contracts; (2) lengthening of umbilical cord through the vagina; (3) sudden trickle of blood
  c. As instructed by physician, checking fundus for firmness, massaging it if so directed
2. *Directing* the mother's pushing to expel the placenta, as the father may relax his coaching.
3. *Continuing* observation of the newborn, for clear airway and maintenance of body temperature.
4. *Maintaining* a supportive environment for the new parents. If appropriate at this time, the nurse gives the baby to the parents to hold (Fig. 9·17). Usually the father holds the baby first, as the mother completes the third stage. If the parents will have to wait until the end of this stage to hold the

fig. 9·16 A job well done. Mother and father see their son at close hand for the first time.

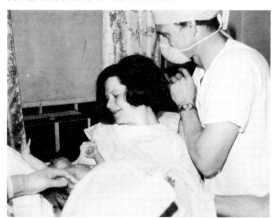

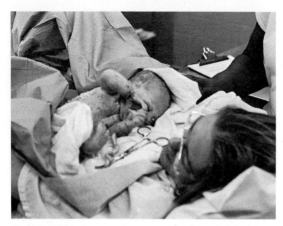

fig. 9·17 Mother needs an opportunity to "claim" her baby by touching and holding.

infant, the baby should be within sight, and the mother assured that she will hold it shortly.

5. *Administering* medications as directed. *Oxytocin,* and/or *methergine,* is commonly given to stimulate uterine contractions and minimize blood loss.

Immediate postpartum period. Elation, a sense of joy and accomplishment, and relief from anxiety—"All is well"—typify the mood of both mother and father.

OBSTETRIC CARE

The physician repairs the episiotomy and any lacerations that may be present, using a local anesthetic. He observes the mother's general condition, particularly in regard to bleeding. The placenta is examined, to be sure that it was delivered intact and that no parts remain in the uterus which would interfere with the important uterine contractions that control bleeding.

MOTHER'S REACTIONS

Soon after delivery, the mother manifests *physiologic reactions.* She often becomes chilled, and may tremble. She is tired and may be very hungry and thirsty.

If the mother is not given the opportunity to hold her baby, she experiences a strong feeling of deprivation and loss. Most progressive hospitals see to it that this opportunity is provided to diminish the sense of loss and increase her feeling of well-being.

More and more women are requesting to breast-feed immediately after delivery. The infant's sucking reflex is very strong at this point; nursing also seems to create strong maternal bonds with the infant, an important aid to the first-time mother (Figs. 9·18, 9·19).

NURSING APPROACH

The nurse's primary responsibility remains the observation of the mother's physical condition. She removes the woman from stirrups, carefully removing her legs simultaneously, makes her comfortable, and observes her for bleeding.

In providing for the mother's physical comfort, the nurse has an opprotunity to provide her with significant gestures of human caring. Once the first hour has passed, during which the nurse is primarily concerned with control of bleeding, the nurse can provide this care.

fig. 9·18 Nurse helps mother with breast-feeding techniques.

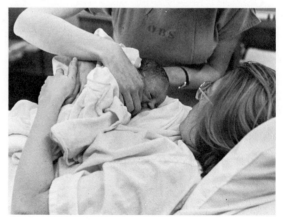

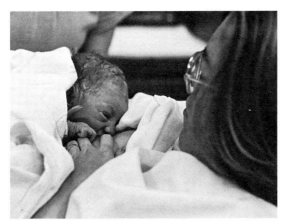

fig. 9·19 Newborn may nurse vigorously immediately after birth.

A sponge bath is not only refreshing but also emotionally comforting and restful. Providing nourishment for both parents also has dual importance. Mothers report attaching great significance to these simple activities, which take so little time and effort.

SUMMARY OF NURSING CARE IN IMMEDIATE RECOVERY PERIOD

1. Observes mother's condition: vital signs, firmness of fundus, amount of vaginal bleeding. Should there be any indication of variance from normal recovery, the nurse firmly massages the uterus and immediately notifies the physician.
2. Provides for mother's comfort:
   a. In the *delivery room*: removes soiled linen, adjusts the delivery table and removes both legs from stirrups simultaneously, provides the mother with a covering and a sterile perineal pad, often gives her a sponge bath, and provides her with a fresh gown.
   b. In *recovery area*: provides warmth for the mother and simple nourishment for both parents, changes perineal pad, observes for distension of bladder, allows parents to remain together, encourages rest.

LABOR SUMMARY

PHASE	TECHNIQUE	COACH
PRELIMINARY (0–many hours) *Contractions*: Mild, 30–40 s long, 20–5 min apart, irregular. *Work*: Early effacement. *Mood*: Excited, ambivalent. Show; membranes "leak" if they break.	Conserve strength. If at night, nap; if daytime, keep busy at light activities. Bland diet as permitted. Small amounts of sweet liquids. Experiment with position.	If at home, help with organizing household, assist general relaxation.
EARLY (2–6 h) *Contractions*: Moderate, 30–45 s long, 10–5 min apart, more regular. *Work*: Effacement and dilation to 4 cm *Mood*: Talkative, comfortable.	Conserve energy. Call doctor; emphasize degree of comfort. Take clear fluids as permitted. As necessary: Use *controlled relaxation*. For control: *Rhythmic chest breathing*, (1) slow rate, 8 bpm, (2) modified rate, 16–20 bpm.	Time contractions and note progress every hour. Support her efforts. Help with relaxation. Monitor breathing techniques.

ACTIVE (2–3½ h)
Contractions: Strong, 50–60 s, 5–3 min apart.
Work: Dilate 4–8 cm
Mood: Very busy, concentrated; intense. If membranes break, contractions increase in strength.

Conserve energy.
For control: *Controlled relaxation, combined breathing pattern—rhythmic chest/shallow.*
If necessary: *Shallow, accelerated-decelerated* with contraction.
Usually go to hospital. Sips of water or ice chips, if allowed.

"Count down" contractions.
Mouth rinses, cool cloth to hands and face.
Touch; stroke arms and legs.
Talk to her; encourage efforts.
Remind: Labor intermittent.
Monitor breathing.

ADVANCED (20–60 min)
Contractions: Erratic, 60–90 s, 3–2 min apart; intense.
Work: Dilate 8–10 cm.
Mood: Irritable, discouraged, overwhelmed.
Physical sensations: nausea, vomiting, chills, trembling, profusely sweating, pressure sensations, difficult to relax.
Special considerations:
Hyperventilation: Tingling, dizzy, light-headed, apprehensive, out of rhythm.
Back labor: Strong discomfort in small of back; difficult to relax; contractions may be erratic; tension increases.

Controlled relaxation
Shallow breathing: pant-blow 3/1, 2/1, 1/1 as contraction demands.
Rectal pressure: 1/1 pant-blow rhythm.
Urge to push: Repeated blows.
Rhythmic chest breathing between contractions.

Give specific directions.
Insist on taking one contraction at a time.
Remind her that baby is almost here.
ENCOURAGE!
Monitor breathing.
If she uses repeated "blowing," summon doctor, R.N.
Remain with her.

Rebreathe exhaled air between contractions.
Prevent: Keep breathing light, rhythmic.
Get off back—lie on side.
Focus on progressive relaxation throughout each contraction.
Apply warm or cold compresses.
Constant pressure to small of back.

Monitor breathing.
Correct technique—cadence, breathe with her.

Talk through contractions.
Assist with techniques.
Apply counterpressure.
Stroke.
ENCOURAGE!

DELIVERY (20–60 min)
Contractions: Rhythmic, 60–90 s, 5–3 min apart.
Work: Descent and birth of baby.
Mood: Refreshed, sense of work.
Physical: Vaginal fullness, pressure in rectum, Burning, stretching.
Episiotomy: painless, "unzipped."

The harder the push, the better it feels.
Expulsion technique.
If instructed to stop pushing at birth of head, *pant-blow.*

Coach efforts:
in, out/in, out/ in, hold,
relax key areas,
push out (count slowly to 10), release air,
in, hold (repeat above).
Several deep breaths at end of each effort.

PLACENTA (10–30 min)
Contractions: Mild.
Mood: Thinking of baby.
Work: Placenta expelled.

Push as directed.
Enjoy baby.

Enjoy baby together.
Praise wife.

bibliography

Castor, Constance R.: *Participating in Childbirth: A Parents' Guide,* 2d ed., Council of Childbirth Education Specialists, New York, 1973.

———, P. Hassid, and J. Sasmor: "The Childbirth Team during Labor," *American Journal of Nursing,* **73**(3):444–447, 1973.

Eastman, N. J., and L. M. Hellman: *Williams' Obstetrics,* 13th ed., Appleton-Century-Crofts, Inc., New York, 1966.

Farill, M. S.: "Adolescent in Labor," *American Journal of Nursing,* **68**:1952–1954, 1968.

Fitzpatrick, E., et al.: *Maternity Nursing,* 12th ed., J. B. Lippincott Company, Philadelphia, 1971.

Friedman, E. A.: *Labor: Clinical Evaluation of Management,* Appleton-Century-Crofts, Inc., New York, 1967.

———: "The Use of Labor Pattern as a Management Guide," *Hospital Topics,* **46**:57–59, 1968.

Kopp, Lois: "Ordeal or Ideal–The Second Stage of Labor," *American Journal of Nursing,* **71**(6):1140, 1971.

Loriner, A. B.: "Danger Signs in the First Stage of Labor," *Hospital Medicine,* 6:115, 1970.

Oxhorn, H., and W. Foote: *Human Labor and Birth,* 2d ed., Appleton-Century-Crofts, Inc., New York, 1968.

Tryon, Phyllis: "Assessing the Progress of Labor through Observation of Patient's Behavior," *Nursing Clinics of North America,* **3**(2):315–326, 1968.

Williams, Barbara L., and Sharon T. Richards: "Fetal Monitoring during Labor," *American Journal of Nursing,* **70**:2384–2385, 1970.

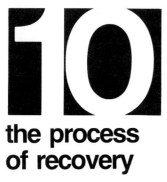

10
the process of recovery

Martha Olsen Schult

The period of time after a woman gives birth until her recovery 6 or 8 weeks later is known as the *puerperium,* derived from the Latin words *puer*, "child," and *parere*, "to bring forth." The two major occurrences of the puerperium are *involution* and *lactation.* The goals of physical care in the puerperium are threefold:

To prevent infection of the bladder, breasts, and uterus

To promote healing and the return to normal of the pelvic structures and perineum

To establish successful lactation if this is the desire of the woman

Involution involves the return of the pelvic reproductive structures, particularly the uterus, to their prepregnant size and position. *Lactation,* the other phase of the puerperium, begins after the delivery of the baby and can extend well beyond the 6- to 8-week period. If a woman chooses not to breast-feed her infant, lactation can be suppressed or interrupted. Breast-feeding will be discussed in detail in Chap. 14.

the uterus

At the time of delivery, the uterus weighs approximately 1000 Gm (2.2 lb). In 1 week it is reduced to one-half this weight, and by the end of the postpartum period, it weighs only 40 to 60 Gm (about 2 oz). The reason this organ can approximate its prepregnant weight and shape is that during pregnancy the *size* of the muscle cells increases while the *number* of muscle cells remains basically the same (Fig. 10-1). During the puerperium, the protein cytoplasm of the muscle fibers undergoes catabolic or autolytic changes. The products of this destructive process are carried off by the circulatory system and excreted as nitrogenous waste in the urine of the patient.

Immediately after delivery the very hard, round, contracted uterus lies between the umbilicus and the symphysis. Later the uterus rises to the level of the umbilicus or slightly above it and remains there for 2 days. After the second postpartum day, the uterus begins its descent into the pelvic cavity. It diminishes quite rapidly in size, weight, and position until the tenth day, when it can no longer be palpated. At this point it is at or below the level of the symphysis pubis.

The uterus, throughout its descent, should remain firm and contracted in order to act as a tourniquet to prevent hemorrhage from the large blood vessels at the placental site. The uterus will contract on its own. However, oxytocics (drugs which act to contract uterine smooth muscle) are often given to the patient following delivery to assist the uterus in this function. Breast-feeding in response to the sucking of the infant also causes the uterus to contract, triggering oxytocin release from the posterior pituitary.

postpartum check

After a period of observation in the recovery room, the patient arrives on the postpartum unit for the remainder of her hospital stay. This is a crucial time in the recovery process. To monitor this period, the nurse will check four factors:

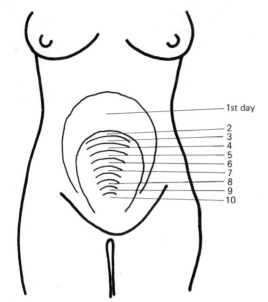

fig. 10·1 Postpartal descent of uterus into pelvic cavity. (*Courtesy of Carnation Company.*)

1st day
2
3
4
5
6
7
8
9
10

Fundus—the position and firmness of the uterus
Lochia—the type and amount of vaginal discharge
Bladder—the amount and timing of voiding
Vital signs—the reflection of postpartum adjustment

FUNDUS

The palpation of the top of the uterus is called the fundus check (Fig. 10·2). It is done to determine the rate of descent and the position and condition of the uterus. The unit of measurement of descent of the uterus is in centimeters and is known as a *fingerbreadth.* Descent is measured and recorded in relation to the umbilicus. The fingerbreadth is the width of a finger, 1 cm (½ in) as it is placed horizontally on the abdomen at the height of the fundus. With *U* indicating the umbilicus, fingerbreadths are recorded in numbers. The usual rate of descent of the uterus is 1 fingerbreadth (1 cm) a day after the second postpartum day.

1/U—The fundus is located 1 fingerbreadth above the umbilicus.
U—The fundus is at the level of the umbilicus.
U/1—The fundus is 1 fingerbreadth below the level of the umbilicus.
U/2—The fundus is 2 fingerbreadths below the level of the umbilicus.

It is important for the nurse to keep an accurate check on the descent of the uterus. Any retardation of the process indicates a problem or complication.

Procedure for Fundus Check
1. Explain reason for procedure to patient.
2. Screen and position patient.
3. Remove perineal pad and have her empty bladder.
4. Lower the head of the bed.
5. Cup hand around the fundus. If firm, do not massage. If "boggy" or soft, gently massage in a rotating manner, and observe for passage of blood clots.
6. Cleanse perineal area, securing a fresh pad.
7. Assist the patient to a comfortable position.
8. Chart findings. For example, fundus firm, 1/U, midline.

The precautions with a fundus check stem

fig. 10·2 Measurement of descent of fundus in finger breadths. (*Photo by Ruth Helmich. Courtesy of the Jamaica Hospital, Jamaica, N.Y.*)

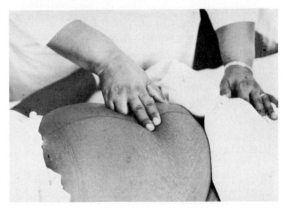

from physiologic changes within the abdominal cavity. With the change in pressure in the abdomen, the bladder easily becomes distended, pushing the uterus up and to the side. Because the uterus must be able to contract to stop bleeding from the placental site, a "boggy," soft uterus out of midline or above the umbilicus is an indication that the bladder is full and that bleeding will occur. Be careful not to knead or massage too vigorously because the uterus may become fatigued or overstimulated. Hemorrhage or undue pain may result. Check for the amount of bleeding and for the presence of clots or any other untoward symptoms.

Immediate Care It is very important that the fundus be checked frequently for the first 24 h. The following schedule suggests fundus checks for the first hours when danger of hemorrhage is greatest.

Every 10 to 15 min × 6 in recovery room; and then
Every 30 min × 6
Every 1 h × 3
Every 3 to 4 h for the remainder of the first day.

Patients can be taught to check their own fundus and will quickly report to their nurse any changes. Involving the recovered patient in her own case is especially helpful when the unit is busy or short-staffed.

Intermediate Care After the first 24 h, the fundus should be checked every 4 h the first postpartum day and once a shift every day thereafter. Any problems regarding the location or quality of contracture of the uterus would require more frequent checks.

LOCHIA

After delivery the decidual lining of the uterus sloughs off as a vaginal discharge known as *lochia.* This discharge includes blood, decidual tissue, epithelial cells from the vagina, mucus, bacteria, and occasionally membranes and small clots. The color of lochia is an indication of the progress of the healing of the placental site. At first the discharge is quite red and bloody. Frank bleeding occurs from the torn vessels of the placental site. As healing takes place and the lining of the rest of the uterus sloughs off, the discharge becomes more serous and now contains leukocytes. Soon the discharge turns pale and diminishes. The first stage is termed *lochia rubra* (red), the second is *lochia serosa* (reddish brown), and the third is *lochia alba* (white).

Immediate Care Check the lochia whenever the fundus is checked. Record the amount on the pad—for example, scant, moderate, or heavy. Note the frequency of the pad change. If it is more often than every hour and the pad is saturated, the patient should be checked for causes of extra bleeding. Record any deviations such as odor, clots, or the absence of lochia. Save any large clots or pieces of tissue for examination by the physician.

Intermediate Care Intermediate care is the same as the immediate care, with the addition of the following instructions for the patient who is changing her own perineal pad and checking her own lochia.

Instruct the patient to notify the nurse or physician if she notices any of the following:

Bright red bleeding beyond the fourth postpartum day
Foul odor
Pain or discomfort in the lower abdominal area
Absence of lochia within the first 2 weeks of delivery
Clots or tissue in lochia
Bright bleeding recurring after lochia alba begins

BLADDER

After delivery, the capacity of the bladder increases because of decreased intraabdominal pressure and the relaxed, stretched

table 10·1

LOCHIA CHARACTERISTICS

RUBRA	SEROSA	ALBA
Bright red	Pink	Creamy-yellow
Bloody	Pinkish-brown Serous	May be brownish
1–3 days postpartum	5–7 days postpartum	1–3 weeks
No odor or slightly "fleshy"	No odor	No odor or stale body odor

abdominal muscles. During the delivery period the bladder and urethra may be traumatized and temporarily paralyzed because of nerve damage or edema. Drugs and anesthesia during the labor and delivery may diminish sensitivity of the bladder or the alertness of the patient. Pain in the perineal area may cause a reflex spasm of the urethra. Psychologically, the patient may fear that voiding may be painful. Lack of privacy, inability to communicate with the nurse, and the discomfort of using the bedpan—all these will contribute to difficulty in voiding. The use of intravenous fluid therapy results in rapid urine formation, especially if fluids were given rather fast during immediate recovery. It is important that the patient void at least once and, more important, that she *empty her bladder* within 6 to 8 h of delivery to prevent:

Atony (loss of muscle tone of bladder)
Stasis of urine, predisposing to infection
Postpartum bleeding from obstruction of uterine descent

Methods used to determine the status of the bladder include checking oral and parenteral intake, checking output since delivery, and palpation of the uterus and bladder (Fig. 10·3).

After the nurse has determined that the bladder is distended or full, she must assist the patient in emptying her bladder. Many methods have been used to help a patient void. Some of the following have helped:

1. Have the patient walk whenever possible. Walking to the bathroom is normal and may trigger voiding.
2. If the patient is unable to walk, place her in a sitting position, either with a commode or on the bedpan.
3. Warm the bedpan and pour measured warm water over the perineal area.
4. Run the water faucet.
5. Provide for privacy. Give the patient fluids.
6. If the patient can walk, sitting in a warm tub often stimulates voiding. A sitz bath, especially the portable variety, may help.

Among the methods that have been used to induce voiding are ice applications to the suprapubic area and hypnosis.

Early ambulation reduces the need to catheterize for retention. If the patient experiences difficulty in voiding, catheterization is done only upon the physician's orders. Catheterization is the *least* desirable method of emptying the bladder because of the possibility of contamination during the procedure. The meatus of the urethra may be edematous and difficult to locate. Explain the procedure to the patient, and drape her. Use a good light source and get some assistance if it seems necessary.

Immediate Care During the first 24 h the patient may need assistance in voiding and emptying her bladder. If she is unable to void within 6 to 8 h of delivery, a Foley catheter may be inserted and left in place until edema or spasm has diminished.

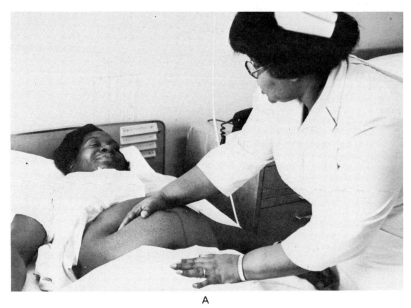

A

fig. 10·3 Bladder check postpartum. A Full bladder has displaced uterus to left. B After woman has voided, fundus is in midline and below umbilicus. (*Photo by Ruth Helmich. Courtesy of the Jamaica Hospital, Jamaica, N.Y.*)

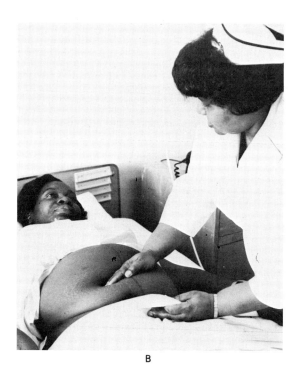

B

Intermediate Care After the first 24 h, when the patient is ambulatory, she generally requires little assistance in voiding. After the second day she may notice *polyuria* (frequent urination). The change in hormonal levels of estrogen and progesterone leads to a diuresis during the intermediate period, when the excess body water and blood volume of pregnancy begin to diminish. An accurate record of intake and output is maintained until the patient is free of problems and the possibility of retention of urine, or residual urine in the bladder.

VITAL SIGNS

The vital signs are a means of checking the condition of the patient after labor and delivery. The cardiovascular status is abruptly changed after delivery because of the removal of uterine pressure, the removal of the placental bypass, and the return to the system of most of the blood previously circulating through the uterus and placenta. These changes will be reflected in the vital signs. Table 10·2 serves as a guide for taking vital signs in the postpartum period.

diet

One of the first needs or desires of the newly delivered patient is for something to eat or drink. She has been without oral intake for several hours, and unless she has received intravenous fluids she is probably dehydrated. With the exceptions below, the postpartum patient is allowed whatever she wishes to eat or drink (1):

The patient who is nauseated, vomiting, or not fully reacting because of a general anesthetic

The patient who must lie flat in bed because of a caudal or spinal anesthetic

The heavily sedated, drowsy, or unconscious patient

The diabetic, cardiac, or toxemic patient (or some other type of patient requiring a special diet)

IMMEDIATE CARE

Just after delivery the patient usually appreciates a cup of tea or coffee, preferably with sugar or honey. Replacement of fluids and electrolytes and the blood volume lost through diaphoresis and through the exertion and fluid loss of delivery are the concern of the nurse. The patient requires adequate fluid intake to help her to void, to maintain a normal temperature, and to maintain adequate nutrition. Encourage her to take fluids slowly to avoid nausea.

INTERMEDIATE CARE

Throughout her hospitalization the patient is encouraged to eat a well-balanced diet to assist her body in the healing regenerative process. Adequate fluid intake is encouraged in order to assist in the elimination of waste products through the kidneys.

rest and sleep

Labor and delivery are strenuous, fatiguing activities. It may be difficult for the patient to rest after the excitement of the delivery, but the process of recovery is based upon adequate rest. Without sufficient rest and sleep her recovery will be retarded and she will become irritable, frustrated, and unable to cope with the situations around her, including the care of the new infant. Her need for rest cannot be overemphasized and must be a nursing priority.

IMMEDIATE CARE

Most of the patient's first day is spent in resting and sleeping after the exhaustion of labor and delivery. Interruptions are frequent because of the necessary checks by the nurse. Nursing activities should be grouped and planned to interrupt the patient as little as possible.

INTERMEDIATE CARE

After the first 24 h, the nurse will be checking the patient less frequently, allowing her more time for sleep and rest. At least half her day should be spent resting in bed. If the patient finds it difficult to sleep in the hospital because of the noise, smells, and hospital routines, nursing intervention may be necessary. A back rub, a warm drink, conversation, altering the environment, or, as a last resort, a sleeping medication will promote a good night's rest. If the telephone is disturbing to daytime rest, it should be disconnected while the patient naps.

visitors

In the first 24 h the visitors are usually limited to the husband, the father of the child, or a member of the immediate family. Visiting time should be brief so that the patient can rest. Should she become lonely for visitors, encourage her to use the telephone to visit.

Visitors throughout the hospital stay should be limited. Depending on hospital procedures, usually the husband, parents, boyfriend, or other members of the family are allowed visiting privileges. Visitors, although they are welcomed by the patient, can be exhausting and not in the best interest of the patient.

weight

At delivery the patient loses approximately 12 to 13 lb. This weight consists of the fetus, placenta, amniotic fluid, membranes, and blood. Contrary to what is general believed, not all patients lose further weight during the first 8 days of the puerperium. In a study of 200 postpartum patients, Sheikh (2) discovered that approximately 28 percent of the patients showed weight *gain* during the first 3 days after delivery. Only 40 percent of the patients showed a weight loss. Breast-feeding patients lost significantly more weight than nonlactating patients. A possible explanation might include the sodium- and water-retaining properties of the hormones used to suppress lactation. (The stress reaction of sodium and water retention and potassium loss found in postoperative patients may possibly explain the weight gained during the first week of the puerperium.) However, unless the patient gained excess weight during her pregnancy, she should return to her pre-pregnant weight by the end of the puerperium. If she gained excess weight, she may have difficulty losing it during the next few months. When weighing the patient, the nurse should check to see that the patient:

Has voided before being weighed
Is wearing a similar weight of clothing each day
Is weighed at the same time each day, usually before breakfast

diaphoresis

Labor and delivery are strenuous activities and many patients perspire freely during this time. In the body's attempt to rid itself of the extra tissue fluids accumulated during pregnancy, the patient may perspire profusely. Diaphoresis may also be caused by the hormonal changes in the body. Many patients experience nocturnal diaphoresis and awake during the night damp with perspiration.

It is important for the nurse to be aware of these physiologic reactions in order to reassure the patient that it is a normal body response.

bowels

The abdominal muscles used in the act of defecation have been stretched and may be flaccid and ineffective in assisting with defecation. For this reason many patients experience difficulty in having a bowel movement in the early puerperium. Some of the means used to reestablish proper bowel function could include the following:

Exercise to tone stretched muscles
Early ambulation
Adequate diet
Adequate fluid intake

Some physicians order stool softeners or laxatives to assist the patient until she is able to resume adequate bowel elimination. Occa-

table 10·2

VITAL SIGNS IN THE POSTPARTUM PERIOD

VITAL SIGN	FREQUENCY	PHYSIOLOGIC AND PHYSICAL CHANGES AND INFLUENCES	RESPONSE OF THE BODY	NURSING RESPONSI-BILITY AND ACTION
Temperature	q4h × 24 h Then qid when temperature is within normal limits	Immediately following delivery patient may experience "chilling" due to exertion, muscle fatigue, decrease in intra-abdominal pressure	Trembling Shivering (usually without elevation of temperature)	Cover with warm blanket Administer warm beverage Take and record temperature A significant and morbid temperature is considered any elevation over 100.4°F for any two consecutive days (excluding the first day) (1) Report any temperature elevation because it may indicate infection
		The patient may be excited or anxious	Slight temperature elevation	Attempt to calm the patient by means of a warm drink conversation, a warm bath, a back rub
		Dehydration from inadequate intake and/or excessive output	Slight temperature elevation	Increase fluid intake
Pulse	q15min × 4—then q½h × 6 qh × 3 then q4h qid	Decrease in the circulating volume of blood Cessation of pressure on the heart from the enlarged uterus Resting position of the patient	Slowing of the pulse	Take pulse rate Record pulse Note: it is within normal limits for the pulse to be slower than usual A rapid pulse may indicate hemorrhage (or phlebothrombosis) and should be reported
Respirations	Same schedule as for pulse	Decreased pressure on lungs and diaphragm from decreased size of uterus	Breathing easier and slower	Take respiratory rate Record

table 10·2 (continued)

VITAL SIGN	FREQUENCY	PHYSIOLOGIC AND PHYSICAL CHANGES AND INFLUENCES	RESPONSE OF THE BODY	NURSING RESPONSI-BILITY AND ACTION
		Medications—anesthetic or analgesic effect	Respirations may be depressed	Check patient, until she is reacted and awake, for signs of respiratory distress
Blood pressure	q15min × 1 h	Physical exertion of labor and delivery	Slight temporary increase in bp	Take bp
	q¹/₂h × 6	Sudden increase in blood volume		Compare with previous readings
	qh × 3	Medications—anesthetic or analgesic effect	Rise in bp or in fall bp	Record
				Be alert to medications and their effect on patient
	Then q4h until stable	Normal decrease in circulating blood volume begins	Slight drop in bp may occur	Check bp
	Then bid until patient discharged	A sudden loss of blood at delivery and after will dramatically affect bp	Sharp drop in bp	Check bp and amount of bleeding, degree of fundal contraction

sionally the doctor orders an enema to eliminate straining or pain for the first bowel movement. A patient with hemorrhoids may require stool softeners, enemas, local medication, sitz baths, compresses, or suppositories to reduce pain and swelling and to assist with elimination.

bath

After the strenuous activity of labor and delivery, the patient, tired and perspiring, will probably welcome a sponge bath. The bath will remove body secretions, discharges, and odors, and will be gently soothing.

IMMEDIATE CARE

The initial bath is given by the nurse either in the recovery room or on the postpartum floor. The patient may require special mouth care because of the special breathing techniques performed during labor and delivery or the drying action of scopolamine.

The patient may be drowsy and not reacting normally because of residual effects of analgesia or anesthesia. If the patient is not awake or alert enough when the nurse bathes her the first time, the nurse will have to teach her about the following hygienic care when she is alert:

1. Wash her hands. Then, with a clean washcloth, wash her breasts first. Start with the nipple and wash in a circular motion away from the nipple if she is breast-feeding.
2. Wash the rest of the body in the usual manner.
3. Use a clean washcloth to cleanse the perineal area. Wash the anal area last to prevent carrying organisms to the vagina and the bladder.

INTERMEDIATE CARE

On the second day the physician may allow the patient to take a shower. The same order listed under "Immediate Care" is to be observed when showering. The nurse must reinforce the correct procedure for hygienic care, even though she is not bathing the patient. The nurse should accompany the patient for her first shower to be sure that the shower stall is clean, that the patient has the necessary equipment, and that she is able to manage safely. The emergency signal call-light should be brought to the attention of the patient. The nurse should carry an ammonia "pearl" in her pocket whenever she accompanies a newly delivered mother to a shower or sitz bath. Fainting is not uncommon.

Some physicians are allowing their patients to take tub baths when a bathtub is available on the unit. They believe that immersion of the body in water is more effective in removing the lochia from the perineum and, particularly, from the folds of the labia. The warm water soothes the episiotomy, relieves the edema and soreness of the area, and soothes hemorrhoids if they are present. Water does not enter the vaginal canal, so there is no danger of infecting the uterus from this source. The nurse must accompany the patient for her first tub bath, to check on the cleanliness of the tub, to help the patient into the tub, and to acquaint her with the call-signal light should she need it. On subsequent days, the patient may be allowed to shower or bathe on her own with assistance from the nurse as necessary.

breast care

The non-breast-feeding mother is given hormones to suppress lactation. Occasionally a woman may still experience engorgement, with the breasts becoming enlarged, hard, painful, and warm to the touch. The nurse can employ several measures to relieve the patient's discomfort:

1. Apply an ice pack to the breasts, as ordered by the physician.
2. Support the breasts with a supporting bra or apply a breast binder.
3. Administer a mild analgesic as prescribed by the physician.

Nonlactating mothers should not pump the breasts to relieve engorgement because this only serves to stimulate further production of milk. Engorgement should diminish under these measures within 36 to 48 h (see Chap. 14). Both nonlactating and lactating mothers should be taught breast care to prevent infection and avoid trauma to the breasts; they should understand why the use of a supportive bra is important.

perineal care

During delivery the pelvic muscles are greatly stretched and usually cut by the episiotomy. It is most important that the area be kept as clean and dry as possible to prevent infection.

IMMEDIATE CARE

The initial perineal care routine is carried out by the nurse. When the patient is awake and alert, it is up to the nurse to instruct her in the following points:

1. Removing the perineal pad. Remove the pad from front to back so that the microorganisms in the rectal area are not dragged across the vaginal opening.
2. Flushing the perineal area with warm water or a mild antiseptic solution.
3. Patting dry with gauze or wipes.
4. Securing the perineal pad snugly (to pre-

vent its moving back and forth between the rectum and the vaginal opening).

INTERMEDIATE CARE

Reinforce the instruction that the patient should flush her perineal area every time she goes to the bathroom or changes her perineal pad.

Inspect the perineal area daily by having the patient lie on the same side as her episiotomy, for easier viewing. Because of the edema of the tissue it may be difficult to see the episiotomy. Chart condition, whether sutures are intact, and any signs of inflammation. The episiotomy should heal in 7 to 10 days.

If the patient has pain in the perineal area, there are several ways in which the nurse may alleviate it:

1. Administer compresses, a heat lamp, or a sitz bath as prescribed by the physician.
2. Administer analgesics or local anesthetics, as ordered.
3. Advise the patient to rest on her side and to avoid standing for long periods of time, to eliminate as much strain as possible on the area.
4. Advise patient to relax and contract the perineal-pelvic muscles periodically to stimulate circulation and muscle tone (Kegal exercise).

Should the patient complain of severe pain in the perineal area, she should be checked for a possible hematoma caused by bleeding into the vaginal wall or vulva (see Chap. 22).

afterpains

As discussed earlier, the uterus contracts and retracts in its descent into the pelvic area. In the primipara these contractions are gener-

ally painless. However, in the multipara or the patient whose uterine muscles have been stretched excessively, as in polyhydramnios, or multiple pregnancies, the uterus has lost some of its tonicity. For these patients the contractions may be painful. The pain usually subsides in 4 to 7 days. Mild analgesics are given as prescribed (see Chap. 18).

Lactating patients may be aware of the contractions when the infant nurses because of the sucking stimulus to oxytocin release.

activities

Just as early ambulation aids in bladder and bowel elimination, it also hastens the recovery of the postpartum patient. Ambulation stimulates circulation and helps to prevent thrombosis. It also helps the body to retain and regain muscle tone. The patient regains her strength sooner without harming her episiotomy or interfering with her vaginal discharge.

IMMEDIATE CARE

The patient remains in bed until she is fully recovered from the effects of any analgesics or anesthetics she may have received. Unless otherwise indicated the patient should be out of bed initially 4 to 6 h after delivery for a short time with assistance, perhaps to the toilet. While she is in bed, raise the head of the bed and have her turn frequently, to assist in the draining of the lochia.

INTERMEDIATE CARE

After the first day, the patient is allowed out of bed at will . However, do not relinquish your functions simply because the patient is now out of bed. Your role as teacher, planner, and observer is necessary for the out-of-bed patient as well. See that the patient rests, has an adequate diet, and does not stand for long periods.

exercise

The exercises the mother may have practiced during the antepartum period will be useful in helping the body and muscles regain strength and tone. Exercise promotes circulation and helps to reduce the possibility of thrombosis. The physician directs the program of exercise for the patient. The following schedule is suggested in the psychoprophylaxis method of preparation for childbirth (PPM) (see Chap. 7 for review and diagrams).

Day of delivery—Kegal exercise
Postpartum day 1 (P.P. 1)—Kegal exercise and pelvic tilt—bid
P.P. 2—Kegal exercise, pelvic tilt, abdominal isometrics, chest breathing
P.P. 3—Same as 2—add head tilt
P.P. 4—Same as 3—add back exercise-arch
P.P. 5—Same as 4—add modified situp

Additional exercises are illustrated in Fig. 10·4.

The postpartum period is a crucial time in the recovery process for the patient. The nurse must keep in mind the goals of postpartum care:

To prevent infection
To prevent hemorrhage
To promote healing

The aspects of care of particular concern for the nurse are:

The uterus-fundus
Lochia
Voiding
Vital signs
Nutrition

Patients are discharged between the second and fifth days after delivery. The nurse must teach the patient about fundus check, lochia check, perineal care, and bath hygiene including breast care, so that the patient can continue her care at home.

fig. 10·4 Postpartal exercises. (Note: Each exercise is to be repeated four times, twice daily, with a new exercise added each day.)

A *First day:* Breathe in deeply; expand the abdomen. Exhale slowly, hissing; draw in abdominal muscles forcibly.

B *Second day:* Lie flat on the back with the legs slightly apart. Hold arms at right angles to the body; slowly raise the arms, keeping the elbows stiff. Touch hands together and gradually return arms to their original position.

C *Third day:* Lie flat on the back with the arms at the sides. Draw the knees up slightly. Arch the back.

D *Fourth day:* Lie flat on the back with the knees and hips flexed. Tilt the pelvis inward and contract the buttocks tightly. Lift the head while contracting the abdominal muscles.

E *Fifth day:* Lie flat on back with the legs straight. Raise the head and one knee slightly. Then reach for, but do not touch, the knee with the opposite hand. Alternate with the right and left hand.

F *Sixth day:* Slowly flex the knee and then the thigh on the abdomen. Lower the foot to the buttock. Straighten and lower the leg to the floor.

G *Seventh day:* Raise first the right and then the left leg as high as possible. Keep the toes pointed and the knee straight. Lower the leg gradually, using the abdominal muscles but not the hands.

H *Eighth day:* Rest on the elbows and knees, keeping the upper arms and legs perpendicular with the body. Hump the back upward. Contract the buttocks and draw the abdomen in vigorously. Relax, breathe deeply.

I *Ninth day:* Same as seventh day, but raise both legs at the same time, etc.

J *Tenth day:* Lie flat on the back with the arms clasped behind the head. Then sit up slowly. (If necessary, hook feet under furniture.) Slowly lie back.

(*Courtesy of R. C. Benson, Handbook of Obstetrics and Gynecology, 4th ed., Lange Medical Publications, Los Altos, Calif., 1971.*)

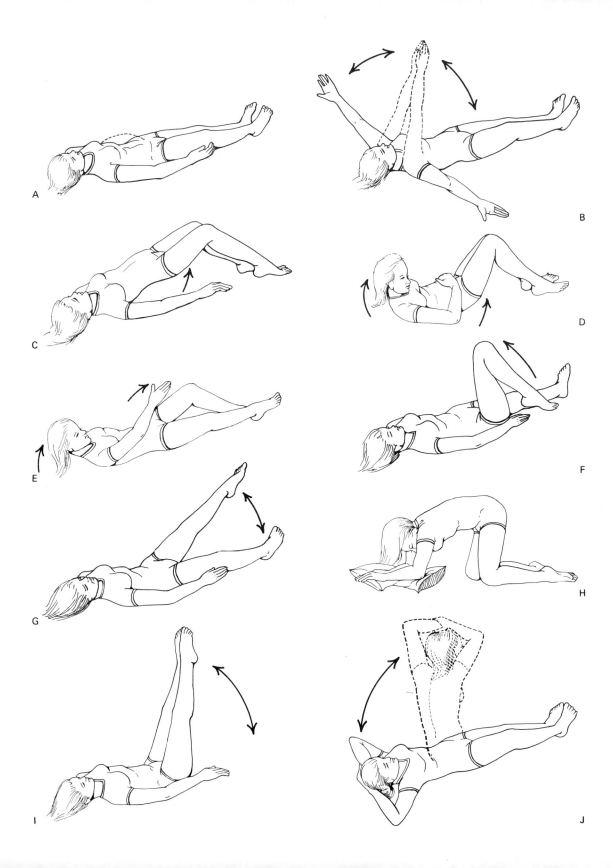

A

B

C

D

E

F

G

H

I

J

references

1. *The Manual of Standards in Obstetric-Gynecologic Practice,* The American College of Obstetricians and Gynecologists, Chicago, 1965.
2. Ghulam N. Sheikh, "Observations of Maternal Weight Behavior during the Puerperium," *American Journal of Obstetrics and Gynecology,* **113**(2):244–250, 1971.

bibliography

Anderson, Edith H.: "Today's Parents and Maternity Nursing," in Betty S. Bergersen et al. (eds.), *Current Concepts in Clinical Nursing,* vol. 1, The C. V. Mosby Company, St. Louis, 1967, pp. 355–364.

Benson, Ralph C.: *Handbook of Obstetrics and Gynecology,* 4th ed., Lange Medical Publications, Los Altos, Calif., 1971.

Fitzpatrick Elise, et al.: *Maternity Nursing,* 12th ed., J. B. Lippincott Company, Philadelphia, 1971.

Hellman, Louis M., and Jack A. Pritchard: *Williams' Obstetrics,* 14th ed., Appleton-Century-Crofts, Inc., New York, 1971.

Hogan, Aileen I.: "The Role of the Nurse in Meeting the Needs of the New Mother," *Nursing Clinics of North America,* **3**:337–344, 1968.

Hytten, Frank E., and Isabella Leitch: *The Physiology of Human Pregnancy,* 2d ed., Blackwell Scientific Publications, Ltd., Oxford, 1972.

The Manual of Standards in Obstetric-Gynecologic Practice, 2d ed., The American College of Obstetricians and Gynecologists, Chicago, 1965.

Rich, Olive J.: "Hospital Routines as Rites of Passage in Developing Maternal Identity," *Nursing Clinics of North America,* **4**:101–109, 1969.

Rubin, Reva: "The Neomaternal Period," in Betty S. Bergersen et al. (eds.), *Current Concepts in Clinical Nursing,* vol. I, The C. V. Mosby Company, St. Louis, 1969, pp. 388–391.

Rugh, Roberts, and Landrum B. Shettles: *From Conception to Birth: The Drama of Life's Beginning,* Harper & Row, Publishers, Incorporated, New York, 1971.

Salk, L.: "The Critical Nature of the Postpartum Period in the Human for the Establishment of the Mother-Infant Bond: A Controlled Study," *Diseases of the Nervous System,* Suppl., 110–116, November, 1970.

Sheikh, Ghulam N.: "Observations of Maternal Weight Behavior during the Puerperium," *American Journal of Obstetrics and Gynecology* **3**(2):244–250, 1971.

Williams, Barbara: "Sleep Needs during the Maternity Cycle," *Nursing Outlook,* **15**:53–55, 1967.

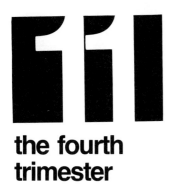

the fourth trimester

Hilda Koehler

initial adjustments

New parents begin to come to grips with being a family at various points in their relationship—some during pregnancy, some at the birth of the baby, some at one of the visiting hours during the hospital stay. For first-time parents, the shift in thinking goes from, "We're a couple," to, "We have a child." For many it is not until the second child that the orientation becomes, "We're a family!"

The first sensations after delivery vary from a matter-fo-fact, "I'm relieved *that's* over!" to a mystical, triumphant sense of achievement. For women who actively participate in giving birth, a rush of maternal feeling may occur as the baby is born, with the mother reaching out her arms to enfold the baby (Fig. 11·1). If the baby is active, crying vigorously but becomes quiet in her arms or demonstrates a readiness to suck and nuzzles onto the mother's nipple eagerly, mother-child rapport seems to become more easily established.

On the other hand, especially to the woman who was not actively involved in the birth of her baby, the newcomer may seem like a very strange creature indeed and a getting-acquainted period is in order. At first the mother may need to familiarize herself with the baby from top to toe, section by section,

exploring with her fingertips in a tentative way (Fig. 11·2). Gradually she will feel more comfortable with the newcomer, and will hold the baby close. Since practically all mothers-to-be expect that they will love their babies immediately when they see them, they are likely to be confused and feel guilty at feelings of strangeness and relative indifference in the presence of the little one. Reassurance that it can sometimes take 3 months or more after the baby comes to begin really to feel like a mother can help ease the strain and start the first stages of this most intimate relationship.

Most new parents need to know that a newborn baby tends to be very groggy, in a "twilight sleep" of his own, after initially being alert and active at birth. If a limp, uninterested, seemingly unresponsive baby is brought in to the mother several hours after birth, she may become anxious about the child's condition; in addition she may feel inadequate as a parent because she cannot rouse him.

The mother's immediate energy level may vary from intense exhilaration and gaiety, especially in those who were "awake and aware" for the birth, to extreme fatigue and a need for restorative sleep. The nurse will find it therapeutic for the new mother to provide her with the opportunity to share her birth experience—and she may find herself caught up in the mother's enthusiasm and joy.

An early visit with the baby's father, or another family member, is important. Not too long a visit, though, because, whether or not she is aware of it, the parturient has worked very hard during labor, and she should be urged to try to rest at this point. Usually these women can only sleep in naps, anyway, many times reliving the childbirth experience during sleep or rehearsing it mentally in the drowsy state between wakefulness and sleep.

Prolonged, difficult labor or emotional/psychologic complications (for example, when a woman is not going to keep her baby

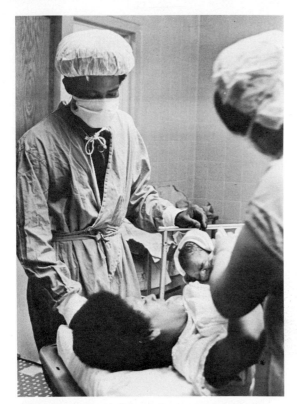

fig. 11·1 Mother holding baby on delivery table. (*Photo by Andrew McGowan.*)

or when there has been an abnormality) may lead her to retreat into sleep for a while. The exhausted new mother needs a milieu in which she can rest undisturbed. It will take a creative, watchful nurse to ensure this atmosphere in a busy hospital with its attendant "routines." Careful planning can minimize the number of times the new mother is disturbed for checking fundus, lochia, voiding, temperature.

If the new father is still present while the mother is resting or delayed in the recovery room, the alert nurse will be sensitive to his needs and suggest appropriate remedies if he seems to need direction. Providing refreshment or a listening ear, or finding a place for him to rest undisturbed temporarily are services for which a new father usually is very appreciative.

taking in-taking hold-letting go

Reva Rubin has described three phases in the puerperium which help nurses to understand the behavior of new mothers and plan their care (1). The first phase, *taking in,* lasts from 2 to 3 days and is marked by behavior which indicates that the mother is trying to absorb her new experience. She eats, she sleeps, she is concerned with the baby's eating and sleeping, and is eager to verbalize to anyone ready to listen. The nurse can help her interpret what has happened, enabling her to integrate and make a cohesive whole out of her new status. The second phase, *taking hold,* lasts about 10 days, and indicates that the new mother is now trying to take some initiative in her responsibility for herself and the infant. What she needs most is support and encouragement. Since she usually questions her competence to take charge of her own life and that of her infant, she may be overzealous in seeking advice and information. Organized teaching programs will be useful during the taking-hold phase—but the teacher/nurse, if she is wise, will avoid the temptation to appear as having all the answers and knowing all the tricks (2). The third phase, *letting go,* signifies that the mother is ready to regard this new baby as truly a

fig. 11·2 Mother exploring baby with fingertips. (*Photo by Andrew McGowan.*)

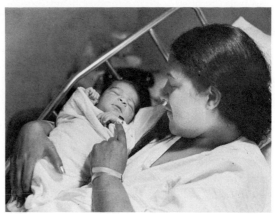

person separate from herself. Some women find this transition harder than others, for some derive great pleasure in considering the baby an extension of themselves.

Differing styles of maternity in-patient services are used throughout the United States today. They range from a rooming-in plan, in which the mother and father assume complete care for the infant, with professional help and guidance available as needed, to the standard central nursery, with the baby being brought out to the mother so that she may feed him only on a periodic basis. Somewhere in between is the flexible family-centered maternity care system, in which new parents participate in the baby's care as much or as little as they wish, with individual assessment made of both the baby and the parents' abilities by the professional staff, and a planned educational program for new parents. Recently there is impetus, which springs from the expressed desires of parents, to have a "father's hour" in those institutions without rooming-in or family-centered maternity care plans. During "father's hour," the father can handle, play with, and perhaps feed his offspring, with supervision nearby (Fig. 11·3).

Whichever situation the nurse is in, her support and anticipatory guidance can determine whether the adjustment period at home will be filled with anxiety and frustration or with an operational "Let's-learn-together!" approach, leavened with a sense of humor. If the same person is caring for both mother and baby throughout the course of the hospital stay, there are innumerable opportunities to fit teaching and anticipatory guidance into the natural pattern of care. In standard maternity care, a team plan is usually most convenient and effective, with the nursing care coordinator delegating responsibility to the team member most expert or willing to prepare new parents for home going. Depending on the skill and performance of the instructor, lecture/demonstrations, demonstrations re-

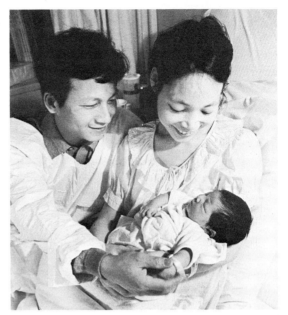

fig. 11·3 "Father's hour": participating in feeding time. (*Photo by Andrew McGowan.*)

turned by the mother or father, filmstrips/films/videotapes, and coffee-klatch discussions all have their place in helping new parents cope with their new 24-hours-a-day, 7-days-a-week responsibility (Fig. 11·4).

postpartum depression

In the intermediate postpartum period (frequently on the third day), there is a distinct possibility that the phenomenon called "after-the-baby blues" may occur. This period of depression can be quite frightening if it is not anticipated. It is thought to be caused by a combination of factors: losing the hormones of pregnancy, which disappear with the expulsion of the placenta; making general physical adjustments to return to the nonpregnant state; and dealing with the reality of the child's truly being here. After-the-baby blues are usually short-lived—48 h at most. Typically, the attention of family and friends has swung from the woman, who enjoyed it during

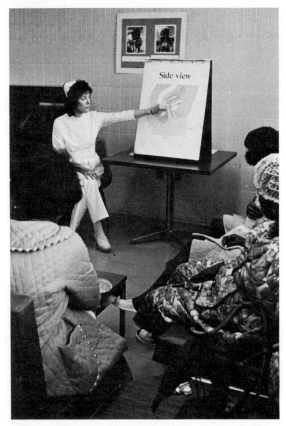

fig. 11·4 Nurse teaching postpartum class on family planning. (*Photo by Nancy Goodman.*)

formance in labor; they may not have met their own expectations of how they should have acted. Changes in the mother's relationship to her spouse, other children, and possibly other family members may give general cause for apprehension.

If a woman begins to be increasingly irritable and anxious, with crying spells, insomnia, somatic complaints, and seclusiveness, the nurse should suspect that her patient has become one of those new mothers (statistically 1 in every 1000) who are unable to withstand these emotional burdens and who develop a psychosis. When a woman disclaims her baby or confides to a nurse that she doesn't like it or if she begins expressing antipathy toward her husband, the nurse should recognize the need for close observation and psychiatric referral (3). Generally, the behavior changes indicating pathologic emotional disturbances arise in the first 6 weeks at home. (Some of these psychoses show symptoms during the antenatal period.) A woman who has had a previous mental disorder, with or without pregnancy, is the most obvious candidate for a postpartum psychosis, and the nurse should be particularly alert in such a case and responsive to the cues of depression.

her pregnancy, to the baby. The baby's father may, without thinking, reinforce her feeling of decreased importance by putting his head into her room and saying, "Hi! I'm going to go see the baby," and not returning until visiting hours are almost over. Obviously this does nothing for the mother's plunging self-esteem!

Some mothers, though they are relieved that they did not die in childbirth and profoundly grateful that the baby is normal, still have a certain amount of grieving to work through. This baby is simply not the "perfect" child they pictured in their fantasies. Some are exploring the impact which complete responsibility for the child will have on their lives. Others may be disappointed with their per-

going home

The first day home with a new baby is exciting, tiring, and bewildering (Fig. 11·5A, B). A sense of humor is invaluable. Even parents who have received a thorough orientation to infant care under the guidance of medical professionals are likely to have surprises in store.

All people experience their babies uniquely. Taking an infant home after childbirth is a human experience so affect laden that it cannot be experienced vicariously. Touching this product of human intimacy,

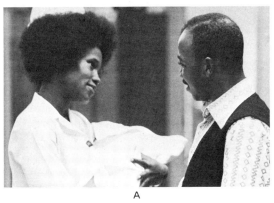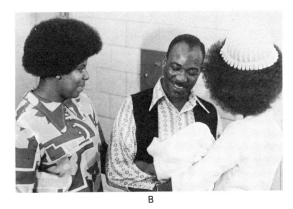

fig. 11·5 Home going—a time for anticipatory guidance. A Father's turn. B Assuming new responsibility. (*Photos by Nancy Goodman.*)

feeling its supplicating tenderness, responding to the urgency of its early bleating helplessness, coming to know its cycles of pain and pleasure, struggling with its phylogenetic heritage of animal needs and impulses, permitting it enough mastery in the external world to insure security while imposing enough limits so that it comes to know reality, these are performances which are necessarily spontaneous and immediate, and no educational procedure can be designed to soften the impact of their newness (4).

So those who have carefully schooled themselves for new parenthood, hoping, perhaps unconsciously, to enter the experience as "old hands," are likely to be disappointed. Nothing can totally prepare a parent for the experience of having a new baby but the experience itself.

Everyone will want to see the mother and child. But new parents should take caution to limit the number and kinds of visitors, especially the length of time visitors stay. The recovering mother and the newborn are particularly susceptible to infection, so any visitors with skin or upper respiratory infections should be asked to wait until they are well before they visit. The new mother should in no way do anything special to entertain the visitors, but, unless forewarned, she may find herself preparing meals for outsiders—and being exhausted! Signals should be arranged in advance between the mother and another family member, so that she may indicate when she is getting weary; the family then says a gracious but firm goodbye to the guests. If the mother doesn't get fully dressed for the first 2 weeks, visitors often are more considerate because they realize she does not have her usual level of energy.

help

Considering how physically weary new mothers are, and all the anxiety involved in having the complete care of a newborn when the baby is home, one of the most useful things a family can do is to arrange for housework help for the first few weeks at least. Dr. Spock says that if there are twins, the family should go into debt, if necessary, in order to ensure adequate domestic assistance (5)! Various sources are possibilities: agencies, family, neighbors; full-time, part-time, rotating help. Most needed is help with cooking, cleaning, shopping, and laundry. Actually, many of these things can be done by new fathers—especially if homemade "TV" dinners are frozen in advance and a flexible schedule prepared which can be consulted after coming home. Many men arrange to take vacation when the baby comes home, which enables them to provide household care. There also are many men who find it very upsetting to leave the house for work, knowing they won't be back for several hours every day—they feel as if they are deserting and not providing the protection and support their new family needs.

Mothers and mothers-in-law are most frequently called on to help; in most cases this works out well, but it is wise for the new mother to establish the ground rules ahead of time; otherwise she may find that grandmother is taking care of the baby and mother is doing the cooking, cleaning, etc. Conflict in styles of baby care between the novice mother and the experienced grandmother are an ever-present possibility; these often are focused on disagreements over how, when, and what the child should be fed. Grandmothers may also have a heightened sense of rivalry with their daughters or daughters-in-law, consciously or unconsciously seeking to confirm to themselves and their sons that they are still the experts. A frank discussion before the baby's birth can open the possibility for these feelings and attempts to minimize their destructiveness when the new mother most needs aid and reassurance.

Similarly, a baby nurse may be magnificently instructive and a real assistance to the family, or she may be possessive and tyrannical, scarcely letting the parents near the baby. Her role and functions should be agreed upon prior to employment.

Often overlooked are teen-agers or senior citizens in the neighborhood who might be free to spend an hour or two periodically just baby-sitting—listening for the baby, allowing the mother to sleep without having to keep one ear attuned for the baby's cry, or allowing her to go for a walk alone for a short time.

The Visiting Nurse Service is a frequently used resource, either because the new parents seek consultation, or because the professionals send a referral before the family is home. Nurses should be aware that referrals are important, especially when there is a premature birth, when a teen-ager gives birth, or when there is an abnormality.

Some parents have the misconception that the visiting nurse is to come in to bathe the baby, prepare the formula, or perhaps check the house for dust. Being able to see the nurse as a helper instead of a policeman and a consultant instead of a homemaker prepares the family for relating to her appropriately. As Yeaworth says, the mother does not need a nurse who demonstrates her own ability in quieting the baby or who offers to take the baby aside and give him a bottle. She needs a nurse who can assess the mother's lack in understanding and information and provide this information while conveying the impression that she views her as a concerned and potentially competent mother (6). "All the technical knowledge is to no avail if the mother sits there and says, 'Yes, yes, I understand.' The only thing that she understands is that, if she says 'yes' to everything, the public health nurse will go away sooner than if she says 'no'" (7).

The following checklist has been found to be very useful. It developed out of the work of Richard and Katherine Gordon.

1. The responsibilities of parenthood are learned: *Get information.*
2. Get help from dependable friends and relatives.
3. Make friends with "experienced" couples.
4. Don't overload yourself with unimportant tasks.
5. Don't move soon after the baby arrives.
6. Don't be concerned with keeping up appearances.
7. Get plenty of rest and sleep.
8. Don't be a nurse to relatives and others at this period.

9. Confer and consult with your friends, family, and each other—*discuss your plans and worries.*
10. Don't give up outside interests, but cut down on responsibilities and rearrange schedules.
11. Arrange for baby-sitters early.
12. Get a family doctor/pediatrician early (8).

jealousy

All previous relationships are open to jealousy when a new member joins the family—husband/wife, parent/child, master/pet. Open discussion is the primary means of minimizing jealousy that a new father may experience, as so much attention is of necessity lavished on the newborn. Frequently the fathers of breast-fed infants may discover hostility toward the baby that surprises them, as expressed by one father who said, "Those breasts are mine, not that baby's!" Comprehending the facts intellectually is entirely different from being able to act without emotions interfering, however. An example of this is the new mother who remarked, "He knows I need rest, and urges me to take naps. But then he asks why his socks haven't been washed!"

If the new father participates in the care of the baby—and men are often far better at burping and quieting babies than women—jealousy is often sublimated through this sharing of responsibility. Unfortunately, cultural conditioning or fear of doing damage to the seemingly fragile newborn tends to make some men resist being included. Previous experience during a "father's hour" at the hospital, or in rooming-in or a family-centered maternity care unit, eliminates having to deal with the brunt of these feelings at home, away from professional encouragement and guidance. New mothers may need to be reminded to be sure to leave the new father alone with the child several times a week. He needs to develop his own special relationship with the baby, and her presence can interfere, particularly if she continually makes suggestions as to how to hold, handle, and relate to the baby (Figs. 11·6, and 11·7).

The birth of a son can be particularly stressful for a man who is unsure of his masculinity and his male role. In its extreme this becomes a pathologic fear of closeness with the new, dependent male (9). Added responsibility threatens the security of most husbands, but for some, a new son may be a real competitor (10).

It is not uncommon for a new father's behavior to prompt jealousy in the mother and for the mother to begin to feel that he regards her primarily as the nurturer of his child rather than as his lover/wife. This is accentuated if he continually comes home from work to

fig. 11·6 Father participates in baby care. (*Photo by John Young.*)

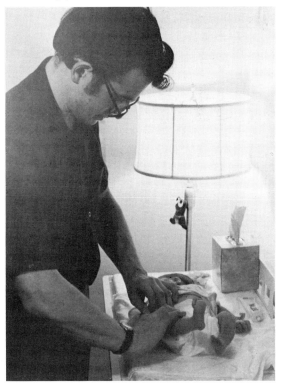

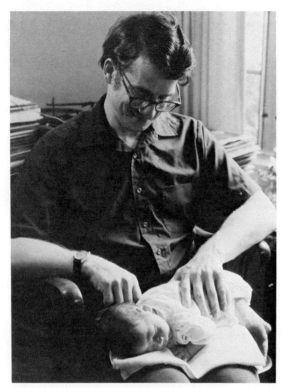

fig. 11·7 Father and son get acquainted. (*Photo by John Young.*)

concentrate on the activity and behavior of the child, neglecting to relate to her as a person.

Other children are sure to be jealous of the new family member, the severity and manifestation of this emotion being peculiarly dependent on the age of the sibling. To the age of approximately four years, when the child's logic begins to be fairly reliable, the new baby is looked upon only and absolutely as an intruder. Saying, "We thought you were so wonderful we decided to have another child," to a two-year-old is equivalent to a husband's telling his wife, "I thought you were such a marvelous wife that I've decided to have another one. Here she is! I'm going to sleep with her one night and you the next."

Early, subtle involvement will help deter-

mine whether the older child(ren) will be an ally rather than a sulking, potential enemy. Dr. Kappelman (11) suggests the following:

PREPARATION BEFORE THE BABY COMES:

1. Include the child in activities related to the coming event, such as shopping, building, painting, redecorating.
2. Plan with the child where s/he will stay during mother's hospitalization. If staying with a neighbor or relative, he might spend the night as a "dry run" in advance of the expected due date. (When mother returns as promised, this reassures the child that s/he had not been abandoned.)
3. Be aware that children can misinterpret things they overhear; parents should be matter-of-fact and positive about the impending hospitalization.
4. If the older child will be going into a new bed, make the transfer as early in pregnancy as possible.
5. If possible, begin toilet training well in advance of the new baby's arrival. Otherwise, delay toilet training until the older child has gotten used to the new baby and the attention given the new baby's bowel habits.
6. Consider buying (and wrapping) inexpensive items and storing them for later use when visitors arrive gift-laden for the newcomer.

WHEN THE NEW BABY ARRIVES:

1. Try to understand that the older child needs to express his continued dependency and need for attention. Explaining gently and frequently the positive aspects of "growing up" helps prevent regressive behavior.
2. When guests arrive with gifts for the baby, besides giving the older child the tucked-

away surprises at intervals, let him/her have the fun of pulling the wraps from the baby's gifts, especially if the older child is two or three years old.

3. Consider giving the older children a special gift when the baby is brought home from the hospital, specifying this as the newcomer's "thank you" for making everything ready for him.

4. Remember that older children still need physical attention—snuggling, rocking, hugging. This extra assurance helps convince the child that love can be expanded to fit two or three or more children.

5. Let the child "help" with the baby: this helps him/her feel important. However, don't overdo it to the point that the older sibling feels like the baby's slave ("I'll never get to *play*, ever again . . .") (Fig. 11·8).

6. Alert other important people in the child's life—grandparents, friends—to be particularly sensitive to him/her at this upsetting time. Prevent any anger or hurt that might get displaced on the baby.

7. If there is a change in the expected plan for the newborn, deal with the older child's fears kindly and realistically. For example, if the baby is premature, try to have a Polaroid picture taken to show to the older child.

8. Take advantage of books that express the message of the problems the older child experiences in living with the new arrival: *Peter's Chair* and *A Baby Sister for Frances* (Harper & Row) and *The Very Little Girl* and *The Very Little Boy* (Doubleday), for example (11).

parental roles

Two obstacles are common to new parents as they seek to assume their new responsibilities. The first is a feeling of inadequacy, which can lose much of its devastating effect if a professional can remind them that they are not inadequate but merely inexperienced.

The second obstacle besetting new parents is the feeling of being trapped, followed by a feeling of resentment of the baby. Husbands often need help in understanding how claustrophobic and confining being with a baby 24 h a day, 7 days a week, can be. Good, thoughtful planning can eliminate much of this frustration in new mothers.

Mann lists the following as the most important and frequently played roles of parents:

1. Loving, cherishing, enjoying, caring for, giving
2. Observing, listening, inquiring, learning, understanding, accepting
3. Allowing, permitting, consenting, approving, encouraging, praising
4. Sharing, feeling with, playing with, working with, talking with, and even thinking with
5. Guiding, directing, controlling, requiring, leading, disciplining, socializing
6. Informing, teaching, demonstrating, explaining, helping set experience into a set of values and standards

fig. 11·8 Siblings. (*Photo by Karen Gilborn.*)

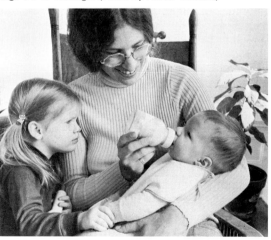

7. Trying to prevent troublesome emotions, such as fear, anger, or hostility; and when these cannot be prevented, helping the child get rid of or manage them (12)

Surely these are formidable responsibilities. Professionals should give all possible assistance to parents so that they may fulfill their roles smoothly—even if it takes the simple form of affirming their competence and goodwill.

postpartum and interconceptional care

Most obstetricians instruct new mothers that they should obstain from intercourse the last few weeks of pregnancy, and that nothing should go into the vagina until after the check-up 4 to 6 weeks postpartum; that is, no douching, no tampons, and no sex. For the first 3 weeks after the baby is born, when the woman is having at least some lochia alba, following those instructions is important in preventing infection. Usually, too, the episiotomy area is healing and is tender. But after 3 weeks, when the episiotomy is healed and there is no vaginal discharge, the issue of whether to resume vaginal intercourse may become a live one. Although the couple may have been using other techniques of sexual pleasure, it may have been two or three full months since the couple has enjoyed intercourse and it is understandable if they will want to resume that part of their relationship. Women seem to divide clearly into two groups: those who are most eager to resume sexual intercourse and those who are completely uninterested. Frequently this subject is not discussed by any of the professionals who come in contact with the couple; but resuming intercourse certainly deserves as much attention as how to prepare formula!

If the woman is breast-feeding, vaginal secretions and lubrication may be greatly diminished because of the hormones that maintain lactation; sterile lubricants can be used to facilitate the comfort of love play and penetration. For some women, full, leaking breasts will be accompanied by a let-down reflex during orgasm. This may not only make the traditional position impossible, but may make for a very liquid experience if a towel is not used. Breast-feeding women are unlikely to ovulate for the first 8 weeks if they are giving the baby no other food, so that chances of conception are rare (13). However, if one becomes pregnant, one is 100 percent pregnant, so contraception should be used.

If a woman is bottle feeding, the couple should know that she may ovulate before she resumes having periods, at 4 to 6 weeks. More and more women who plan to use contraceptive pills are beginning to use them on leaving the hospital. But not everyone is so protected.

Women using contraceptive pills or an intrauterine device will receive a thorough physical examination each time they come for a follow-up visit, usually at least annually. Many women are tempted not to return for their postpartum checkup; they feel well and consider it a trip for no useful purpose other than keeping their chart's paperwork in order. The nurse is in a key position to impress the mother that a postpartum examination is not simply "routine." Valuable data as to the woman's general well-being, as well as confirmation that the reproductive organs have resumed proper nonpregnant position and function, can set the woman's mind at rest, as well as give her family confidence in her ability to do her nurturing tasks. If conditions such as slight anemia or cervical erosions exist, they can be treated before they become major problems. At this visit, the effectiveness of the body-toning exercises that the woman should have been doing can be assessed and further instructions given as necessary. The nurse or the physician can teach or reinforce the necessity and method of breast self-examination and the wisdom of interconceptional health maintenance, including a Papanicolaou smear.

In past years the health checkup was considered even more of a waste of time than the postpartum examination. But with the renewed emphasis on preventive medicine, plus the impact of the Women's Movement, more and more women are taking advantage of gynecologic services before their condition demands a visit. With the expected coming of a national health care system within the next few years, women from all socioeconomic levels will use health maintenance facilities, not the least important of which is early prenatal care and complete postdelivery care.

references

1. Reva Rubin, "Puerperal Change," *Nursing Outlook,* **9**(12):753–755, 1961.
2. Betty S. Bergersen et al., "Adapting Postpartum Teaching to Mothers' Low-income Life-styles," chap. 27 in *Current Concepts in Clinical Nursing,* The C. V. Mosby Company, St. Louis, 1969, pp. 280–291.
3. Elizabeth M. Seward, "Preventing Postpartum Psychosis," *American Journal of Nursing,* **72**(3):529, 1972.
4. David Mann et al., *Educating Expectant Parents,* Visiting Nurse Service of New York, New York, 1961.
5. Benjamin Spock, *Baby and Child Care*, Pocket Books, Inc., New York, 1968.
6. Rosalee C. Yeaworth, "Maternity Nursing—Challenging or Routine?" *Nursing Clinics of North America,* **6**(2):247, 1971.
7. Marguerite W. Bozian, "Nursing Care of the Infant in the Community," *Nursing Clinics of North America,* **6**(1):93, 1971.

8. R. E. Gordon et al., "Factors in Postpartum Emotional Adjustment," *Obstetrics and Gynecology,* **25**(2):158–166, 1965.
9. Arthur D. Coleman and Libby Lee Coleman, *Pregnancy: The Psychological Experience,* Herder and Herder, Inc., New York, 1971, p. 164.
10. Ibid., p. 165.
11. Murray M. Kappelman, *What Your Child Is All About*, Reader's Digest Press, New York, 1974.
12. Mann, op. cit., p. 102.
13. T. J. Cronin, "Influence of Lactation upon Ovulation," *Lancet,* **2**:422, 1968.

bibliography

Bergersen, Betty S., et al.: "Adapting Postpartum Teaching to Mother's Low-income Life Styles," chap. 27, in *Current Concepts in Clinical Nursing,* The C. V. Mosby Company, St. Louis, 1969.

Bordon, D.: "Puerperal Psychosis," *Nursing Times,* **68**(20):615, 1972.

Boston Women's Health Book Collective, *Our Bodies, Ourselves,* Simon & Shuster, Inc., New York, 1973.

Bozian, Marguerite W.: "Nursing Care of the Infant in the Community," *Nursing Clinics of North America,* **6**(1):93, 1971.

Coleman, Arthur, D., and Libby Lee Coleman: *Pregnancy: The Psychological Experience,* Herder and Herder, Inc., New York, 1971.

Good, Raphael S.: "The Third Ear: Interviewing Techniques in Obstetrics and Gynecology," *Obstetrics and Gynecology,* **40**(5):760, 1972.

Gordon, R. E., et al.: "Factors in Postpartum Emotional Adjustment," *Obstetrics and Gynecology,* **25**(2):158, 1965.

Kappelman, Murray: "Welcome to the New Baby!" *Family Health,* November, 1972, p. 9.

Kitzinger, Sheila: *The Experience of Childbirth*, 3d ed., Penguin Books, Inc., Baltimore, 1972.

Rozdilsky, Mary Lou, and Barbara Banet: *What Now?: A Handbook for Parents Postpartum*, Magic Machine, Seattle, 1972.

Rubin, Reva: "Puerperal Change," *Nursing Outlook*, **9**(12):753, 1961.

Seward, Elizabeth M.: "Preventing Postpartum Psychosis," *American Journal of Nursing*, **72**(3):520, 1972.

Shaywitz, Sally E.: "Catch 22 for Mothers," *The New York Times Magazine*, Mar. 4, 1973, p. 50.

Spock, Benjamin: *Baby and Child Care*, Pocket Books, Inc., New York, 1968.

Sweeney, Bernadette: "Family Centered Care in Public Health Nursing," *Nursing Forum*, **9**(2):169, 1970.

Yeaworth, Rosalee C.: "Maternity Nursing—Challenging or Routine?" *Nursing Clinics of North America*, **6**(2):247, 1971.

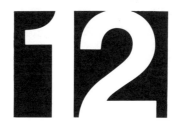

observations of the newborn

Janet S. Reinbrecht

The fetal organ systems usually function efficiently as long as the mother provides a healthy uterine environment. At term (around 38 weeks or 266 days after conception) the fetal systems, not unlike a space ship, must stand at "ready" for "blast-off." They must be ready in order to make the marked changes that occur at birth. The sudden exit from the warm, weightless, fluid environment to a cold, dry, and pressurized atmosphere makes the transition abrupt and hazardous.

The demands upon the neonate are many as the relative security of fetal life ends with the first breath and cutting of the cord. The newborn begins a long process of adapting to a new phase of life. It is both a joy and a responsibility to assist in the nurturing of another of God's intricate and unique creations. To accomplish the awesome task better, the nurse must become familiar with the behavior and normal characteristic changes which indicate how smoothly the adjustments are occurring.

The first 28 days of life, referred to as the *newborn,* or *neonatal, period,* are highly critical. Many physiologic adjustments are required if the neonate is to survive outside the uterus. The critical nature of these adjustments is supported by mortality and morbidity rates.

In the United States, more than two-thirds of

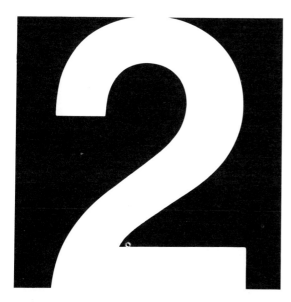

the healthy infant

the deaths in the first year of life occur in the first 28 days after birth. The importance of a smooth adjustment in the *first 24 h* is attested to by the fact that more human beings die in this short period of time than at any other time of life.

the first twenty-four hours

The transition from fetal to neonatal life is not predictable. Although many babies make the transition very efficiently, every newborn must be assessed individually. He must be observed closely to determine if he has made the transition smoothly. The nursing goal is *anticipatory* and *preventive* care. The nurse must anticipate the stressors involved in the reorganization of the baby's metabolic processes, and must act accordingly to prevent additional stress because of chilling or exposure to infection.

The influences of prenatal environment, the labor forces, the trauma of birth, plus possible congenital conditions, affect the transition to postnatal life. Knowledge about these factors can help minimize possible complications. The first 24 h are the most crucial, since at this time, shock, hemorrhage, convulsions, and respiratory distress may occur with lightning speed. There is a higher incidence of death in these hours than at any other period of the first 4 weeks.

Initially the baby appears alert and cries lustily. He may even suck hungrily on his fist. Breast feeding at this time tends to be very satisfying to the mother because the baby sucks well and usually has his eyes open. Generally a mother finds greater satisfaction in seeing her baby with his eyes open; he seems more a real person. By about 30 min after birth, he begins to settle down, with slower heart and respiratory rates. His temperature begins to fall. (To keep his temperature from dropping too low, any bathing

should be avoided during this time.) He falls into a deep sleep which may last from 2 to 4 h.

Following this first period of sleep, the baby again becomes active. His heart and respiratory rates may fluctuate, depending upon the extent of his activity. At this time the nurse takes his temperature. This may be the time when he passes his first stool, *meconium,* before or after insertion of the rectal thermometer. Be alert for mucous secretions that may interfere with the established respiratory pattern. A healthy baby may be able to cough and swallow the mucus, if it is not excessive. However, gentle suctioning of the mouth may be necessary.

Positioning is an important assist to the baby's ability to handle the oral secretions. The best positions are on the side and abdomen. Only if mucus is excessive, the stomach may need to be aspirated to remove accumulated swallowed amniotic fluid. After the stomach contents have been removed, the infant should be placed on his abdomen, with his head lower than his feet, for postural drainage. Gentle patting over the lung bases will aid drainage. If any mucus remains in the mouth, the baby can be turned over for aspiration of the nasopharynx. Finally, he should be placed on his side with his head slightly elevated. Continue to observe him at least every 15 min.

Heretofore, the most accepted position for the newborn has been with head down. Though this may prevent aspiration of mucus, it may contribute to increased cerebral edema. The head-elevated position allows for better expansion of the lungs with descent of the diaphragm.

The second period of activity may continue for 2 to 5 h. Short periods of apnea may be observed, but they are not necessarily related to the amount of oral mucus. During this period, the baby may again exhibit sucking behavior suggestive of hunger. Initiation of his first feeding, whether from breast or bottle, is appropriate at this time.

Whether he feeds or not, the infant's heart and respiratory rate will probably stabilize. His temperature should be leveling off to normal. He will begin to establish a variable pattern of sleep, waking, and feeding if this transition progresses smoothly. Though all babies follow this general pattern during the first 24 h, each baby does so with variations, depending upon the amount of time he requires to achieve stabilization. The influences mentioned earlier will affect the pattern of adjustment. Wide divergence from the above pattern should alert the nurse to possible, yet-undetected, problems.

physiologic characteristics

Birth is a critical event, followed by highly complex physiologic changes. The circulation of the baby must make complex hemodynamic adjustments after the cessation of fetal circulation. The beginning of respiration creates another major transition. Changes also are required in the functioning of the hepatic, genitourinary, and gastrointestinal systems, as well as in the reorganization of the metabolic processes.

CIRCULATORY SYSTEM

Prior to birth, several major shunts are functioning which are unique to fetal circulation (Fig. 12·1). One of these shunts, called the *foramen ovale,* is an opening of the septal flap between the right and left atria of the heart. This shunt allows some blood to flow directly from the right atrium to the left atrium. Another shunt, the *ductus arteriosus,* carries blood from the pulmonary artery to the aorta.

When the cord is clamped and the placental circulation no longer is functioning, there is a rise in the blood pressure and a fall in the

oxygen saturation of the baby's blood. The first breaths open up the vascular bed of the lungs. This increased flow of blood in the lungs balances the effect of the rising blood pressure because there is reduced vascular resistance in the lungs. This lowered resistance allows the flow of blood to increase and assists in reversing the direction of the flow in the ductus arteriosus. Now the blood flows from the aorta to the pulmonary artery.

Meanwhile, the increased pulmonary blood flow raises the pressure in the left atrium. There is reduced pressure in the right atrium because the flow of blood into it has slackened after the placental circulation ceases. Both these factors help to force the septum functionally to close the foramen ovale.

Though the functional changes are sudden at the time of birth, the anatomic changes are more gradual. The fetal blood vessels slowly are transformed, as they are no longer functioning. Varying lengths of time are within normal limits for complete transformation of these fetal structures, as seen in Table 12·1.

BLOOD

During intrauterine life, the number of red blood cells (RBC) needed by the fetus is higher than required after birth. The large number of RBC is essential to assure an adequate level of oxygenation in the fetus. The extra cells are broken down, and most of the hemoglobin is stored in the liver for reuse. At birth, the average RBC count is about 5.5 to 6.0 million cells per cubic millimeter; the hematocrit average is between 46 to 50 percent; and the average hemoglobin is between 16 to 18 Gm/100 ml. In the first 2 days of life, the RBC count may rise from 1 to 1.5 million cells, and the hemoglobin from 1 to 2 Gm. However, after the first 2 days of life, the RBC count and the hemoglobin may begin to decrease, with the hemoglobin dropping most rapidly. All infants have some elevation of

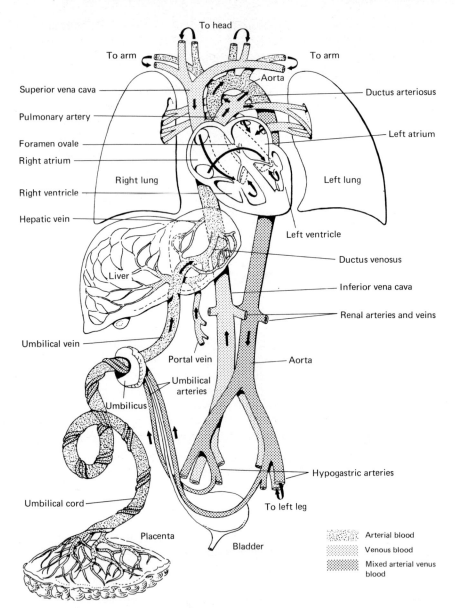

To head

To arm

To arm

Aorta

Superior vena cava

Ductus arteriosus

Pulmonary artery

Foramen ovale

Left atrium

Right atrium

Right lung

Left lung

Right ventricle

Hepatic vein

Left ventricle

Ductus venosus

Inferior vena cava

Liver

Renal arteries and veins

Umbilical vein

Portal vein

Aorta

Umbilical
arteries

Umbilicus

Umbilical cord

Hypogastric arteries

To left leg

Placenta

Bladder

Arterial blood

Venous blood

Mixed arterial venus
blood

fig. 12·1 Fetal circulation. (*Courtesy of Ross Laboratories, Clinical Education Aid.*)

bilirubin as a result, but not all of them show jaundice during this period (see Chap. 29).

The vitamin K supply is close to normal levels at the time of birth. However, it will fall in the next 2 to 3 days, causing a deficiency in the clotting factors, such as prothrombin, which must have vitamin K in order to be manufactured in the liver. To prevent a deficiency from developing, an intramuscular injection of a vitamin K_1 preparation is administered to the newborn soon after birth. Though

table 12·1

ANATOMIC CHANGES IN THE FETAL STRUCTURES AFTER BIRTH

FETAL STRUCTURES	INFANT STRUCTURES	RANGE IN WHICH CHANGE IS COMPLETED
Foramen ovale	Fossa ovalis	Several weeks to 1 yr
Ductus arteriosus	Ligamentum arteriosum	Several weeks to 1 yr
Ductus venosus	Ligamentum venosum of the liver	1–2 mo
Umbilical arteries	Lateral umbilical ligaments	2–3 mo
Umbilical vein	Ligamentum teres of the liver	2–3 mo

some institutions give the mother vitamin K during labor, it is generally felt that this method is not as reliable to assure that the newborn will receive an adequate amount.

RESPIRATORY SYSTEM

Before birth, respiratory movements occurred frequently, with the result that the fetus has fluid in the lungs. Therefore, at birth, the alveolar spaces in the lungs may be filled with fluid. This fluid adds to the resistance of the lungs to inflation. As respiration is established, the resistance to inflation decreases. Excess fluid in the trachea must be removed to allow the rapid increase in oxygen inhalation for maximum saturation of the baby's blood. The fluid left in alveolar spaces is reabsorbed during the first few days.

GASTROINTESTINAL SYSTEM

In the fetus, the functioning capacity of the gastrointestinal system was more limited than that of the circulatory or urinary systems. As early as the fourth month of intrauterine life, the fetus swallowed amniotic fluid. The muscle action, though weak, aids in the formation of fecal matter, called *meconium.* The intestinal tract was not required to digest or absorb food; nevertheless, it is able to assume these functions with relative ease.

With some exceptions the enzymes necessary for the digestion of simple foods are present at birth. A pancreatic amylase deficiency exists and persists for several months. Lipase also is deficient. Therefore, the baby is able to absorb proteins and carbohydrates, but poorly absorbs fat.

GENITOURINARY SYSTEM

In utero, the kidney function is primarily carried on by the placenta. At birth, the kidney must begin to function as an excretory and a regulatory organ. Renal functions, such as glomerular filtration and concentration of urine, are limited. When the organ is under stress, its efficiency is decreased even further. Maturation of the kidney function is a gradual process. Care must be taken to limit the solute load and keep the fluid intake high (see Chap. 28).

The first voiding may be just after delivery. It should be charted, because some infants then do not void for a number of hours. An insufficient amount of fluid intake may cause the urine to appear dark yellow as well as leave a deposit on the diaper that looks like brick dust and is frequently mistaken for blood. Nevertheless, the amount of urinary output may not decrease because the baby is unable to concentrate urine efficiently. Because the baby continues to urinate frequently, it is possible to miss the fact that the baby is becoming dehydrated. Since the infant has difficulty concentrating fluids, it is important to begin giving fluids 3 to 6 h after birth.

table 12·2
ASSESSMENT OF GESTATIONAL AGE

FEATURE	DESCRIPTION	WEEK OF APPEARANCE*
Sole creases	Anterior only transversed	36 or under
	Anterior two-thirds covered	37–38
	Sole covered with creases	39 or over
Breast nodule	2 cm in diameter	36 or under
	4 cm in diameter	37–38
	7 cm in diameter	39 or over
Scalp hair	Fine and fuzzy	38 or under
	Coarse and silky	39 or over
Earlobe	Without cartilage	36 or under
	Some cartilage	37–38
	Thick cartilage	39 or over
Genitalia	Testes in inguinal canal, few rugae	36 or under
	Testes in scrotum, rugae extensive	38 or over

*Measured from the first day of the last menstrual period (LMP).
Source: Adapted from Robert Usher, Frances McLean, and Kenneth Scott: "Judgment of Fetal Age, II. Clinical Significance of Gestational Age and an Objective Method for Its Assessment, *Pediatric Clinics of North America*, **13**:835, 1966.

physical characteristics

An appraisal of the physical appearance of the newborn demands the acute attention of all the examiner's senses and the ability to interpret accurately what the senses have registered.

RELATIVE SIZE

An easily observed fact is the small size of the baby. A closer look reveals significant relationships between parts of the body and between the baby and an adult. The baby's head is one-fourth his total length, but the adult's head is only one-eighth his total height.

The size of the newborn may give a false impression of gestational age. A more accurate assessment of maturity can be made by observing five key features of the baby: the sole creases, breast nodule, scalp hair, earlobes, and genitalia. The relative development of each of these features is briefly shown in Table 12·2. Further details about these features are discussed in Chap. 30.

MEASUREMENTS

Various factors contribute to the weight and length of the neonate. Gestational age has already been mentioned. Some maternal factors influencing these measurements include the mother's nutritional status at conception and her dietary pattern throughout the pregnancy. Recent studies show that the greater the increase in maternal weight the larger, and usually healthier, the infant (1). The mother's health prior to conception and during pregnancy can contribute either negatively or positively to the environment in which the fetus develops. Both father and mother contribute genetic factors which determine, to some degree, the height and weight of their offspring.

The following figures refer to the majority of newborn infants born in the United States. Approximately 90 percent of the full-term babies born in this country weigh between 2500 and 4600 Gm (5.5 to 10 lb). Their length runs between 45 and 55 cm (18 to 22 in) (see Table 12·3).

POSTURE AND POSITION

When a baby is lying on his side, quietly, his posture may closely resemble his intrauterine position. That is, a baby who was delivered in an occipitoanterior (OA) position is most likely to assume a posture of partial flexion. The nurse can note the extension of the knees and flexion at the hips of the baby whose delivery was a frank breech. The posture gives a clue as to the baby's posture in utero and helps in understanding the residual effects of that posture if the feet seem unusually tight against the inner ankle. The arms are flexed at the elbow so as to give a boxer effect. As a result the baby's fists are often in an eye or the mouth and the face becomes easily scratched. Most of the action seems to be in the shoulders.

MOVEMENT AND MUSCLE TONE

The healthy newborn's muscle tone usually is good; it can be tested by trying to extend an extremity. If the infant is awake and alert, he will vigorously resist the pull. The neonate's extremities move symmetrically in an alternating pattern, if there has been no injury or congenital deformity. Medication given to the mother during labor and the anesthetic

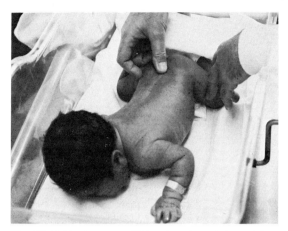

fig. 12·2 Newborn can lift head and turn it from side to side. (*Photo by Ruth Helmich: courtesy of the Jamaica Hospital, Jamaica, N.Y.*)

used at delivery can depress the baby's responses.

Usually the baby can lift his head when he is in a prone position (Fig. 12·2). If his responses are not depressed, he will turn his head to one side when he is placed upon his stomach and may try to raise himself with his hands as if doing a pushup. He will lift and turn his head if it is held against your shoulder, but he cannot support his head when held in a semisitting position (Fig. 12·3). He will try to bring his head along as you pull him from a flat position to a sitting one. However, his head will soon lag and begin to fall back as you bring him higher off the mattress. A firm hold on the buttocks and under the head and shoulders will give him a sense of security and keep the head from dropping back (Fig. 12·4).

HEAD: BONES, SUTURES, AND FONTANELS

The head is extremely important, since it makes the most severe adjustment to the pelvic cavity. The skull comprises eight bones. Figure 12·5 illustrates the relationship of these bones and the membranous spaces, called *sutures,* which separate them. The

table 12·3

THE AVERAGE NEWBORN

MEASUREMENTS	AVERAGE
Weight	3400 Gm = 7.5 lb
Height/length	50 cm = 20 in
Head circumference	33 cm = 13 in
Chest circumference	30 cm = 11.75 in

Source: *Maternal Nutrition and the Course of Pregnancy, Summary Report,* U.S. Department of Health, Education and Welfare, Publication (HSM) 72-5600, 1971, p. 8.

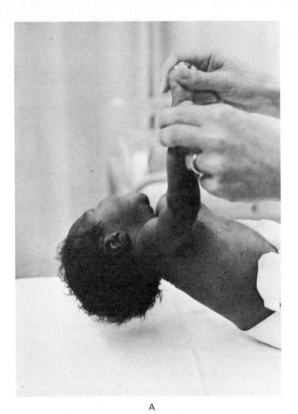

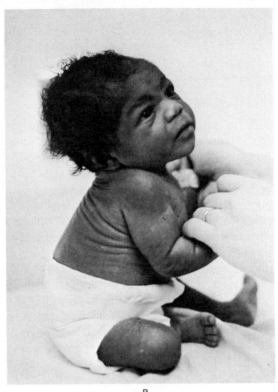

A

B

fig. 12·3A Pulling to sit. B Sitting. Note head lag. (*Photo by Mary Olsen.*)

bones of the roof and sides of the cranial vault develop from membrane, whereas most of the skeleton develops from cartilage (2).

The sutures meet, forming *fontanels,* or irregular spaces enclosed by membranes. Two of these fontanels—the anterior and the posterior fontanels—are used as landmarks during labor. These two fontanels also provide indices for evaluating normal growth of the head (Fig. 12·5).

The anterior fontanel is a diamond-shaped space at the junction of the sagittal, coronal, and frontal sutures. Its approximate size is 2.5 cm anteroposteriorly, and 1.25 cm laterally. The pulsations of the cerebral vessels may be felt through the membrane. Normally, the fontanel should feel soft and flat. Persistent bulging and tenseness may indicate high intracranial pressure, as in babies with hydrocephalus or meningitis. A depressed fontanel may be indicative of dehydration and malnutrition. Hold the baby in a sitting position or erect to evaluate fontanels; these positions permit more accurate interpretation of palpation. The anterior fontanel may begin closing as early as 6 months after birth, but its complete closure should not occur before sixteen to eighteen months of age.

The posterior fontanel is situated at the junction of the sagittal and lambdoidal sutures. It is more difficult to feel. To locate it, begin by identifying the wedge or apex of the triangular occipital bone. This bone is slightly depressed below the level of the two parietal bones posteriorly. The tip of the wedge can be felt at the very end of the sagittal suture. It is triangular and measures 1 cm or less at the base. It closes usually by 6 weeks to 3 months after birth.

Caput Succedaneum and Cephalhematoma The degree of difficulty in identifying the suture lines and fontanels depends upon the degree of molding and edema present. A swelling known as *caput succedaneum* involves that area of the scalp presenting during labor and delivery. The hemorrhage and fluid are in the subcutaneous tissue overlying the skull. The edema is seen at the time of birth. In fact, it may be felt on vaginal examination, particularly in a long labor. The edema is caused by sustained pressure on the scalp veins by the dilating cervix. The cervical pressure on the scalp veins obstructs the venous return. The edema will be more pronounced after a long labor. Localized discoloration may be detected. The

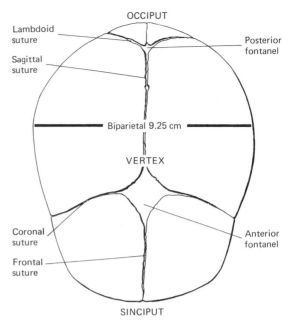

fig. 12·5 Anterior and posterior fontanels. (*Courtesy of Ross Laboratories, from "Mechanism of Normal Labor."*)

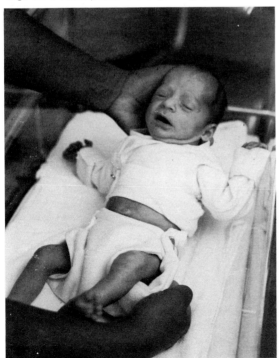

fig. 12·4 Hand placement for picking up infant.

swelling feels soft and has no clearly defined margins. It will pit under digital pressure.

In several days the swelling will subside. The mother will appreciate an explanation about the baby's strange head shape and why it feels so odd. Help her to observe the decrease of swelling from day to day.

In other presentations, the edema will be noted at the point where the presenting part was encircled by the dilating cervix. The genitalia and buttocks will be edematous following a breech delivery. The shoulder and upper extremity may be involved in a shoulder presentation. There may be general or localized discoloration.

In contrast to caput succedaneum, *caphalhematoma* usually does not appear until 24 to 48 h after birth. Cephalhematoma is a bump caused by hemorrhaging ruptured blood vessels lying between the surface of a cranial bone and the periosteal membrane covering that bone. Therefore, it has definite margins

table 12·4

DIFFERENTIAL DIAGNOSIS CAPUT SUCCEDANEUM AND CEPHALHEMATOMA

CAPUT SUCCEDANEUM	CEPHALHEMATOMA
Present at birth	Appears usually 24 h after birth
May be seen on any part of infant's body that presented in labor	Seen only on the head, usually over parietal bone(s)
May cross suture lines	Never crosses suture lines
Decreases in size after birth	Increases in size before decreases
Fluid usually absorbed in 36 h	May persist for weeks
Is diffuse; pits on pressure	Is circumscribed; does not pit
No treatment	Usually no treatment

because the hemorrhage is confined to the limits of the cranial bone by the membrane. Points of difference are summarized in Table 12·4. The diagrammatic sketches illustrate the origin of the hemorrhages in each condition (Fig. 12·6).

The baby is in no grave danger from either condition. On rare occasions, massive hemorrhage may cause a significant drop in the baby's hematocrit. Such a severe hemorrhage usually occurs when the cephalhematoma is bilateral (Plate 4F). The alert nurse will detect signs of distress (see Chap. 28). Most authorities do not relate cephalhematoma to skull fractures. However, when systematic skull x-rays were performed on every baby with cephalhematoma, the fracture rate was 25 percent (3). The mother must be reassured about her baby's progress. En-courage her to handle the baby and show her how to recognize evidences of his normal behavior.

Molding The scalp swelling may hide the degree of molding. It can be identified by palpating along the sagittal suture running between the parietal bones (refer to Fig. 12·5). By running your finger along this suture you should be able to feel the presence, or absence, of the overlapping of one parietal bone over the other. Follow the parietal bone in front of the ears to the coronal suture. Here you may detect overriding of the frontal bone by the parietal. Similarly, the occipital bone may be felt under the parietal bone near the posterior fontanel. These changes in the shape of the head are known as *molding*; they allow the head to adapt to the changing diameters of the pelvic cavity. Both the

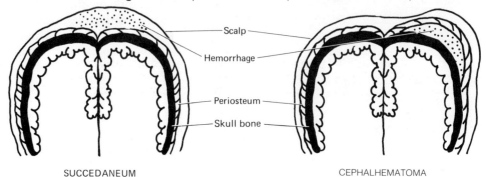

fig. 12·6 Comparison between caput succedaneum and cephalhematoma.

SUCCEDANEUM   CEPHALHEMATOMA

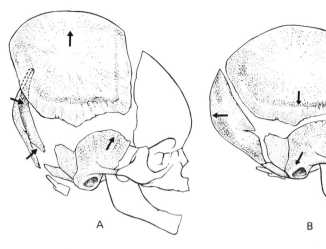

fig. 12·7 Molding during the birth process causes: A Overlapping and movement of cranial bones. B Reexpansion of cranium on third day with return to normal positions. (*Courtesy of Mead Johnson Company.*)

amount of molding and the overriding depend upon the position of the fetal head, the duration and severity of the intrapartal pressure, and the size of the pelvic cavity (Fig. 12·7A, B; Plate 4E).

Hair A small amount of fine downy hair, called *lanugo,* may be found on the shoulders, back, forehead, and temples of a mature newborn (Fig. 12·8). By the end of the first week this hair is usually completely shed. Certain familial characteristics may be brought to light by the mother or other relatives when a baby has additional facial hair or some hair persists in certain areas of the body. In some families the girls may have excess hair extending in front of the ears like sideburns. In other cases, mothers need to be reassured that the facial hair is probably temporary. In a premature baby the lanugo will remain longer, depending upon his gestational age.

SKIN

Color Changes in the color of the newborn may be rapid and of varying significance. At birth, color is one of the five variables on the Apgar score. It can tell much about the ade-

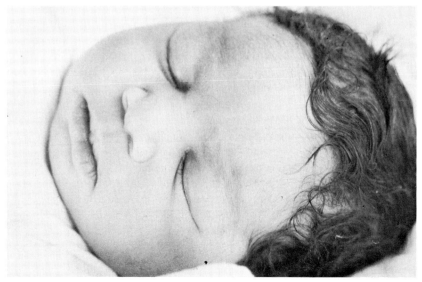

fig. 12·8 Lanugo. (*Photo by Ruth Helmich: Courtesy of Booth Memorial Medical Center, N.Y.*)

table 12·5

APGAR NEWBORN SCORING SYSTEM†

SIGN	SCORE		
	0	1	2
Heart rate	Not detectable*	Below 100	Above 100
Respiratory effort	Absent	Slow, irregular	Good (crying)
Muscle tone	Flaccid	Some flexion of extremities	Active motion
Reflex irritability	No response	Grimace	Vigorous cry
Color	Pale*	Blue*	Pink*

†If the natural skin color of the child is not white, alternative tests for color are applied, such as color of mucous membranes of mouth and conjunctiva, color of lips, palms, hands, and soles of feet.

Source: Used by permission of Dr. Virginia Apgar, with recent modifications, indicated by asterisk.

quate functioning of the heart and lungs (Table 12·5).

Initially, the newborn shows some degree of cyanosis. It is the rare baby who is delivered crying and pink. Within 1 min after birth the neonate may continue to have *acrocyanosis* (blueness of the extremities) while the face and body have become pink. By 5 min of life, most babies are pink all over.

The reddish-pink color of the newborn's skin is caused by the fact that the blood vessels are closer to the skin surface than in an older person. One obvious reason for this is the smaller amount of fatty tissue in the newborn, especially the premature infant and low-birth-weight baby. Evidence of the proximity of the vessels to the skin surface is noticeable when the baby cries. The increased exertion speeds up the heart rate, and the color of the skin becomes darker pink as the blood flow to the periphery increases (Plate 3).

The mechanism causing color changes is similar in all babies. However, the significant differences in appearance caused by familial

and racial pigmentation must be carefully observed. The Caucasian baby may vary from a pale pink to a red or dark pink; the black baby may appear pale pink to a pinkish brown; the Oriental baby may resemble a shade of tea rose; the Latin baby may have an olive tint or a slight yellow cast to his skin.

Because of immature peripheral circulation, the newborn at times may show signs of *circumoral cyanosis*—local blueness around the lips. The normal color of the lips of the black baby is gray, while that of the Caucasian baby is pink. A heightening of the normal color may be your clue to increasing cyanosis, e.g., a gray-blue in a black baby.

Even after a normal respiratory pattern has been established, the baby may develop acrocyanosis if he becomes chilled from exposure to cool or wet air. This is important to remember when he is being examined or receiving a bath. He must not be exposed too long, nor should his environment be allowed to become too cool (Plate 4G).

Skin Turgor Another aspect of the baby's skin must be observed—its elasticity, or *turgor.* Use your thumb and index finger to grasp the skin and subcutaneous tissue over the baby's abdominal wall. By grasping at least an inch of the skin, then squeezing, releasing, and allowing it to fall back into place, you can test the elasticity. The healthy baby's skin will immediately return to its original place and no residual marks will be seen. On the other hand, poor turgor is frequently seen in "small-for-dates" infants whose skin remains suspended and creased for a few seconds after being released. It is one means of estimating the newborn's state of nutrition and hydration. Poor turgor suggests that the baby was malnourished in utero.

Vernix Caseosa A cheesy substance, *vernix caseosa,* began to form on the fetus about the fifth month in utero. This thick white material covers the fetal skin and "may have the important function of protecting the skin from constant exposure to the amniotic fluid" (4). The amount of vernix on the newborn varies with gestational age. The postmature newborn may have none or only a very minute amount under his fingernails and in the folds of the groin, where it is normally found in the term baby (Fig. 5·3).

Edema The presenting part of the baby at the time of delivery normally will be edematous (caput succedaneum), but generalized edema usually is not seen unless an abnormality is present. Edema frequently is hard to recognize. The absence of wrinkles at the wrists and ankles is highly suggestive. If your finger impression can be left in the skin, the presence of edema is suspected. However, edema of the genitalia is common in both sexes. It may be more pronounced in the boy baby after a breech delivery (see Chap. 26).

Mongolian Spots At first glance, mongolian spots may be mistaken for bruising because of the bluish-gray pigmentation of the deep skin layer. The gray areas appear over the sacrum and buttocks and may also extend up the back and down the extensor surface of the extremities. You may expect to see this kind of pigmentation in Asians, Southern Europeans, and blacks. The coloration spontaneously disappears anywhere up to four years of age (Plate 4D).

Birthmarks (Nevus) A number of benign birthmarks may be present on newborns, and mothers often become very much concerned about them. Stork's beak mark, a reddish pigmentation at the base of the skull and the sacrum, is a very common mark on light-skinned Caucasians. Like mongolian spots, it fades as the child gets older. Other raised marks may shrink with the changing size of the infant. Any birthmark that is disfiguring or contains vulnerable blood vessels that might be injured is noted by the physician for follow-up (Plate 4C).

EYES

Frequently a baby will spontaneously open his eyes if he is held in a semi-Fowler's position away from direct light. Observe for any hemorrhage, clouding of the cornea, opacity of pupils, and size of cornea. Pressure on the fetal head during delivery may result in impairment of the venous return and rupture of capillaries in the sclera. This *subconjunctival* hemorrhage can be seen in the sclera but is of no pathologic significance. It usually disappears spontaneously within a week. On the other hand, retinal hemorrhage may be indicative of subdural hematoma.

Edema of the eyelids frequently occurs during the first 2 days after delivery. It occurs more commonly when silver nitrate 1 percent is instilled into the eyes, but antibiotic ointment may cause a local reaction.

If you are unable to make the baby open his eyes spontaneously, you must be very gentle in the force that you use. Practice on your own eyes, placing the index finger over the upper lid on the bony prominence and the next finger on the bony surface below the eye. As you are pressing on the bony surface, spread your fingers apart so that the eye is exposed. In this way, you avoid putting any pressure on the eyeball itself, as well as avoiding eversion of the eyelid.

The color of the eyes most frequently seen is gray-blue in Caucasion babies, black or brown in black babies, and green-blue in the Orientals. *Nystagmus* (spasmodic movement of the eyes, either rotary or from side to side) occurs because of poor coordination of the eye muscles. True nystagmoid movements are rare in the newborn and, if persistent, may indicate some kind of intracranial damage. If nystagmus occurs each time the infant tries to focus after the first few months, the infant should have a thorough ophthalmologic examination. *Ptosis* (drooping of the eyelid) is hard to detect until the baby tries to open his eyes. It is sometimes associated with the use of forceps, in which case it will generally be transitory. It may also be due to edema; as the edema subsides, the eyelid begins to function normally.

Some newborns look cross-eyed because of the wide flat bridge of the nose. *Pseudostrabismus* is not unusual and will change in appearance as the infant matures.

EARS

The ears should be in the same plane as the angle of the eyes. If the tops of the ears are lower than the eye level, it suggests the possibility of a rare congenital anomaly.

NOSE

Newborns are nose breathers. Any obstruction to the nasal passages may cause mild to severe respiratory distress. You must be alert to the presence of mucous secretions and develop acute hearing with regard to expiration noises. If you are attuned to these noises, you may detect if the baby is inspiring air through his nostrils. Choking noises should warn you to look for possible causes of distress, such as nasal passages filled with mucus, or not patent as in *choanal atresia* (see Chap. 28).

Tiny cysts called *milia* are commonly seen over the bridge of the nose. These cysts are a result of obstruction in the sebaceous glands. They will disappear in a short time without treatment. The mother must not attempt to squeeze them (Fig. 12·9).

MOUTH

A clear view of the mouth and pharynx is most important but extremely difficult to attain (Plate 4A). Stimulate the baby to cry before depressing the lower jaw. Examine both the hard and soft palates, so as accurately to confirm their intactness. Either palate may be cleft, even in the absence of cleft lip. Sometimes only the uvula is cleft (see Chap. 28).

Epstein's pearls, or retention cysts, are small papular structures on either side of the hard palate. No significance is attached to them, and they usually disappear spontaneously after a few weeks or 2 or 3 months.

Occasionally a baby is born with precocious teeth, usually the lower incisors. You

fig. 12·9 Milia (plugged sebaceous glands on nose and chin). Note newborn's mouth with sucking pads. (*Photo by Ruth Helmich: Courtesy of Booth Memorial Medical Center, N.Y.*)

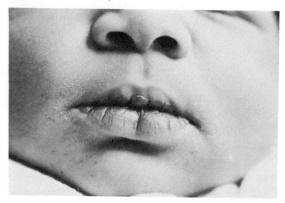

might overlook one if it is covered with membranous tissue because it will appear pink rather than white. When a white tooth is visible and loose, it is best to have it removed immediately to prevent its being aspirated. Be sure to reassure the mother that this is neither uncommon nor dangerous.

Tongue-tie occurs rarely, but mothers need help to understand what is normal. The *frenulum* of the tongue consists of a sharp thin ridge of tissue that has its origin in the midline of the base of the tongue. It attaches itself to the underside of the tongue at varying points toward the tip. When the attachment is closer to the tip of the tongue than to the back, a groove or concavity may be seen at the tip of the tongue when it is extended out of the mouth. The shortness of the frenulum leads to the term, *tongue-tie*. It rarely interferes with feeding or causes a speech impediment later on. Rarely is it necessary to clip the frenulum, although relatives may be overconcerned about the possible need for this procedure. Again, reassure the mother and help her to withstand the pressure of family, well-meaning though they may be.

Symmetry of the mouth should be observed. When the baby cries or yawns, look for any drooping or drawing down of one corner of the mouth. This indicates some degree of facial paralysis. Note the presence of bruising on the same side as the paralysis. If forceps were used during delivery, then the paralysis may be transitory and full recovery will be noticed in 3 to 5 days.

The amount and type of mucus are important guides to esophageal normalcy and respiratory adjustment. A normal amount of mucus will give the newborn a minimal amount of trouble so long as the baby is healthy. But one must not have a false sense of security about what is normal. Bubbly or frothy mucus may lead one to suspect a tracheoesophageal fistula (see Chap. 28). An attempt to aspirate the stomach may be thwarted because the catheter curls up rather than passing into the stomach. If this occurs, be sure not to let anyone feed the baby until he is thoroughly examined by a pediatrician.

NECK

The neck normally appears short in the newborn. Abnormalities may be webbing below the ears or excessive folds at the nape of the neck.

THORAX

The chest usually appears almost circular, with the xiphoid cartilage protruding as if broken. This normal appearance is due to its weak attachment to the body of the sternum. This protrusion usually disappears in the first 2 or 3 weeks.

Clavicles A clavicle may be fractured during delivery. To detect a fractured clavicle, use your thumbs. Starting at the neck, run your thumbs along the clavicle to feel for any irregularity or projections. Crackling noises, termed *crepitus,* may be heard when the arm is moved. The Moro reflex response may be absent on the side of the fracture. The fracture heals without difficulty, and the only treatment may be to immobilize the arm on the affected side.

Respirations Visual observations of the chest movements will assist in assessing the adequacy of respiratory efforts. There should be symmetry of the size and motion on both sides of the chest. The respiratory movement will be mostly diaphragmatic, which will be evidenced by the rise and fall of the abdomen. The thoracic cage remains relatively still. The average *respiratory rate* varies between 30 and 60 respirations a minute. Fluctuations in the rate are common in the newborn, who responds to stress by increasing his oxygen requirements. And his short periods of apnea, followed by several deep gulping breaths, are not abnormal in the healthy newborn if they do not persist indefinitely. As already stated, the newborn is a nose breather, which influences his ability to eat and breathe. He may need to pause more frequently in the early feedings as he perfects his pattern of breathing and swallowing.

Heart Rate The heart rate varies in newborns because it is affected by stimuli. When the infant is asleep, the rate may be as low as 80 beats per minute. An average pulse rate is 120 to 130 but may jump to as high as 160 to 180 when the baby is very active or crying.

Breasts Examination of the breasts in the first 24 h focuses upon the areolar development, as a sign of maturity. Sometimes one may see pink spots below or toward the midline. These may be *supernumerary* nipples without any glandular tissue. In both the male and the female babies, enlargement of the breasts may be seen. The condition is due to the stimulation of the breast tissue by the maternal hormones. The baby's breasts may become hard and swollen, a condition known as *engorgement,* and they may even begin to secrete milk. Under no circumstances should the breasts be squeezed or compressed. The swelling will subside in a week to 10 days. Normal sponge bathing is the only care required.

ABDOMEN

The baby's abdomen normally protrudes, giving it the appearance of distension. In observing the newborn, it is important to try to note whether the distension is increasing or decreasing as the feeding pattern is being established. Patency of the anus can be detected by insertion of a rectal thermometer.

The *cord* will appear bluish white right after being clamped and cut. Quickly it will begin to dry and become shriveled and black. It may remain moist around the base of the stump where it is attached. Usually the cord stump will detach after the first week of life.

BACK

Even though the back may visually appear normal (Fig. 12·2), it is important to run a finger down the vertebral column to detect any unusual depressions. The pelvic flare, or hip line, is assessed for symmetry. In the lower part of the back, the "diamond" formed by the sacral protrusion and the depressions laterally to the protrusion can be measured for symmetry to detect possible hip abnormality. The crease between the gluteal folds is examined to find any sinuses or cysts.

GENITALIA

Male The maturity of the baby will influence the genital development. The term baby will have a well-developed scrotum hanging loose. The testes will be descended into the scrotum. The scrotum may be edematous and darker in color than later on.

Observation of the penis is important in locating the source of the urinary flow. *Hypospadias* describes the condition in which the urethral meatus opens on the ventral portion of the gland. The external meatus of the penis is covered by the *prepuce,* the foreskin. A degree of narrowing of the foreskin, *phimosis,* is normal, and it is nonretractable for the first 4 to 6 months (Fig. 12·10).

Female A frequent appearance in term babies is the prominence of the labia minora compared with the labia majora. The size of the clitoris varies, sometimes making it difficult to determine the baby's sex. Sometimes a *hymenal tag* appears as an additional segment of the hymen. This tag protrudes from the floor of the vagina and is usually gone after 2 or 3 weeks. Also frequently seen in the first week of life is a mucoid discharge. It is a milky white, but sometimes it is tinged with blood. It may be frightening to the mother, who needs to understand its normalcy. The same hormones which cause the breast

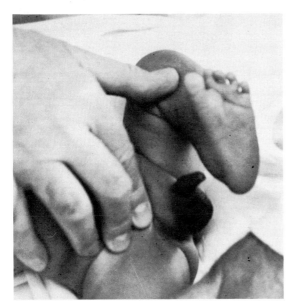

fig. 12·10 Examination for undescended testes. (*Photo by Ruth Helmich.*)

engorgement also cause this uterine discharge.

EXTREMITIES

In observing the movement of the extremities, you must be particularly alert to the symmetry of movement. Does any one extremity lag or not move at all? If one extremity does not move as the others do, a fracture may be suspected or a dislocation. The fingers and toes are counted to discover *polydactyly,* an extra digit. Sometimes a very rudimentary digit is attached by a thin pedicle. If the pedicle is ligated with a silk suture, the digit will drop off in a few days.

Abduction of thighs helps to pick up possible dislocation of the hip, or congenital dysplasia. The baby should be on his back; his thighs are then flexed one at a time, outward and downward toward the table or bed. If one or the other thigh cannot be abducted easily, the diagnosis is fairly certain. Another indication of this diagnosis will be a consistent sharp click heard during abduction of one side. Of less significance, unless these other signs are present, is the presence of extra creases high on the thigh on the affected side (Fig. 15·4).

REFLEXES

Specific reflexes need to be provoked for assessment of the baby's neurologic status.

The *grasp* reflex is normally strong and can be elicited by placing a finger across the newborn's palm at the base of the fingers (Fig. 12·11). The *plantar* reflex in the foot is similar; it can be observed as you stroke the sole just below the toes. The digits curl around the object (Fig. 12·12).

Rooting, sucking, swallowing, and gagging reflexes constitute an important group of interrelated responses essential for adequate nutritional intake. *Rooting* can be activated, if some hunger exists, by rubbing one's finger gently over the baby's cheek, lips, or corner of the mouth. Instantly he tries to keep in contact with the finger. The recently fed baby, or one that is lethargic, may merely purse his lips.

Like rooting, *sucking* in the alert baby is almost automatic when something touches his lips. The first feeding helps you to assess

fig. 12·11 Grasp reflex. (*From* Neurological Examination of the Newborn. *Courtesy of Kenneth Holt, M.D.*)

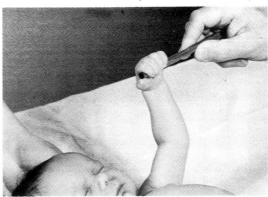

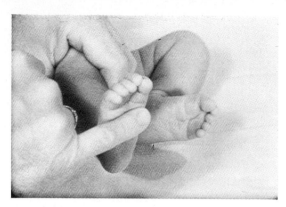

fig. 12·12 Plantar reflex. (*From* Neurological Examination of the Newborn. *Courtesy of Kenneth Holt, M.D.*)

the ability of the baby to *swallow*. You may anticipate some slowness in swallowing if the baby is having trouble handling his mucous secretions.

Certain responses of the baby are described as *protective* reflexes. The *Moro* reflex, sometimes referred to as the startle reflex, demonstrates the baby's awareness of equilibrium (Fig. 12·13A and B). The best time to test for its presence is when the baby is resting quietly. If his crib is jarred or a sharp noise is made nearby, he will respond by stiffening his body, drawing up his legs, and flinging his arms up and out, then gradually bringing the arms forward as if to embrace something. And he may begin crying. Both sides of the body should perform equally, symmetrically. Otherwise some injury is suspected.

Other protective reflexes include blinking, yawning, coughing, sneezing, drawing back from painful stimuli, fighting restraints, and hiccuping.

Navigation-type reflexes are evident early and then are lost again before actual crawling and walking take place. If the baby is placed on his abdomen, he may attempt push-ups or pull his knees up and try to crawl, or both. When he is held upright so that his soles touch the bed or table, he will make stepping

movements if he is not too sleepy or too excited (Fig. 12·14).

CRYING

The baby's only language is crying. Rather than responding negatively to his vocal attempts, the nurse would do well to know the many meanings the baby's special language can convey. To name only a few translations, the cry may mean hunger, thirst, pain, discomfort (such as a wet diaper or cramped position), the feeling of being too hot or too

fig. 12·13 Moro reflex. A In position for checking the Moro reflex. B Arms begin to move toward the body; note finger position. (*Photos by Beverly Hemlock.*)

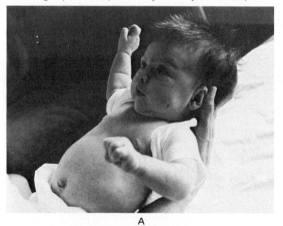

A

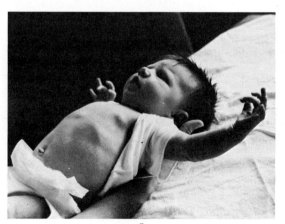

B

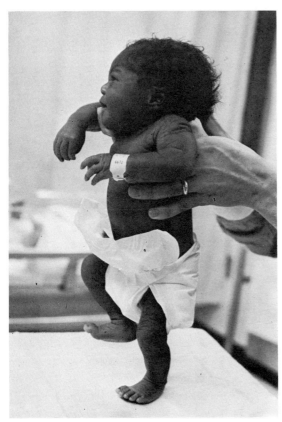

fig. 12·14 Stepping reflex in two-day-old infant. (*Photo by Mary Olsen.*)

cold, boredom, or loneliness. In the first 2 weeks of life, the same cry can mean any one of the above. Learning to check on what the cry means must be by trial and error, as the baby learns to give slightly different inflections to the cry. The mother soon learns to distinguish the cries if she listens and then checks their possible meaning (Chap. 16).

references

1. *Maternal Nutrition and the Course of Pregnancy, Summary Report,* U.S. Department of Health Education and Welfare Publication (HSM) 72-5600, 1971, p. 8.
2. Jack Davies, *Human Developmental Anatomy,* The Ronald Press Company, New York, 1963, p. 254.
3. N. Kendall and H. Woloshin, "Cephalhematoma Associated with Fracture of the Skull," *Journal of Pediatrics,* **41**:125–132, 1952.
4. Davies, loc. cit.

bibliography

Abramson, H.: *Resuscitation of the Newborn,* 2d ed., The C. V. Mosby Company, St. Louis, 1966.

Amiel-Tison, C.: "Neurological Evaluation of the Maturity of Newborn Infants," *Archives of Diseases of Children,* **43**:8, 1968.

Auld, P. A. M.: "Resuscitation of the Newborn Infant," *American Journal of Nursing,* **74**(1):68, 1974.

Brazie, Joseph V., and L. O. Lubchenco: "The Newborn and Premature Infant," chap. 3 in C. Henry Kempe, Henry K. Silver, and Donough O'Brien (eds.), *Current Pediatric Diagnosis and Treatment,* Lange Medical Publications, Los Altos, Calif., 1972.

Cohen, A. N., and W. A. Olson: "Drugs That Depress the Newborn Infant," *Pediatric Clinics of North America,* **17**:835, 1970.

Dahn, L. S., and L. S. James: "Newborn Temperature and Calculated Heat Loss in the Delivery Room," *Pediatrics,* **49**:504, 1972.

Desmond, M. M., et al.: "The Clinical Behavior of the Newly Born," *Journal of Pediatrics,* **62**:307, 1963.

Drillen, C.: "The Small-for-dates Infant: Etiology and Prognosis," *Pediatric Clinics of North America,* **17**:9, 1970.

Freeman, M., W. Graves, and R. Thompson: "Indigent Negro and Caucasian Birth Weight and Gestational Age Tables," *Pediatrics,* **46**:9, 1970.

Helmuth, J. (ed.): *Exceptional Infant: The Normal Infant,* vol. I, Brunner/Mazel, Inc., New York, 1967.

Johnson, C. F., and E. Opitz: "Unusual Palm Creases and Unusual Children," *Clinical Pediatrics,* 12:101, 1973.

Korones, S. B.: *High-risk Newborn Infants: The Basis for Intensive Nursing Care,* The C. V. Mosby Company, St. Louis, 1972.

Lubchenco, L.: "Assessment of Gestational Age and Development at Birth," *Pediatric Clinics of North America,* **17**:125, 1970.

Popich, G. A., and D. W. Smith: "Fontanels, the Range of Normal Size," *Journal of Pediatrics,* **80**:749, 1972.

Roberts, J.: "Suctioning the Newborn," *American Journal of Nursing,* **73**:63, 1973.

Scanlon, J. W.: "How Is the Baby?: The Apgar Score Revisted," *Clinical Pediatrics,* **12**:61, 1973.

Stern, L.: "The Newborn and His Thermal Environment," *Current Problems in Pediatrics,* **1**:3, 1970.

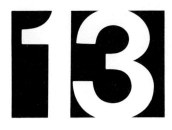

newborn care

Janet S. Reinbrecht

immediate care in the delivery room

The anticipated moment has come. This event of birth culminates a long history involving hurdles and potential problems for the new life. The nurse is aware that the new baby will require assistance in making a safe adjustment to extrauterine life. Three major areas of concern guide her preparation for the baby's birth:

Maintenance of a clear airway
Provision for warmth and a dry skin
Protection from injury and infection

Generally the newborn will be held with his head lower than his feet at the level of the mother's perineum. In this position, the mucus, blood, and any amniotic fluid that may be present will be drained away from the baby's respiratory tract. A soft bulb syringe should be in the delivery table pack to be used in gently removing excessive fluid first from the oropharynx and then from the nostrils (Fig. 13·1).

If the newborn cries and begins breathing immediately, this initial suctioning may be adequate. The cord will be cut and clamped. When the baby is ready to be handed over to the nurse, she should have a warm blanket ready to receive him. Just after birth, the usual position for placing the baby in the warm crib is head down, at a 15° Trendelen-burg angle. Close to the crib should be additional mechanical means for resuscitation and oxygen, should these be necessary. For most babies, respirations will be initiated within seconds to a minute after birth.

KEEPING THE BABY WARM

The nurse will have seen to it that a receiving crib has been heated prior to delivery. The baby should be dried thoroughly before being placed into the crib and wrapped in a warm blanket. Chilling occurs quickly from evaporation of the baby's wet skin. Control of heat loss assists the baby in conserving his energy in metabolism for the establishment of adequate respiration and absorption of the oropharyngeal secretions (Fig. 13·2).

PREVENTION OF INJURY AND INFECTION

The nurse sees to it that all the supplies used for the new baby are medically clean. Hand-washing technique must be carefully followed. The newborn has passive immunity to whatever specific diseases the mother has had. But this immunity will not be protective against the organisms encountered at the time of birth and immediately thereafter. The danger of infection is increased if any abrasions resulted from passage through the birth canal.

The eyes are especially susceptible to infection, particularly to gonorrheal infection. A prophylactic ointment or eye drops are required by law in the United States. Some institutions continue to use silver nitrate, 1 percent solution, a drop in each eye, followed by a flushing with distilled water. Other institutions use a broad-spectrum antibiotic eye preparation. Because it is important to the mother to see into her baby's eyes, some hospitals are delaying the eye instillation until after the baby has been admitted to the nursery if the mother is not awake to see her baby in the delivery room. Once the prophy-

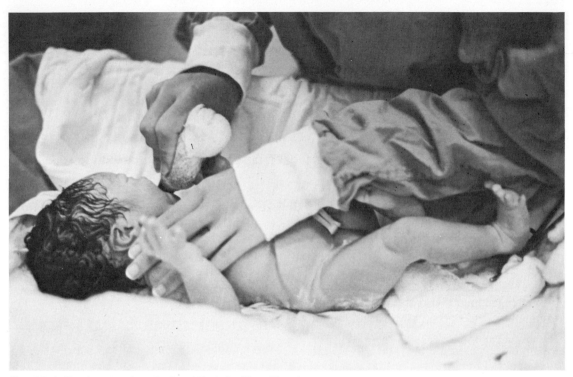

fig. 13·1 Oropharyngeal suctioning. (*Photo by Mary Olsen.*)

fig. 13·2 Newborn with temperature probe attached to abdomen to monitor temperature constantly. (*Photo by Mary Olsen.*)

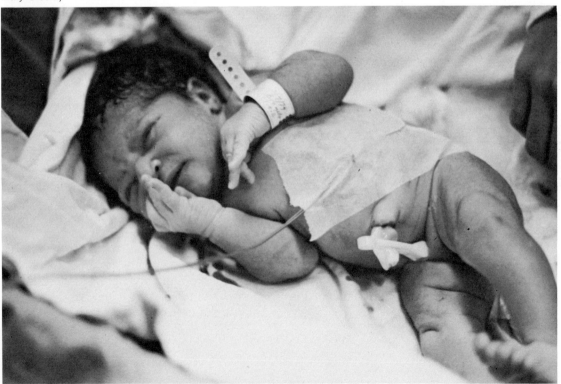

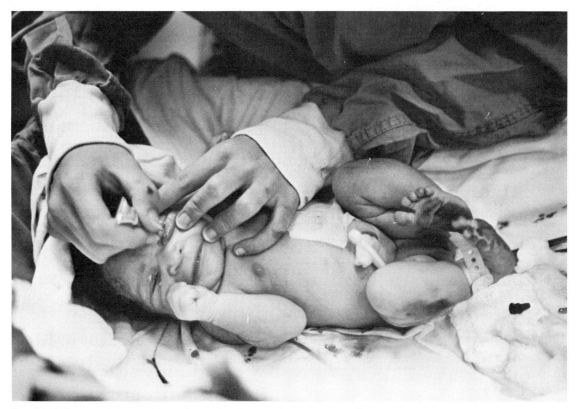

fig. 13·3 Eye prophylaxis with erythromycin ointment. (*Photo by Mary Olsen.*)

lactic medication has been instilled, the eyes begin to react and become swollen and puffy. Then it becomes more difficult for the baby to open his eyes (Fig. 13·3).

Vitamin K Frequently an intramuscular injection of vitamin K₁ is administered to the baby in the delivery room or the nursery (see Chap. 19).

IDENTIFICATION

The identification of the baby takes place in the delivery room before either mother or baby leaves the room (Fig. 13·4). It is accomplished in two ways:

1. The name of the mother is attached to the baby. Usually it is accomplished by the use of bracelets for mother and baby

fig. 13·4 Attaching arm band. (*Courtesy of Hollister, Inc.*)

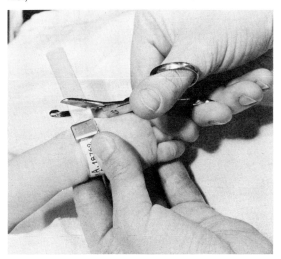

which contain the identical information: mother's full name, the baby's sex, the date and time of birth, and the same code number.

2. The baby's footprints and a print of the mother's index finger are placed on a record which stays with the baby's chart (Fig. 13·5A, B, C, D).

If you show the mother her baby after you have taken the footprints, be sure to explain to her why the feet look inky.

TRANSFER TO THE NURSERY

The transfer of the newborn to the nursery depends on his condition. Should he be in need of special attention immediately, he may be transferred to a transitional or intensive care nursery without delay. If his condition is stabilizing, he probably will be transferred as soon as his identification has been processed. The vitamin K injection and eye treatment may be performed in the delivery room or delayed until he is admitted to the nursery.

It is important for the nurse to have pertinent information to give to the nursery personnel. This information should include the type of labor, type of delivery (including whether or not forceps were used), kinds of medication received by the mother and any anesthetic given, the Apgar score of the baby, and the general condition of both mother and baby after delivery, as well as any anomalies noted in the baby. When a report is given to the nursery nurse, she will be able to anticipate what specific observations she must make on this particular baby.

preparation for the newborn

A crib should be warmed before the baby is expected in the nursery. Supplies for the baby are stored in the crib unit and should include the following items:

Baby soap, lotion
Clothes: shirts and diapers
Crib covers: blankets and sheets
Cotton balls
Lubricant
Thermometer in a container
Towels

For admission, additional equipment will be utilized. The following equipment should be ready, medically clean, for appraisal of the newborn.

Alcohol wipes
Capillary tubes
Finger pricks
Hemosticks
Ophthalmoscope
Otoscope
Stethoscope
Syringes and needles of various sizes
Tape measures (disposable)
Tongue depressors

Although the baby may have appeared to make a satisfactory immediate adjustment at the time of birth, he requires close observation. Anomalies at first not visible may show up in the first 6 h. Planned assessment may provide essential clues to potential trouble areas; the initiation of immediate intervention may then prevent irreparable damage. An attitude of watchfulness with a conscious *pattern* for assessment will assure the baby the best chance of maintaining the adequate adjustment made at birth.

PERTINENT INFORMATION

To assist in the maintenance of the newborn's adjustment to his new environment the nursery nurse should be familiar with the baby's prenatal and intrapartal history. The care provided will depend upon knowing some basic facts, including the following:

1. *General health of the mother,* especially any maternal conditions which might have

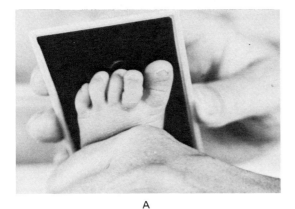

A

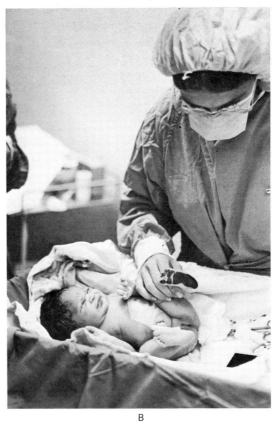

B

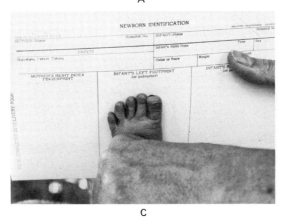

C

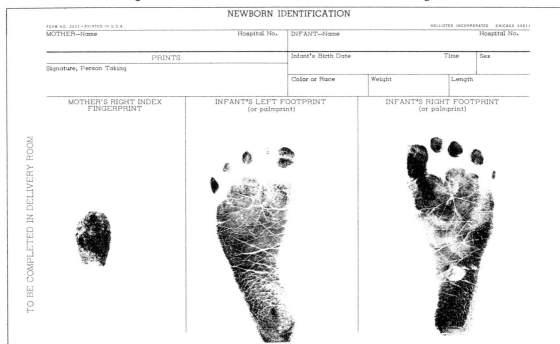

D

fig. 13·5 Identification process. A Footprint pad. B Inky foot. C Printing. D Mother's right index fingerprint added.

affected the fetal development, such as toxemia, Rh-negative blood type with rising antibodies, or anemia.

2. *Approximate gestational age,* which indicates the degree of maturity of the newborn and his ability to sustain his body functions (Chap. 11).

3. *Specific types of medication taken by the mother prenatally* which may influence the baby's progress, such as ACTH, synthetic progestins, and hallucinogenic drugs or narcotics (Chap. 18).

4. *Medications received by the mother during labor and delivery,* as there is growing evidence that certain medication affects the behavior of the baby, interfering with his reflexes and inhibitory responses.

5. *Time of rupture of the membranes,* since the earlier the rupture, the more likelihood of severe molding and possible cephalhematoma, along with tearing of the *tentorium cerebelli.* In addition, there is danger of infection from prolonged rupture of the membranes and frequent vaginal examinations as well as manipulations when the fetus is being monitored.

6. *Type of delivery, including all operative procedures,* which could be cause of injury to the baby.

7. *Apgar score and specific behavioral responses at birth* that indicate the normalcy of the infant's adjustment. If the mother nurses the infant in the delivery room, that, of course, suggests adequate sucking reflex and alertness following delivery.

8. *Findings of the gross physical assessment in the delivery room,* so that the nursery nurse can compare the admission observations with the description given in the delivery room.

initial care and assessment

Placing the baby in a prepared warm crib minimizes body temperature loss. If the im-

mediate condition of the baby is satisfactory, confirm the identity of the baby with the delivery room nurse, and record. Review the significant aspects of the prenatal history and the labor and delivery facts referred to above. Should the baby's condition warrant immediate attention, have the delivery room nurse assist until such a time as it is safe for the review of the factors contributing to the baby's present status.

An initial rectal temperature is taken to determine the amount of assistance the newborn will need to maintain or recover a normal temperature. A baby's normal temperature range lies between 36.7°C (98°F) and 37°C (98.6°F) rectally. The shock of birth and the new atmosphere may cause the newborn's temperature to drop as low as 35°C (95°F) rectally. The restoration of the temperature to 36.7°C may take up to 4 h. The time of the first temperature should be recorded (Fig. 13·6).

The full-term baby, normally, is capable of maintaining a stable body temperature, if the stressors are kept to a minimum. A warm crib will not be of much value unless the environment directly surrounding the baby also is warm, is free from draughts, and does not fluctuate. This means that the baby must be protected from exposure to cool air during physical examinations, tests, and x-rays.

fig. 13·6 Taking rectal temperature. (*Photo by Ruth Helmich.*)

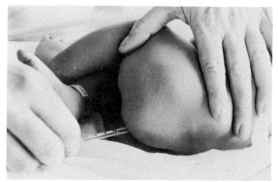

Should the baby require any tests or treatments, heat can be provided by special heat lamps; he should be kept dressed as completely as is feasible. Be sure the lamp has warmed the area to be heated *before* placing the to-be-exposed baby under the lamp. Another temperature check should be taken upon completion of the test or examination. Comparison of the temperature before and after the procedures may help to evaluate both the baby's heat-regulating mechanism and the adequacy of the heat provided.

If no specific anomalies or distress signs have been noted in the delivery room or since admission, the nurse should proceed to check the other vital signs, keeping the baby warm all the time.

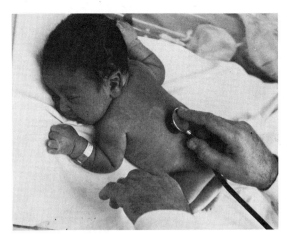

fig. 13·7 Listening for respiratory sounds. Note blanching of skin from slight pressure of stethoscope. (*Photo by Ruth Helmich.*)

APICAL PULSE

The pulse rate of the newborn ranges between 120 and 140 beats per minute. It is best to check the pulse rate by auscultating the apex beat. Because the baby's heart is higher than that of the adult, the bell of the stethoscope should be placed at the fifth intercostal space at the left sternal edge. The intensity of sound may vary, so that sometimes the maximum sound may be above the left nipple. The second sound is somewhat higher than the first. Because of the rapid beat the nurse needs to take time to adjust to the rhythm before starting to count. The activity of the baby will be reflected in the changes in heart rate. These changes occur quite rapidly, and care should be taken not to startle or overstimulate the baby while trying to locate the sound.

RESPIRATIONS

The normal newborn respirations are almost entirely abdominal and quiet. For this reason care must be taken to keep the baby warm while noting the respiratory rate. The rate may be irregular in the first few hours but then should stabilize. Should the irregularity persist beyond the first several hours, one would suspect respiratory difficulties resulting from persisting acidosis or depression of the respiratory center by drugs (Fig. 13·7).

The normal range lies between 30 to 60 breaths per minute, with the average around 40 per minute. The rate and rhythm are easily influenced by stimuli such as heat fluctuations, and will vary with activity, e.g., when the baby is eating or crying, as well as sleeping.

Since the respiratory movements of the newborn are accomplished by the coordination of the diaphragm and the abdominal muscles, there is little thoracic activity. Consequently, respiratory movements may be curtailed if pressure is placed upward on the diaphragm. This is why care must be taken in positioning the baby. The abdominal organs could put pressure on the diaphragm if the baby is left in a position with the head lower than the rest of the body, with the result that the respirations could become unnecessarily shallow. The baby is more subject to the danger of this type of diaphragmatic pressure after feedings, if he is placed in the Trendelenburg position.

CORD

The condition of the cord should be noted on admission. It should be free from oozing and should be firmly clamped. There should be no pressure from the cord clamp at any point on the surface of the abdomen. The stump should be examined for the correct number of vessels (three), especially if this had not been checked in the delivery room.

PENIS

Care should be taken in examining the penis to see if the urethral opening is in the normal location on the tip, rather than on the dorsal or ventral surface. If either of the latter conditions exists, circumcision will be postponed until time of the surgical repair.

ANAL PATENCY

The patency of the anus can be best determined at the time of checking the rectal temperature. The normal placement of the thermometer and patency of the anus can be noted simultaneously.

daily observations

The observations described below are aimed at developing skill in recognizing the normal variations in the newborn's appearance and behavior. Continual assessment of the appearance and behavior helps the caretakers to discern healthy progress or evidence of developing problems. Assisting parents to recognize these same variations will contribute to a healthy parent-child environment, free from much anxiety due to ignorance.

Some very basic factors indicate that a baby is progressing in a healthful manner.

1. A clear, pink-tinged skin most of the time
2. Muscles which are strong and resistant when extended, as with a leg or an arm, and a firm palmar grasp
3. A vigorous kick
4. A lusty cry to tell how he feels
5. An eager sucking response, when hungry, to food that is offered
6. Normal stools
7. Peaceful sleep

If the baby has these characteristics he will undoubtedly be growing normally. The nursing goal is to give anticipatory and preventive care to the normal newborn and his parents.

Observations, in systematic patterns, of the baby's appearance and behavior must be made and recorded. Only by written records can information be compared and progress assessed. It is *dangerous* and irresponsible to assume that a baby is progressing normally if there is no record of any observations on the chart. In fact, the lack of any notation may mean that no observations have been made. Be *specific, concise, and consistent*, to permit the best comprehension of the implications of the facts recorded. For example, when the temperature is recorded, a notation should indicate the time and reason for checking the temperature. For the newborn, time is the number of minutes after birth. The amount of exposure from the time of birth to the taking of the temperature should be noted.

Each day a complete assessment of the newborn's condition should be carried out by the nurse and recorded. A description of newborn patterns has been outlined in detail in Chap. 12. A simplified outline to follow ensures accuracy and uniformity in observations. The practice of carefully adhering to an outline could reduce the neonatal mortality and morbidity rates. Relationships between prenatal and intrapartal management and the condition of the newborn might become more apparent.

Head Note the shape and molding; presence of cephalhematoma and its size; tension of the fontanels; appearance of the eyes for hemorrhage, discharge, and inflammation; symmetry of the facial muscles when the baby cries; amount of mucus; and any spots suggestive of thrush.

Chest Observe the chest movements for any intercostal muscle action which is indicative of distress; note respiratory rate and regularity of respirations. Be alert for breast engorgement and any discharge from the nipple. Take the pulse rate and compare each day's findings.

Abdomen Be alert for distension of the abdomen (including before and after feeding), changes in the cord indicative of healing or interference with normal drying, and inflammation, discharge, or odor at cord site.

Skin Note and describe accurately its condition, its color, rashes, dryness, peeling, mottling, cracking, or bruises.

Temperature Take the temperature initially soon after delivery, and then at intervals to be certain that it is becoming stabilized. Daily records are usually taken but are of minimal value in the case of a normal infant. Suggestive behavior indicates the need to check the baby's temperature, to detect either hypothermia or any elevation.

Weight Compare the initial weight with the daily weights while the baby is in the hospital. The significance of the weight is in relation to the feeding pattern. The expected loss of 5 to 10 percent is more readily found when the baby is not given anything by mouth for 12 or more hours after birth. If the baby is on demand feeding the loss will be less (Fig. 13·8).

Feeding Pattern The baby's hunger is a more accurate guide to feeding patterns than the artificial schedules imposed by most hospitals. The important observations to make are the strength of the suck, length of time needed to satisfy his hunger, retention of the milk, contentment with the feeding (as evidenced by quiet wakefulness or sleep after the feeding), and the type of milk taken—

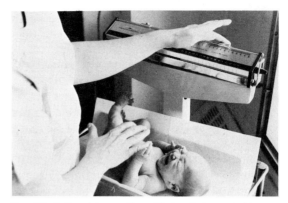

fig. 13·8 Careful guarding of baby during weighing. (*Photo by Ruth Helmich.*)

breast or formula. Be alert to the mother's behavior during feedings to see if she is comfortable and conveys a sense of comfort and relaxation to the baby, as these can affect the infant's feeding behavior.

Muscle Tone Compare the reflex responses for symmetry, vigor or the lack of it, the amount of resistance to manipulation, and the type of response to stimulation, including a description of the kicking in various positions.

Cry Note the pitch of the cry, and the baby's behavior at the time of crying; e.g., whether the baby cries while frantically sucking or while straining, or whether he cries softly while his body remains flaccid. Describe the baby's response to the type of attention given; e.g., when the baby's wet diaper is changed, note whether he becomes quiet and content. This indicates normal behavior and is as important to note as the abnormal, such as excessive and unrelieved crying.

Urine Note the frequency, color, and presence of crystals. Peach-colored crystals indicate uric acid but are not pathologic. Failure to void must also be noted.

Stools Progressive changes in the baby's stools are indicative of the baby's general health status and intestinal functioning. *Meconium*, the first stool of the newborn, may have started forming as early as the sixteenth week of intrauterine life. It is sticky and dark green to almost black, as a result of its constituents: bile pigments, fatty acids, mucus, blood, epithelial cells, and amniotic fluid. As the baby begins to ingest milk, the color, consistency, and frequency of the stools change. Record the color, consistency, and time of noting the stool to indicate the frequency and pattern of the change.

Usually, by the third postnatal day, the transitional stool appears as green-brown to yellow-brown in color and looser than meconium, with some mucus. Subsequently, the breast-fed baby has stools which are soft, semiliquid, and yellow, possibly with a sour odor. In contrast, cow's milk produces a firmer, paler stool, similar to putty. There is a characteristic, offensive odor to the stool of formula babies.

The frequency of the stools depends upon the type and number of feedings. The number of stools each day may vary from one to eight and be within normal limits; and the color and consistency provide the clues to abnormality. The size of the feedings influences the consistency of the stools. Overfeeding can produce loose stools, as the baby is unable to digest throughly all the milk forced upon him. For this reason it is thought that breast-fed babies are more likely to be better fed, because the baby determines the amount of his intake since his mother cannot see the number of ounces he is or is not taking. The responses of the baby to the feeding are a better guide to his required intake than the number of ounces he takes.

If the stool appears green, this fact should be noted so that it can be seen whether this is a one-time occurrence or persists. A green stool that is watery causes concern that the baby may have an intestinal infection. The physician must be notified immediately. Any color or consistency differing from those described above demands attention without de-

lay, as the newborn condition can deteriorate rapidly without immediate intervention.

Genitalia In girls it is important to observe for irritation, swelling, vaginal discharge, bleeding, mucus, and hymenal tag. For boys it is important to note the size, retractability of the foreskin or healing if he has been circumcised, scrotal swelling, and descent of testicles (Fig. 12-10).

Circumsion Cultural and religious backgrounds influence parental decisions regarding circumcision. Many nursery services assume that the male child will be circumcised before discharge. Parents must give their consent and sign a surgical permit. The nurse will learn about the various views on circumcision if she takes time to listen to the parent's response to the question, "Do you want your baby circumcised before you leave?" For the Jewish baby, there will be a ritual circumcision on the eighth day after birth. European families are less likely to have their sons circumcised. Moslem families do not circumcise their sons. An uncircumcised father usually will teach his son how to keep his penis clean, thus preventing infection. When no cultural preferences exist, the psychologic implications of not having the boy circumcised may be important to consider.

Because pain may be less intense during the early weeks of life, this appears to be the best time to perform the operation. The operation consists of surgically removing the foreskin of the penis. Cleansing of the glans is thus made easier, and there is less danger of developing an infection of the glans and prepuce, so that unless there are family preferences, most babies are circumcised.

The baby should not be fed within an hour or so of the operation. Just before the operation the baby is restrained so as to immobilize him. He dislikes this curtailment of his freedom even more than the operation. He should not remain restrained long before the operation, as he may become unduly exhausted

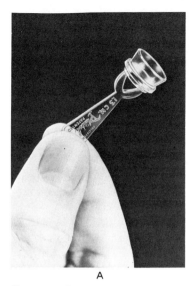
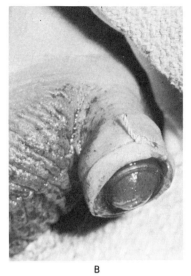
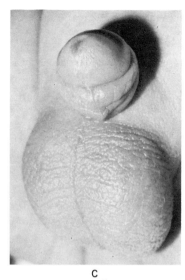

| A | B | C |

fig. 13·9 Circumcision. A Using Hollister plastibell. B Suture around rim of plastic controls bleeding. C Plastic rim and suture drop off in 7 to 10 days. (*Courtesy of Hollister, Inc.*)

just from crying before any surgery is performed. He should be kept warm by being comfortably covered above the groin. The area of operation should be heated and free from temperature fluctuations.

The operation is a sterile procedure requiring sterile gloves, instruments, gauze, wipes, draping towels, petroleum jelly dressing, and a solution for preparing the skin. The Gomco clamp helps to minimize the bleeding and prevent the removal of more than the foreskin. The method using the Hollister plastibell is illustrated in Fig. 13·9. After the operation the petroleum jelly dressing is applied to aid in the healing. It is then important to watch the dressing for signs of postoperative bleeding. The baby may be released from the restraints as soon as the operation is completed and the dressing is in place (Fig. 13·10).

The baby will need comforting; he may even be very hungry, and feeding him may be extremely soothing. The mother will be quite concerned and anxious about the operation. Therefore, she may be greatly relieved if she is able to see that he is feeding. Both mother

and baby will receive the reassurance they need.

daily care

WARMTH

The importance of minimizing the heat loss in the newborn by maintaining a consistent tem-

fig. 13·10 Petroleum jelly gauze dressing is kept on circumcision for 24 h and then removed (Gomco method). (*Photo by Ruth Helmich.*)

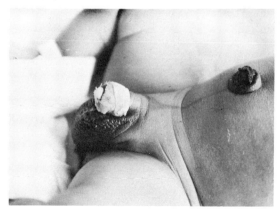

perature in the nursery has been emphasized. The heat loss in the newborn is greater from radiation and convection than from evaporation. Nevertheless, care must be taken to protect the baby from heat loss during any bathing, including diaper changes. The baby's clothing should be for cover and protection from heat loss but, except in emergency situations, not for overcoming the problems of an unstable environment. Overdressing can be as taxing to the newborn's heat-regulating mechanism as too cool an environment.

PROTECTION FROM INJURY

Because the newborn has little immunity against the pathologic organisms in his setting, protecting him from infection must be uppermost in the minds of those caring for him. The importance of hand washing cannot be overstressed. Removal of as many organisms from our hands as possible by friction lessens the number of organisms transmitted to the delicate and often bruised skin of the baby. When there is a personnel shortage, the danger posed to newborns by anyone who works in the nursery when he has signs of upper respiratory infection, rashes, or even a sore throat may frequently be ignored. Personnel need to rally to one another's support to encourage that proper care be given every staff member when he is ill and that the work load be shared while he is absent. The properly cautious person should not be made to feel guilty for practicing preventive health.

Keeping the baby clean is another way of guarding against infection. Bathing the baby daily keeps him clean and provides an excellent opportunity for a thorough assessment of his appearance and behavior. Proceeding cephalocaudally, in the normal manner of bathing, one can readily make the observations outlined previously.

Whatever technique for bathing is used, the nurse should include the mother as soon as possible in the care of her baby. As the mother begins to perform caretaking acts for her baby she begins to feel closer to him. In this way she begins to establish a bond which reinforces the reciprocal behavior of mother and baby. If the bathing, as well as any other care, is kept relaxed and free from rigid routines, the mother will be less likely to be fearful of handling her baby and making mistakes. If she is relaxed, the unique parent-infant relationship between these two individuals has a better chance of an early start. The father should be given the same opportunities to handle this child. We must remember that each person has to have the freedom to establish his relationships in his own way and within his own timing.

Special attention to the eyes will help prevent infection from continuing unchecked. Early detection of any discharge from the eye(s) makes it possible to initiate treatment before irreparable injury has occurred. Clean, clear water is used for the eyes and face.

Naturally, we know the baby is not likely to become really "dirty" while in the nursery. However, the folds of the neck, the axillae, and the creases of the arms and wrists may become messy from milk or lint. If left indefinitely, dried milk or lint could cause irritation to the baby's sensitive skin. Besides at the time of the bath, the nurse should be sure to clean the baby thoroughly after each feeding, especially if he regurgitates.

The approach to cord care varies among institutions. The basic principle underlying whatever technique and solution are used is the same—the cord must be kept clean and dry. Asepsis must continue after the cord separates until the navel is completely healed.

In the baby girl the labia minora appear unusually large because the labia majora are underdeveloped. The vaginal discharge is mucoid and may be slightly blood-tinged in the first week of life. As in the adult female, care must be taken to prevent the introduction of any contaminants into this rich media for rapid bacterial growth.

Gentle cleansing of the vulva with baby oil or lotion on a cottonball will remove the secretions without undue irritation. Use a single swipe with each cottonball. It may take several days to remove the vernix caseosa from between the labia. A little cleansing with each diaper change is better than a prolonged rubbing at any one time. In the cleansing process one should apply the principle of wiping from front to back, from the cleanest area to the least clean, even when there is no stool. Extra care is required to keep any excessive amount of feces from being spread toward the vagina.

The genitalia of boy babies vary in size. The swelling of the scrotum will decrease in the first week, although at times it may seem that there is an excess of fluid. Cleansing of the area includes washing the scrotum and the glans of the penis. However, the foreskin should *not* be forcibly retracted. An adequate cleansing of the secretion, *smegma,* around the glans of the penis can be accomplished by gently pulling back on the foreskin, and then returning the skin to its original loose position. The foreskin must be quickly returned to the original position before it tightens and cuts off the circulation, resulting in edema of the penis.

If the boy is not going to be circumcised, the nurse will want to help the mother learn how to push the foreskin back gently until it slips back easily. The earlier the mother learns, the more she will be able to care for her son comfortably and safely at home. The doctor may dilate the prepuce to allow ease of retraction in the first week and prevent any danger of swelling.

The groin and buttocks are inspected for possible skin irritation resulting from feces or urine. If clear water removes the stool completely, that is fine; the area should then be thoroughly dried by patting. Sometimes a little (baby) oil may be used to help remove the last signs of stool. It should be used sparingly so as not to leave a film upon which bacteria may grow.

Because newborns are very susceptible to skin irritation, the baby requires dress appropriate for the environment. Disposable diapers are likely to keep the buttocks warm enough to develop a rash, especially if the room is quite warm. Cleansing the baby's bottom with clear water, drying thoroughly and keeping the diapers off for a short period of time will help clear up most rashes quite quickly.

Heat rash around the neck and in the groin may develop very quickly even when the baby has been too warm only briefly. Therefore, it is important to dress the baby to fit the environment, rather than constantly adjusting the room temperature. When the buttocks are being exposed for healing, a cover over the crib may prevent heat loss and an ordinary lamp can give enough heat to maintain an even temperature around the baby.

Changing the baby's position after the wet diaper has been replaced with a clean one can help reduce prolonged pressure or friction in any one area of the body. When the baby is on his abdomen, his knees may become irritated from his kicking or rubbing while trying to find a comfortable position for sleep. Continuous rubbing may cause abrasions which can lead to infection.

EMOTIONAL AND COMFORT NEEDS

The baby responds to the stimuli in his environment and seems to be alert to the special rhythm of the mother. An early opportunity to be with mother helps to develop a mutual attitude of trust and pleasure. The mother learns to relieve the infant's hunger, to make him comfortable after changing the diaper or his position, and to note whether he is too hot or too cool. Natural impulses of parents to cuddle, fondle, and generally offer themselves through touch are to be encouraged.

Privacy with the baby allows the parents to become uninhibited in their efforts to reach out to the baby. Continuation of these efforts to meet the needs of the baby depends upon the parent's feeling that the baby is responding and desires the exchange of emotions to continue.

tests

COOMBS' TEST

When the mother is Rh-negative, umbilical cord blood should have been sent to the laboratory directly from the delivery room. The Rh type and blood grouping will be determined, and a direct Coombs' test will be made. Other tests will include those for hemoglobin level, serum bilirubin level, erythrocyte count, nucleated red blood cell count, and reticulocyte count. The Coombs' test will reveal the presence of maternal anti-Rh antibodies attached to the red blood cells of the Rh-positive baby. The nursery nurse will want to know the result of the Coombs' test so that she will know whether to expect clinical signs of hemolytic disease of the newborn. The report will indicate if the Coombs' test is negative or positive for antibodies.

BILIRUBIN

A bilirubin level determined at birth helps to guide in interpreting later tests. Evidence of a rising bilirubin level can be detected by a watchful nurse, who can learn to observe the slightest color change in an infant's skin in sunlight or under a fluorescent light. In one infant a serum bilirubin level under 10 mg/100 ml of blood may be physiologic hyper-bilirubinemia, while in another it will indicate a pathologic condition. A baby who becomes lethargic, whose cry begins to turn shrill, and who sucks poorly may be developing jaun-dice of the nuclear masses of the brain. Treatment needs to begin immediately (see Chap. 29).

Jaundice usually progresses from the face down the body, eventually becoming visible on the palms and soles. Treatment should have been started before the full progression has developed. To detect jaundice the nurse should pick a firm surface of the body and apply a firm pressure with the thumb to the area, causing the skin to blanche. As the underlying color returns, it will become apparent, whether it is a pinkish or yellowish.

PHENYLKETONURIA (PKU) TEST

Before the baby is discharged blood will be taken, usually from his heel, and placed upon special blotting paper. Since phenylketonuria is a metabolic disorder, it is essential for the baby to have been receiving milk before this test. Even so, a baby with phenylketonuria may have a negative result on the initial test. Another test should be done at least a month after birth.

discharge procedures

The nurse assumes the responsibility for making certain that the mother and baby are ready for discharge. Before leaving the hospital the mother and the baby should have complete physical examinations, by the obstetrician and pediatrician respectively. In preparation for the physical examination it is wise to have the results of the tests available for the doctor, to add to the facts guiding the decision to discharge the baby or to keep him for further observation. It will save much heartache if the date of discharge of the baby can be decided before the time of the mother's discharge. It adds to the mother's separation problems if when she is ready for homegoing she learns that she is to go without the baby.

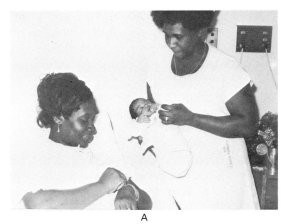

A

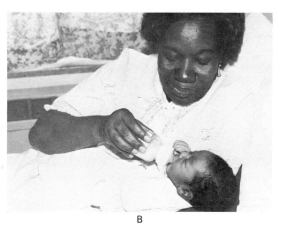

B

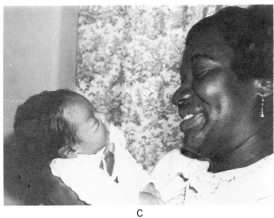

C

fig. 13·11 The critical nursing function of helping to establish a satisfying feeding pattern. A Identifying mother and baby by band number. B Being sure that the mother's position is comfortable. C Allowing time for mother and baby to get acquainted. (*Photos by Ruth Helmich; courtesy of Jamaica Hospital, Jamaica, N.Y.*)

At some time during the postpartum period plans for medical supervision of the baby should be discussed with the mother. If there will be no family or private physician, the nurse may give her information about the most convenient well baby clinic. Instructions as to how to make contact with the clinic should be given.

Follow-up by the visiting nurse needs to be arranged before discharge so that the parents understand the reason for the visit and what the financial cost if any, will be. The nurse should not hesitate to enlist the help of the community nurse if there is a specific advantage to continuing some special assistance the family needs.

The ideal situation would be for the mother, and even the father, to have had an oppor-

tunity to participate in the care of the baby throughout the hospital stay. When this has not been done the nurse will help smooth the baby's adjustment to home by sharing her observations of his behavior so that the mother will know what to anticipate. If there is any special problem, a complete report should be sent to the nurse who will make the home visit (Chap. 15). Because questions arise after the family is back home, the community nurse can help to interpret changes in behavior from that observed in the hospital.

homegoing

Preparation for the discharge of the mother and baby from the hospital begins with the mother's admission. She has the right and the responsibility to follow her own progress and that of her baby very closely. Therefore include her, and the father, in care and assessments as soon as possible.

The first time the nurse brings the baby to her, the mother should be encouraged to become intimately acquainted with her child.

Even the father should have an opportunity privately to become acquainted with his child. Unwrapping the baby may stimulate the parent to become curious and ask questions. Encourage touching and looking at specific features to assist in overcoming hesitancy and fear of harming the baby. A demonstration of how the baby grasps an extended finger helps to validate a comment about how strong the baby is and lessen the idea most parents have of the extreme fragility of a newborn (Fig. 13·11A, B, C).

Mary Fowler suggests that a mother cannot really begin to assume responsibility for the new baby until she has "claimed" him. In order to claim this baby she must separate him from her "fantasy baby" of pregnancy. Only by careful scrutiny, examination of every detail, can she claim him as her own. And possibly, only after claiming him is she ready to internalize any instructions about his care. Therefore, it seems clear that mothers and fathers must be given the opportunity to see and thoroughly to feel what their baby is like as early after delivery as possible. The caretaking acts such as bathing and feeding may flow more easily from the parents who have claimed this child as theirs and who reach out for ways to establish a meaningful relationship. Homecoming will become a less frightening experience, and the frantic calls for help may decrease.

bibliography

Abramson, Harold: *Symposium on the Functional Physiology of the Fetus and Neonate,* The C. V. Mosby Company, St. Louis, 1971, 182 pp.

Arnold, Helen W., Nancy Putnam, Betty Lou Bernard, Murdina M. Desmond, and Arnold J. Rudolph: "Transition to Extrauterine Life," *American Journal of Nursing,* **65**(10):77–80, 1965.

Bowes, Watson A., Jr., Yvonne Brackbill, Esther Conway, and Alfred Steinschneider: "The Effects of Obstetrical Medication on Fetus and Infant," *Monographs of the Society for Research in Child Development,* (137) **37**(4):1970.

Buchanan-Davidson, Dorothy: "What Can We Learn from Meconium?" *American Journal of Nursing,* **65**:103–107, 1965.

Craig, Margaret E.: "Normal Neonatal Behavior Patterns: The First Week of Extra-uterine Life," *Bulletin of the American College of Nurse-Midwives,* **15**:93–110, 1970.

Dahm, Lida S., and L. S. James: "Newborn Temperature and Calculated Heat Loss in the Delivery Room," *Pediatrics,* **49**:504–514, 1972.

Eppink, Henrietta: "An Experiment to Determine a Basis for Nursing Decisions in Regard to Time of Initiation of Breast Feeding," *Nursing Research,* **18**:292–99, 1969.

Fowler, Mary: "Psychological Needs in the Puerperium," in Ann Clark (ed.), *Maturational Crisis of Childrearing,"* University of Hawaii Press, Honolulu, 1971, pp. 40–43.

Galloway, Karen: "Early Detection of Congenital Anomalies," *Journal of Obstetric, Gynecologic, and Neonatal Nursing,* July–August, 1973, pp. 37–39.

Hervada, Arturo R.: "Nursery Evaluation of the Newborn," *American Journal of Nursing,* **67**:1669–1671, 1967.

Keitel, H. G.: "Preventing Neonatal Diaper Rash," *American Journal of Nursing,* **65**:124, 1965.

Klaus, Marshall, et al.: "Maternal Attachment: Importance of the First Post-partum Days," *New England Journal of Medicine,* **286**:460–663, 1972.

Lutz, Linda, and Paul H. Perlstein: "Temperature Control in Newborn Babies," *Nursing Clinics of North America,* **6**:15–23, 1971.

Moore, Mary Lou: *The Newborn and the Nurse,* Saunders Monographs in Clinical Nursing No. 3, W. B. Saunders Company, Philadelphia, 1972.

Silverman, William A., and Priscilla Parke: "The Newborn, Keep Him Warm," *American Journal of Nursing,* **65**(10):81–84, 1965.

Solomon, Lawrence M., and Nancy B. Esterly: "Neonatal Dermatology. I. The Newborn Skin," *Journal of Pediatrics,* **77**:888–894.

Towell, Molly E.: "The Influence of Labor on the Fetus and the Newborn," *Pediatric Clinics of North America,* **13**:575–598, 1966.

"Where Babies Get a Running Start," *Medical World News,* May 11, 1973, pp. 60–61.

Whitner, Willamay, and Margaret C. Thompson: "The Influence of Bathing on the Newborn Infant's Body Temperature," *Nursing Research,* **19**:30–36, 1970.

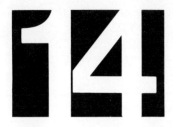

infant feeding

Beatrice Lau Kee
and
Jane Wilson

The food intake of young children is to provide for their rapid linear growth and increase in weight; their nutritional needs are influenced also by the maturation of their gastrointestinal tracts and by the changes in muscle development and coordination.

The infant in his first year of life undergoes the most rapid period of growth outside the fetal period. He usually triples his birthweight and doubles his length by the first birthday. Nutrients provided for the infant must meet the demands of this rapid growth as well as maintain the health of the tissues.

The gastrointestinal tract takes time to mature. Structurally, the stomach is small and the intestinal mobility fairly rapid, causing the stomach to empty within 2 to 2½ h at first. Later the infant can go 3 to 3½ h without symptoms of hunger. Enzyme development is not yet fully mature, so that the infant's ability to digest certain foods is hindered. Sucking, swallowing, and gag reflexes must be coordinated, allowing the infant to suck about 10 to 12 times a minute while breathing 35 to 40 times a minute. Quite an intricate task!

The newborn has the capacity to digest human milk. When cow's milk is substituted, it must be modified to change the curd tension. Fresh cow's milk in a cup and semisolid foods are gradually added to the diet as the infant becomes able to digest this milk and to swallow without sucking. When teeth develop, muscle coordination has reached a point at which the child is able to assist in feeding himself.

If infant feeding is based on maturation processes, questions about timing of new foods are easily answered. The nutritional adequacy of an infant's diet can be evaluated by making various observations. A steady increase in weight and length and developmental ability to perform the tasks of his age will show that he is well nourished. Healthy tissues and normal amounts of subcutaneous tissue indicate good nutrition. Elimination should be normal, and the child should have a good balance of rest and activity.

the infant from birth to six months of age

The nutrient needs of the newborn infant are based upon the number of calories he requires to gain at the normal rate. The other nutrients, such as protein, minerals, vitamins, and fluids, are calculated in proportion to the caloric content of human milk. These figures for an infant from birth to one year of age are found in Table 14·1.

Calories The newborn infant from birth to six months of age requires 117 kcal/kg body weight, about 54 kcal/lb. To calculate the caloric need, multiply the weight in kilograms by 117, or the weight in pounds by 54. Thus an infant weighing 3.5 kg would need 410 kcal each day.

Protein The amount of protein listed in the Recommended Dietary Allowances for an infant from birth to six months is 2.2 Gm/kg, or 1.0 Gm/lb. To calculate the protein needs of an infant, multiply his weight in kilograms by a factor of 2.2, or his weight in pounds by a factor of 1. An infant weighing 3.5 kg will need 7.7 Gm protein daily.

Fluids The amount of fluid needed by the infant depends on his caloric requirements.

table 14·1

RECOMMENDED DIETARY ALLOWANCES FOR INFANTS DURING THE FIRST YEAR OF LIFE

	0 TO 6 mo (0.0–0.5 yr)	6 TO 12 mo (0.5–1.0 yr)
Weight	6 kg (14 lb)	9 kg (20 lb)
Height	60 cm (24 in)	71 cm (28 in)
Kilocalories	kg × 117	kg × 108
Protein, Gm	kg × 2.2	kg × 2.0
Fat-soluble vitamins:		
Vitamin A, IU	1400	2000
Vitamin D, IU	400	400
Vitamin E, IU	4	5
Water-soluble vitamins:		
Ascorbic acid, mg	35	35
Folacin, μg	50	50
Niacin, mg	5	8
Riboflavin, mg	0.4	0.6
Thiamine, mg	0.3	0.5
Vitamin B_6, mg	0.3	0.4
Vitamin B_{12}, μg	0.3	0.3
Minerals:		
Calcium, mg	360	540
Phosphorus, mg	240	400
Iodine, μg	35	45
Iron, mg	10	15
Magnesium, mg	60	70
Zinc, mg	3	5

Source: Adapted from *Recommended Dietary Allowances*, 8th rev. ed., National Research Council, National Academy of Sciences, Washington, 1973.

He needs about 1.5 ml for each kilocalorie, because the waste products of metabolism, excreted through the kidneys, need adequate fluid in which to be dissolved. If the proportion of waste products from protein and calcium and electrolytes is too high in proportion to fluid output, the high renal solute load can be dangerous to the infant.

Fluid needs can also be calculated directly in proportion to the infant's weight. He should receive 165 ml or 5.5 oz/kg, (75 ml or 2.5 oz/lb). An infant weighing 3.5 kg should receive about 19 oz fluid a day.

If the nurse knows the caloric, protein, and fluid needs of an infant, it is then possible to determine how these nutrient needs can be met by the infant's diet. At three months of age, when the infant begins to receive additional foods in his diet, the milk intake may be no higher or may even be less than during the first 2 months.

the infant from six to twelve months of age

The recommended dietary allowance for an infant from six to twelve months of age is 108 kcal/kg and 2.0 Gm protein per kilogram. The growth rate is slowing; thus the caloric and protein levels are diminishing. If an adult weighing 55 kg received the caloric intake of a newborn, he would take in 6000 kilocalories per day!

obesity

Recent studies have found that the incidence of obesity is higher among formula-fed infants than breast-fed infants. It seems to be easier to force an infant to finish the bottle even when he is not hungry than to overfeed him with breast milk. A mother who breast-feeds has only the awareness that the infant is satisfied and therefore does not coax him to drink more.

Obesity is an excess of adipose tissue in the body. In early childhood when body cells multiply rapidly, overfeeding will cause excessive formation of fat cells. As the child grows, these fat cells will also grow in size. If obesity is corrected by diet, the fat cells can only shrink in size; they will never disappear. To prevent obesity in adulthood, it is best to prevent it in early childhood.

malnutrition

Malnutrition is defined as faulty nutrition, implying either under- or overnutrition, in any degree. However, this term is most commonly used to refer to severe undernutrition. Undernutrition, an inadequate supply of any of the basic nutrients to the cells, involves more than a lack of proper food. It can also be a result of failure to digest, absorb, or metabolize nutrients from normal amounts of ingested food. The underlying cause of malnutrition must be discovered and corrected if possible before adequate nutritional intake will be effective.

Although undernutrition is not now a major health problem in the United States, the nurse may see some severely malnourished infants in the hospital. Their diagnoses may range from malabsorption syndrome, nutritional failure, failure to thrive, or marasmus. In countries where protein foods are scarce, kwashiorkor may be a major problem.

Marasmus—protein-calorie malnutrition—may be either a primary or secondary deficiency. Primary deficiency refers to a lack of intake of a nutrient; a secondary deficiency is due to the inability of the body to digest or utilize nutrients properly. Examples of primary deficiency are infantile scurvy from lack of vitamin C, and kwashiorkor, from protein-deficient diets. Secondary malnutrition may be due to celiac disease, parasitic infection, or intestinal obstruction, among other causes. Marasmus is usually found in younger children and is characterized by gross underweight and retarded growth, with atrophy of subcutaneous fat and muscle mass. The skin is wrinkled and has poor turgor. Body temperature will be below normal, as metabolism slows and body fat is metabolized. Diarrhea and vomiting are common, quickly upsetting fluid and electrolyte balance.

Kwashiorkor is found especially in poverty areas of the world and usually becomes evident after weaning. The basic lack of protein foods in the diet, caused by poverty or ignorance, is too often accompanied by parasitic intestinal disease, to further complicate recovery. The most obvious signs of kwashiorkor are edema of the abdomen and depigmentation of skin and hair. Growth is retarded, and muscular atrophy, liver enlargement, mental apathy, and lethargy are found. The children of the Biafran conflict demonstrated to the world the effects of malnutrition. Since brain growth is so rapid during the first years of life, protein malnutrition will prevent a child from developing to his potential.

breast feeding

ANATOMY AND PHYSIOLOGY OF THE BREASTS

The breasts, or mammary glands, are two accessory organs of reproduction located on each side of the anterior chest wall. In the adult they extend from the second to the sixth or seventh rib and laterally from the sternum to the anterior axillary border. Though the size

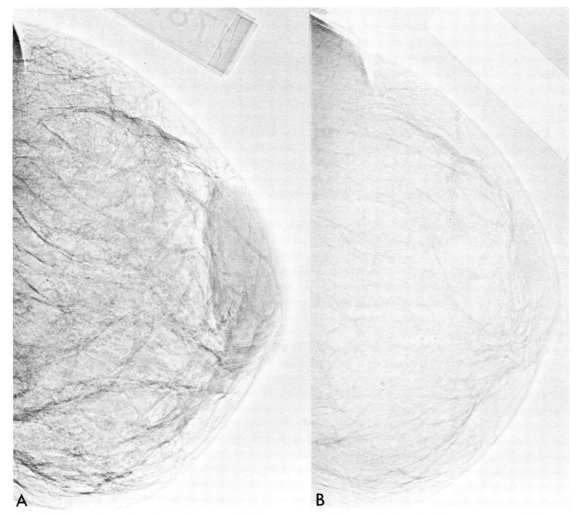

fig. 14·1 Zeroradiographic views of a breast. A Showing general increase in density during pregnancy. B Six months after cessation of lactation. (*Courtesy of John N. Wolfe, M.D.*)

and shape vary a great deal among individuals, generally they are dome-shaped and have an average weight of 100 to 200 Gm. During lactation they increase two to three times in weight.

These glands are composed of adipose, glandular, and fibrous tissue, and are separated from the ribs and chest muscles by connective tissue. They are supported by bands of fibrous tissue called *Cooper's ligaments*. The glandular tissue radiates out from the nipple, forming 15 to 20 lobes. Spaces between the lobes are filled with adipose tissue, and the lobes are connected by fibrous tissue. Each lobe is divided into smaller lobules, which contain many *acini,* the acini constituting a layer of epithelium richly supplied with capillaries. The various elements of the milk are formed in this layer. Out of each lobule comes an excretory duct, the *lactiferous duct,* joining into a single main channel that becomes enlarged near the nipple to form a reservoir, the *sinus lactiferus* (Fig. 14·1).

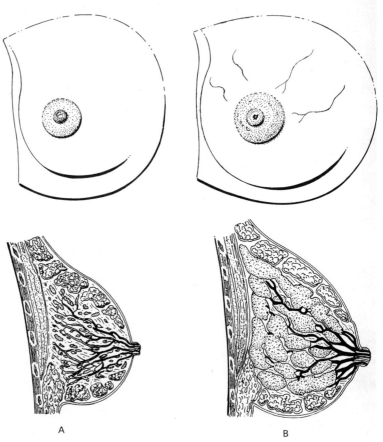

fig. 14·2A Cross section of the breast. B The lactating breast. (*Courtesy of Ross Laboratories, Clinical Education Aid No. 10.*)

The lactiferous ducts open at the tip of the nipple. The nipple, composed of fibromuscular tissue, is small, pigmented, and cylindric. It may be flat or may project outward for a few millimeters, and becomes erect on stimulation. The circular pigmented area around the nipple is called the *areola*. Many sebaceous glands, known as the *tubercles of Montgomery,* secrete fatty substances that lubricate and protect the nipple tissue.

BREAST CHANGES DURING PREGNANCY

Feelings of fullness and tenderness in the breasts are among the first signs of pregnancy. The following are the changes most no-

ticeable after the second month of pregnancy (Fig. 14·2):

The breasts increase in size (some almost double in size).

The nipples become erect and prominent.

The areola becomes larger in diameter and more darkly pigmented.

The blood vessels enlarge, and darker bluish veins can be seen under the skin.

The tubercles of Montgomery become enlarged and more noticeable.

A thin, yellowish, watery fluid, *colostrum,* can be expressed from the breasts from about the fourth month on.

All these changes are brought about by the

two major hormones of pregnancy, estrogen and progesterone. Estrogen is responsible for general breast and milk duct growth; progesterone causes the maturation of the lobular-alveolar system. The secretion of milk is inhibited during pregnancy by high levels of these two hormones. When estrogen and progesterone blood levels rapidly decrease after delivery of the placenta, the leuteotropic hormone (LTH), also called *prolactin,* is released from the anterior pituitary gland to begin the production of milk.

MECHANISM OF LACTATION

When the infant is put to the breast, the sucking stimulus at the nipple transmits nerve

fig. 14·3 Sucking reflex control of oxytocin secretion and milk letdown. (*From A. Vander, et al.,* Human Physiology, *McGraw-Hill Book Company, New York,* 1970.)

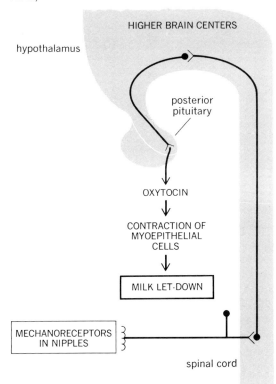

impulses to the spinal cord and brain, causing release of oxytocin from the posterior pituitary gland. Oxytocin stimulates the anterior pituitary gland, which releases LTH, which in turn stimulates the production of milk. Oxytocin also causes contraction of the acini, forcing milk expulsion into the ducts. The sucking of the baby during nursing draws the milk out of the lactiferous sinuses. The whole process is called the *letdown reflex* (Fig. 14·3). Some mothers may actually feel it as a tingling sensation; others feel nothing. Usually the first outward sign of the letdown reflex is the dripping of milk from one breast as the baby nurses from the other. The reflex may be triggered when a mother hears her baby crying or just sees him, particularly before a feeding. The letdown reflex can be inhibited by pain or emotional stress in the mother.

Oxytocin, released as a result of the sucking stimulus, causes the uterine muscle to contract strongly. For the first few days after birth, mothers will often complain of uterine cramps while they are breast-feeding.

PRENATAL PREPARATION FOR BREAST FEEDING

The prenatal period is the ideal time to discuss breast feeding with the mother. The advantages of this method of feeding can be presented in prenatal classes, with each mother being given an opportunity to express her feelings and to ask questions. There are many myths in our society about breast feeding: that it spoils the figure; that a woman with small breasts cannot produce enough milk; that breast milk is too thin for the baby; that breast feeding is too complicated; etc. Some women are embarrassed by the idea of breast feeding; others find it repugnant. Much depends on the woman's feeling of comfort with her own body. Often a woman will find resistance on her husband's part. Open discussion at home or in the childbirth education class may reduce his concerns. If he remains ada-

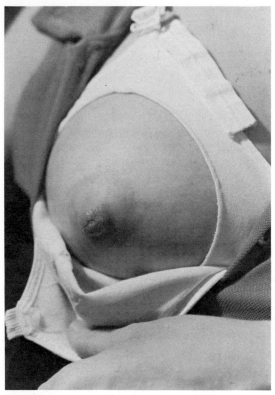

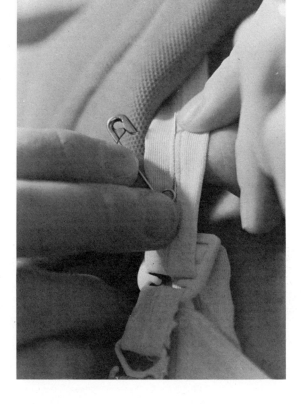

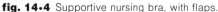

fig. 14·4 Supportive nursing bra, with flaps.

mant, she probably should not breast-feed because tension over this issue can reduce her ability to produce milk.

Nipple and breast care Opinions differ widely on the importance of prenatal nipple care and whether or not it has any effect on successful breast feeding. It is certain, however, that positive thinking and looking forward to the experience help. If the mother is given routine, practical instructions on how to care for her breasts and nipples during her pregnancy, this may stimulate her interest in breastfeeding and give her a positive attitude toward it. Once the breasts enlarge, support is needed. Breast tissue will stretch if not supported during pregnancy and the lactation period. A variety of supportive brassieres is available; nursing brassieres can be used during pregnancy (Fig. 14·4).

Daily washing of the breasts and nipples is the only care that is necessary during most of the prenatal period. Soap should be used sparingly, if at all. Beginning in the eighth month, a small amount of colostrum should be hand-expressed from the breasts daily. The mother learns now how to express fluid from the ducts and can later help prevent painful engorgement when lactation begins (Fig. 14·5).

Daily gentle "pulling out" of the nipple during the last few months of pregnancy is also recommended. A treatment for flattened nipples, it also helps to toughen the nipple and prevent soreness from developing during nursing. Inverted nipples are relatively uncommon; unless they are noticed and treated during pregnancy the mother will have difficulty with feeding the infant. The inverted nipple retracts when pressure is applied to it between the thumb and forefinger, and folds back into itself. The most effective treatment is the use of breast shields during pregnancy, worn daily for as many hours as possible. The shields fit over the nipples and exert a mild suction which helps draw out the nipple. A hand breast pump used several times a day will also help to correct inversion.

THE PROCESS OF BREAST FEEDING

When the baby is brought to his mother for the first feeding, she may be truly overwhelmed with feelings of wonder and joy, mixed with those of tremendous anxiety over her responsibility for such a helpless, tiny creature. She needs not only emotional support, but positive, clear instructions on how to manage breast feeding. Even if she does not ask, the nurse should be prepared to spend time with the mother for the first feeding, to help her handle her baby, and to help start him nursing. The mother will need privacy while breast feeding to enable her to relax so that the letdown reflex can effectively function.

Positioning The mother should nurse her baby in the position most comfortable for her. If she has had a cesarean section or is sore from the episiotomy, the side-lying position may be most comfortable. If the mother chooses to nurse while sitting up in bed, a pillow can be placed under the baby so that she doesn't have to hold him completely. Some women are comfortable in the tailor-sitting position; others prefer to sit in a straight-back or rocking chair. The mother should support her breast with her free hand, holding the breast just above the areola between her second and third fingers so that the breast does not press against the baby's nose and hinder his breathing (Fig. 14·6). The whole of the areola should be in the baby's mouth so that the milk reservoirs above the nipple are compressed by the baby's lips (Fig. 14·7). Sucking only on the

nipple will produce no milk and causes sore nipples.

The nurse should show the mother how to use the baby's natural *rooting* reflex (Fig. 14·8)—a slight touch on the baby's cheek will cause him to turn in that direction and open his mouth to take the nipple. This reflex needs to be understood, because if the mother touches any part of the baby's face while holding his head, he will keep turning his head in the direction of the touch and will become confused and frantic when he doesn't find the nipple.

The baby's sucking causes a strong suc-

fig. 14·5 Expressing milk. The thumb and forefinger are placed on either side of the nipple at the edge of the areola. Thumb and finger are squeezed together, with care being taken not to slide down toward the nipple. The hand is rotated so that all the milk ducts are reached.

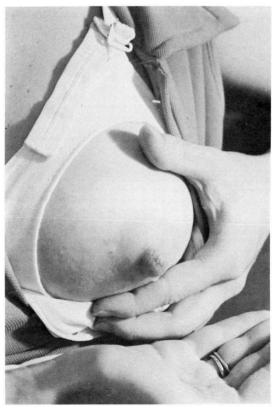

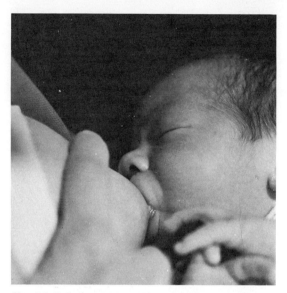

fig. 14·6 Baby sucking. (*Photo by John Young.*)

tion, which should be broken before taking the baby from the breast. The mother can press down on the breast, thus letting air into the baby's mouth, or place a fingertip into the corner of his mouth and gently press it open (Fig. 14·9).

Bubbling All babies swallow some air while sucking, and need several opportunities to burp during and after a feeding. Babies can be bubbled half-way through the feeding or when they appear to slow down. (Figure 14·10 shows several methods of holding an infant to bubble him.) During burping, small amounts of undigested milk may be regurgitated with the air. Mothers usually term this "spitting up." Regurgitation is due to air swallowed during sucking, and also to the fact that the cardiac sphincter at the entrance of the stomach is not fully closed in newborn infants. An infant who regurgitates frequently can be placed on his right side with his head and trunk in an elevated position or placed in an infant seat for 15 or 20 min after a meal.

Mothers may confuse simple regurgitation with actual vomiting, when a larger amount of sour, partly digested milk is thrown up. It is important for the nurse to teach the mother the difference between the two. Mothers have been known not to report vomiting because they didn't want to bother the pediatrician. Since babies become dehydrated quickly, true vomiting is always a symptom to be reported.

Length of Feeding Periods Feedings the first day are limited to about 5 min at each breast. The time period is increased slowly, so that by the time milk replaces colostrum on the third or fourth day, the nursing time is about 15 min. Mothers tend to let the baby suck for long periods as the thrill of actually being able to feed, touch, and be so close to their infants supersedes any teaching on gradual extension of time in feeding. Extended sucking causes sore nipples, and since most of the milk is taken in the first 10 min, any extra time is for emotional satisfaction for mother and baby. Once feeding is established, the most important principle in breast feeding is to *empty at least one breast at a feeding*. Complete emptying causes a fresh influx of milk, whereas partial emptying inhibits new production.

Feeding Schedules It often happens that when the baby is brought to the mother in the hospital, he is asleep and resists all efforts to awaken him. The obvious solution is to feed

fig. 14·7 The proper positioning of the infant's mouth on the breast. (*Courtesy of Ross Laboratories, Clinical Education Aid. No.* 10.)

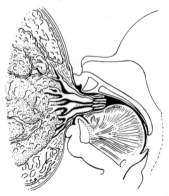

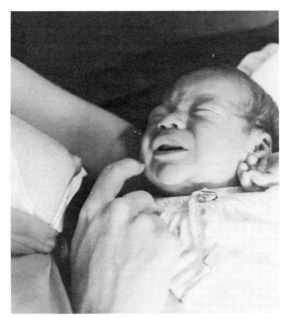
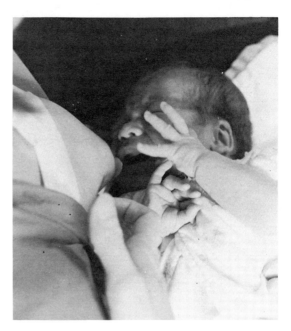

fig. 14.8 Rooting reflex. (*Photos by John Young*)

fig. 14.9A Grasping nipple. B Releasing suction after feeding.

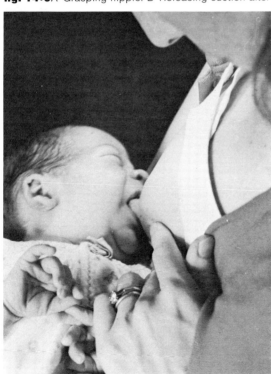
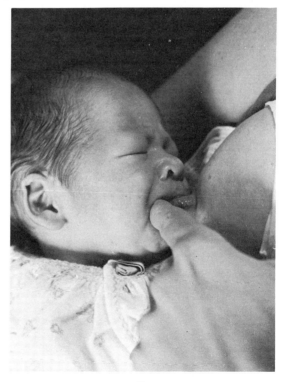

A   B

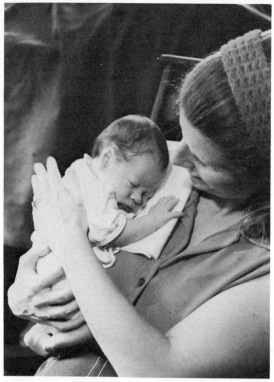
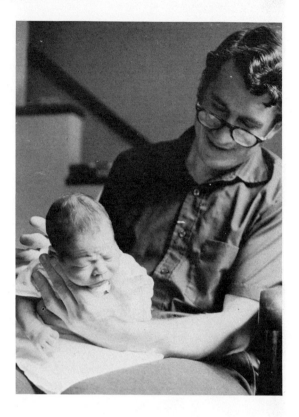

fig. 14·10 Two ways of bubbling the baby.

him when he is hungry. Unfortunately, most hospitals still adhere to a 4-h schedule, even though early breast feeding is best on a 2- to 3-h schedule. Rooming-in allows for self-regulatory demand feedings. Breast feeding is much more easily established in such a situation. Night feedings are important in the hospital. Many mothers who are bottle-feeding their infants request to sleep while the baby is fed in the nursery, but the lactating mother must carry on her frequent feedings to get lactation well established.

SUCCESSFUL BREAST FEEDING AT HOME

In the 2 to 3 days that the mother and baby are in the hospital, breast feeding is usually only tenuously established. In the hospital the mother usually has the support of the hospital

staff and the assurance from others that her baby is doing well. When she goes home, she may be very much on her own and may lose confidence in her ability to feed her baby. Feelings of self-doubt may be fostered by relatives and friends who have not breast-fed and question if the baby is getting an adequate supply.

Before the mother goes home, the nurse should instruct her on several points, as anticipatory guidance. The mother should be instructed about the physiology of the let-down reflex and the need for emptying the breast at a feeding. The factors that diminish the milk supply can be discussed: fatigue, poor nutrition and inadequate fluid intake, and anxiety. If, in concern, the mother gives a supplemental bottle of formula, the breast-feeding process is due to fail, as the baby will take a bottle nipple more easily than the breast. Lack of the stimulation provided by enough sucking to empty the breast will decrease the supply, and the cycle of normal production will quickly cease. Of course, after breast feeding is thoroughly established, the mother may use a bottle for a feeding when she is out of the house for dinner or a visit. She will become uncomfortable, perhaps, but the baby will be well fed and the milk supply will not be hindered.

The mother needs to know the names of books with information on breast feeding, and she should be informed of organizations that can be helpful to her. La Leche League (1), an organization dedicated to the promotion of breast feeding, has excellent literature available and in most parts of the country has members ready to help new mothers if they need support and guidance. The Visiting Nurse Service is available in many areas: if the nurse senses that the mother will need further support at home, she can make a referral to the V.N.S.

maternal nutrient needs during lactation

In order to breast-feed her infant successfully, the mother must eat appropriate foods in adequate amounts, to produce milk as well as to maintain her health. The recommended dietary allowances for lactation (2) are determined in proportion to the amount of milk produced each day, the average being 850 ml (see Table 4·4).

Calories For every 100 ml milk which the mother produces, she should consume about 130 kcal over and above her usual base-line caloric intake. An average yield of 850 ml milk provides 650 kcal to the infant. Calories from the mother's food intake can be converted to breast milk calories at 80 percent efficiency. The maternal fat which is stored during pregnancy can also provide 200 to 400 kcal each day for up to 6 months of lactation. Therefore an additional 500 kcal is needed to provide for lactation and the gradual restoration of normal body composition.

Protein Human milk contains an average of 1.2 Gm protein in 100 ml milk. Assuming that the average production is 850, with maximum amount of 1200 ml, protein needs just for lactation are considered to be about 15 Gm daily. A margin of safety is considered in the allowances because protein quality varies in foods. To be completely safe, an allowance of 20 Gm protein over the normal intake is recommended daily during lactation.

Calcium and Other Nutrients An additional intake of calcium is recommended during lactation. Drinking two extra cups of milk over the baseline requirements will meet the calcium recommendations for lactation. If the mother finds that she cannot drink that much milk, the nurse should work with her to discover what milk-based foods she could include. An addition of 1000 IU of vitamin A is recommended. This need can be met by adding dark green and deep yellow vegetables daily to the diet. Recommendations for iron and for vitamins C and D are the same as for pregnancy.

Fluids If 850 ml milk is produced by the lactating woman, she should receive at least that amount of fluids over and above her normal intake. The two extra cups of milk needed to meet the calcium needs will provide about half these fluid requirements.

SUGGESTED MEAL PLAN
DURING LACTATION

Milk	4 cups
Meat and meat substitutes	6 oz daily, 2 to 3 servings
Vegetables, fruits Include:	4 servings
Dark green or Yellow	1 serving daily

Vitamin C source	1 serving daily
Bread or cereal	4 or 5 servings
Fluids	6 to 8 cups daily in addition to milk

Additional foods to make up the caloric requirements should be wholesome not such nonnutritional foods as sodas, fats, and candies.

A mother will often ask if there are any foods which should be omitted during lactation. Some sources recommend that she refrain from chocolate or fried foods because they might affect her milk and thus the infant. There seems to be no physiologic reason for avoiding these foods as long as she receives other adequate nutrients in her diet.

The nutritional quality of human milk has no direct relationship to the nutritional status of the mother. The composition of mature human milk varies among women of similar backgrounds, in the same woman from one time of day to another, and in the same woman from one breast to another. If the mother is breast-feeding one infant who gets the full amount of milk she produces, these changes of quality are not significant. If the nutritional intake of the lactating mother is not adequate, the *total quantity of the milk produced is decreased,* rather than the *quality.*

Cost Breast milk is not free milk. The cost of lactation is related to the cost of additional foods that the mother needs during lactation (3).

the advantages of breast feeding

The nutrients of human milk are in the right proportion for a human infant.

Purchasing of formula and bottles is not necessary.

No formula preparation is needed.

Milk is always available.

The tendency to overfeed the infant and thus predispose him to obesity in later years is lessened.

While breast-feeding, the mother holds the baby close, thus providing warmth and pleasure as part of the food intake experience. She receives physiologic benefits, promoting involution.

common feeding problems

Sore nipples are very common; they are most likely to occur in fair-skinned women and in those who let the baby suck too long at first. Soreness usually starts about the third postpartum day and may be present in one or both of the nipples. The nipple will look cracked and sore, and may begin to bleed. Treatment consists mainly of keeping the nipple dry by exposure to air; the mother should be instructed to leave down the flaps of the nursing bra and to wear a loosely fitting gown to allow the air to circulate. The doctor may order short periods of sun lamp treatment to promote fast healing. Topical medications such as lanolin or Massé cream help to relieve soreness. Preparations containing alcohol are excessively drying and painful and should not be used. Nursing should be done for short, frequent periods so that the breasts do not become engorged. To relieve the pain and enable the letdown reflex to function, many doctors recommend an analgesic such as aspirin approximately $1/2$ h before feeding. If the pain is severe, a nipple shield can be used: the mother holds the shield over the breast and the baby sucks the rubber nipple.

Engorgement of the breasts occurs to some extent with all nursing mothers as lactation begins, but it is most common with the first baby. It begins with tenderness and distension which are due to the first formation of milk in the acini and a rush of blood and lymph to the tissues. The breasts become hard, hot, and heavy, and feel lumpy. If the newly formed milk is not removed, the flow becomes obstructed and the breasts become red, swollen, and extremely painful. This swelling flattens the nipple, thus compounding the problem of nursing.

If the amount of engorgement appears to be only moderate, some milk should be hand-expressed just before feeding, making the nipple and areola softer and easier for the baby to grasp. After the baby has finished nursing, the breasts should be completely emptied by hand. When engorgement is severe, between feedings a firm binder or bra will give support. The doctor will order ice packs and analgesia. Discontinuing breast feeding is an extreme measure and should never be necessary if the nurse is alert and the mother has been taught how to recognize and relieve engorgement.

Severe engorgement can be prevented to a large extent by frequent feedings whenever the breasts begin to feel full. One breast should be emptied at every feeding by massaging the breast as the baby nurses. The mother should be encouraged to tell the nurse whenever her breasts feel overfull; she can then feed the baby or express her milk by hand until she feels comfortable.

With early discharge from the hospital, engorgement is likely to occur after the mother and her baby have returned home. Postpartum teaching becomes very important at this point.

Mastitis is an infection in the breasts, most commonly caused by *Staphylococcus aureus*. It results from entry of the bacteria through a cracked or sore nipple, and occurs most often in the third or fourth week post partum. The symptoms are an elevation of temperature, an increased pulse rate, and pain in the breast. Pain and swelling become localized in one area of the breast, then spread as cellulitis to the surrounding breast tissue. In some cases an abscess may form.

Treatment consists of administration of antibiotics and analgesics, and rest for the mother. The breasts should be supported with a firm bra. The application of ice packs will help to relieve the pain and swelling. A deep abscess may require needle aspiration or incision and drainage. Before the advent of antibiotics, mastitis was an indication to stop breast feeding. This is no longer necessary. Continued breast feeding will reduce engorgement and contribute to a quick recovery. With early treatment, symptoms will be gone within 24 h (4).

contraindications to breast feeding

Chronic illness in the mother is the main contraindication to breast feeding. Diseases such as tuberculosis, kidney impairment, cardiac insufficiency, severe anemia already place enough stress on the mother.

Acute illness or infection during the postpartum period may also lead to a temporary or complete cessation of breast feeding. Unless contraindicated by her physician, the mother's wishes should be followed. To maintain a flow of milk during her illness, a breast pump may be used. The infant would be given a premodified milk formula for the duration of the illness.

Breast feeding should be discontinued if the mother becomes pregnant again. Ovulation begins again in the nonlactating woman about 36 days after delivery, with the first menses occurring regularly following the woman's usual pattern. When the mother is lactating, the probability of ovulation during the first 9 weeks is nearly zero, according to Perez (5), but it may occur any time after that even though the woman continues breast feeding. Because ovulation is unpredictable, and women vary widely, lactation should not be considered an effective method of contraception beyond the first 6 weeks after delivery.

BREAST MILK AND JAUNDICE

In fewer than 1 percent of breast-feeding mothers, a factor is secreted in milk which seems to inhibit the reduction of bilirubin to a more water-soluble, more easily excretable form. The result is an elevated level of indirect bilirubin in the infant, who is already dealing with physiologic hyperbilirubinemia (see Chap. 29). The physician will usually prescribe extra water for the infant and may ask the mother to discontinue breast feeding, placing the infant on formula for 3 or 4 days. By 5 days of life, the infant should be able to metabolize bilirubin adequately and may be returned to breast milk. The mother who wishes to resume feeding may use a hand or electric pump on the breast while the infant is receiving formula (6). Prevention of jaundice may be possible by giving extra fluids to the breast-feeding infant in the first few days of life.

DRUGS AND BREAST MILK

An excellent discussion about the feasibility of drugs passing into the breast milk, passing the blood/milk barrier, is found in Catz and Giacoia (7). The knowledge of the effects of drugs ingested by the mother is incomplete at this time. Catz states:

> It has become apparent that a number of drugs should not be given to the mother while she is nursing. Included in this group are atropine, anticoagulants, antithyroid drugs, antimetabolites, cathartics (excluding senna), dihydrotachysterol, iodides, narcotics, radioactive preparations, bromides, ergot, tetracyclines, and metronidazole (Flagyl).

Caution seems to be the clue to the use of the other drugs not yet proved harmful.

PASSIVE IMMUNITY

Some investigators have speculated that there is a related mechanism of transfer, in which maternal antibodies are passed to the infant through breast milk. Although colostrum is rich in antibodies, most of them are inactivated in the gastrointestinal tract and are useless to the infant. Many of the studies supporting the concept of passive immunization were done on animals in which passive immunity is acquired mainly through the milk (8). What passive immunity is present seems to be acquired through the placental transfer, not through breast milk (9).

the formula-fed infant

There is little evidence to show that the bottle-fed baby in modern Western society fares any differently than the breast-fed baby (8). Artificial formulas produced today are safe and, when used as directed, produce strong, healthy babies. The mother who chooses to bottle-feed her baby is not depriving her child, and she should not be made to feel guilty about it. In underdeveloped areas of the world, where poor facilities for sterilization and inadequate refrigeration exist, a baby must be breast-fed to survive. In some cultures the diet is so unsuitable for infants that the mother must breast-feed for two or more years.

Since most mothers in our society know something about bottle feeding, the nurse might assume that a woman will feel comfortable giving her baby a bottle for the first time, and she may fail to give enough support and attention. The mother who bottle-feeds, as well as the one who breast-feeds, needs instruction on how to hold and burp her baby and how to recognize when he has had enough.

The baby should be held closely with his head in a slightly elevated position in the crook of the mother's arm, as in breast feeding, so that he feels warm and secure while he feeds (Fig. 14·11). It is fairly common to see mothers or nurses, as they bottle-feed small babies, hold the baby out away from them on one knee with a hand behind the baby's head while the baby's arms flail around insecurely. The baby receives the milk but misses out on the comforts of cuddling. Feeding should always be a social time. Studies have been done to measure the impact of the mother's methods of feeding on

fig. 14·11 Satisfying a baby by bottle. (*Photo by Karen Gilborn.*)

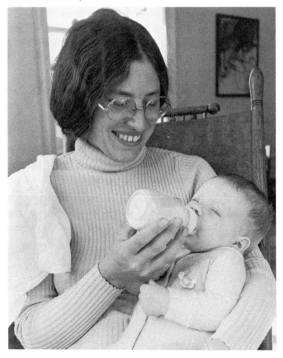

the infant's adjustment and ability to perform certain developmental tasks (9). Consistency, socialization, and play are important aspects of feeding. In line with the findings on the importance of giving pleasure during feeding, the nurse should instruct the mother not to prop a bottle, for that would isolate the infant from contact with his mother. Infants should be fed *before* going to bed for naps or the night sleep for two reasons: (1) The taking of food should not be connected with separation from mother in a dark room. (2) Infants sucking slowly on milk as they lie flat in bed tend to get more inner-ear infections, as this position allows milk to enter the eustachian tube more easily. If the baby wants the security of something to suck on as he falls asleep, the mother can provide a safely constructed pacifier.

It is much easier to hurry an infant through a bottle feeding. The mother should understand that food time must be as relaxed as possible. A baby needs the satisfaction of sucking, the socialization of being held and cuddled, and a mother who enjoys this time as much as the baby does. A mother does well to limit those who help her with feeding during the first few months so that the baby is not confused by multiple methods and styles of feeding. To many a busy mother this emphasis may sound too nearly ideal, but nurses should try to convey the importance of food and feeding in the infant's development.

CONTENT OF FORMULA

Cow's milk is the usual substitute for human milk, but it must be modified to meet the needs of the newborn human infant. Because of the high ratio of casein to whey in cow's milk, the curd formed in the stomach is difficult for the newborn infant to digest. Boiling the milk changes the curd tension so that it is smaller and softer. Cow's milk is also more concentrated in protein and calcium and has less carbohydrate than human milk; therefore it must be diluted with water and have carbohydrates added to make it resemble human milk.

Only evaporated milk and premodified commercial formulas are recommended for infant feeding. Fresh whole milk can be given to an infant after he is four or five months old. In some cultures, fresh milk is a status symbol in newborn feeding and mothers insist on using it. If they persist, nurses should instruct them to boil the milk before diluting it and adding sugar. Condensed milk is canned milk with a large amount of sugar added. This is *not* suitable for infant feeding, because the proportion of carbohydrates is too great. Infants fed on condensed milk become very obese before their first birthday. Obesity is a mark of health in some Latin cultures, and untutored mothers may feel very proud of their obese condensed-milk-fed infants.

Skim milk of any kind is not suitable for the newborn infant because, if enough milk is given to provide the calories needed, the amount of calcium, protein, and electrolytes would be so high that the renal solute load would be too great for the infant. Skim milk has half the calories of whole milk because most of the fat is removed. Essential fatty acids are necessary to maintain the health of infants. Essential fatty acid deficiency is manifested by eczema-type lesions. If the infant is obese, some pediatricians recommend skim milk after the infant is six or seven months old and is receiving meats and vegetables.

Premodified Milk Formula Commercially prepared formula has the butterfat removed and vegetable oils added to provide a larger proportion of unsaturated fatty acids. The exchange of vegetable oils for the butterfat does not seem to benefit the infant's serum cholesterol levels, but is used to provide a greater proportion of the essential fatty acids,

linoleic, linolenic, and arachidonic acids, that are found in human milk. An advantage to the mother of this substitute is that the vomitus of modified formula does not have the sour odor that is present in milk containing butterfat. Milk is diluted to lower the concentration of protein and calcium, and lactose or dextrose is added to raise the carbohydrate level. Multivitamins are added. Some formulas have added iron and are used with infants with anemia or who have a low birth weight.

Premodified milks come in four different formats. Concentrated formula must be diluted with an equal part of water. Ready-to-use formula is sold in large cans, small (4-oz) cans, and prefilled disposable bottles. Because most hospitals send the mother home with a 24-h supply of disposable bottled formula, a new mother may think that that is the format she must use. The nurse must be sure to discuss methods of feeding and preparation of formula with the mother before homegoing. For the convenience of disposable bottles, the cost becomes three or four times as much as the concentrated formula, and much more than home-prepared evaporated milk formula.

As long as vitamins are given to babies receiving evaporated milk, there is no real difference in the growth rates of children whether they are breast-fed or given premodified or evaporated milk formulas.

Milk Substitutes If the infant is found to be allergic to cow's milk, a formula of goat's milk or a soybean-based milk may be ordered by the physician. Formulas based on meat are also available. The substitutes have to be extensively modified to provide the necessary nutrients. They are available in drug and grocery stores and will always cost substantially more than standard formulas.

Evaporated Milk Formula and Its Preparation Canned evaporated milk has been used for many years. The process of evaporating and canning milk lowers the curd ten-

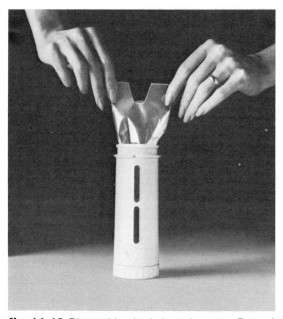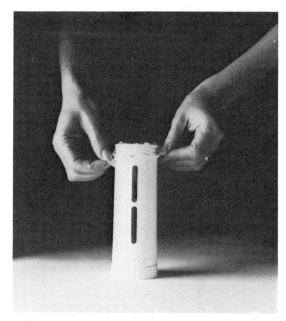

fig. 14·12 Disposable plastic bags in nurser. Parts of the bottle setup which come in contact with the baby are boiled; nipple, screw ring. Bags are sterile and disposable. (*Courtesy of International Playtex Incorporated.*)

sion and makes the milk bacteriologically safe. It can be stored at room temperature and requires no refrigeration until the can is opened. It is fortified with 400 IU vitamin D per quart of reconstituted milk. Ideas on formula preparation differ, but to balance evaporated milk, it must always be diluted with two parts of water and sugar or corn syrup must be added for extra carbohydrates. Since water in most areas of the United States is considered to be essentially safe, some pediatricians are recommending only medical asepsis in formula preparation: clean bottles and nipples and clean tap water mixed with milk fresh from a can. In these cases, where there is any question of poor refrigeration, contamination of bottles or nipples by flies, pets, litter, or other children, the mother should still be instructed in boiling bottles and nipples for the first 3 to 4 months, and preparing only one bottle at a time. Many women prefer and feel more comfortable with the disposable plastic bag Nurser (see Fig. 14·12), with which it is necessary to boil only nipples and the dispenser.

The American Academy of Pediatrics Committee on the Fetus and Newborn continues to recommend the terminal heat method for preparing evaporated milk formula:

The recommended method of formula preparation is the one in which heating is applied after the formula is bottled. This is often referred to as the "terminal sterilization method," although it is not technically sterilization. It is more properly called the "terminal heat method."

Equipment needed:

Baby bottles (heat-resistant type)
Bottle caps or nipple covers
Nipples
Large kettle or bottle sterilizer with wire rack (if wire rack is not available, a clean cloth in the bottom of the large pot can be used)
Saucepan or pitcher with a pouring lip

Measuring cup
Measuring spoon
Long-handled spoon
Funnel
Bottle brush with stiff bristles and long
   handle
Can opener

Procedure:

1. Wash hands.
2. Wash all equipment clean with hot soapy
   water, including the work surface. Use
   brush to wash bottles; milk curd is hard to
   remove without a brush.
3. Wash top of can of milk and rinse well.
4. Measure the amount prescribed by the
   physician of water, milk, and sugar or
   syrup into saucepan or pitcher. Stir with
   spoon.
5. Pour into bottles in prescribed amounts.
6. Put nipples and bottle caps or nipple
   covers on bottles, then loosen bottle
   caps.
7. Place bottles on wire rack or clean cloth
   in the bottom of the large pot. Add 3 or 4
   in water.
8. Cover the pot and turn on heat. After
   water in pot reaches boiling point, let it
   boil for 25 min. (In some areas, the local
   health departments may recommend that
   the boiling time be shortened because
   the water supply has been tested and
   found to be very pure.)
9. Turn off heat. With the cover on, let the
   entire pot cool slowly, undisturbed, until
   the entire unit is lukewarm. (The slow
   cooling of the formula prevents the milk
   from thickening, often a cause of clogged
   nipples.)
10. Remove bottles, tighten bottle caps, and
    place bottles in the refrigerator.

After each feeding the bottles and nipples
should be rinsed and soaked in cold water.
This will facilitate washing prior to the next
use.

Sample formula:

$$8 \text{ oz evaporated milk } 44 \text{ kcal per oz}$$
$$16 \text{ oz water}$$
$$\underline{1 \text{ tbsp corn syrup} \qquad \underline{24} \text{ kcal per tbsp}}$$
$$24 \text{ oz formula} \qquad = \underline{\quad} \text{ kcal in 24 oz?}$$

For an infant of what weight would this
formula be prescribed (117 kcal/kg)? Would
additional fluid be needed to meet daily
requirements?

TEMPERATURE OF FORMULA

For many years, the formula was heated before being given to the baby. In hospitals,
formula in disposable bottles is given at room
temperature and studies have been done on
infants fed refrigerated cold milk. There is no
difference in growth rates of infants fed
formulas that are warm or cold. If the mother
prefers to serve lukewarm formula, she
should immerse the bottle in warm water just
prior to the feeding. Warm milk is a good
medium for bacterial growth, so it is wise not
to let the formula remain at room temperature
too long. If the mother is in a location without
refrigeration, she can mix one bottle of evaporated milk or premodified milk and feed it
immediately. The opened can of milk should
be covered and used within 1 day.

introduction of additional foods

Feeding an infant with a spoon involves a
whole new system of swallowing. Until the
second or third month when the *retrusion
reflex* disappears, this protective mechanism
keeps him from inadvertently swallowing
harmful foreign objects. Mothers observe this
reflex as the baby appears to spit out any
food offered by spoon (Fig. 14·13). The stimulus to swallow is triggered in the early weeks
after birth by the touch of the nipple at the
back of the tongue, as swallowing is intricate-
ly coordinated with breathing.

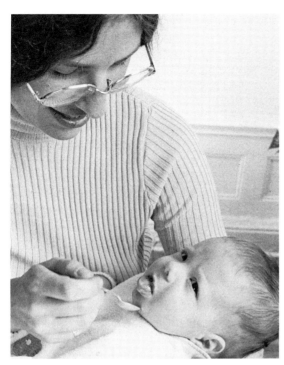

fig. 14·13 Spoon feeding while retrusion reflex is still present. (*Photo by Karen Gilborn.*)

An infant pushing cereal or fruit out of his mouth in spite of mother's cooing and coaxing is not demonstrating a dislike of the taste. The spoon must be small enough to enter the mouth and touch the back of the tongue, and the cereal must be thick enough to be "wiped off" the spoon on the way out of the mouth.

Studies have shown that infants most willingly accept cereal at $2^{1}/_2$ to $3^{1}/_2$ months, vegetables at 4 to $4^{1}/_2$ months, and meats and meat soups at $5^{1}/_2$ to 6 months. There seems to be no nutritional advantage in introducing foods on an earlier schedule. Although impatient mothers often ask the pediatrician to begin at 3 or 4 weeks, it is best to follow the physiologic pattern of gastrointestinal maturation.

Some physicians feel that early introduction to a mixed diet enables the infant to adjust to a variety of foods at an earlier age. There seems to be no nutritional advantage to this, although it is known that infants who have an exclusively milk diet after six months of age may be subject to iron-deficiency anemia.

By the time the infant is six or seven months old, he is usually eating foods from each of the four basic food groups. As he matures, the texture changes from strained to mashed or chopped foods. Puddings, toast, teething biscuits, and bite-sized pieces of cooked vegetables and fruits are added gradually. By the first birthday most infants are weaned for meals from the bottle to a cup, although they have "comfort" from bottles well into the second year.

USE OF COMMERCIALLY PREPARED FOODS

Commercially prepared strained foods have been subject to many criticisms. Ingredients are added to improve flavor (the manufacturer always visualizing the mother tasting a bite and telling the baby that it tastes good) and to stabilize the product. The nutritional benefits of additives are questionable (12). Fruits and fruit juices are sweetened with sugar, which not only adds nonnutritional calories but also develops a desire for sweet foods in the infant. Salt is added to many foods. Since infants are not born with an awareness of how salty or sweet a food should be, these flavors begin to be learned in the very early months after birth. The role of sodium sensitivity in individuals with hypertension in later life does not support the use of excess salt in baby foods.

Since most infants in our society continue to be fed commercially prepared foods, the nurse can advise the mother to wean the infant to lightly seasoned, chopped table foods as soon as his digestive tract permits it. Other mothers will be willing to prepare puréed foods for their infants by using a blender or a sieve.

Fruit Juice and Vitamin C By three to four

weeks of age, especially if evaporated formula is used, it is necessary to supplement the food intake with ascorbic acid, because vitamin C is lost in the pasteurization process. Premodified milk has multivitamins added; human milk contains a small amount of vitamin C.

Orange juice is a good source of vitamin C. If there is any problem with sensitivity to orange juice, grapefruit juice may be used. Pineapple, apple, and prune juices are not as good sources of the vitamin, but can be used later when the baby is taking a variety of foods and fruits.

If fresh fruit is used, it should be washed before the juice is extracted and strained. If canned juice is used, the top of the can should be washed before opening. The juice should be diluted in half when first introduced. After a few days this is not necessary; the amount is slowly increased over 2 or 3 weeks until the baby is accepting 2 oz of undiluted juice each day.

Fruits Cooked, strained fruits may be prepared by mashing them with a fork or using the blender; or they may be purchased as baby food. Popular fruits are apples, peaches, pears, or apricots. The mother may start with a choice of any of these.

Cereals When cereal is first introduced to infants, it is best to add a little formula to make the consistency very thick. Some mothers, to speed the meals, will add cereal to the formula. If that is done, a larger hole in the nipple or a cross-cut nipple must be used. Rather than continuing this practice, as soon as feasible the mother should teach the baby to eat from a spoon. When fruits and cereals are added to the diet, it is no longer necessary to continue the use of sugar or corn syrup in the evaporated milk formula as these foods provide the extra carbohydrates.

Vegetables Strained vegetables are added to the diet after the baby learns to accept fruits and cereals. Fresh, frozen, or canned vegetables (the mildly flavored ones such as peas, carrots, and green beans) may be puréed in the blender, or sieved. Commercially prepared strained vegetables can be used until the infant is about six months old, when he graduates to mashed or junior foods.

Eggs Cooked egg yolks are usually given to the infant before meats are introduced. The egg yolk should be cooked over hot water until the yolk is thickened but not hard. The protein of cooked eggs is more easily digested. Raw eggs should not be given to children because of the danger of salmonellosis, always a possibility in uncooked eggs. Egg whites are not usually given in the first year because infants do not tolerate the albumin in their immature gastrointestinal tracts or may have an allergic reaction.

Meats Infants may be given canned strained meats or meats strained at home. Lamb, chicken, liver, and beef seem most easily digested. To prepare meats at home, the mother should use tender, lean meat. Scrape a little lean, raw meat and cook it at a low temperature with a *little water.* A blender could also be used to purée cooked meat. If fish is used, the mother should be sure it is mildly flavored and boneless. When the child is over six or eight months old, canned fish such as tuna or salmon can be used if the oil is drained off.

The timetable for introduction of foods varies from region to region. Remembering that for many years, infants did not begin on additional foods until well near their first birthday, the mother should not compare and contrast her pediatrician's choice of schedule with her neighbor's. The mother may feel pressured by advertising or may feel that she has to buy the most expensive product, as equaling the best. The nurse can instruct the mother in following the growth patterns of the child, and in:

Ensuring that formula is prepared and stored in a medically aseptic way

Providing adequate fluid intake for the infant, especially during hot weather

Introducing one food at a time to test for response

Giving vitamins and adding foods as the pediatrician prescribes

Correlating development with infant ability to participate in feeding himself

Providing the baby with stimulation, pleasure, and play while he is being fed

Enjoying her infant during the whole process of feeding him

references

1. *The Womanly Art of Breastfeeding*, 2d ed., La Leche League International, Franklyn Park, Ill., 1963.
2. National Research Council, *Recommended Dietary Allowances*, 8th ed., National Academy of Sciences, Washington, 1973.
3. "Economy in Nutrition and Feeding of Infants," *American Journal of Public Health*, **56**:1756–1784, 1966.
4. M. Reynolds, "Disorders of Lactation and the Mammary Gland," in Nicholas Assali and Charles R. Brinkman (eds.) *Pathophysiology of Gestation*, vol. I, Academic Press, Inc., New York, 1972.
5. Alfredo Perez, "First Ovulation after Childbirth: The Effect of Breastfeeding," *American Journal of Obstetrics and Gynecology*, **114**:1041, 1972.
6. Lawrence M. Gartner and Melvin Hollander, "Disorders of Bilirubin Metabolism," chap. 8 in Nicholas Assali and Charles R. Brinkman (eds.), *Pathophysiology of Gestation*, vol. III, Academic Press, Inc., New York, 1972.
7. Charlotte S. Catz and George P. Giacoia, "Drugs and Breast Milk," *Pediatric Clinics of North America*, **19**(1):151–165, 1972.
8. A. J. Schaffer, *Diseases of the Newborn*, 3d ed., W. B. Saunders Company, Philadelphia, 1971, p. 632.
9. J. A. Knowles, "Excretion of Drugs in Milk: A Review," *Journal of Pediatrics*, **66**:1068–1080, 1965.
10. Virginia A. Beal, "Breast Feeding and Formula Feeding of Infants," *Journal of the American Dietetic Association*, **55**:31–37, 1969.
11. Roberta S. O'Grady, "Feeding Behavior in Infants," *American Journal of Nursing*, **71**(4):736, 1971.
12. Thomas A. Anderson and Samuel J. Fomon, "Commercially Prepared Strained and Junior Foods for Infants," *Journal of the American Dietetic Association*, **58**:520–526, 1970.

bibliography

Brewer, T.: "Nutrition and Infant Mortality," *Pediatrics*, **51**:1107, 1973.

Brown, Roy C.: "Breast Feeding in Modern Times: A Review," *American Journal of Clinical Nutrition.* **26**(5):556, 1973.

Castle, Sue: *Complete Guide to Preparing Baby Foods at Home*, Doubleday & Company, Inc., Garden City, N.Y., 1973.

Countryman, Betty A.: "Hospital Care of the Breast-fed Newborn," *American Journal of Nursing*, **71**:2365–2367, 1971.

Craig, W. S.: *Care of the Newly Born Infant*, The Williams & Wilkins Company, Baltimore, 1969.

Dodds, Janice M., Joan P. MacReynolds, and Donough O'Brien: "Normal Nutrition," chap. 4 in C. Henry Kempe, Henry K. Silver, and Donough O'Brien (eds.), *Current Pediatric Diagnosis and Treatment*, Lange Medical Publications, Los Altos, Calif., 1972.

Fomon, Samuel J.: *Infant Nutrition*, W. B. Saunders Company, Philadelphia, 1967.

How the Nurse Can Help the Breastfeeding Mother, La Leche League International,

Franklyn Park, Ill.

Ladas, Alice K.: "How to Help Mothers Breast Feed," *Clinical Pediatrics,* **9**:702, 1970.

MacMahon, Brian, T. M. Lui, and C. R. Lowe: "Lactation and Care of the Breast: A Summary of an International Study," *Bulletin of WHO,* **42**:185–194, 1970.

Nutrition in Pregnancy and Lactation, Report of a WHO Expert Committee, Tech. Rep. Ser., no. 302, World Health Organization, Geneva, 1965.

Pryor, Karen: *Nursing Your Baby,* Harper & Row, Publishers, Incorporated, New York, 1963.

Spock, Benjamin: *Baby and Child Care* (rev.), Pocket Books, Inc., New York, 1968.

Vorherr, Helmuth: "To Breast-Feed or Not to Breast-Feed?" *Postgraduate Medicine,* June, 1972, pp. 127–134.

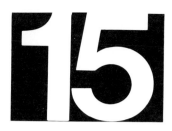

home care of the mother and baby

Joyce Hanna Nave

After the baby and mother are discharged from the hospital, a nurse may visit the family in the home. In some communities, all babies are visited by a nurse from the local public health or visiting nurse agency; in other communities, only mothers and babies with problems or potential problems are seen. The hospital nursery, or the doctor, makes the contact with the agency, giving a brief summary of the obstetric history, doctor's orders, and the reason for referral. The nurse who makes the referral, keeping in mind that mothers and babies who seem to be doing very well in the hospital may not manage as well at home, should err on the side of over-referring rather than underreferring. In some situations, the nursery nurse, pediatric nurse practitioner, or office or clinic nurse may visit the newborn and his family at home.

The parents should be told that a nurse will be visiting to examine the mother and baby and to answer any of the parents' questions. Since occasionally parents may interpret the visit as criticism of their ability to care for the baby, the explanation for the visit should be as matter-of-fact as possible.

the role of the nurse

The nurse who visits in the home has an important role. The mother and baby have been discharged from the protective and artificial environment of the hospital. If all goes well, they will not be seen by a physician for another 4 to 6 weeks. The nurse is present at a crucial time for the health of the mother and baby, and in the adjustment of the family to a new member. Her role is unique in that she is practically the only health care professional who sees the family in their own home setting, and thus truly has the opportunity to work with the family as a unit.

The primary role of the nurse is to evaluate the health status of the mother and baby. She also may teach specific techniques, offer emotional support, give anticipatory guidance, or work with the family as they solve social problems connected with providing adequate care to the child.

To appraise the situation adequately the nurse learns to make observations, to develop her awareness and listening skills, and to ask questions which will give her necessary information about the family. After recording her observations, she develops a set of priorities, with a focus for each visit. Although she asks similar questions and makes similar observations in each home, the nurse's services will not be utilized in the same way in every situation. In one home the need may be to help the parents gain a sense of balance after the disrupting event of having a baby. In another home, the presence of rats or lack of refrigeration may be the focus of concern, or perhaps the nurse may find that a baby with diarrhea is severely dehydrated and requires immediate medical attention. Thus the nurse's role varies as she perceives the needs of the family. The number and spacing of visits vary also according to the situation. Usually frequent, short visits during the first crucial days at home are most meaningful to the family.

nursing appraisal of the mother

It is often best to begin the visit by directing attention to the mother, as she needs support and recognition, too. Assess the mother's physical condition, her emotional state, and her need for knowledge in the caring of the newborn.

THE PHYSICAL CONDITION

Lochia Record the amount, color, and whether there is a strong odor. If there is any deviation from normal, check the *fundus.* Lochia may increase when the mother is first home if she takes on too many tasks or must climb stairs frequently. If the flow is heavy, emphasize the importance of rest, and check the *pulse* and *blood pressure.*

Episiotomy Ask if the "stitches" are uncomfortable. If so, examine the perineum for evidence of infection.

Temperature While recording the temperature be alert to other signs of infection—headaches, pain, nausea, burning upon urination, or pain in the lower extremities.

Breasts Breasts should be soft and comfortable. If not, examine for signs of cracking or infection. Engorgement may occur after the mother gets home; the first early visit should include assessment of progress of breast condition.

Rest Ask the mother how many hours of actual sleep she is getting, and if she has any help at home. *Anorexia,* an increased *pulse,* and frequently *postpartum blues* are indications of lack of rest.

Exercise A gradual (not sudden) return to normal activity should be encouraged. A young mother who has no help, several young children, and lives in a four-flight walk-up apartment several blocks from the nearest grocery store will probably be forced to resume more activity than is good for her, whereas a primipara with plenty of household help may not get enough exercise. You may teach the mother specific exercises to strengthen the muscles of the abdomen and perineal floor (refer to Fig. 10·4).

Diet In the activity of the first days home, the mother may not be up to preparing meals or may "just forget" to eat. Ask her what she has been able to prepare or if anyone has brought meals to her. Further evaluate the diet and teach as necessary.

Elimination Constipation is a frequent problem. The mother should have had a soft movement since delivery. If not, dietary measures (fluids, roughage), exercise, and a cathartic may be necessary.

Postpartal Examination After securing the date and place of the examination, discuss the importance of the postpartal checkup.

EMOTIONAL SUPPORT

Bringing home a new baby is a time of tremendous emotional upheaval for a family. The nurse, by her presence during a crucial period in the development of parent-child relationships, may influence these relationships by the kind of support and guidance she gives. By asking a few questions, she expresses her interest and identifies problem areas for further discussion. Some areas of discussion may be:

1. Has the mother had previous experience caring for newborns? Does she feel comfortable caring for this baby?
2. What are the father's feelings about this baby? If the mother is unwed, or separated, does she see the baby's father at all? Does he offer financial or emotional support?
3. Does she have any help at home? Is there a grandmother or another relative present in the home? What kinds of help do they offer, and how does the mother feel about the kind of help they give?
4. What are the medical plans for the baby? What would she do if the baby were sick?
5. How have the older children reacted toward the baby? If there has been sibling rivalry, how has the mother handled it?
6. Does she feel that she is "getting back to

her old self"? Or does she feel too much is being asked of her at this time? Has she ever felt like crying?

7. Is she having difficulty managing financially?

NEED FOR KNOWLEDGE IN THE CARING OF NEWBORNS

The nurse needs a great deal of sensitivity in teaching parents how to care for their newborn. Since information will be utilized only when it meets the parents' needs, it is necessary to explore what kinds of need there are. Often, parents need to learn skills, such as giving the baby a bath, taking a temperature, preparing a formula, or caring for a diaper rash. In the teaching of such skills, however, strive to strengthen the parents' confidence in themselves, building on the strengths and knowledge they already have, and be aware that there may be more than one right way to do a task. Be very tactful when dealing with ritualistic practice, as ritual serves the purpose of giving the parents confidence. Such practices as the use of a "bellyband" (a strip of cloth) over the umbilicus may be important in helping the parents feel that they are doing the best for their baby. As long as the practice is safe (e.g., the band is applied loosely and the umbilicus is clean and dry), it may be ignored. In general, parents need not so much advice on what they ought to do, as information on what to expect of young infants. The most frequent questions seem to concern the baby's crying and sleeping patterns and feeding behavior.

The nurse should also *anticipate* what kind of information the parents are likely to need as the baby grows. You may find pamphlets very helpful tools. But reading materials should be used with care, and reading levels assessed. Find out whether the parents *do* acquire information by reading, and review the pamphlet with the parents. On your next visit, ask what was found helpful and why.

nursing appraisal of the home

The environment has far-reaching effects on a baby's physical health and emotional and social development. It is often the area in which the nurse feels she has the least amount of control. Yet, if a nurse is observant of problems in the home environment and has made herself aware of community resources for help, it may be the area where she will see the greatest change. When evaluating the home it is important that the nurse not prejudge the family on the basis of her own standards, and that she look for the effect the environment actually has on the baby and his family.

HEAT AND COLD

The temperature of the environment may adversely affect a newborn. You would suspect that a home is too cold when the newborn's skin is mottled, cool, or dusky, or when the baby is cyanosed around the mouth or extremities. The parents, especially if they are unfamiliar with the requirements of a northern climate, may need to be taught how to dress a baby warmly enough. However, even a warmly bundled baby seems to suffer cold stress in the chronically cold environment found in much substandard housing. You may be able to work through community agencies to secure a more suitable environment for the baby.

More frequently you will find babies who are overdressed, especially during warm weather or in a too hot, too dry, apartment. Sometimes babies are exposed to too much sun or are too close to hot stoves or radiators. Help the parents to understand their baby's needs.

FILTH

Many, many children thrive in apparently filthy surroundings, and many dirty babies grow up to be healthy, happy adults. Although the nurse must be careful not to prejudge the family on the basis of their housekeeping, she must also be aware that a dirty, smelly baby may be a clue to parental neglect. Tactfully, work with the parents to evaluate their knowledge of diapering and bathing and their feelings about this baby.

INFESTATION

Infestation of rats, mice, flies, and *roaches* occurs frequently in substandard and occasionally in good housing. Their source (garbage, holes in walls, etc.) must be located and eradicated if possible; for this the services of the board of health may be available. The family should be taught good sanitation practices. Rats, which have been known to bite babies, and flies, which may carry disease on their sticky legs, are more of a health hazard than mice or roaches.

COMMUNICABLE DISEASE, CROWDING

Since the newborn's resistance to communicable disease is low, the presence of an ill family member or the crowding of many people into small living quarters may be a health hazard.

SAFETY

The neonatal period is an excellent time to begin discussions of safety, as the parents usually have many fears and concerns about their baby at this time. Discussions may center around the following: never leaving the baby alone ("not even for a minute") on a high surface or alone in a house, adequacy of fire exits and existence of a fire safety plan, approved baby safety car beds, buying a crib with slats close enough together to prevent the baby from strangling himself when he is older by locking his head between the crib slats. Offer guidance in anticipation of the baby's growing needs (see Table 17·2).

EQUIPMENT

Families seem to manage in the most difficult environments with the sparsest of equipment. Some equipment, however, is essential. Refrigeration (or some means of keeping food cold), a tall covered pot, bottles and nipples, a bottle brush, and measuring spoons are essential for formula preparation. If the formula is prepared one feeding at a time or if one of the commercially prepared formulas is used, the family may get by with a little less equipment. If bottles need to be purchased, urge the family to buy the more easily sterilized glass bottle in the 8-oz size. Diapers, shirts, and something with which to bundle the baby (blankets and sweater) are also essential. A newborn may sleep in a drawer or cardboard box temporarily. If income is limited, a full-size crib is a better buy than a cradle, as it will be utilized for a longer period of time by the infant.

nursing appraisal of the newborn

IMPORTANCE OF THE NEONATAL PERIOD

The first month of life is the most hazardous period of time an individual ever faces. Problems arise during this period that never arise again. Serious disorders affecting an individual's entire future (e.g., congenital dysplasia of the hip) may often be corrected if discovered during this period. An illness which may be minor in an older child (such as diarrhea) may be life-threatening to a newborn.

With each hour of life, the baby's chances are better. By the time of discharge, the doctor has screened the baby and the most critical period of the first 28 days is over. The average baby will not be seen again until his first checkup, at about six weeks of age.

However, changes occur rapidly in the newborn, and not all problems are detected before discharge. Who is there to detect possible problems and bring them to the attention of the physician? Sometimes the *parents* make important observations. When the family is fortunate enough to have a *nurse* visit, she lends her knowledge and experience to this important task.

THE NURSE'S ROLE IN INFANT APPRAISAL

During the visit, every newborn should be carefully appraised. Most parents are concerned about whether their baby is all right and feel reassured when a nurse takes the time to examine him. Utilize this opportunity to answer questions and explain minor variations that may concern the parents. More importantly, an apparently normal newborn may have slight deviations from normal that are discovered during the infant appraisal. These deviations *may* be an important clue to a serious disorder.

One of the most difficult tasks is determining the significance of an observation. Making your judgment is complicated by the fact that during the newborn period there is a tremendous range of normal variations, and the line between normal and abnormal is poorly defined. It is helpful to remember that the further from normal the observation is, the more significant it is. A good understanding of the problems newborns may have is essential. Acquaint yourself thoroughly with the more common newborn problems—respiratory distress, feeding problems, diarrhea, dehydration, thrush, skin rashes.

When you appraise the infant, look at him systematically—head, chest, perineum, etc. Don't ignore anything that seems unusual to you. Record your observations. Examine the baby under good lighting, *especially* when noting his color. Keep the baby warm. Most importantly, maintain an alert concentration during the examination of the infant, so that nothing of significance will be overlooked.

SYSTEMATIC APPRAISAL OF THE NEWBORN

Head The scalp should be clear, with no pustules or crusty yellow patches. The fontanels and sutures should be checked, and their size recorded. The neck should move easily from side to side (Fig. 15·1). Measure head circumference (Fig. 15·2).

EYES The eyes should look approximately the same when compared with each other. The cornea should be clear and the sclera

fig. 15·1 Checking anterior fontanel.

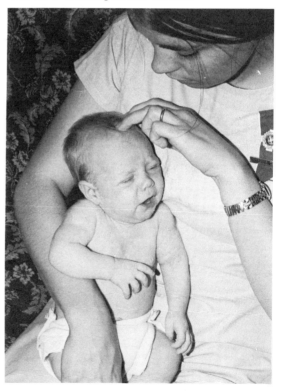

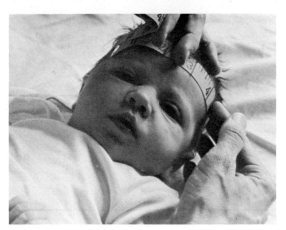

fig. 15·2 Head measurement by nurse at home. (*Photo by Beverly Hemlock.*)

white or a very light bluish white. Many times, an epicanthal fold is normal. However, if it is present, look for other signs of Down's syndrome (incurving fifth finger, simian line, "floppy" muscle tone, etc.) There should not be a large amount of eye discharge after the first week, nor should there be a continual flow of tears down the cheek.

NOSE The nose should be clear. A "runny" or "stuffy" nose is often due to a cold environment and may be the first sign of a respiratory infection. A "stuffy" nose may interfere with feeding or breathing. If the baby has a stuffy nose, evaluate the respirations carefully (see Chap. 28). Upper respiratory infections, though common, may be serious in a newborn.

EAR The appearance of the external ear differs considerably from one individual to another. Even so, observe carefully, as malformed ears may be the first clue to many anomalies, particularly defects of the genitourinary system. Look for very low-set ears, protruding ears, lacks of folds on the auricle, or extremely small or large ears. Compare one ear to the other. Look behind and in front of each ear for dimples (these sometimes extend more deeply into a sinus tract), papules, or growths.

MOUTH Look inside the mouth with a flashlight. Note whether the mucous membranes are moist (one of the best indicators of hydration and to be noted on every visit). Look closely at the anatomic groove on the palate (see Plate 4B). The palate should be joined at this groove from the very front of the hard palate way back into the soft palate, and the uvula (the soft fleshy mass hanging down from the back of the soft palate) should not be double or divided in two (see Fig. 28·11). White patches or flecks on the tongue and buccal mucosa which look like milk but cannot be scraped off are caused by a common infection (thrush). Thrush often travels (Plate 4C) through the gastrointestinal tract and causes a severe diaper rash.

The lips should be pink. The baby should move both sides of the face symmetrically.

Chest and abdomen Skin color should be noted; one should look especially for pallor, jaundice, and cyanosis. These often-subtle changes may be signs of serious disorders, such as anemia, infections, or congenital heart disease. Jaundice may first appear as a muddy color in the sclera; pallor and cyanosis may first appear in the nailbeds or around the mouth or extremities (Plate 3A through D).

The skin turgor should *always* be tested.

Describe and report rashes or pustules carefully, recording when and where they first appeared. Pustules and vesicles should be reported to the physician and hospital nursery at once, as they may represent *Staphylococcus* or *herpes simplex* infections. Do not confuse these pustules with the small papules of milia or erythema toxicum (see Fig. 12·9). Learn to identify the normal birthmarks so that you will recognize the unusual (Plate 4C, D).

A birthmark should be reported under any of the following conditions:

1. If there is any *change in size or shape—* especially if it seems to be growing.

2. If there is any *change in color or appearance* other than just fading away.
3. If there seems to be a *lump or tumor* near or under the birthmark.
4. If the birthmark seems to *pulsate or to be formed of blood vessels.*
5. If the birthmark is *large and extensive.*
6. If the birthmark is *over the nose and cheeks* (butterfly area).
7. If the birthmark *follows the distribution of a nerve* (for example, the fifth cranial nerve).

THE UMBILICAL CORD The umbilical cord dries up after a few days and should drop off in about a week. Occasionally it does not drop off for as long as 3 weeks, but this is acceptable as long as there is no sign of bleeding or infection. Sometimes the umbilicus is a little wet and there is a tiny oozing of blood when the cord drops off, but by the next day the umbilicus should be dry. Other than this, any bleeding is abnormal.

Once the cord is off you may observe a normal navel, an amniotic navel, a skin navel, or an umbilical hernia. A *normal* navel has the same appearance as the surrounding skin. The skin in an *amniotic* navel does not extend to the base of the cord, and amniotic membrane covers the skin at the base. This type of cord may be wet for a few weeks as granulation tissue forms and the cord gradually heals, leaving a scar. Because the area is wet, it is very important to keep it free of organisms that may cause a serious infection. Many physicians advise dabbing the area with alcohol, which acts as an antiseptic and drying agent. In a *skin navel,* the skin extends up the side of the cord and a little stump remains. This is often confused with an *umbilical hernia,* a soft swelling in the umbilical area covered by skin which protrudes when the baby cries or strains. As the child grows and uses his abdominal muscles more, the skin navel and the umbilical hernia will become less prominent. Coins, bellybands, or Band-Aids will not keep the umbilicus from protruding. If the parents insist on using these measures, make sure the umbilicus is clean and dry and that there is no sign of infection or sloughing skin.

With the exceptions described above, the umbilicus should be dry. No odor or inflammation should be present. Because the umbilicus may serve as a portal of entry to a serious systemic infection, early recognition and prevention of an umbilical infection are important.

Advise the mother to sponge-bathe the baby until the cord has dropped off and the area is dry and healed. It is also a good practice to diaper the area so that the wet diaper is folded down away from the umbilical area.

Vital Signs Check the pulse apically for a full minute, noting the rate and rhythm. A pulse over 170 or below 70 may merely reflect the baby's activity. Record it again in a few minutes. It is rarely significant unless it persists (Fig. 15·3).

More importantly, the respirations should be counted and carefully observed for one full minute, with note taken of any signs of respiratory distress such as retractions, nasal flaring, cyanosis, or expiratory grunting or groaning. The earliest and most consistent sign of respiratory distress is a rapid or

fig. 15·3 Checking apical heart rate.

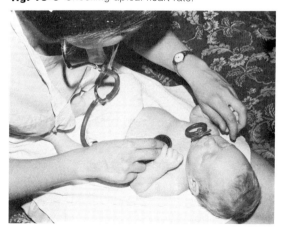

increasing rate. Since respiratory failure is the most common cause of morbidity and mortality in the neonatal period, a thorough appraisal of the respirations is extremely important on each visit to a newborn. Any baby having difficulty in breathing should be seen without delay by a physician.

Parents often express concern about the various noises newborns make. Other than the expiratory grunt associated with severe respiratory distress, these noises, grunts, crowing sounds, etc., are normal for newborns. Occasional sneezing is also normal in newborns; repeated sneezing is often caused by dust or insufficient clothing, or it may be the first indication of a respiratory infection. Hiccuping is also normal and has no significance.

Fever is not as reliable an indicator of illness in the newborn as it is in the adult. A temperature over 37.5°C (99.8°F) usually indicates dehydration; often it is the first sign. However, serious infections may occur even when the temperature is normal or subnormal. Overdressing or underdressing may be reflected in the temperature reading also.

Perineum The testes of the male infant should appear fairly equal in size. If he has been circumcised, check the site for bleeding or signs of infection.

Urine should be amber in color, clear, have an ammonia odor, and be passed at least five times in 24 h.

Loose, frequent, greenish stools, especially in the breast-fed baby, are no cause for concern. On the other hand, breast-fed babies may, by two or three months of age, have stools only every 2 to 3 days. If the stools are watery, frequent, and explosive, check for signs of dehydration and obtain a complete feeding history; this type of stool usually indicates diarrhea.

Straining with each stool is normal. If the stool is soft, straining does not mean that the baby is constipated, although it may indicate that the baby has flatus and needs to be bubbled. Stools that are very hard require further investigation; often an incorrectly mixed formula or too early feeding of solids is responsible.

Diaper rash is a common problem. It is usually cleared up by gentle, consistent washing of the skin and by exposure of the skin to warm air. Petroleum jelly and other moisture-proof barriers, which are helpful in *preventing* a rash from developing, may *aggravate* an existing rash by keeping air from reaching and healing the area. Use of waterproof pants should also be discouraged, as they keep the area warm and damp and prevent the drying and healing action of the air. Baby powder may clog the pores. The skin may be sensitive to a variety of irritants—soaps used on the skin or in the laundry, baby lotions, disposable diapers, drugs or food ingested by the baby or by the breast-feeding mother. If the rash does not heal quickly, or if pustules, blisters, or white patches are present, an infection is likely. Diarrhea, a serious problem in itself, may cause a severe rash.

Extremities Fractures and paralysis are usually detected before the baby leaves the hospital (see Chap. 12). Occasionally the first clue is a report from the mother that a baby does not move an extremity, or cries when an extremity is moved or when he is placed in a certain position. Follow this up by comparing the length and movement of one extremity with its mate.

Since limitation of abduction of the hips may not appear until the baby is three to six weeks old (1), check for possible congenital dysplasia of the hip at intervals (see Fig. 15·4A and B). If anything suggests congenital dysplasia of the hip, demonstrate to the mother how to double-diaper the baby until the baby can be seen by a physician.

Abnormal positions of the foot are common. Most of these "straighten out" in time, but it does no harm to teach the mother to *gently* "overcorrect" the foot (that is, gently move it

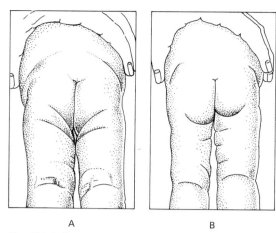

fig. 15·4 Congenital dysplasia of the hip. A Normal gluteal and popliteal skin creases. The displacement of the head of the femur, due to laxity of the hip capsule and ligaments, occurs after birth; it is more common in females and in the left hip. B Abnormal skin creases in congenital dislocation of the right hip, showing asymmetry of skin folds and apparent shortening of the right hip. (*Courtesy of Mead Johnson Laboratories.*)

to and a little beyond the normal position, without forcing it) several times a day until a physician can evaluate it.

Behavior Patterns Each baby has his own individual personality. In the early weeks, the expression of this personality is pretty much limited to his crying, sleeping, and feeding behavior. Parents are faced with the task of learning what this new baby's behavior is like, and developing a beginning relationship with him. This adjustment may be relatively easy for some parents and babies, but for many it is difficult. Parents need to be reassured that day by day, they will get to know their baby's habits and it will be easier to interpret his behavior.

Certain behavior may concern parents. A fussy baby who continues to cry after the parents have tried all the usual measures may be very upsetting to the whole household. The nurse can encourage the parents to vent their feelings, and can give specific suggestions that may help (see "Colic," Chap. 17). On the other hand, the parents of a baby who sleeps

most of the time may worry that something is wrong. The information the nurse gives to the parents will help them appreciate normal differences in babies.

As different as babies are, be watchful for extremes in behavior. Investigate a baby who is lethargic, difficult to arouse, unusually irritable or jumpy, or who has frequent tremors or twitchings or an extremely high-pitched cry. As you handle more babies you will develop a sixth sense of what is and what is not normal neonatal behavior.

Reflexes, Muscle Tone Checking the reflexes and muscle tone give a fairly precise estimation of health, especially if there is some question in your mind about the normalcy of the baby's behavior.

You should be able to obtain good Moro, grasp, and stepping reflexes from every newborn during the first month (Fig. 15·5).

A baby with good muscle tone sticks his buttocks and head up slightly when in the prone (face-lying) position, and moves his arms and legs vigorously when crying. If you hold the baby, you may detect an abnormal muscle tone by the way the baby feels; a hypotonic baby always feels very limp and floppy, while a hypertonic baby always feels very stiff (Fig. 15·6).

Feeding Feeding is another aspect of behavior that may give the nurse vague but significant clues to the health of the infant and to the emotional interaction between parent and baby. Feeding a baby is a skill that takes time to learn, both for the parents and for the baby. It takes time for the baby to learn to coordinate his sucking, swallowing, and breathing, and to satisfy his hunger. It also takes time for parents to interpret a baby's cry, the faces he makes while eating, his way of signaling when he needs to be "bubbled" or is finished eating. During the first few days at home, as parents and baby learn to interact with each other, there are apt to be problems related to feeding. The nurse will want to assess whether the feeding experience is a

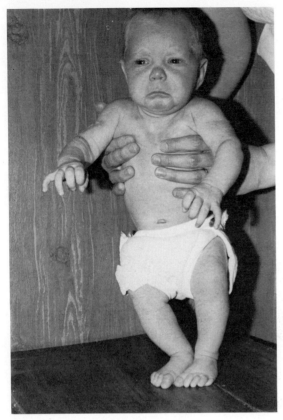

fig. 15·5 Eliciting stepping reflex.

satisfactory one for both parent and baby, whether the amount of formula is appropriate for the infant's size and age, and whether the formula is prepared correctly (Fig. 15·7).

Asking the mother specific questions about the baby's feedings may reveal a lot about her attitude toward the baby. If she is unable to answer any questions at all, she may be overburdened, be rejecting the baby, or be of limited intellectual capacity. An overanxious mother is often extremely talkative. When feeding problems seem to exist, it is worthwhile to plan to observe a feeding. Usually the solution then becomes quite clear; perhaps the nipple hole is too large, causing the baby to choke, or too small, tiring the baby too quickly, or perhaps the nipple simply

needs to be inserted further into the baby's mouth.

Also, obtain an estimate of how much the baby is eating, and whether this amount is appropriate. Ask how often the baby feeds, how many ounces he drinks (or how long he nurses), if he cries when hungry, if he seems satisfied after the feeding, and if the feeding is retained. Overfeeding usually occurs when every cry is interpreted as a hunger cry. Underfeeding may occur as a result of neglect or because of inexperience. Some babies need to be awakened for feedings. Undernutrition may also occur if the newborn is being fed solid food, which he cannot utilize, instead of the milk that he needs, and it also occurs with certain diseases. Dehydration can occur very quickly in an infant as a result of decreased intake (underfeeding) or increased output (vomiting, diarrhea). Because dehydration is so very serious and if untreated may result in death, it is important to check the mucous membranes and skin turgor, frequency of voiding, and temperature on each visit.

Make sure the formula is being prepared correctly. Review the formula preparation in detail with the mother. Observe the equipment and ingredients used. Many feeding problems are due to simple errors in prepara-

fig. 15·6 Eliciting the Landau response to check muscle tone.

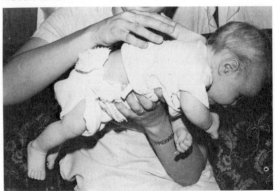

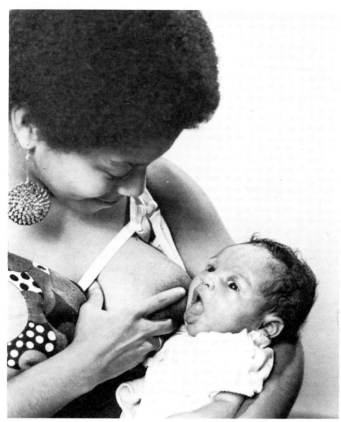

fig. 15·7 Breast feeding at home. (*Photo by Lester Bergman in D. Vietor and M. McCutcheon,* Care of the Maternity Patient, *McGraw-Hill Book Company, New York, 1971, p. 493.*)

tion; e.g., forgetting to add sugar, or using too much water. Try to spot these mistakes before they become a serious problem.

Be alert for problems such as coughing and choking while eating, refusal of several feedings, or vomiting after every feeding. Vomiting should be differentiated from spitting up (see Chap. 17). These problems may be signs of a more serious disorder.

Finally, subtle changes in behavior are one of the most frequent ways in which newborns signal when they are ill (2). Since newborns may have a serious illness with few or no clinical symptoms, a general vague "feeling" on the part of the parents or the nurse that the baby is not all right may be the only clue to illness. Although you may not be able to be specific, report this feeling to the physician. Early signs of illnesses ranging from infections to neurologic damage are often detected in just this way. This may be one of the most important observations you make as you provide home care for the mother and infant.

The nurse who visits the family in their own home has a unique but complementary role to that of the nurse who functions in the hospital setting. She continues the important observation and teaching tasks begun in the hospital. She also serves as a valuable resource person to the hospital personnel and to the physician, because she has been in the home and can assess and report on the home situation. She has made herself aware of the resources of her community so that she can utilize them to support the family better. As the need arises, she becomes an advocate for the family in securing improved health care for the new infant and the other family members.

references

1. Waldo Nelson, Victor Vaughan, and James McKay, *Textbook of Pediatrics,* 9th ed., W. B. Saunders Company, Philadelphia, 1969, p. 1354.
2. Mary Lou Moore, *The Newborn and the Nurse,* Saunders Monographs in Clinical Nursing, W. B. Saunders Company, Philadelphia, 1972..

bibliography

Adams, Martha: "Early Concerns of the Primigravida Mother Concerning Infant Care Activities," *Nursing Research,* Spring, 1963.

Barness, Lewis: *Manual of Pediatric Physical Diagnosis,* 3d ed., Year Book Medical Publishers, Inc., Chicago, 1971.

Chin, Peggy L.: *Child Health Maintenance,* The C. V. Mosby Company, St. Louis, 1974.

Deutsch, Helene: *The Psychology of Women,* Grune & Stratton, Inc., New York, 1945.

Hayes, Una: *A Developmental Approach to Case Finding,* U.S. Department of Health, Education and Welfare, Public Health Service Publication 2017, 1969.

Heider, Grace M.: "What Makes a Good Parent?" *Children,* **7**(6):207–212, 1960.

Hellman, Louis M., and Jack A. Pritchard: *Williams' Obstetrics,* 14th ed., Appleton-Century-Crofts, Inc., New York, 1971.

Hodgman, Joan: "Clinical Evaluation of the Newborn Infant," *Hospital Practice,* May, 1969, pp. 70–86.

Illingworth, Ronald: *The Development of the Infant and Young Child,* 4th ed., The Williams & Wilkins Company, Baltimore, 1970.

Kempe, Henry, Henry Silver, and Donough O'Brien: *Current Pediatric Diagnosis and Treatment,* 2d ed., Lange Medical Publications, Los Altos, Calif., 1972.

Lytle, Nancy: *Maternal Health Nursing,* William C. Brown Company Publishers, Dubuque, Iowa, 1967.

Nelson, Waldo, Victor Vaughan, and James McKay: *Textbook of Pediatrics,* 9th ed., W. B. Saunders Company, Philadelphia, 1969.

Schaffer, A. J., and M. E. Avery: *Diseases of the Newborn,* 3d ed., W. B. Saunders Company, Philadelphia, 1971.

Silver, Henry, Henry Kempe, and Henry Bruyn: *Handbook of Pediatrics,* 9th ed., Lange Medical Publications, Los Altos, Calif., 1971.

Ziai, Mohsen, Charles Janeway, and Robert Cooke: *Pediatrics,* Little, Brown and Company, Boston, 1969.

Ziegel, Erna, and Carolyn Conant Van Blarcom: *Obstetric Nursing,* 6th ed., The Macmillan Company, New York, 1972.

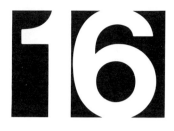

psychology of infancy

Philip E. Wilson

How does the new baby display the psychologic and emotional qualities which are considered "human"? Is he aware of pride, love, hope, justice, envy, guilt, disgust, and anger? His humanity lies in his potential to develop all these feelings—the human emotions—and to take action upon them and control them.

It may be difficult to imagine what is in the mind of a newborn, yet consistent observation with accurate recording of what infants do and how they react at different ages has given us much insight and evidence from which we can conclude what the infant perceives, knows, and appears to understand.

In seeking understanding of the psychology of the first year of life, the following questions need to be answered: by what means does the infant begin to comprehend the world around him? Can the infant begin to build a relationship from birth? Why is one consistent relationship so important? Why is separation so harmful to both mother and infant? How well does the infant's perceptual system work? Why does the infant believe that he is the cause of everything that goes on around him? Why does an infant feel that mother is a part of himself and, later, that mother knows everything he feels? Why does an infant cry? What are the effects of adequate and inadequate mothering? As we seek to answer these questions, we will discuss the psychologic processes and tasks of the first year.

establishing mother-infant bond

The psychology of infancy must necessarily include the psychology of the mother-infant unit. The positive feelings within the mother after she has given birth serve the purpose of beginning the maternal-infant bond. Many patterns of handling a baby are built upon the first spontaneous desire to hold the baby immediately after birth.

Thus, every effort should be made in the delivery room to allow time for the mother and the father to meet their infant. Klaus has noted that emotional bonding (the feelings of attachment to the infant) increases even in those witnessing the delivery (1). It is of great importance to encourage parent attachment by allowing the father to be present, and by ensuring that the mother is awake to witness her infant's entry into and response to the world.

The feelings of pride in accomplishment, joy that the baby is "normal," and relief that the delivery is over underlie her initial reactions to the infant. The infant is not able to respond in very direct ways to the mother's cuddling and exploring movements, but if the infant is not crying, is able to open its eyes and suck the proferred milk, the mother is satisfied that the infant "likes her." The cycle of mother-infant response is thus set up and a rhythm established.

The first days immediately after the baby's birth are perhaps more important to the establishment of the mother's relationship with the baby than the baby's with the mother. They both need time to gaze at each other, to touch and explore. The mother needs the assurance that she can meet the infant's needs. If the baby can remain with her continually from birth, her positive feelings of coping and the continual expression of caretaking help to assure the formation of a fulfilling relationship.

Separation of the infant from the mother causes her to repress her feelings, because of the frustration experienced at not being able to express her maternal desires. A prolonged separation immediately after birth, because of illness or immaturity in the infant, or infection and poor recovery in the mother, will interfere with the establishment of the maternal-infant bond (1).

The subtleties around the process of breast feeding give a clear example of how separation interferes with the development of the mother's relationship with her new baby. Breast feeding comes as another step in the process of holding and handling the new one. Nervousness and fears are overcome when the mother can capitalize on her initial positive emotional response to her infant, but this response can be utilized by the mother only if she has early consistent contact with her infant. The mother and baby both must go through the *process* which leads up to the baby's taking the nipple and beginning to breast-feed. The mother needs to have ample opportunity to acquaint herself with her child and to present the breast in an unhurried and relaxed fashion. The infant also must go through the process of connecting his "rooting" reflex to the actual nipple he is looking for. All infants look for or "root" for the breast, but even with this instinctual reflex working, it takes time—trials and errors—to work out the pattern for breast feeding. The nursing staff also has the opportunity of teaching the mother about breast feeding in the optimum setting, if the mother and baby are consistently together.

If the baby is brought to the mother only on the hospital's nursery schedule, then the mother and baby do not have the leisurely opportunity to go through the handling process which leads up to breast feeding.

Any hospital routine which separates mothers and their infants, unless for medical reasons, is requiring the mother to shut off her feelings like a water tap. Each time these feelings are pushed down, when the infant is taken away, they are in part repressed, and fears and doubts amplified in the baby's absence. Put in this position, the mother feels that she has to prove herself in the time allotted to her. The mother should *never* have to feel that she is competing with the hospital staff about the care or needs of her own baby. Instead she must be reassured that they are there to help and to instruct her as necessary. She should never have to feel that she is scheduled according to the hospital's time clock but should be able to request her infant for a visit, or be able to choose rooming in, to care for the infant at all times.

The nurse's role is one of supporting the new mother as the relationship is established with her infant. Teaching is especially important so that the inexperienced mother can become confident enough to enjoy handling her infant.

development of the infant's perceptual system

During the first few days of life the infant experiences his first "perceptions" of the world and begins to develop many of his basic feelings on which all other experiences will be built. Initially, the infant does not have a fully developed sensory system, and perceptions are not received with the same intensity, clarity, or understanding that they later will be, but the system does operate and begins to provide the initial input to the infant's mind. With repetition, perceptions are organized into the earliest memories. How the infant responds depends on the significance of the stimulus to him. Significance develops with experience and "memories." Because of the routine and physical gratification involved with feeding, its significance is great and is organized into memories of satisfaction and pleasure. These memories then make feeding even more important. Sensations in the infant's mouth and stomach while feeding are of such intense gratification that they become the unconscious symbolic essence of feeling satisfied and thus become the basic feeling of satisfaction throughout the infant's later life.

The sensory system parallels the development of all the body's voluntary systems. Initially being uncontrolled and unrefined, the motor reflex system is immature in human young and takes physical maturation and experience in order to develop. The immaturity of the perceptual system protects the infant by screening out much of what goes on about him (2). As the infant gains experience, the system develops, giving him more perceptual material, thus making it possible to select perceptions on a voluntary basis. As the systems develop together, the infant can both more clearly understand the world and effectively react to it.

TACTILE AND MOTION

Perceptions of motion and touch are perhaps the most important of all sense impressions for the brand new infant. Rocking and motion are sensations of equilibrium sensed in the inner ear. The awareness of motion is already acute at birth, having been present for months in utero. Infants respond to rocking and motion as well as to tactile sensations of warmth, closeness, and snugness with pleasure.

VISUAL

The infant's initial visual impressions are unfocused, and every object is strange, unfamiliar, and without meaning. Objects and faces float in and out of view and focus as if by magic. Everything is new and only somewhat significant, and must be moving, bright, or flashing in order to capture attention.

Gazing, really "looking," gradually devel-

ops. Soon after birth a baby begins to pick out single objects from the whole clutter of stimuli around him (3). Typically, the infant will stare transfixed at something like a picture on the wall, not seeing the picture itself but fixing on the square shape which is seen as a single object of contrasting color. Faces become familiar objects by about 6 to 8 weeks (4). Perceived as sets of eyes and noses, faces take on the significance of special pleasure as they are associated with being held or fed.

SOUND

Sound is at first filtered out. The infant reacts only to soothing hums and frightening bangs. Other sounds are just part of the background and are meaningless to the infant. Sounds gradually gain significance and meaning when associated with care givers, food, and pleasure. Language of the mother is important from the beginning as a pleasant background to feeding. Infants respond to the higher tones, and sometimes are startled by deeper male voices. Groundwork for verbal ability begins to be developed long before words appear (see Table 17·1).

beginning of the infant's relationships

The infant is totally dependent; all his needs must be met by his care givers. The infant is totally dependent also upon his parents to introduce him to the world and to allow him to perceive the world as a place of gratification and relative harmony, with frustrations, but with hope of relief from tension as well. If parents are not able to be supportive during this period, he may learn to perceive the outside world as a place of hostility and indifference, hopelessly frustrating.

Child studies have shown that continuous loving contact between the infant and his mother provides stimulation and gratification for the infant which has an observable effect on his physical and psychologic development (Fig. 16·1). If a relationship is not begun immediately, not only is progression interrupted but other experiences which have intervened have to be overcome before a relationship can become well established. Salk (5) has pointed out that the child is stimulated and gratified through cuddling and simple play. He gives response and begins to subtly "understand" the personal warmth his mother transmits to him through her body and tender gestures. He begins to direct some attention toward the outer world through gratification of needs (Fig. 16·2).

Without gratification, the infant concentrates *only* on his inner needs and particularly

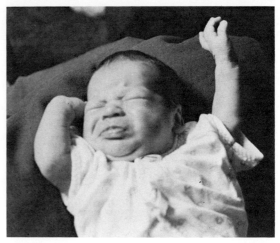

fig. 16·2 A big stretch after eating. What is he feeling or thinking? (*Photo by John Young.*)

fig. 16·1 Feeding time brings satisfaction to mother and infant. (*Photo by John Young.*)

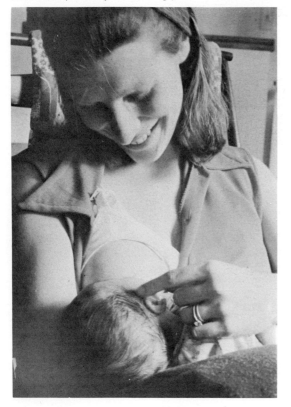

the demands of hunger. Left for long periods without personal contact, or left to cry it out, when either food or other forms of attention would reduce discomfort, the infant learns not to expect anyone to satisfy his needs. As a result, he can develop *autistic* symptoms, or self-involvement to the exclusion of the outside world.

The infant's mind is preoccupied with his own needs and the belief that in some magical way the outside world is connected to his inner world. Each infant reacts as if he is the center of the world, all activity revolves around his needs and wishes, he is the only real person, all others do his bidding. Simply, there is nothing more central than his own existence. The infant believes that he causes everything to happen and everything which goes on around him, and every person, especially mother, is an extension of himself. If her face appears above the crib it is because he magically caused it to appear.

The infant's belief that he and his mother are magically connected is his first understanding of a relationship. For instance, during the interval of crying which immediately precedes a late night feeding, a baby believes that his mother feels everything that he feels and is therefore able to know exactly what he needs and wants. From his viewpoint, his stomach hurts, he feels it, mother feels it, she comes, and changes and feeds him. He cannot imagine that mother is not connected to himself as his stomach is. After all, he does not know yet how his stomach works and assumes that it belongs to him; he makes the same assumption that mother and everything else are extensions of himself.

WHY THE INFANT CRIES

All crying in infants is a response to their need to *discharge tension*. The infant who wakes up in the night for his late feeding does not cry to attract mother's attention, but cries to discharge immediately the tension which has built up in his nervous system from hunger spasms or other causes. This discharge is accomplished through the motor reflex system of crying. As an infant grows and matures he develops more sophisticated motor reflex systems. Babies cry because they have needs which cause tension, and for no other reason. Since they feel they magically communicate with mother and that she automatically "knows" their every need, then crying does not need to be done to attract attention or communicate, but only to release tension.

However, some parents feel that an infant is "after" attention, is deliberately disturbing them, or is in some way plotting against them. The infant's crying may interfere with sleep so much that the parents become angry and feel the child is deliberately crying to get even with them. These feelings are simply the parents' feelings, not the child's. Babies cry often at irregular and interfering times. But they cry out of their needs; they have no ability to develop any other motive, especially one of revenge. If a baby cries excessively, his parents should discuss it with their pediatrician (see Chap. 17). Possibly, the condition can be helped, or possibly the parents will have to tolerate having the household upset by their new arrival. Whatever the case, it should be made clear that the baby is not punishing them.

THE PERCEPTION OF FEELING

While the infant is developing a relationship to his mother, he is learning the way his mother *feels* toward him. Later on as his ability to perceive and remember develops, he will remember particular things about their relationship, but initially he only reflects and remembers mother's *feeling* tone. If the child has an adequate mother who can provide the necessary emotional atmosphere, then the early impressions are of warmth, tenderness, comfort, and the satisfying milk that mother gives. If the child has an inadequate mother who is unable to provide a healthy emotional tone, then the early impressions are of isolation, frustration, coldness, and as a result "undersirable" milk. Even food can be given in such a way as to make good milk *seem* bitter.

Even at a very early stage, unhealthy mothering can greatly affect the child's development, because the feelings at this stage will be carried with him the rest of his life. Because basic feelings are so essential to personality makeup, the adult who has not had a satisfying infancy has the mark of infancy always with him. Some children continue to be "babies"—to act in babyish ways—until they reach adolescence. In adolescence they either do not rebel at all or overreact and become destructive in their desire to be independent. As adults they are very dependent and cling to friends, their spouses, or parents. Thus, it is necessary first for infants to have relationships. That is most basic. Then the healthier the person is to whom they relate, the healthier their development will be (Fig. 16-3).

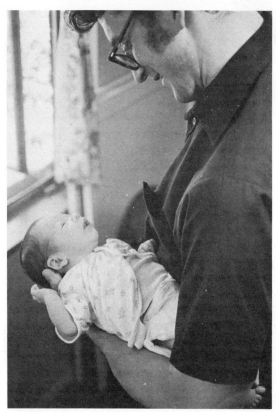

fig. 16·3 Security with father, too. (*Photo by John Young.*)

THE PSYCHOLOGIC TASK OF SEPARATION

To become a person the baby must go through a process of separation and individualization in his own psychologic development. The process begins while the baby is completely physically dependent on his parents and is fearful of any separation. After the child's first birthday his unquenchable need to explore drives him toward independence. By the age of two the child has begun his rebellion, armed with the word "no," which he fires at anyone in range. In the third and fourth years, the child's understanding greatly expands and he is capable of much more independence. Normally the same theme of individualization and separation is again the major developmental concern years later in adolescence. People who have not been allowed to develop normal independence because of overprotective parents will stay concerned their entire lives with the psychologic tasks of individualization and separation, as is shown by those who never "cut the apron strings."

Because the infant believes that his mother magically understands all his needs, their relationship becomes quite exclusive, and separation brings a traumatic sense of loss for the child. The early memory impressions of mother are based on the usual and consistent feeling tone mother transmits to the infant. Within a few weeks the baby begins to recognize the routine which leads up to feeding in particular. A change in this routine or in the type of tenderness which mother usually displays has meaning to the child. During the first several months as the baby grows older and develops a greater store of impressions about the outside world, his sense of security comes in part from being able to connect past impressions with what happens to him at any particular moment—the repetition of the familiar—and from being able to build on his impressions, adding to what he already knows. Separation interrupts what is familiar and disturbs the basis the infant uses in perceiving the outside world.

At approximately eight months the baby is able to focus his eyes well enough and is able to recall visual memories sufficiently to identify mother from other people by her facial features, making their relationship completely exclusive. It is at this point when *separation anxiety* begins to operate and will be a major concern into the third year. Separation anxiety is the overwhelming fear and sense of loss the child feels when he is separated from his mother in particular. The child has pinned his security to the one person who has provided consistent care, the tenderness, warmth, and love which are so gratifying. When the child has the ability visually to confirm mother's well-established relationship, and when the child is visually separated from mother (except in terms of the usual routine, i.e., before naps, etc.), then he experiences an agonizing and panicky sense of loss. Father and others can be of help to the child in comforting him, but no one can really take mother's place.

Within the normal routine, the child suffers enough mini-separations and frustrations to develop a certain degree of tolerance, but long, unprepared-for separations must be handled with great understanding. Occasional separation with a familiar baby sitter can add the sense that life is not perfect, but not consistently terrifying either. Parents who use a totally strange baby sitter or who sneak out of the house when their baby is not looking, sabotage the child's beginning attempts at handling his anxiety. Separation, like anything else, should be handled openly. It is better for a child to cry over his parents' leaving when they straightforwardly wave and say "bye-bye," than when he misses them and vainly searches the house for them. If mother is going to have to leave her baby or young child, the person (including father) who will be substituting for her should spend time beforehand with the child to build some familiarity with him.

Should the infant under one year of age have to be hospitalized, it is just as important for his mother to be with him as when he is older.

AN EXAMPLE OF CROSS-CULTURAL MOTHERING PATTERNS

In different cultures, basic mothering patterns vary greatly and offer alternative methods for consideration. In particular, one mothering pattern of the Kikuyu tribe of central Kenya in East Africa, stands out as strikingly different from Western styles. Infants and babies are almost at no time put down, either to sleep or for any other reason, but rather are consist-

ently carried, usually tied on their mothers' backs, and therefore are rarely deprived of physical contact with their mothers. The reasons for this are simple. Traditionally, in a Kikuyu hut there is no "nursery." Baby's bed is that part of mother's bed between mother and the wall. Because of the excellent weather and agricultural tasks of the household, much of the day is spent outside, not inside. The child has no problem in adapting to sleeping on mother's back; being quite used to riding around *in* mother, he has no new feeling when riding *on* mother. This continuation of a pleasurable, relaxing, known experience in the midst of a world of unknown experiences offers security.

The question which may be raised here is who really has the advantage—the infant who sleeps in his own room, in a beautiful crib, surrounded by cuddly teddy bears, or the infant who sleeps feeling the warmth and motion of his mother's back? The first situation is the outgrowth of a highly materialistic society. The other is still part of a highly personal society where only now the emphasis is shifting from living things (people, cows, sheep, crops, etc.) to material things (money, radios, cars, etc.). The traditional Kikuyu mother is using her own warmth and physical contact as a part of her relationship to her child. Western society tends to be much more "hygienic" and materially oriented, perhaps to the detriment of the development of physical and emotional relationships. To have relationship there must be *contact*. There is a tendency to intellectualize the meaning of "contact," but in fact it necessitates large amounts of time spent together—the mother and the baby getting the "feel" of each other.

One method to provide more physical contact has been tried in our society by mothers who use the cloth back carriers (for infants and babies) to carry their babies around the house. Use of such a carrier makes it very easy to put to sleep an infant who is satisfied but a little uppity; the mother simply puts him on her back and gets on with her duties. By the time the dishes are done, baby is asleep and can be easily lowered into his crib.

the infant without a family: comments on foster care and adoption

Many infants do not become a part of the family into which they were born. These infants are placed in either adoptive or foster homes. For a variety of reasons many parents are unable to care for or bring up a child to whom they have given birth. The reasons for the parents' or mother's inability to care for the child are as widespread and varied as the situations and personalities of the people themselves. Some parents or individual mothers recognize that given their circumstances, they are inadequate to care for a baby or raise a child, at least at this time in their lives. Other mothers, because of social pressures, problems of drug addiction, or mental illness, either give up or abandon children. But, of course, there are many reasons other than these why children are given up either temporarily or completely.

For a mother to recognize that she is unable to care for and raise a child because of whatever circumstances, and to plan so that the child will be provided with good parents, requires great maturity and courage. Such an individual needs the understanding and support of the nursing staff with whom she will deal at the time of delivery and immediately after.

The infants who go into either adoptive or foster home placement frequently remain in the hospital nursery longer than other infants. The nursing staff has a special responsibility to these children, as to those who are left longer because of medical reasons, to supply the missing personal attention, warmth, and comfort that an enthusiastic and loving mother would normally provide. Even in a brief stay, the infant faces the risk that all infants who are institutionalized face. Although all their physical needs may be met, they have great need for psychologic stimulation in the form of tender and playful handling. Studies have shown that infants in institutions without personal contact, given adequate food and comfortable but unstimulating surroundings, are retarded in their physical and psychologic development, and in extreme cases may even die (6).

Every nurse who establishes some type of relationship with an infant risks her own feelings of attachment to the child. Nurses who have gone through the experience of extending themselves to an infant left for several weeks in the hospital have suffered with their own normal feelings of separation and loss and must grieve when the infant has had to leave. Though these feelings are painful, normal signs of separation, they are also the proof that the infant has had the giving relationship that will help him to approximate a normal experience.

Some children who leave the hospital will go into adoptive homes. *Adoption* is the legal placement of a child with suitable adoptive parents to whom the state gives full responsibility for the child, with the child becoming an actual legal member of the family. Adoption requires either that the child's biologic mother has voluntarily given up her legal rights to the child or that a court has terminated her rights, usually on the basis of abandonment. After a period of placement, usually of a year, the adoption is legally finalized in the courts, and in most states a new birth certificate is issued showing the adoptive parents as the only parents. At this point, there is *complete protection* against removal of the child from home because of claims to the child made by another party. Once the child is adopted, the adoptive parents are entirely responsible for the child's life, as in a natural birth. Adoption assures the child of having continuing family relationships throughout his life. These relationships can begin as soon as the infant leaves the hospital, sometimes 1 or 2 weeks after birth, but possibly later.

Other babies leave the hospital's nursery for foster homes. If the biologic mother chooses not to give up her rights to the child and remains at least somewhat interested in the child so that abandonment cannot be proved (even though possibly the biologic mother can in no way care for the child herself, for whatever reasons), then the child is placed in a foster home. Often foster care is used for children who could be adopted but for whom adoptive homes are difficult to find because the children are older, of a minority race, have medical problems, etc. *Foster care,* then, is defined as a method of child care in which the child is placed with a family which is given major responsibility for the child's care. Legal responsibility for the child is assigned to a state agency or a state-licensed private agency. Foster homes are usually administered directly through these agencies. Foster parents are paid through the agency a monthly rate plus medical and other expenses. A social worker is assigned to each home to give professional assistance in the raising of the children. The social worker works with the biologic parent toward resolution of the uncertainty of the child's status by proving abandonment, voluntary surrender of the biologic mother's rights to the child, or return of the child to the biologic mother.

The distinction, then, between a child who can be placed in an adoptive home for adoption and a child who is placed in a foster home for extended care is usually a legal one. The child must be "free" for adoption, which means that there is no parental claim to the child. Biologic parents may voluntarily surrender their rights to the child by signing affidavits stating that this is their wish. Or

biologic parents can be sued in court and have their rights to children severed. However, in most states, the judicial systems favor the "blood bond" over the "psychologic bond" that the child has to the family with whom he lives. Courts tend to protect biologic parents' rights to their children even if the biologic parent plays no part whatsoever in the child's life, except perhaps to pay perfunctory annual visits to the child. Complete abandonment of the child by his biologic parents constitutes the one consistent grounds on which the courts of the various states usually sever parental rights.

If the biologic parental rights remain intact while the child lives with a foster family, then many psychologically damaging conflicts are intrinsic to the situation. The foster parents find it difficult to commit themselves totally to the child because of the possibility that he will be removed from their home to be returned to his biologic parents. The child at first does not understand the situation in which he finds himself, and then is confused by the burden of two sets of parents (one set of which he knows as his "real" parents but whom in fact he hardly knows); later the child is in conflict because of the uncertainty of not knowing where his identity and allegiance really lie. Finally, the biologic parents are also frequently in conflict over the situation, torn between their own feelings of guilt over not being able to take their child and their sense of inadequacy which reminds them that they probably never will be capable of caring for their own children.

The foster care situation is difficult from the foster parents' viewpoint because the legal uncertainties make them insecure in their feelings of love for their foster children. Many foster parents who commit themselves fully to children placed in their care suffer agonizing loss when the child is removed from their home. Even for the child who remains in the foster home, there can be deep emotional conflicts around such matters as visits from the biologic parents. Foster parents must be unusually strong parents to be able to reach out to the child and explain the very mixed feelings which are involved in this situation.

The present trend in the legislative and judicial systems is to give the children themselves and their foster parents more rights in court. Presently, children, even infants, are being assigned their own lawyers to protect their rights, and to guarantee that the best possible living situation is available to them in terms of both their psychologic and physical development. Every state has its own laws concerning foster care, but as an example of progressive legislation, New York State has given foster parents who have had a child in their home for two or more years the right to a hearing prior to the removal of the child from the home for any reason. This is a step toward protecting the *psychologic bonds,* the delicate, fragile feelings of relationship, between the foster child and foster parents. Foster care needs to be further restructured legally to guarantee that the "psychologic parents" of the foster child will have the fullest possible opportunity to develop normal family relationships and—most important—that the child will have the fullest opportunity to feel that he is a secure and wanted member of a family.

Compared with other forms of child care, foster care is the most excellent way devised by our society of taking care of the child who can't be brought up by his biologic parents. In a foster home, a child relates to a complete family and has the possibility of close relationships on an individual basis. Even in the present legal situation, it is possible for a child to enter a foster home immediately after birth and to remain as a member of the family throughout his childhood and adolescence, although, unfortunately, this usually does not happen. The infant who enters a foster home will be able to relate to one consistent mother with whom he can form the comforting, satisfying, and stimulating relationship which

every baby must have in order to be able to go on to more mature levels of psychologic development.

references

1. Marshall Klaus, et al., "Maternal Attachment: Importance of the First Postpartum Days," *New England Journal of Medicine,* **280**:460, 1972.
2. R. Spitz, *The First Year of Life, A Psychoanalytic Study of Normal and Deviant Development of Object Relations,* International Universities Press, New York, 1965, p. 36.
3. Burton L. White, *Human Infants' Experience and Psychological Development,* Prentice-Hall, Inc., Englewood Cliffs, N.J., 1971, p. 16.
4. Spitz, op. cit., pp. 50–51.
5. Lee Salk and Rita Kramer, *How to Raise a Human Being,* Random House, Inc., New York, 1969, p. 12.
6. Selma Fraiberg, *The Magic Years,* Charles Scribner's Sons, New York, 1959, p. 40.
7. Joseph Goldstein, Anna Freud, and Albert J. Solnit, *Beyond the Best Interests of the Child,* The Free Press, New York, 1973, pp. 37–39.

bibliography

"Adoption—Some Answers to the Doctor's Dilemma," *Contemporary OB/GYN,* vol. 1, no. 1, 1972.

Brenner, Charles: *An Elementary Textbook of Psychoanalysis,* Doubleday Anchor Books, Garden City, N.Y., 1957.

Essentials of Adoption Law and Procedure, Social Security Administration, Children's Bureau Publication 331, 1949.

Fenichel, Otto: *The Psychoanalytic Theory of Neurosis,* W. W. Norton & Company, Inc., New York, 1945.

Freud, Anna: *Psychoanalysis for Teachers and Parents,* Emerson Books, Inc., New York, 1963.

Goldstein, Joseph, Anna Freud, and Albert J. Solnit: *Beyond the Best Interests of the Child,* The Free Press, New York, 1973.

Hymovich, Debra P., and Martha Underwood Barnard: *Family Health Care,* McGraw-Hill Book Company, New York, 1973.

Ritz, Jean P.: "Termination of Parental Rights," *New York University Law Review,* **32**(3):1957.

Spock, Benjamin: *Baby and Child Care,* Pocket Books, Inc., New York, 1957.

White, Burton L.: *Human Infants' Experience and Psychological Development,* Prentice-Hall, Inc., Englewood Cliffs, N.J., 1971.

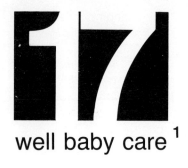

well baby care [1]

Jane Corwin Reeves

Nurses are functioning in a new role in well baby clinics and private pediatricians' offices across the country. They are taking more responsibility for assessing the infant's condition, administering the proper tests, giving immunizations, and counseling the mother on common problems. It is the nurse who may see the well baby both in the home and in the clinic. The nurse is the one who takes the history and does a physical examination, screening the infant for deviations from normal patterns. On subsequent visits, the infant's progress is followed to make sure that he is getting proper nutrition and developing normally, and that both mother and baby are coping with the changes of the first year.

Observation is an important tool in approaching the mother with her infant. Look and think. Look and compare with normal ranges of activity and behavior. Observe the mother's "body language," how she holds the baby—does she cuddle him, hold him like a sack of potatoes, set him down on a table and walk away? If she is tense, do you see a corresponding tension response in the infant? How does the mother respond when the baby cries, and how when he disregards her verbal commands? Are her commands reasonable for his age level? Does the baby look

[1]Grateful appreciation to Henry K. Silver, M.D., for his teaching and for his inspiration.

well? If not, why not? Is he happy, sad, fussy, solemn, crying, fretful? Is he fat, thin, pale, rosy? How old does he appear by his size and by his activity? Even the first 5 min of contact with the mother and the baby can give a great deal of information which will help in the assessment of the child's level of development and its relationship and meaning to the mother.

observation based on growth and development

Silver defines growth and development as follows:

> *Development* signifies maturation of organs and systems, acquisitions of skills, ability to adapt more readily to stress, and ability to assume maximum responsibility and to achieve freedom in creative expression. *Growth* refers to a change in size resulting from the multiplication of cells or the enlargement of existing ones (1).

All that nurses do in assessment is based on principles of development and growth. An understanding of the normal ranges of growth and development is a basic tool for the nurse in comparing each child with others. Wide variations are possible, and skill in interpreting differences will come as experience is gained with many infants. Brazelton, in *Infants and Mothers* (2), has made an interesting comparison between the "average" baby, the "quiet" baby, and the "active" baby. He states that each new mother must find her own way as a mother with her own special baby. Each is stuck with the other's unique ways of reacting. He further states that the idealized suggestions of authorities may be entirely wrong for a particular mother and child. Especially nurses working in cultural situations different from their own must avoid the pitfalls of an authoritative approach based on textbook ideals, and yet must be

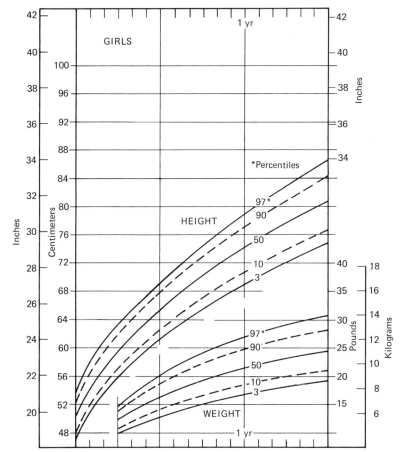

fig. 17·1 Height and weight for girls (Harvard data), 3, 10, 50, 90, 97 percentile ranges. (*From Kempe, Silver, and O'Brien*, Current Pediatric Diagnosis and Treatment, *3d ed., Lange Medical Publications, Los Altos, Calif.*, 1974.)

able to bring some clear suggestions to the mother when problems are observed.

The basic principle to communicate to mothers is well stated by Silver.

Development and growth are continuous dynamic processes occurring from conception to maturity and take place in an *orderly* sequence which is approximately the same for all individuals. At any particular age, however, wide variations are to be found among normal children which reflect the active response of the growing in-

dividual to numberless hereditary and environmental factors (1) (Figs. 17·1, 17·2).

Nurses can pick up problems early in many cases if they have a basic understanding of how a baby develops. The focus of development is at the center of the head and trunk, and moves downward and outward, *cephalocaudal* and *proximal-distal*. The infant smiles before he begins to coo, and holds his head steady before he reaches for an object. The baby who sits well alone will have already mastered the task of turning over. He must be

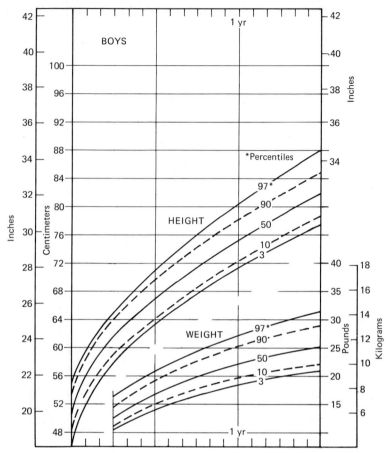

fig. 17·2 Height and weight for boys (Harvard data). (*From Kempe, Silver, and O'Brien,* Current Pediatric Diagnosis and Treatment, *3d ed., Lange Medical Publications, Los Altos, Calif.,* 1974.)

able to stand alone before he can walk. Changes also involve refinement of motor control. This can be seen clearly in the newborn's aimless movements, which change rapidly to an ability to grasp larger objects and then to use the pincer grasp of thumb and forefinger around a Cheerio or raisin.

DENVER DEVELOPMENTAL SCREENING TEST

Frankenburg and Dodds formulated the Denver Developmental Screening Test (3) as a tool which can be used to pick up develop-

mental lags. Some developmental problems can be corrected by introducing new experiences into the infant's world, but sometimes lags indicate something more serious. For instance, the baby who does not turn to the sound of a voice or respond to the bell by the age of five months may have a serious hearing problem.

Cautions in the use of the DDST by nurses are given by Roberts (4). The tool is for preschool screening only, and its validity rests there. However, nurses have used it in a variety of ways—to alert parents and students to the dynamics of child growth and development, for referral, and for evaluation of follow-up. The tool should not be adapted, and its purposes should be kept clear. Frankenburg adds that it is not an intelligence test but a screening instrument to determine whether the development of a particular child is within the normal range (3) (Fig. 17·3).

Instructions for Use Generally, in the first year the test utilizes the nurse's observation skills, rather than giving verbal directions for infant responses. Involving the mother in the test is one way of recognizing her unique contribution and provides a good opportunity for teaching. The parent must participate if the child refuses interaction with the observer. The parent also participates by reporting behavior (R = passes test according to report of parent) (see Fig. 17·4).

Begin the evaluation by drawing a line through the chart at the chronologic age (for a premature child, subtract the number of months premature from the chronologic age). Administer pertinent items—the footnotes give specific directions. The significance of the test lies in the comparison of the child with himself as the months go by, and in a comparison of the child with the norms demonstrated on the bar graph. Each marking on the bar means that a certain percentage—25, 50, 75, or 90 percent—of the age group had a successful performance. If the child does not pass what 90 percent of his peer group passes, it is considered significant and reportable. An overall pattern is gained by administering the test at every well baby visit.

STIMULATION

During the test, the nurse can explain how the baby develops and how the mother can help. She can ask what the baby is doing that is new. She can talk about what is normal for his age and what the mother should watch for over the next month or so. The nurse should explain what the test shows. An infant low in social development may not be getting enough *stimulation.* Sometimes a mother does not know that it is important to talk to a baby. She needs to know that although the infant cannot understand what she says, he will enjoy the sound of her voice and begin forming the language that he will speak the following year (Table 17·1). Infants can learn from the earliest days of life and therefore need stimuli and sound, conversation, and colors. For example, a cradle gym over the crib can be easily and inexpensively made with elastic, colored yarn, brightly colored chewable objects. There are safe things that are common to every home: plastic spoons, wooden spoons, yarn, empty thread spools, clothespins, cardboard boxes, paper bags, pots and pans. Add to this blocks, teething ring, a soft toy with no movable parts, a rattle, a squeaky toy, and the infant will be kept busy his whole first year. Advertising has given the impression to mothers that they must buy expensive toys or their children will be deprived. Often these "bought" toys are too advanced, require only passive response, and may even be unsafe. The nurse does well to have examples of inexpensive toys on hand. Use imagination in helping mothers be economical and creative (Fig. 17·5).

SAFETY

The nurse is aware of the time when the baby will probably start to crawl, and can begin to talk with the mother about potential home hazards. A discussion on lead-free paint is very important, whether or not the mother is planning to refinish furniture or toys. Ask her about falling plaster and paint chips in the house before the baby starts to crawl. If a visit to the home is possible, there will be time for a check with the mother about electrical outlets, poisonous detergents, bleaches, and other hazards in the environment. Guidance should be offered in *anticipation* of the time of development of these new skills. In talking with a mother, use growth and development

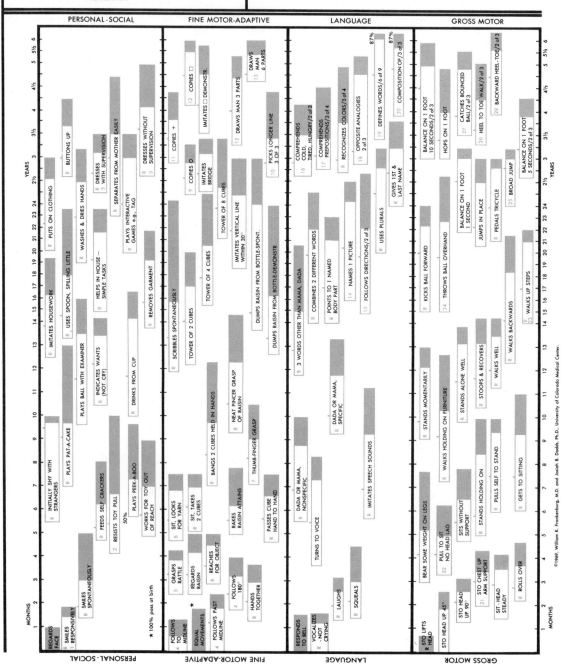

Denver Developmental Screening Test

1. Try to get child to smile by smiling, talking or waving to him. Do not touch him.
2. When child is playing with toy, pull it away from him. Pass if he resists.
3. Child does not have to be able to tie shoes or button in the back.
4. Move yarn slowly in an arc from one side to the other, about 6" above child's face. Pass if eyes follow 90° to midline. (Past midline; 180°)
5. Pass if child grasps rattle when it is touched to the backs or tips of fingers.
6. Pass if child continues to look where yarn disappeared or tries to see where it went. Yarn should be dropped quickly from sight from tester's hand without arm movement.
7. Pass if child picks up raisin with any part of thumb and a finger.
8. Pass if child picks up raisin with the ends of thumb and index finger using an over hand approach.

  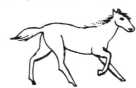 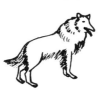

9. Pass any enclosed form. Fail continuous round motions.
10. Which line is longer? (Not bigger.) Turn paper upside down and repeat. (3/3 or 5/6)
11. Pass any crossing lines.
12. Have child copy first. If failed, demonstrate

When giving items 9, 11 and 12, do not name the forms. Do not demonstrate 9 and 11.

13. When scoring, each pair (2 arms, 2 legs, etc.) counts as one part.
14. Point to picture and have child name it. (No credit is given for sounds only.)

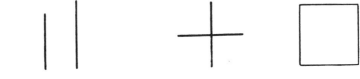

15. Tell child to: Give block to Mommie; put block on table; put block on floor. Pass 2 of 3. (Do not help child by pointing, moving head or eyes.)
16. Ask child: What do you do when you are cold? ..hungry? ..tired? Pass 2 of 3.
17. Tell child to: Put block on table; under table; in front of chair, behind chair. Pass 3 of 4. (Do not help child by pointing, moving head or eyes.)
18. Ask child: If fire is hot, ice is ?; Mother is a woman, Dad is a ?; a horse is big, a mouse is ?. Pass 2 of 3.
19. Ask child: What is a ball? ..lake? ..desk? ..house? ..banana? ..curtain? ..ceiling? ..hedge? ..pavement? Pass if defined in terms of use, shape, what it is made of or general category (such as banana is fruit, not just yellow). Pass 6 of 9.
20. Ask child: What is a spoon made of? ..a shoe made of? ..a door made of? (No other objects may be substituted.) Pass 3 of 3.
21. When placed on stomach, child lifts chest off table with support of forearms and/or hands.
22. When child is on back, grasp his hands and pull him to sitting. Pass if head does not hang back.
23. Child may use wall or rail only, not person. May not crawl.
24. Child must throw ball overhand 3 feet to within arm's reach of tester. (8-1/2 inches)
25. Child must perform standing broad jump over width of test sheet.
26. Tell child to walk forward, heel within 1 inch of toe. Tester may demonstrate. Child must walk 4 consecutive steps, 2 out of 3 trials.
27. Bounce ball to child who should stand 3 feet away from tester. Child must catch ball with hands, not arms, 2 out of 3 trials.
28. Tell child to walk backward, 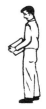 toe within 1 inch of heel. Tester may demonstrate. Child must walk 4 consecutive steps, 2 out of 3 trials.

DATE AND BEHAVIORAL OBSERVATIONS (how child feels at time of test, relation to tester, attention span, verbal behavior, self-confidence, etc,):

fig. 17·3 Denver Development Screening Test. (*From William K. Frankenburg, and Josiah B. Dodds, University of Colorado Medical Center.*)

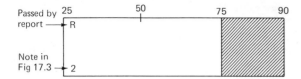

Passed by
report
Note in
Fig 17.3

fig. 17·4 DDST bar graph. R = passes on basis of mother's report; 2 = footnote number; shaded areas indicate the ages at which 75 to 90 percent of children can pass the test item. Failure to perform an item that can be done by 90 percent is significant and should be reported.

as the basis of instruction; the mother will then have a basis for understanding her own infant's progress. Table 17·2 relates teaching about stimulation of the baby and safety factors to the developmental changes in the infant.

immunization

Active immunization of children provides an effective means of disease prevention and health maintenance. The schedule for active immunization given in Table 17·3 is recommended for healthy infants. It is intended as a *guide* to be used with any needed modification to meet the requirements of an individual or a group. Immunization is a dynamic field in which the continuing changes require constant evaluation.

The generally recommended age for beginning routine immunizations of normal infants is two months; the first vaccines given are diphtheria and tetanus toxoid combined with pertussis vaccine (DTP), and trivalent oral poliovirus vaccine (TOPV). Measles vac-

table 17·1
NORMAL SPEECH AND LANGUAGE DEVELOPMENT

AGE	SPEECH	LANGUAGE
1 mo	Throaty sounds	
2 mo	Vowel sounds ("eh"), coos	
2½ mo	Squeals	
3 mo	Babbles, initial vowels	
4 mo	Guttural sounds ("ah," "goo")	
7 mo	Imitations of speech sounds	
10 mo		"Dada" or "Mama," nonspecifically
12 mo		One word other than "Mama" or "Dada"
13 mo		Three words
15–18 mo	Jargon (language of his own)	Six words
21–24 mo		Two- to three-word phrases
2 yr	Vowels uttered correctly	Approximately 270 words; use of pronouns
3 yr	Some degree of hesitancy and uncertainty common	Approximately 900 words; intelligible 4-word phrases
4 yr		Approximately 1540 words, intelligible 5-word phrases or sentences
6 yr		Approximately 2560 words; intelligible 6-7-word sentences
7–8 yr	Adult proficiency	

Source: By permission from C. H. Kempe, H. K. Silver, and D. O'Brien, *Current Pediatric Diagnosis and Treatment*, 3d ed., Lange Medical Publications, Los Altos, Calif., 1974.

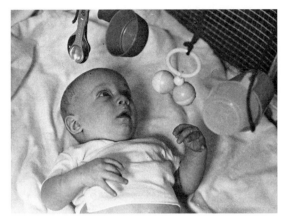

fig. 17·5 Homemade cradle gym over baby's crib. (*Photo by Mary Olsen.*)

cine is most effective when given at or after one year of age, because all the maternal antibody has dissipated by then. If measles vaccine needs to be given by six months of age because of the prevalence of the disease, a repeat dose should be administered after the first birthday (5, 8).

Parents should be fully informed about the immunization proposed. They should know the antigens to be administered, the reasons for their use, and the associated reactions which might occur. Antigens should be injected deep into the muscle mass, preferably into the midlateral thigh muscle; caution should be used about the deltoid or the upper outer quadrant of the buttock (6). Until the child is walking, the gluteus medius muscle is not well developed. In an older child, if injection is given in this area it should be toward the ventrogluteal area. During the course of primary immunizations each injection should be made at a different site (5).

minor problems of the first year

The most important tool in dealing with problems of the first year is the skill of listening. Listen to what the mother says even if it does not fit with what is seen or known. Mothers are more often right than wrong. The mother may sense that the baby is "not quite the same" in activity or mood some time before the child shows symptoms of illness.

COLIC

Many infants experience colic during the first 3 months of life. Often associated with first children, it has been thought due primarily to tense mother-infant interaction. Closer study, however, shows that there are many causes of colic. A baby who appears very much distressed after feeding, who draws his legs up to the abdomen and cries incessantly, has some underlying disorder.

Birdsong (7), in his discussion of infantile colic, identifies five problems to be differentiated and treated:

1. Pain caused by anal fissure leads a baby to hold back his stool, causing further discomfort. The crying-air swallowing-distension-pain-crying cycle is typically seen with this baby.
2. Stenosis of the anus, causing somewhat the same symptoms as those under (1).
3. Allergy to milk or orange juice.
4. Improper feeding techniques—underfeeding, overfeeding, too rapid feeding, poor burping.
5. Parental insecurity, resulting either in overstimulation, so that the baby becomes very fatigued, or in parental neglect.

The pattern varies, but the baby may cry for 4 h or more without letup, often in the late afternoon or very early morning. The anxiety level (perhaps even hostility) of the parent adds to the problem of quieting the baby. Incidentally, a normal baby averages 2 h of crying out of 24.

Suggestions that have been tried (with varying degrees of success) to help parents comfort crying babies are as follows:

Feeding Techniques Place the infant on the right side, head and trunk elevated, after

table 17·2

SUMMARY OF DEVELOPMENT CORRELATED WITH ANTICIPATORY GUIDANCE

AGE, mo	DEVELOPMENT	STIMULATION	SAFETY
1 (Fig. 17·6)	Smiles	Hold, smile at, talk to. Something to watch over crib.	Protect from falls. Flat hard mattress, no pillow, blankets tucked in. Leave on side or abdomen after meals.
2	Coos, gurgles.	Responds to voice. Talk to infant. When he is awake, have him with people.	Strap into infant seat. Protect from falls.
3	No head lag; head up 90°	Responds to singing, talking, people. Becoming sociable.	As above.
4 (Figs. 17·7 to 17·9)	Reaches.	Cradle gym over crib. Will play with small blocks, "squeeze toys," soft toys, rattles, teething rings.	Keep sharp, small, dirty, harmful objects away. Lead-free paint on toys.
5	Rolls over.	Allow more room. Put him on floor or in playpen with toys.	Protect from falls. Never leave alone in bathtub.
6	Sits alone.	Can be put in high chair to eat. Likes to sit in laps. Needs lots of "lapping."	Does not sit securely. Fasten into high chair.
7 (Fig. 17·10A, B)	Crawls.	Needs freedom and room to crawl.	*Dangerous time:* Detergents, bleaches up; open light sockets covered; cords out of reach; stairs with gates. Baby can be taught how to crawl backward down the stairs.
8	Pincer grasp.	Likes nesting boxes. Is happy picking up Cheerios from high-chair tray.	Will pick up and eat the tiniest things—pins, dust, pills.
9 (Fig. 17·11)	Pulls to stand.	Sociable. Likes to be out of crib and playpen.	Crib sides up. Mother to start turning pot handles in.
10	Cruises.	Needs people, blocks, pots and pans, and safe rooms.	Valuables removed from low tables. Check for hazards.
11 (Fig. 17·12)	Stands alone.	As above.	As above.
12	Walks.	Needs to hear something besides "No"—music, conversation, etc.	Check yard, house, stairs for hazards. Watch him.

Note: Babies vary. It is perfectly normal for a baby to begin to walk at 18 months.

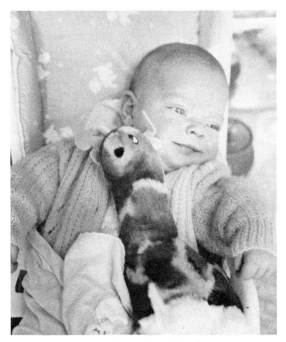

fig. 17·6 Social smile at six weeks of age.

fig. 17·7 A four-and-one-half-month-old infant with good head control, beginning to sit with a straighter back. (*Photo by Mary Olsen.*)

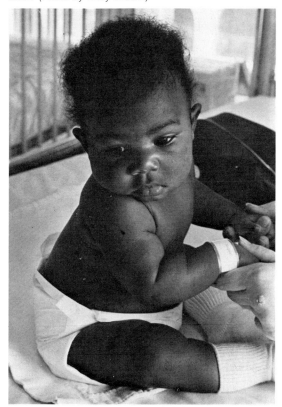

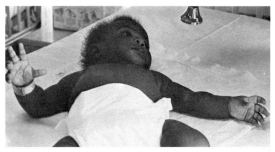

fig. 17·8 A four-and-one-half-month-old infant alerting to the sound of the bell. (*Photo by Mary Olsen.*)

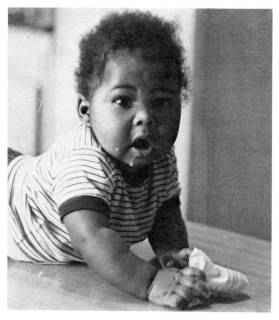

fig. 17·9 At four and one-half months of age, this baby demonstrates 21 on the DDST. He reaches for everything to put it into his mouth, and lifts chest off the table with support of forearms.

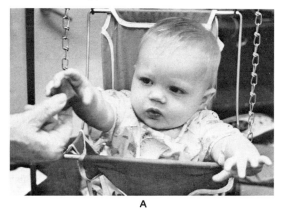

A

fig. 17·10A At seven and one-half months of age, this baby reaches equally well with either hand, but may still be palming objects.

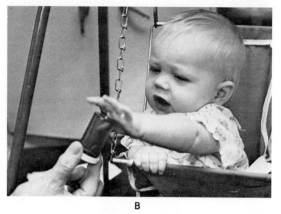

B

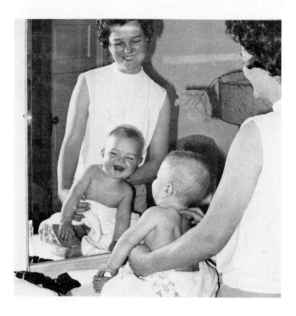

fig. 17·10B This infant enjoys jumper, conversation, bright unbreakable toys, and mother. (*Photos by Mary Olsen.*)

fig. 17·11 At nine and one-half months of age, bath time is a wonderful time for playing with one's mirror image. (*Photo by David Dickason.*)

fig. 17·12 Watch out for the practicing eleven-month-old—he can reach objects that may seem safely out of reach, and he is *determined*. (*Photos by Mary Olsen.*)

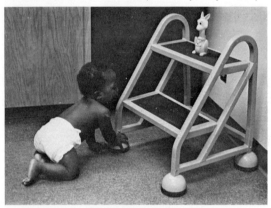

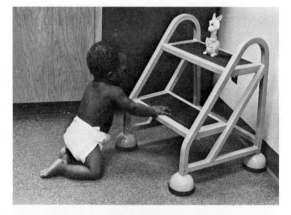

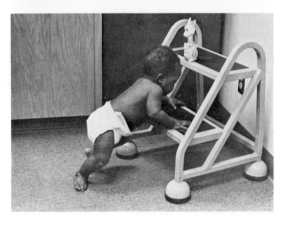

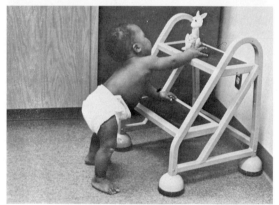

table 17·3

ROUTINE PEDIATRIC VISITS

AGE, mo	IMMUNIZATIONS	TESTS	REVIEWED ON EACH VISIT
1	Immunizations explained	DDST explained	Appetite Activity
2	DPT no. 1, trivalent OPV	Phenylketonuria DDST administered	Sleep Immunizations
3			Elimination Illness exposure
4	DPT no. 2, trivalent OPV		Allergies Fainting
6	DPT no. 3, trivalent OPV	Urinalysis Hematocrit	
8		DDST	
10		DDST	
12	Measles vaccine alone or given as measles-rubella, or measles-mumps-rubella vaccine	Tuberculin test DDST	

Note: DPT, diphtheria-pertussis-tetanus; OPV, oral polio vaccine; DDST, Denver Developmental Screening Test.
Source: Immunization Schedule, from *Report of the Committee in Infectious Diseases*, 17th ed., American Academy of Pediatrics, Evanston, Ill., 1974.

feeding. Burp thoroughly before, during, and after feedings. Follow physician's orders regarding change in feedings. Check nipple holes, allow more sucking time, try a pacifier. Observe stools and report any changes to physician.

Comfort Measures Place a carefully filled *warm* water bottle under abdomen, swaddle baby tightly in baby blanket for feeling of snug pressure and security.

Noise Make some kind of soothing steady noise—turn on water faucet, run vacuum cleaner, play music, ride around in car.

Steady motion Simulate the movements of the uterus, by rocking or carrying baby around in arms or strapped to mother or father in a "back-pack" baby carrier.

The nurse can give one of these simple instructions to the mother at each phone call for help. Sympathetic support will make a great difference in her ability to handle this difficult period. The parents do need a great deal of support, and they need to be reas-

sured that they are *not* the cause of the crying and that they are not harming the baby in some unknown way. Myths about all cases of colic being caused by the mother's tension have aggravated the anxiety of mothers unnecessarily. Attention must be directed toward diagnosing the cause and giving the mother positive steps to take during the process.

THE COMMON COLD

During the first year, infants can be expected to have one or two colds, although the problem does not usually begin until the baby is several months old. There is very little fever normally, although there may be sneezing, coughing, and a runny nose. If the baby looks sick, has a fever over 38.5°C (101°F), has any difficulty with respirations, has a bad cough or a congested chest, is refusing food, or is pulling at his ears, then the problem is more serious than a simple cold (Fig. 17·13).

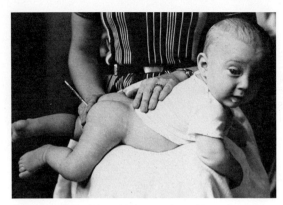

fig. 17·13 Position of infant during taking of rectal temperature. (*Photo by Mary Olsen.*)

The nurse should inquire about the humidity in the house; if it is low, she can advise the parents to purchase a cold steam vaporizer. Cold steam is very effective in keeping the lining of the nose moist, without the danger of the baby's being burned. The mother should be reminded to keep the baby out of drafts and warmly dressed in winter. He should be kept indoors for several days, and at least for 2 days after a fever goes down. With a cold, he can stay on his usual diet but may not have an appetite. Sufficient fluids should be given in the form of juice, water, and milk. One of the difficulties for a baby with a cold is sucking and swallowing with a stuffy nose. Being a nose breather, he may not be able to breathe while trying to take fluids. The doctor may order a small rubber ear bulb syringe to suction out nasal mucus. The mother should be taught the correct way to use the syringe. Finally, with a cold the baby will adjust to his own rest needs. Playing quietly is more restful to an infant than enforced bed rest.

SPITTING UP/VOMITING

Spitting up involves a small amount of liquid (which may look like a large amount when splashed on mother's dress) and is never a sign of abnormality. The cause is mechanical; e.g., milk comes up with an air bubble or when the baby is bounced after feeding. Some babies spit up a great deal the first year and, for some unknown reason, have very little colic.

Vomiting is the bringing up of a large amount of food, which gushes forcefully out of the mouth and sometimes from the nose. It occurs occasionally in most babies and is of no concern unless it is frequent. Vomiting may be caused by sucking on soft nipples, or nipples with holes that are too large; by eating too much and/or too often; or by a formula that disagrees with the baby. It could also be an indication of a bowel obstruction, or a symptom of a generalized illness. In these cases the baby would probably look sick, refuse solid food, or have other major symptoms such as repeated vomiting with every feeding, fever, or diarrhea (Fig. 17·14). *Note*: Any time the nurse is concerned about the baby, or he is presenting more than *one* major symptom, the physician's advice should be sought.

What to ask the mother:

1. How much is spit up, when, how often? To determine the amount, ask if it would fit into a teaspoon, tablespoon, cup, or bowl.
2. Does the baby look sick?
3. Is he dehydrated? Is he passing urine in his normal manner? Is his mouth moist?
4. Is he having any diarrhea? Are his stools hard?
5. Is he gaining weight normally?
6. Is he eating normally? A baby who is eating well is less likely to be seriously ill.

Once the nurse has determined that the problem is spitting up, she can make a few suggestions:

1. Burp the baby well and more frequently.
2. Keep him in an upright position for a few minutes after he eats.
3. Don't bounce him after meals.
4. Give solids with liquids, as spitting up lessens when solids are added.

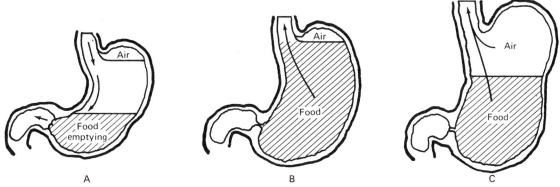

fig. 17-14 Regurgitation, vomiting, and stomach emptying. Normal emptying of stomach (A), overeating or over-distention (B), and swallowing air while crying or nursing (C) may cause regurgitation or vomiting. (*Courtesy of the Carnation Company.*)

RASHES

Tender baby skin appears very susceptible to irritation. Mild rashes are quite common. Sometimes rashes are a sign of illness. The resistance of the skin is lowered with fevers and systemic disease. The other symptoms should be noted—temperature elevation, feeding response, stools, and state of irritability. Any fluid-filled vesicles or pustules are serious and may indicate a staphylococcal infection, herpes simplex, or impetigo neonatorum.

Cradle Cap is a form of seborrheic dermatitis which results in yellowish oily scales on the scalp. There may be a rash on the forehead, cheeks, and shoulders. It is prevented by scrubbing the scalp, including the soft spot, with soap and water each day at bath time. It is much easier to prevent than to cure. If it is present, suggest mineral oil rubbed into the scalp at bedtime for several nights to loosen the crusts. The scalp must be scrubbed the next morning with soap and water and a fine-tooth comb used to loosen crusts. Most mothers wash the scalp lightly and superficially, being afraid of "hurting the soft spot." The nurse can demonstrate on the back of the mother's hand to show what is meant by *firm* scrubbing. If the condition persists, medication can be prescribed.

Diaper Rash (Diaper Dermatitis) The skin becomes reddened and then breaks down because of chemical irritation by the urine and feces. Often occurring infancy even though diapers are changed at reasonable intervals, diaper dermatitis can be treated best by gentle washing with soap and water and then exposure to the air. Before reapplication of diapers, a thick coat of zinc oxide or Desitin ointment can be applied. The best prevention is to use plain water for cleansing after each stool or voiding, and then to coat the perineal area liberally with plain petroleum jelly. Disposable, flushable diaper liners will help the washing problem so that strong detergents may be eliminated.

The mother needs to check out the infant's responses to the type of detergent, bleach, or water softener being used. Double rinsing or using sodium borate in the wash or 2 cups of vinegar in the final rinse will help overcome irritating ammonia. Some babies with sensitive skin may not be able to tolerate plastic waterproof pants or disposable diapers. A change in diet may add a new element in the stool or urine that irritates skin. After all these factors have been checked, or should any ulceration occur, call the physician.

Heat rash (Miliaria Rubra) Some infants develop rashes when too warm. Face, neck, trunk, and diaper area are the first to break out with reddened pustules. Cooling the infant with a tepid bath or a change to lighter clothing will improve the rash.

How the mother dresses her baby is an important topic in a well baby visit. Most mothers tend to overdress, even in summer. A baby is *at least* as warm as an adult. The baby should be kept out of drafts. In summer he does very well in a diaper and short-sleeved shirt. Long-sleeved undershirts are practical in the winter. If they extend over the hands, they can be sewn closed at the ends for the first few weeks so that the baby cannot scratch himself. The mother does not need to purchase fancy clothes, as she will probably be given several outfits. (An important safety note: All clothes should be flame retardant!) There are many booklets which discuss the number of diapers and shirts needed, the kind of clothing advisable, nursery equipment required, etc., and the nurse should acquaint herself with several good ones. These can be discussed with the mother and then handed to her for reference at home.

Monilia If the mother has *Candida albicans,* the infant may become infected at home. Thrush, with white patches on a reddened tongue and mucous membrane is the most common sign, but a diaper rash can be infected as well. The rash will change in appearance, developing well-defined areas with scalloped edges. There will be a grayish hue and an oozing, wet look. Medication such as Nystatin or Amphotericin B must be ordered by the physician.

CHANGES IN STOOLS

Diarrhea is defined as more frequent bowel movements which become loose and watery. The causes can be viral or bacterial (are there other cases in the household?); upper respiratory infection; starvation; allergy to composition of the milk; or new foods. Observe the consistency of the stool, which should not be watery, greenish, or explosive, or contain blood, pus, or mucus.

The nurse needs to get an accurate history about the following:

1. Duration, frequency in the past 12 h, amount (does it fill the diaper?), consistency, and color. Any solid material present?
2. High fever.
3. Vomiting.
4. Weight loss (estimated).
5. Moisture of the skin and mucous membranes.

Diarrhea can quickly become a major problem. If the child looks sick, has another major symptom, or is refusing food and liquid, the nurse should contact the physician.

Constipation A constipated baby has hard, dry stools. Young breast-fed babies normally have three to five stools per day; bottle-fed babies have slightly fewer. Later, breast-fed babies may have a stool every other day. The author found many mothers who complained that their babies were constipated in the first month of life. After careful history, it was discovered that the stools were not hard, but because the baby grunts, pulls his legs up, and gets red in the face, the mother feels the baby is in pain from constipation. The mother's remedy often was to use a laxative or soap chips in the rectum, either of which does get results; i.e., the baby does not grunt or get red in the face when he passes his stool. She should be informed that a baby normally will appear to use his whole body to strain in passing a stool.

It is important for the nurse to support the mother, but also to help her understand what constipation is and the best way to treat it when it occurs. If the nurse determines that the baby is constipated, she should:

1. Check the rectum for a fistula
2. Determine the amount of fluid the baby is getting in his diet

3. Check his general intake—types of liquids, recent new foods
4. Ask about major changes at home which might upset the baby and his routine
5. Find out if the baby has an established pattern of elimination

Simple remedies parallel those for adults— more fluid in the diet, more activity, a regular schedule. Between six and twelve months of age, the infant may be trying to hold the stool in, a developmental change that must be appreciated by parents. More complex remedies must be prescribed by the physician. Caution the mother not to use a laxative or an enema on the infant as her dosage may be too large. The physician may order barley malt extract or a stool softener for truly constipated infants.

SLEEP PROBLEMS

The pattern of sleep cycles varies from month to month for the infant. Sleep becomes a problem for the parent who does not understand the new development which changes the baby's pattern.

Infants typically go through three to four cycles of sleep, with a period of deep sleep in the middle of each cycle. They wake to a semialert state, at which time they may make noises, move about, practice rolling over, rock or bang their heads on the crib sides. After some activity, they slowly settle back into the conditioned position for sleep.

It takes sensitivity to know when to intervene or when the baby should go through this process on his own. If the crib is in the parents' room, sleep for them is impossible. Mothers are alert to unusual sounds and will wake even if the infant is in another room. If the mother offers food or toys after about three months of age, her participation becomes part of the baby's sleep pattern and the infant will incorporate these actions each night. Taking the baby to bed with the parents may be an important way to quiet an upset infant, but can quickly become a hard-to-break habit.

Because we live at such a fast pace, babies tend to become overtired and fussy. In some cases, the mother's life is so full that she does not have time to give the baby naps or to put him in bed each night at an early hour. A regular schedule works best with infants. Some babies need a great deal of sleep; others manage very nicely on 10 or 12 h/24 h. It is better for the mother to plan her schedule around her baby's nap times so that as soon as he becomes fussy she can put him to bed. Babies are lulled by a steady sound; if a fussy baby is not going to sleep, the sound of the vacuum or running water will have a soothing effect on him. A baby who gets enough sleep and enough to eat is generally a happy baby. Happy babies are nice to have around.

WEANING

Nutrition is covered in Chap. 14. This chapter will deal briefly with weaning, which occurs gradually as other foods are added.

A baby can be successfully weaned when he can (1) grasp with both hands, (2) reach, and (3) sit well. Babies will often lose interest in breast feeding after 7 or 8 months; others will continue longer. The mother who is breast-feeding can wean directly to a cup. A bottle-fed baby will often hold on to his night bottle until well into his second or even third year. He gets satisfaction from sucking, and it will do no harm if only a small amount of milk or juice is given. To begin weaning the baby, the mother should put a small amount of milk in the bottom of a shallow, sturdy, flat-bottomed cup. A training cup with two handles is ideal. The baby will tip it over, bang it, suck on it. This is part of the learning process (Fig. 17·15). Each baby is different in how quickly he gets used to drinking from a cup and how ready he is to hold the cup himself. One baby refused to hold his own bottle or

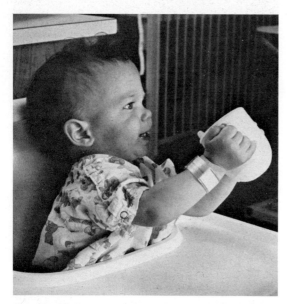

fig. 17·15 Baby using weaning cup. (*Photo by Mary Olsen.*)

cup until well after the first birthday. In such a case, the mother can still offer milk in a cup. The amount of milk the baby consumes may decrease until he gets used to drinking from a cup. However, juices and water can be offered from a bottle to give the baby adequate fluids.

TOILET TRAINING

This subject would not ordinarily be discussed in a chapter on the first year of life. However, some mothers are determined to toilet-train before one year of age, and the nurse can make it easier on both mother and baby. Ask the mother when she plans to toilet-train her baby and how quickly other members in the family have been trained. Slow learners run in families. Boys are harder to train than girls. Bowel movements are more easily caught than urine. If she is determined to train the baby before he is twelve months old—eighteen months is the first age to consider it seriously—make sure he can sit well, and then ask about his elimination pattern. A

baby who has a bowel movement at the same time each day is easily trained. Have the mother put him on the potty with his diaper on for several days for 10 min each time. Praise him if he does something. Then try him without the diaper. Strongly discourage the mother from scolding him if he has no result, and from punishing him if he soils his diaper.

TEETHING

Eruption of teeth usually begins at six to eight months of age for the lower central incisors, and at seven to ten months for the upper central incisors. Teething never causes high fevers, diarrhea, or ear infections, though it may predispose an infant to an infection. Mothers will sometimes attribute an infection to teething and will not consider the baby to be sick. If a baby is having difficulty, a teething ring, dry toast, and plenty of fluid may help. Sometimes the physician will order paregoric for the gums, or "baby aspirin" at bedtime, so that both mother and baby can get some sleep. Once the teeth are through the gums, there is no pain. It is suggested by dentists that the mother brush the new teeth with a soft terry cloth daily. A delay in dentition may be part of the family history and therefore normal for the infant. Delayed dentition may also be associated with hypothyroidism, rickets, and some types of mental retardation.

THUMBSUCKING

There is a picture of a seventeen-week-old fetus in utero sucking his thumb. Since most infants need to suck something, mothers may need help to be more relaxed about thumbsucking. A child can suck his thumb without harm to himself until his permanent teeth come in; only then might the teeth and jaw become crooked. Prolonged bottle sucking sets up a pattern of tongue thrusting and so has a similar effect. Once the child starts to kindergarten, the peer pressure to stop sucking his thumb is very great.

SPOILING, LIMIT SETTING, ROUTINES

Our adult lives are built around certain routines that help to give us structure and stability. Infants, too, need the structure and security of routine. After the first few weeks, either the infant or the mother is on some sort of schedule. Usually the two compromise in the adjustment period. Eating, sleeping, bath time, and play will usually fall into a pattern. The problem of spoiling comes up very often. Some mothers feel that holding the baby will spoil him, and so do not give him the love and affection he needs. The baby who is held often is not necessarily spoiled. Babies need lots of "lapping." The spoiled infant is the infant who demands and gets attention when the mother is busy and does not *want* to hold her baby at that time. As the pattern repeats itself, the baby is learning how to manipulate his mother.

The child by nine months of age can understand what "no" means but does not have the ability to develop the necessary internal controls to prevent the next episode. The mother should remove from his environment whatever she does not want him to poke, touch, explore, or eat.

The parents need to consider carefully what direction they want to take with their child, since children imitate adult behavior (9). The nurse can suggest basic principles of limit setting, which, of course, also apply beyond the first year.

1. Parents should decide together what is off limits.
2. They should agree on reasonable and appropriate discipline.
3. Consistency is the most important common denominator. When parents are not in agreement, or punish only sometimes, or punish too harshly the child becomes confused and does not know what is expected of him.
4. Even children under one year will test the limits to see if the parents are serious about them.
5. It is a sign of love to the child that the parent is willing to provide *external* controls. The infant does not have them innately, but can begin the learning process before the end of his first year of life.

mothers

NORMAL MOTHERS

Mothers come in a variety of sizes, shapes, personality types, and experiences. They enjoy their babies and have reasonable expectations of their infants at different age levels. Each of these mothers has needs of her own which should be met if she is going to be able to give love, affection, and care to her baby. Before the baby arrived people were concerned about the mother, but now the attention is centered on the new arrival. At the same time, the mother's schedule is crowded with bottles, diapers, and sleepless nights. She does not have as much time for her husband, which may cause problems in their relationship. It has been said that it takes 6 months for a family to adjust to every new arrival. The first baby is probably the greatest shock to the family, and both parents experience a variety of emotions, not all of which are positive. There are several things the nurse can do in the very early visits. She can find out how the mother is feeling and what has been the hardest area of adjustment. The nurse can find out when the mother last got out of the house, and when she and her husband have been out together without the baby. If the mother and her husband have not had uninterrupted time together, the nurse could help her think this situation through in terms of time and budget.

BATTERING PARENTS

It may be difficult to understand how some parents can throw their baby against the wall, or hit him hard enough to cause bruises and broken bones. In recent years this problem has become more evident, but that does not mean it is occurring more frequently. Professionals are more aware of its existence and so are more likely to identify it. It does not occur just among the underprivileged. The tragedy of battered children crosses all economic and social lines. Certain observations should alert the nurse:

1. The history and physical findings do not agree.
2. There are bruises where no bruises should be.
3. The baby is poorly cared for—unclean, with severe diaper rash, etc.

If the nurse is suspicious, she can make certain remarks, ask certain questions to help her understand:

1. "It must be very upsetting when he cries."
2. Concerning a ten-month-old: "He should *know* that he shouldn't touch this."
3. Concerning a young infant: "It must be hard to control him. How do you discipline him?"
4. "How were you disciplined?"

In asking these questions, the nurse should ask herself:

1. Are the answers appropriate for the age of the child? For instance, a normal mother would not think of using physical punishment on a two-month-old.
2. Are the mother's actions being done with loss of control?

table 17·4
A SUMMARY OF TEACHING POINTS AT WELL BABY VISITS

1 TO 6 mo	EVERY VISIT
Discuss:	Sleep
Sleep patterns	Feeding, appetite
Breast feeding, bottle feeding	Elimination
How to start solids, new foods	Activity
Stimulation, safety	Illness exposure
Problems:	Allergies
Teething	Immunizations
Thumbsucking	Denver Developmental
Spoiling	Screening Test (DDST)
Sibling rivalry	
Mother's adjustment and level of fatigue	

6 TO 12 mo	EVERY VISIT
Discuss:	Sleep
Sleep patterns	Appetite
Feeding habits	Elimination
Weaning	Activity
Stimulation, safety	Illness exposure
New developments:	Allergies
Different safety levels	Immunizations
Limit setting	DDST
Temper tantrums	
Pica	
Toilet training	

The author found that mothers who are prone to battering do want outside help. In one case, the mother would call and ask to bring her baby in when she felt she could no longer "take it." Once the problem is identified, the doctor, social workers, and other nurses can be helpful in preventing a tragedy. It is important for professionals to get together and discuss their feelings and attitudes toward such parents. It is not so much that a woman is a "bad" mother, or a man is a "bad" father, as that a battering parent lacks that which helps most parents retain control when angry.

summary

What is gained in well child care is greater than the sum of its parts. Much of what has been said has more than an element of common sense. Well child care has a great deal to do with prevention of problems and helping parents to cope better with the changes in their baby. The stress has been on interaction with the mother, because she is the one who usually brings the baby in for well baby visits; however, the whole family is involved in the healthy development of an infant. As more and more neighborhood clinics and health centers open across the country, the nurse will play an increasingly important part. She can add a dimension of concern and creativity in helping families adjust to the arrival of a new member (Table 17·4).

references

1. Henry K. Silver, "Growth and Development," chap. 2 in C. Henry Kempe, Henry K. Silver, Donough O'Brien (eds.), *Current Pediatric Diagnosis and Treatment,* Lange Medical Publications, Los Altos, Calif., 1972, p. 8.

2. T. Berry Brazelton, *Infants and Mothers,* Delacorte Press, Dell Publishing Co., Inc., New York, 1969, p. xviii.

3. William K. Frankenburg, "Denver Developmental Screening Test," *Journal of Pediatrics,* **71**:181–191, 1967.

4. Paula Roberts, personal communication, Nov. 30, 1973.

5. *Report of the Committee in Infectious Diseases,* 17th ed., American Academy of Pediatrics, Evanston, Ill, 1974.

6. Ernest W. Johnson and A. D. Rapton, "A Study of Intragluteal Injection," *Archives of Physical Medicine and Rehabilitation,* Vol. 46, February, 1965.

7. McLemore Birdsong, "Infantile Colic," chap. 73 in Harry C. Shirkey (ed.), *Pediatric Therapy,* 3d ed., The C. V. Mosby Company, St. Louis, 1968.

8. Vincent A. Fulginiti, "Immunization," chap. 5 in C. Henry Kempe, Henry K. Silver, and Donough O'Brien (eds.), *Current Pediatric Diagnosis and Treatment,* 2d ed., Lange Medical Publications, Los Altos, Calif., 1972.

9. T. Berry Brazelton, op. cit., p. 113.

bibliography

Alexander, Mary, and Marie Scott Brown: "The Why and How of Examination," *Nursing '73,* July, 1973, p. 25.

———: "Part 2: History-taking," *Nursing '73,* August, 1973, p. 35.

———: "Part 3: Examining the Skin," *Nursing '73,* September, 1973, p. 39.

———: "Part 4: The Lymphatic System," *Nursing '73,* October, 1973, p. 49.

Andrews, P. M.: "The Pediatric Nurse Practitioner: Growth of the Concept," part 1, *American Journal of Nursing,* **71**:504–506; "Examining the Role," part 2, **71**:507–508, 1971.

Bozian, Marguerite W.: "Nursing Care of the

Infant in the Community," *Nursing Clinics of North America,* **6**(1):93, 1971.

Brinton, D.: "Pediatric Experience in Ambulatory Care Setting," *Nursing Outlook,* June, 1972, pp. 390–393.

Charney, E., and H. Kitzman: "The Child-Health Nurse (PNP) in Private Practice," *New England Journal of Medicine,* Dec. 9, 1971, pp. 1353–1358.

Chin, Peggy L.: *Child Health Maintenance,* The C. V. Mosby Company, St. Louis, 1974.

Feely, W. J.: "Pediatric Nurses Teach Patients," *Bedside Nurse,* June, 1972, pp. 10–15.

Freeman, B. L., et al.: "How Do Nurses Expand Their Roles in Well Child Care," *American Journal of Nursing,* **72**:1866–1871, 1972.

Gersh, Marvin: *How to Raise Children in Your Spare Time,* Fawcett Publications, Inc., Greenwich, Conn., 1966.

"Please Nurse! Help Prevent Child Abuse," (round-table discussion led by Howard Bitton, M.D.), *Nursing Update,* **4**(4): 1973.

Porter, Luz S.: "On the Importance of Activity," *Maternal-Child Nursing Journal,* **2**(2):85, 1972.

Taylor, C.: "The Pediatric Nurse Associate in a Rural Setting," *Maine Nurse,* September, 1971, p. 10.

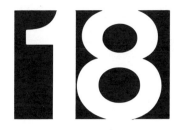

18

pharmacologic factors in pregnancy: maternal factors

Martha Olsen Schult
and
Sister Theresa Thomas

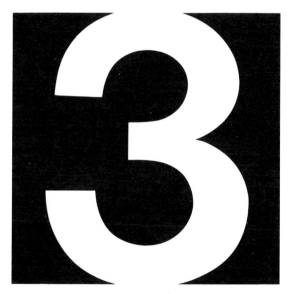

pharmacologic factors in pregnancy

Americans consume exorbitant amounts of sleeping medications, barbiturates, amphetamines, antacids, laxatives, antibiotics, and vitamins. When taken according to prescribed amounts most drugs are considered "safe" for the adult human body. However, many of the drugs considered safe to the adult body can have devastating effects on the unborn baby. The Thalidomide tragedy of 1961–1962 is an example of such an effect; considered a "harmless" sleeping medication and taken by pregnant women, Thalidomide caused thousands of babies to be born with *phocomelia*—the absence of limbs (Fig. 18·1A and B).

Much research is being conducted to try to discover the effects of drugs on the fetus at various points in its development. A few effects of drugs on the fetus are known. For example, aspirin has the potential for causing gastrointestinal bleeding in the fetus. Large doses of phenobarbital can cause neonatal bleeding, and some vitamins taken in excess can harm the fetus. Every drug ingested or inhaled by the pregnant woman crosses the placental barrier in varying concentrations and has the potential for disturbing or altering

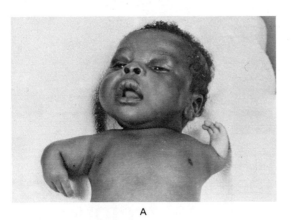
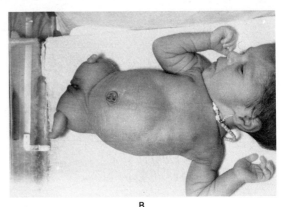

A   B

fig. 18·1A Phocomelia with absence of the upper extermities. (*From D. Bergsma (ed.),* Birth Defects: Atlas and Compendium, *The National Foundation—March of Dimes, White Plains, N.Y., with permission of the editor and contributor.*) B Phocomelia with absence of the lower extremities. (*Courtesy of Marvin L. Blumberg, M.D., the Jamaica Hospital, Queens, N.Y.*)

the growth pattern of the fetus. For this reason, all pregnant women should be warned against taking *any* medication unless it is prescribed by the physician.

nursing responsibilities in the dispensing of medications

Lengthy discussions of the medical and legal aspects of dispensing medications can be found in pharmacology textbooks. However, there are a few important points that every maternity nurse and nurse-citizen should keep in mind.

As health educators, nurses must be aware of their responsibilities to warn their friends, family members, and neighbors who are pregnant of the dangers of self-medication, regardless of the drug, and to encourage the pregnant woman to seek prenatal care and medical advice.

Pregnant women should especially be discouraged from taking any medications during the first *trimester,* when organogenesis is taking place. Unfortunately, most women are not aware that they are pregnant until the second or third month of pregnancy. By that time any harmful drug or disease may have

taken its toll on the fetus before its existence was recognized. For these reasons any woman who even suspects or has any reason for suspecting pregnancy should be shielded from x-rays, stay apart from sick children and adults, and take no drugs without consulting a physician.

Many women have associated childbirth with pain. Either they have experienced previous birth with tension and pain, or they have heard other women's stories. Fortunately, prepared childbirth provides the opportunity to change the cultural anxiety about childbirth. Courses to "decondition and recondition" thinking patterns regarding childbirth do not eliminate the discomfort of labor contractions, but they help the woman to react positively, helping herself throughout the labor and delivery with specific maneuvers and breathing patterns to lessen the discomfort. When she does require medication, it is usually a smaller dose than if she were not prepared and helped to break the fear-tension-pain cycle that grips so many women in labor. (When a woman and her partner work with her contractions and are not overwhelmed by them and frightened by their severity, she can bear the pain, for the most part, benefiting herself and her unborn baby.)

During the postpartal period the patient is often given medications to contract the uterine musculature and help prevent hemorrhage. Medications are also given to suppress lactation or relieve pain. In a few hospitals the postpartum patient is given the responsibility for taking her own medications. Her physician orders a packet of drugs containing analgesics of differing strengths, sleeping medications, or tranquilizers. These drugs remain at her bedside with instructions for their dispensing. The medications are there whenever she needs them. Many patients discover that they do not require as much medication as they had anticipated. Knowing that the drugs are there seems to offer the patients a sense of security. This innovation is releasing the nurse from one function and, it is hoped, freeing her to spend more time with the patient.

prenatal period

VITAMINS, MINERALS

One of the major contributing factors to illness during pregnancy is the lack of good nutrition prior to pregnancy as well as during pregnancy. One of the major teaching responsibilities of nurses is to help patients understand the necessity for good food habits and to guide them in choosing and preparing foods.

Helping the patient to understand how important proper nutrition is for her own health and particularly the health and growth of her baby may do more than merely telling her she should eat properly every day. But even with encouragement, repetition of teaching, and help many patients do not get their necessary daily vitamins and minerals and may need vitamin supplement therapy.

No vitamins or minerals should be taken without the direction of the physician. Without this precaution, women who have been on fad diets may take "therapeutic" doses ten times more potent than prenatal doses. Especial care should be taken to prevent ingestion of excessive amounts of fat-soluble vitamins A and D, which have been linked to fetal anomalies.

Some of the supplemental vitamins and minerals prescribed during pregnancy include the following:

Natabec Kapseals—multivitamin and mineral supplement with iron (ferrous sulfate) and calcium

Natabec R_x Kapseals—same as Natabec Kapseals plus folic acid

Natalins tablets—multivitamins and folic acid, iron, and calcium

Ferrous sulfate, U.S.P., B.P., 200- and 300-mg enteric-coated tablets of iron

Ferrous gluconate, N.F., B.P. (Fergon)—tablets, 300 mg iron

Vitron-C—ferrous fumarate, 200 mg, and ascorbic acid, 125 mg

Iron dextran injection, U.S.P., (Imferon), 50 mg iron per ml

Any patient receiving iron orally should be informed that dark greenish-black stools are to be expected. Some patients experience constipation or a laxative effect when taking iron. Although this is a side effect of iron, if the iron is begun on a low dose and gradually brought to the normal level, most women can adjust to it. Occasionally, the pregnant woman may have to discontinue the medication for several days and then restart (see Chap. 21 for complete discussion of anemia). When liquid iron preparation is ordered, it should be given through a straw, well diluted to prevent staining of the teeth. Iron preparations should not be given with milk as it prevents the absorption of iron. Iron preparations can also be administered before meals or between meals for maximum absorption.

Intramuscular iron is prescribed for the

woman who does not respond to oral iron therapy. Improperly injected, iron dextran stains the subcutaneous tissue for 6 to 12 months. Deep intramuscular injection by the "Z-track" technique (with a long-enough needle to reach muscle) is necessary to prevent staining. This is performed as follows:

1. Use a double-needle technique (one needle to draw up medication, another for injection).
2. Add 0.5 ml air to syringe *after* measuring dose. (Air provides a "plug" to seal off medication in muscle.)
3. Before injecting, twist skin away from site (always use the gluteus medius muscle).
4. After insertion, aspirate. (Iron is dark brown; therefore, increase in the volume in the syringe is the only indicator of the presence of blood.) Inject slowly.
5. Wait 10 s, remove needle, allow skin to return to normal location.
6. Do not massage the site.
7. Rotate sites to avoid tissue injury (never inject in deltoid or vastus lateralis muscles).

The daily calcium requirement for pregnant women is 1200 mg. Since fetal bone formation requires extra calcium, every expectant mother should drink at least 1 qt milk per day. However, many pregnant women do not like milk. For this reason physicians sometimes prescribe calcium during pregnancy as a nutritional supplement. Calcium tablets are also prescribed for women who experience muscle spasms and who therefore have their milk intake curtailed because milk contains phosphorus as well as large amounts of calcium.

The following drugs contain calcium:

Natabec Kapseals—with calcium carbonate, 600 mg
Natalins—with calcium carbonate, 625 mg
Calcium gluconate, U.S.P., B.P., 300-mg tablets

Calcium lactate, N.F., B.P., 300- and 600-mg tablets

Calcium is also available in powdered form.

Other specific vitamins or minerals may be ordered by the physician according to the particular dietary deficiency or blood sample results.

ANTIEMETICS

A common discomfort of pregnancy is the nausea, with vomiting, known as "morning sickness" and occurring in approximately 50 percent of all pregnant women. Before any drugs are prescribed for morning sickness, all other avenues of relief should be explored (see Chap. 4). If an antiemetic is needed, it should be used judiciously during the first 6 to 8 weeks of organogenesis.

Two of the several antiemetics prescribed for morning sickness are:

Tigan—capsules, 250 mg; suppository, 200 mg; ampuls, 200 mg/2 ml for intramuscular injection
Bendectin—tablets, two at bedtime

Tigan is a well-tolerated antiemetic. Much research has been conducted on its effect on the developing embryo. Though there is no conclusive evidence that it is completely safe for the fetus, neither has it been proved harmful to mother or infant. The nurse should inform the patient that she may experience some drowsiness, and ask her to report any allergic symptoms such as a rash to her physician.

Bendectin is a combination of Bentyl, Decapryn, and pyridoxine HCl. Because the tablets are specially coated to produce a long-acting effect, when given at night they are beneficial in the morning when spasms of nausea are most often experienced. Because of the antihistamine component of Bendectin, patients should be cautioned about drowsiness. Any adverse symptom such as diarrhea, rash, or excessive vomiting should be reported to the obstetrician. Bendectin is a researched drug and is primarily prescribed for nausea and vomiting of pregnancy.

LAXATIVES

Constipation is a common complaint during pregnancy. When counseling with a pregnant woman regarding her dietary habits, the nurse should encourage her to include roughage in her meals, as well as ample fluids, in an effort to increase bulk and lubricate the bowel. This, along with exercise, usually will prevent constipation. Again, the advisability of avoiding medications can be stressed to the pregnant woman.

Some of the most commonly prescribed laxatives and stool softeners include:

Milk of magnesia U.S.P., 30 ml (1 oz) orally at bedtime
Colace—capsules (50- and 100-mg dioctyl sodium sulfosuccinate as a stool softener)
Peri-Colace—capsules (100 mg Colace, 30 mg Peristim, a mild stimulant laxative)
Senokap DSS—capsules, (senna and dioctyl sodium sulfosuccinate)

Mineral oil should not be prescribed for the pregnant woman as it interferes with the absorption of the fat-soluble vitamins A, D, E, and K.

DIURETICS

Diuretic drugs are rarely used during pregnancy. When used they are prescribed to relieve accumulated body fluid causing edema of the feet and legs. Generalized edema of the body due to preeclampsia warrants close obstetric supervision and medical intervention. Diuretics would only mask symptoms for these patients and may be harmful. (See Chap. 23 for discussion of preeclampsia.)

The use of any diuretic drug in pregnancy requires that the benefit be weighed against possible hazards to the mother and child. Some of the hazards to the infant include thrombocytopenia, neonatal jaundice, and reduced serum electrolyte levels.

Some of the drugs which act as diuretics are:

Chlorothiazide, N.F. (Diuril)—tablets (0.25-mg) and oral suspension, 0.25 Gm/5 ml
Hydrochlorothiazide, U.S.P. (Hydrodiuril) —tablets, 25-mg and 50-mg
Chlorthalidone, U.S.P. (Hygroton)—tablets, 50- and 100-mg

When a patient's condition warrants the use of a diuretic, ample fluid intake and the dietary intake of potassium should be encouraged. The amount of urinary output should be noted, and the patient should be told to report any vomiting, diarrhea, pallor, shortness of breath, dizziness, vertigo, rash, or oliguria.

Precaution: Infant depression, lethargy, and electrolyte imbalance (hyponatremia) may result from use of these drugs for antepartum patients near term.

HYPNOTICS

Restlessness and inability to sleep during the last trimester due to the large, protruding abdomen and other discomfort may warrant the use of hypnotics.

Some of the hypnotics used to induce sleep include:

Chloral hydrate, U.S.P. (Noctec), 250 mg capsules, 1 to 2 capsules at bedtime. Noctec, one of the oldest hypnotics, provides restful sleep for pregnant patients. It has been used with benefit to alcoholics and the elderly, as well as with children! Although it may be habit-forming, it is considered a mild hypnotic because patients can be aroused with little effort and seldom complain of a "big head" or hangover as an aftereffect.

Sodium secobarbital (Seconal), 100- to 200-mg capsules, may be given orally or rectally. Intramuscular and intravenous preparations are prepared in single-dose ampuls. Seconal is a quick-acting hypnotic or sedative. It produces degrees of drowsiness and depressed reflexes, according to the amount of barbiturate given. Large dosages may cause dangerous depression of the respiratory system.

Sodium pentobarbital, (Nembutal), 100- to 200-mg capsules may be given orally or rectally. It is a short-acting barbiturate and is used to induce sleep and relaxation. It acts as a depressant of the central nervous system of the body; consequently, overdosage can be detrimental.

Phenobarbital, U.S.P. (Luminal), 30- to 100-mg tablets. This drug acts as a depressant of the central nervous system, producing a long-lasting and quieting effect on the individual. With reduced dosages given several times a day it is possible to produce a sustained sedative or quieting effect on the nervous system. (All barbiturates may be habit-forming and also are likely to produce aftereffects ("hangover") if a sufficient time of rest has not ensued.)

When administering sedatives or hypnotics, nurses should see that external stimuli that interfere with rest and/or sleep are removed from the immediate area of the patient. These include loud talking, bright light or sunlight, offensive odors, and food odors that stimulate the olfactory and salivary glands. In the hospital setting all barbiturates must be accounted for and signed for in the narcotic book.

Nurses must provide safety for the patient under sedation. Some patients may not need side rails, but others may; nurses should astutely exercise judgment concerning this question when administering sedatives or hypnotics.

As with all drugs, nurses should be alert to any adverse effects such as rash, diarrhea, gastrointestinal disturbances, or respiratory depression. Hypnotics and sedatives can cause hyperactivity in some individuals, instead of having a quieting effect and producing rest.

TRANQUILIZERS

In the 1950s a whole new category of drugs called *tranquilizers* was introduced. Their ability to reduce anxiety and depression, as well as their side effects, without impairing mental ability and without being habit-forming, has aided tremendously in reducing the need for using habit-forming drugs, such as the barbiturates.

Some tranquilizers prescribed during pregnancy are:

Triflupromazine hydrochloride (Vesprin), 10-, 25-, and 50-mg tablets, acts on the central nervous system and can also be prescribed as an antiemetic during pregnancy.

Chlordiazepoxide, N.F. (Librium) 5-, 10-, and 25-mg capsules, relieves anxiety and tension, has a quieting effect, and is a muscle relaxant.

Diazepam, N.F. (Valium) 2-, 5-, and 10-mg tablets, is a muscle relaxant and generally reduces the anxieties produced by tense situations. (Animal studies on the use of Valium and Librium in rats showed defects produced in neonates. However, there is no conclusive evidence of these teratogenic effects in human beings.)

Nurses should carefully instruct patients that tranquilizers can cause drowsiness and that for this reason they should not operate a car or machinery after using them.

labor period

Although labor is a normal physiologic process for the healthy female, it does involve a degree of stress and discomfort, and for these reasons certain tranquilizers and analgesics have proved useful.

When the nurse is administering any drugs to the laboring mother, bed rails should be up, and the patient should be informed of the sensations to be expected from the drug, especially if it has a quick-acting effect such as light-headedness, vertigo, or nausea.

Once a drug has been administered, the nurse must check frequently to ascertain whether the desired effect is occurring and the patient is benefiting from the drug. The monitoring of vital signs of the mother and fetus can be an indication of the action of the drug. With sedatives and analgesics, the nurse may expect a slight decrease in blood pressure and pulse, a slowing of respiration in the mother, and a slight slowing of the fetal heart rate.

Because of the intimate dependence of the fetus upon maternal circulation, whatever drug effect the mother experiences is also experienced by the infant. The "placental barrier" is not a barrier to most analgesia, sedation, or anesthesia. Furthermore, the infant receives the maternal dosage, and if he is separated from the maternal processes of drug metabolism and excretion before the drug is excreted, he will be born with an excessive dose of the particular drug in his system. Therefore, there are no substances to relieve maternal pain and anxiety, by central action on the brain, which do not affect the fetus as well.

Thus, if drugs are to be used, the problems to be considered in every case are both the dosage and the timing of the dose.

The primary factors affecting the type of medication chosen during labor are the monitoring of the fetal heart rate, as reflecting fetal condition, and the progress of labor as judged by the length, strength, and frequency of contractions.

NARCOTIC ANALGESICS

Narcotics are used during labor to produce analgesic and hypnotic effects in the patient by means of central nervous system depression. The sensation of pain is alleviated or reduced but not obliterated completely.

Two of the more commonly used narcotic analgesics are:

Meperidine hydrochloride, U.S.P. (Demerol) 25 to 100 mg, intramuscularly (IM) or intravenously (IV)
Alphaprodine hydrochloride, N.F. (Nisentil) 20 to 40 mg, subcutaneously (or IV)

A rarely used narcotic is:

Morphine sulfate, U.S.P. 8 to 15 mg IM

Meperidine is used for women in labor to produce analgesia and relaxation. Aside from nausea in some patients, there are few maternal side effects provided dosages are calculated to meet the needs and tolerance of each patient. Demerol usually does not interfere with contractions. A large intravenous dosage may cause contractions to be less frequent for a period, but the work of the uterine muscle will continue, causing dilation and effacement of the cervix. Nurses should be alert to this factor and carefully note other signs of progress so that they are not surprised by a delivery when the patient suddenly appears to awake from the medication. When Demerol is used in conjunction with Phenergan or Vistaril, the dosage is usually halved, as tranquilizers potentiate the analgesic effect.

Meperidine is less potent than morphine. However, if it is administered 1 to 3 h before delivery, the high level in the maternal circulation may unduly depress the infant. This depressant effect is exaggerated in an immature infant born before term. Meperidine has been demonstrated to reduce significantly the cord blood oxygen level, and, therefore, it appears to contribute adversely to the normal biochemical asphyxia present at birth. Recent research indicates that meperidine metabolites have a somewhat toxic effect on fetal nerve tissue; therefore, high doses, even if given early in labor, are not recommended. Since meperidine has a duration in the body of about 4 h, the margin of safety is rather narrow. Brackbill and associates are studying the long-term effects of obstetric medication on infant learning responses. Certainly, obvious signs of depression are seen in the nursery when a sleepy baby does not suck well for several days, when there is an excessive amount of mucus during the first 24 h of life, and when the infant does not respond to tests with quick reflexes.

Nisentil (administered subcutaneously) produces a rapid-acting analgesia with a short duration. The adverse effects resemble those of morphine. Therefore, Nisentil is usually ordered concomitantly with Lorfan to counteract respiratory depression. Its action lies somewhere between that of meperidine and that of morphine.

Morphine sulfate is a most powerful central nervous system depressant. It has only rare use in obstetrics—e.g., to put to rest the overtaxed uterine muscle when *hypertonic uterine dysfunction* occurs or *Bandl's ring.* It is also used to control convulsions of eclamptic patients until appropriate treatment can be instituted.

Morphine crosses the placenta rapidly to depress the respiratory center of the fetus. If the drug has been used within 4 h of delivery, apnea may be present at birth and resuscitation then necessary.

TRANQUILIZERS (Ataraxics)

Anxiety along with anticipation frames the emotional state during labor. Tranquilizers have proved to be useful adjuncts during the labor process by alleviating the patient's anxiety without impairing her mental acumen.

Some of the more commonly used tranquilizers are:

Hydroxyzine hydrochloride (Atarax, Vistaril), 25 to 100 mg, IM, IV
Promazine hydrochloride, N.F., B.P. (Sparine), 25 mg, IM, IV
Promethazine hydrochloride, U.S.P., B.P. (Phenergan), 25 to 50 mg, IM, IV
Diazepam, N.F. (Valium), 2 to 5 mg, IM, IV

Vistaril, Sparine, and Valium potentiate the effects of a narcotic, relieve anxiety and apprehension, and reduce postanesthetic nausea and vomiting. Phenergan is a potent antihistamine and when used with meperidine produces extra sedation, as well as having an antiemetic action.

SCOPOLAMINE

Scopolamine, U.S.P., 0.2 to 0.6 mg (gr 1/320 to 1/100), IM or IV, is an anticholinergic commonly used as a preoperative medication to dry secretions of the oropharyngeal passages. In obstetrics, scopolamine is not used primarily for this action but for a side effect of *amnesia*; when it is combined with a narcotic analgesic the result is *twilight sleep.* The number (formerly great) of patients receiving twilight sleep has diminished in the last few years because of noted side effects.

Scopolamine lasts longer in the body than a narcotic and, as the analgesic effect diminishes, can cause excitation, delirium, and restlessness. Because of amnesia and lack of conscious control, patients may become difficult to manage; they must be kept under close observation, and in some cases restrained. Many women are frightened by the stories they may have heard about "wild talking" under twilight sleep; others react with satisfaction to "not remembering a thing." As more public education about childbirth becomes available, most women may prefer to be awake for their deliveries. Twilight sleep may be useful for a small number of extremely frightened patients.

Scopolamine raises fetal and maternal heart rates and smooths out the normal beat-to-beat variations on the monitor record (Chap. 27); it thus can seriously mask fetal distress. Extreme thirst is the chief complaint of the mother. For these reasons, the use of this drug is decreasing.

METHADONE

When a mother admitted to labor and the delivery unit is on a methadone maintenance program, it is most important that the nurses be aware of her special needs. She is not usually given additional analgesia but may be given an ataraxic or regional anesthesia for pain. She may temperamentally be less able to tolerate the frustration and work of labor and thus need extra support.

Since methadone is usually dispensed from the clinic on a daily basis, the postpartal patient may become very anxious about receiving her medication. The physician must make arrangements with the methadone clinic to have the medication delivered to the postpartal unit. Be careful not to discuss the patient's methadone program with anyone but her doctor and the other nurses involved with her care. Many methadone clients have not discussed the methadone program with their families or friends and may not want them to know about it. It is important that the nursery nurse and the pediatrician be informed in order to give adequate treatment to the baby.

Methadone is transmitted, as are other drugs, across the placenta to the baby, and can seriously depress the respirations of the baby at birth. The seriousness of the withdrawal or the effects of the drug on the baby depend on the amount of the drug and the length of time that the baby has been receiving it.

SEDATIVES, HYPNOTICS

Occasionally, sedatives have been used instead of other drugs for a woman in the early stages of labor. They do not have an analgesic effect, but a sedative one. The barbiturate passes promptly to the fetus, causing respiratory depression; if it is administered, therefore, it should be given very early in labor so that it may be metabolized by the mother before birth takes place.

Two of the more short-acting barbiturates utilized in early labor are:

Seconal (sodium secobarbital)—orally, IM or IV
Nembutal (sodium pentobarbital)—orally, IM or IV

Barbiturates produce drowsiness and calm, and they dispel anxiety. Because of this, nurses should see that external stimuli that interfere with rest and/or sleep are removed from the area of the patient. Such stimuli include noise, bright lights, loud talking, offensive odors, and food odors.

OXYTOCICS

Oxytocin injection, U.S.P. (Pitocin and Syntocinon) (10 units/ml,), act on the smooth muscles of the uterus to stimulate contractions. From 3 to 10 units are diluted in 500 or 1000 ml of Ringer's lactate or 5 percent dextrose in water. In order to have absolute control of the amount infused intravenously, a D_5W intravenous solution should be started and the oxytocic added to a piggyback solution, i.e., the oxytocic is added to a second intravenous solution which is connected via a special insert to the first intravenous solution. The oxytocic solution is always controlled and titrated by the physician, the rate of administration increasing very slowly. As the uterine muscle begins to contract, the rate is adjusted according to the frequency, duration, and intensity of the contractions. As much as 40 drops/min may be given to stimulate beginning contractions; as time elapses the muscle will become more sensitive to the oxytocic solution and the rate of administration must be slowed or the oxytocic discontinued as the status of labor warrants. (See Chap. 25 for nursing responsibility during induction.)

Ideally, infusion machinery such as the *Sage intravenous infusion pump,* the *Ivac peristaltic pump,* or the *Harvard pump,* made for minutely controlling the rate of infusion of intravenous solution and/or medication, is much more accurate than the "drip" method.

Constant monitoring of the fetus is very important. Contractions lasting 1 min or more, and more frequent than 2 min apart, will impair placental circulation and cause hypoxia in the fetus. These *hypertonic contractions* may cause the uterine muscle to tear, rupture, or become exhausted.

anesthesia

The word *anesthesia* indicates that the part affected will have *no sensation.* Anesthetics may provide local or regional numbness with loss of sensation to pain, or they may result in generalized muscle relaxation and loss of sensation because of varying degrees of central nervous system depression.

LOCAL ANESTHESIA

For obstetric use, a local anesthetic can be injected into the tissues around the area to be anesthetized. *Local infiltration* provides a pain-free area for an episiotomy or repair of lacerations. A few minutes for absorption must be allowed before the procedure begins. Mild reactions include dizziness, palpitations, and headache. The mother may be apprehensive about episiotomy repair as she will sense the tugging and pulling of the surrounding tissue and will expect to feel pain, an anxiety similar to that experienced during dental work. A simple explanation that she will have these sensations may help her to relax during suturing.

REGIONAL ANESTHESIA

Regional anesthetics block a group of nerves leading to a region of the body. Medication is injected into or around a nerve pathway or at the plexus of the nerve.

Paracervical Block The paracervical block anesthetizes the hypogastric plexus and ganglia and provides relief from the pain of cervical dilation, especially during the active phase of labor. The injection is made through the vagina at each side of the cervix; care is taken to aspirate before injecting because of the increased supply of blood vessels in the lower uterine area.

Anesthesia is effective for 1 to 2 h. Untoward effects are seen as fetal bradycardia, because of the rapid transfer of the drug across the placenta. Thus careful monitoring of the FHT (fetal heart tone) is essential after paracervical block. Recovery to the normal rate should take place within 5 min. Should a fetus demonstrate persistent bradycardia—longer than 15 to 18 min—a cesarean section may be indicated for fetal distress (Fig. 18·2).

Pudendal Block The pudendal block is an effective regional anesthetic for the second stage of labor and for the delivery. The pudendal nerve plexus lies just above and behind the ischial spine, and the nerve itself supplies sensation to the whole perineal area. A block done just before delivery is effective throughout the delivery and episiotomy repair.

Untoward effects are not seen in the infant. This safe method of anesthesia may not be completely effective for the mother if the injection is slightly out of place. A time period of 5 to 10 min after injecting the anesthetic is preferred to allow for complete numbing of

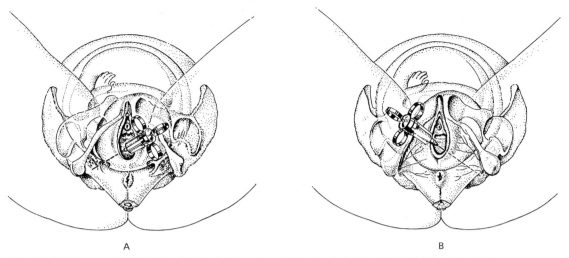

fig. 18·2 A Paracervical. B Pudendal block. (*From* Anesthesia in obstetrics. *Clinical Education Aid No.* 17; *courtesy of Ross Laboratories.*)

the area. Recovery will take place within an hour.

Peridural Anesthesia Peridural anesthesia (outside the dura) is that administered into the bony spinal canal without the needle penetrating into the spinal fluid itself. The local anesthetic surrounds the nerves as they exit from the spinal cord. Signs of effective anesthesia will be seen as the sensation diminishes in the uterus, cervix, and perineum. The lower extremities become tingly and flushed as vasodilation results. Motor control is weak but not absent in the legs.

Because of vasodilation, blood may pool in the extremities, causing maternal hypotension. The immediate treatment is to elevate both legs, in order to return blood to the central circulation. The patient is then turned on her side to reduce uterine pressure on the veins of the pelvic area. Intravenous fluids to maintain adequate blood volume and oxygen by mask to ensure fetal oxygenation are part of the available treatment for hypotension. Fetal bradycardia may result from the primary effect of the drug or as a result of maternal hypotension. Other effects may be dizziness, nausea, and a pounding heart.

CAUDAL ANESTHESIA The injection is made through the opening at the lower end of the sacrum, the *sacral cornua*. The patient must be in a knee-chest position or in a lateral Sims's position. After positioning and explanation, the anesthesiologist inserts a long needle into the caudal space. A test dose of 3 ml anesthetic solution is injected, and the patient is observed for changes in vital signs or any untoward response, for 5 min. The full dose is then administered slowly and the needle withdrawn. At this point, if a continuous caudal anesthetic is planned, a plastic catheter is threaded through the needle and then taped in place after the needle is removed. The continuous method allows a smaller, more frequent dose to be administered throughout the active and advanced active phases and the second stage of labor.

A caudal anesthetic may be administered after the active phase of labor has begun. The anesthesia provides a complete lack of awareness of cervical and uterine discomfort. The mother will not sense a full bladder, nor know when to push during the second stage. The lack of sensation of bladder fullness will persist into the recovery period.

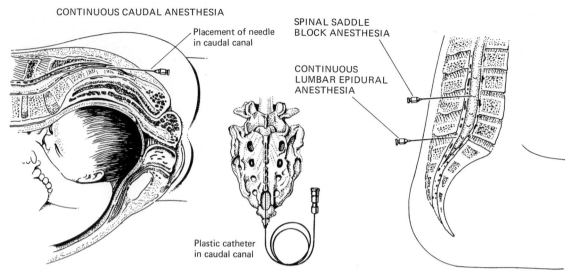

CONTINUOUS CAUDAL ANESTHESIA

Placement of needle
in caudal canal

SPINAL SADDLE
BLOCK ANESTHESIA

CONTINUOUS
LUMBAR EPIDURAL
ANESTHESIA

Plastic catheter
in caudal canal

fig. 18·3 Caudal and epidural anesthesia and saddle block. (*From Clinical Education Aid No. 17; courtesy of Ross Laboratories.*)

EPIDURAL ANESTHESIA The insertion site for an epidural anesthetic is through the lower lumbar area. The patient is positioned on her side, with her neck flexed and knees drawn up to the abdomen. The lower part of the back is prepared as for a spinal tap by cleansing with antiseptic solution. Local infiltration into the superficial tissues with anesthetic precedes the insertion of a long spinal needle into the epidural space. (Aspiration of fluid indicates that the needle has punctured the dura.) A small plastic catheter is then inserted through the needle and the needle withdrawn. The catheter is taped in place to allow the anesthesiologist to administer small amounts of anesthetic into the space at intervals throughout labor and delivery (Fig. 18·3).

Recovery care for the patient who has had an epidural anesthetic is similar to that for the patient who has had a caudal anesthestic. The patient is checked for all the signs of diminishing anesthesia, toe temperature, ability to maintain a normal blood pressure when sitting up or standing, and a return of complete sensation and an ability to control her legs.

The patient may sit or stand when control has returned to her extremities, but the nurse should watch for postural hypotension, fainting, and difficulty in voiding.

Spinal and Saddle Block Anesthesia The spinal and saddle block (low spinal) are closely related methods of anesthesia but differ in position of the patient, amount of medication, and area affected. The spinal is used for cesarean sections, as it blocks nerves of the lower part of the body to the level of the sixth or eighth thoracic nerve, just below the diaphragm. The patient is positioned on the side, asked to arch the lower part of her back and to flex her neck and knees. The nurse usually stands in front of the patient to help her hold her head and knees in this position. A spinal anesthetic is administered on the delivery table just prior to the operation (Fig. 18·4).

Spinal Saddle Block The saddle block is so named because the parts of the body that would come in contact with a saddle are the parts anesthetized. The saddle block can be administered after the patient has completed effacement and dilation of the cervix. The patient is positioned sitting on the side of the

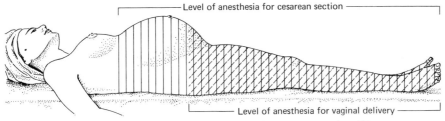

fig. 18·4 Level of anesthesia for vaginal delivery and cesarean section. (*From Clinical Education Aid No.* 17; *courtesy of Ross Laboratories.*)

delivery table, or bed. The nurse should place a stool so that the patient can support her feet, and arm support should also be provided for the patient while she rounds the lower part of her back for the injection. Since the patient is in the descent phase of labor, the position is most uncomfortable (Fig. 18·3).

After a small amount of anesthetic is administered, the patient is kept in a sitting position for about 1 min to allow for the anesthetic to diffuse downward in the spinal fluid. (The anesthetic has been mixed with a glucose solution so that it sinks to the base of the fluid around the cord.) The patient is then placed in a supine position on the delivery table with a pillow to flex the neck. In about 1 min the effects of the anesthetic become evident. It is during this period that careful observation of vital signs is especially important. Hypotension is a frequent side effect of either spinal or saddle block anesthesia, and vital signs should be observed throughout the delivery and into the recovery period (see Fig. 18·5).

Both methods of anesthesia puncture the dura and may result in a "spinal headache." It is thought that the spinal headache is caused by a disequilibrium of spinal fluid pressure due to seepage via the needle puncture site. With administration by a skilled person using a needle with the smallest possible gauge, and with careful nursing care during recovery, very few patients will experience this problem. The patient who has had a spinal anesthetic is kept flat in bed for up to 8 h; she then ambulates carefully, with the nurse

watching for postural hypotension. Personnel on the postpartum unit should be aware of the presence of a patient who has had spinal anesthesia so that they do not inadvertently change her position before she has recovered.

GENERAL ANESTHESIA

General anesthetics are given either by the intravenous route or by inhalation. In effective concentrations they cause unconsciousness by a basic depression of the entire central nervous system. General anesthesia continues to be one of the leading causes of maternal death because of complications such as vomiting and aspiration during anesthesia, and maternal hypotension. Preanesthetic preparation is often not possible for the mother in labor, so that vomiting can be a real danger. Patients who are to have general anesthesia must not be given foods or liquids by mouth during labor, and the last time that food was ingested must be carefully recorded for the information of the anesthesiologist. Digestion and stomach emptying slow naturally during labor, so that even if food and fluids were last taken several hours before admission, the mother may be a poor candidate for general anesthesia.

Perhaps because of this danger, general anesthetics are rarely used today for normal deliveries; when used they are administered just before the actual delivery of the fetal head, and a rather light level of depression is

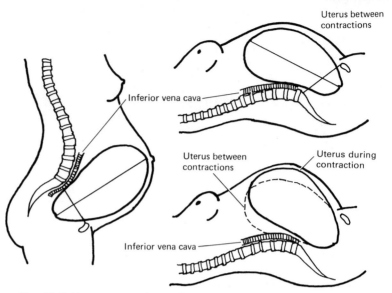

fig. 18·5 Vena cava syndrome. The large uterus presses upon the vena cava as it lies beside the bony spine. When anesthesia relaxes veins, the effect is aggravated. Turning the woman to her side relieves pressure, and blood pressure returns to normal. (*Adapted from John J. Bonica*, Principles and Practices of Obstetric Analgesia and Anesthesia. *F. A. Davis Company, Philadelphia*, 1967, p. 32.)

produced. Because whatever is injected or inhaled will pass quickly into the fetal circulation and depress the fetal respiratory center, anesthesia is induced rather rapidly, with the anesthetist keeping record of the length of time that the infant is subjected to the drug.

Of the available general anesthetics, nitrous oxide, methoxyflurane, and cyclopropane are most commonly used in obstetrics. Precautions against static in the area of inhalation anesthetics and oxygen are set up in each delivery area: conductive shoes; grounded metal fixtures and appliances; conductive rubber matresses and pads on the table. Each person entering the delivery room wears conductive shoes or boots over shoes to reduce the possibility of static sparking.

Recovery Recovery from general anesthetics is gradual and depends upon the depth of anesthesia. The patient should be protected from harm if confusion or restlessness occurs. Side rails are always to be in place. Hypotension is a possibility in re-covery, and pain perception may be distorted. When the patient first requests pain medication, it should be given in half doses, to prevent a possible hypotensive effect. Smooth-muscle activity may be affected, with slowed gastrointestinal motility, and difficulty in voiding as a result.

Vomiting and aspiration are always a danger, even during recovery. Although the patient has had no food or liquids by mouth and perhaps received an anticholinergic drug preoperatively to suppress secretions, suction equipment must always be available. The patient should be on her side or at least with her head turned to the side, so that aspiration will not occur if vomiting takes place.

drugs used postpartally

The processes of involution normally do not require the use of drugs to set them in motion nor to sustain them. If necessary, oxytocics are used to stimulate the uterine muscle, causing it to contract the open sinuses at the site of placental separation from the endometrium, to aid in preventing undue bleeding.

OXYTOCICS

Oxytocin (Pitocin, Syntocinon). From 1 to 2 ml (10 to 20 units) is added to the IV solution left in the bottle after the time of delivery, and the rate of flow is increased to 30 to 40 drops/min, after the delivery of the placenta.

Ergonovine maleate, U.S.P. (Ergotrate), 0.2 mg, orally, intramuscularly, or intravenously. Ergotrate causes the uterus to contract forcibly for a long period. An intravenous or intramuscular injection of ergotrate is given, therefore, *only when it is certain that the placenta is detached* and well into the process of expulsion. Ergotrate may be given orally to sustain the uterine muscle in good contraction for the first 24 h after delivery, 0.2 mg is usually ordered every 4 h for six doses.

Ergotrate has been known to cause elevated blood pressure because of its vasoconstricting (smooth-muscle) effect. Therefore, the drug is *never* administered to patients with hypertension or preeclampsia.

Methylergonovine maleate (Methergine), 0.2 mg, orally, intramuscularly, or intravenously. Its action is similar to that of ergotrate; it is contraindicated in patients with any sign of elevated blood pressure.

Injectable Ergotrate and Methergine should be refrigerated, since they deteriorate with age and exposure to heat and light.

ANALGESICS USED DURING POSTPARTAL PERIOD

Propoxyphene hydrochloride, U.S.P. (Darvon), 65-mg capsules, 1 qid, prn. and Darvon Compound 65 (propoxyphene hydrochloride, aspirin, phenacetin, and caffeine), capsules, 1 qid, prn. Darvon is used for relief of mild to moderate pain in the postpartal patient. Gastrointestinal disturbances, dizziness, headache, and rashes may occur with its use.

Acetylsalicylic acid, U.S.P. (Aspirin), 300-mg tablets, 2 qid. Aspirin is a mild analgesic used in postpartal patients for the relief of pain. It does not produce sedation or euphoria, nor does it disturb the memory. It can produce gastric irritation, and for this reason may be combined with a buffering agent in administration. Some of the side effects include sweating, skin eruptions, and disturbances of sight and hearing. It is often used in combination with other drugs, such as codeine, for synergistic action.

Percodan, a combination of oxycodone, aspirin, homatropine, phenacetin and caffeine, provides relief from moderate and severe pain in the postpartal patient. Since its habit-forming potentiality is greater than that of its relative, codeine, it should be used discretely. Nausea, vomiting, and constipation may occur with its use.

PREVENTION OF BREAST ENGORGEMENT

Mothers who do not wish to nurse their babies may need the aid of a synthetic estrogen to produce sufficient reflex inhibition of the lactogenic hormone to prevent breast engorgement.

Deladumone OB (testosterone enanthate, 360 mg and estradiol valerate, 16 mg), 2 ml deep IM by "Z-track" (see earlier in this chapter, under iron dextran). These drugs, premixed in a single-dose syringe, inhibit the release of lactogenic hormone. The best time for administration is before placental separation during the second stage of labor, but very often Deladumone OB is administered just after delivery or in the recovery room. Because of its thick, viscous consistency, administer it deeply into the upper, outer quadrant of the gluteal muscle, preferably by Z-track technique. Deladumone OB should not be given when malignancy or thrombophlebitis is suspected. Deladumone OB has a delaying affect on weight loss in the first week after delivery, because estrogen inhibits diuresis.

Chlorotrianisene, N.F. (Tace), 12 mg qid for 7 days. Tace is used in the prevention or treatment of breast engorgement. The initial dose should be given within 8 h after delivery. It should not be used where malignancy is suspected.

Ethinyl estradiol, U.S.P.(Estinyl), 0.5-mg tablets, 1 or 2 daily for 3 days, then diminished to two 0.05-mg tablets for 4 days. Estinyl is highly effective in oral usage for the control of postpartal breast engorgement. It may be contraindicated for the patient who has thrombophlebitis.

SEDATIVES

Many mothers find it difficult to sleep the first night after delivery because of overtiredness from a long labor, excitement over childbearing, a strange bed, or the strange noises in the hospital. Because most mothers are in the hospital for only a few days, physicians may prescribe sedatives to ensure sufficient rest and relaxation. *Seconal, Nembutal, chloral hydrate,* or *phenobarbital* may be chosen to provide this desired effect in the postpartal mother.

LAXATIVES

Constipation may be a problem in the postpartal patient. Slowed motility of the bowel during labor, tenderness of the birth tract, and the repaired episiotomy all contribute to the patient's inability to defecate or to her fear of pain upon defecation. *Pericolace, Colace,* and *milk of magnesia* are choices of an effective laxative for the postpartal mother.

IRON

The majority of maternity patients show a slight drop in hemoglobin and hematocrit during pregnancy because of hemodilution. During delivery approximately 200 to 300 ml blood is lost, but usually no anemia results (see Chap. 23). If there has been a greater loss, patients may be given an iron supplement.

VACCINES

Rh immunoglobulin (RhoGAM) is used to build up passive immunization in Rh-negative mothers after delivery of an Rh-positive child. If the Rh mother's serum shows no anti-D antibodies and the infant has a negative reaction to the Coombs test, a single injection is given intramuscularly within 72 h after delivery (see Chap. 29). RhoGAM must be regarded as a transfusion in that the mother's serum is cross-matched with the gamma globulin. The nurse is responsible for cross-checking numbers on the vial with the mother's hospital number to ensure correct identification. The empty vial is returned with the blood bank slip to be held in case of reaction in the patient. Mothers should be completely informed about RhoGAM and its action.

Rubella virus vaccine, live (Cendevax), 0.5 ml subcutaneously (not IM), for active immunization against German measles. Before a woman is given rubella vaccine, she should be given the H.I. (hemagglutinin-inhibition) test to determine her susceptibility to rubella. If she is susceptible, she should be given the vaccine *after,* never during, her pregnancy. It must be emphasized to the woman that she should not become pregnant for 2 months after receiving the vaccine because of possible viral effect on the fetus. Some reliable method of birth control should be utilized to prevent pregnancy until the 2-month period has elapsed. The vaccine can be given any time during the postpartal period. (See Chap. 20 for complete discussion.)

bibliography

Asperheim, M., and L. Eisenhower: *The Pharmacologic Basis of Patient Care,* 2d ed., W. B. Saunders Company, Philadelphia, 1973.

Babson, S. G., and R. C. Benson: *Management of the High-risk Pregnancy and Intensive Care of the Neonate,* The C. V. Mosby Company, St. Louis, 1971.

Baggish, M. S., and S. Hooper: "Aspiration as a Cause of Maternal Death," *Obstetrics and Gynecology,* **43**(2):327, 1974.

Bergersen, B. S., and A. Goth: *Pharmacology in Nursing,* 12th ed., The C. V. Mosby Company, St. Louis, 1973.

Bonica, J. J.: "Obstetric Analgesia and Anesthesia: Recent Trends and Advances," *New York Journal of Medicine,* **70**(7):79, 1970.

Bowes, W., Jr., Y. Brackbill, E. Conway, et al.: "The Effects of Obstetrical Medication on the Fetus and Infant," *Monograph of the Society for Research in Child Development,* (137), **35**(4):1970.

Matthews, A. E. B.: "Drugs in the First Stage of Labor," *Nursing Times,* **63**:648, 1967.

Miller, A.: *Physicians Desk Reference,* Medical Economics, Inc., Oradell, N.J., 1971–1974.

————: "The DES Controversy," *Contemporary OB/GYN,* **3**(1):81, 1974.

Yerushalmy, J.: "The Effects of Smoking on Offspring," *Contemporary OB/GYN,* **1**(5):13, 1972.

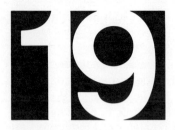

pharmacologic factors for fetus and newborn

Martha Olsen Schult

. . . because of the improved technology in modern obstetrics and the proliferation of drugs, a major obstetric danger may now be medication itself.

Brackbill et al. (1)

The health of the newborn and his future health are influenced by his heredity and by his prenatal environment. Although little can be done to influence genetic makeup, much can be done to influence and modify the environment of the fetus. Good nutrition, good health of the mother, and placing a limit on her drug intake and exposure to toxic chemicals can help to make the fetal environment as safe as possible.

Fetology, the study of the fetus in its environment, is seeking, through extensive research, to determine the effects of nutrition, organisms, disease, chemicals, radiation, and other stresses on the development of the fetus. Amniocentesis, intrauterine treatment such as transfusion, and fetal monitoring are providing clues to the world of the fetus. *Teratology,* the study of the changes in a fetus because of environmental effects, is developing as a separate discipline.

The concept of a "placental barrier" that protects the fetus from maternal ingestants is no longer valid. It must be assumed that whatever drug or chemical the mother takes the baby also receives, and at approximately the same dosage. As long as the fetus is connected with its mother via the placental circulation, the drugs that are transferred to the fetus are returned to her circulation for breakdown and excretion. Metabolism and excretion of nontoxic drugs become a problem only when the child is born with the maternal dosage (or a high percentage of it) in its bloodstream. Its liver, kidney, and enzyme functioning will not be mature enough to handle the metabolism of such high drug levels. This immaturity of the metabolic and excretory functions may cause excessive levels of drugs and their metabolites to remain in the infant's body for many days after birth.

There is no standard dosage of drugs for the newborn, nor any rule for calculating dosages for premature or full-term newborn infants. Empirical evidence, suggestions from the drug companies, laboratory tests, and reports of adverse reactions of a particular drug are but guides for use in calculating dosages of drugs for the newborn. Drug response in the infant is radically different from that in older children and adults. Factors affecting the response in the newborn are linked to the maturity of the body enzymes and the rate of absorption and route of excretion of the drug. It follows that the less mature the infant, the more difficulty there will be with drug dosage and response.

The time during pregnancy that drugs are ingested will make a difference in their effect on the fetus. During the first 12 weeks, organogenesis may be interrupted and basic body structure changed by impinging foreign chemicals. Only since the early 1960s have all new drugs been studied specifically for teratogenic effects, and then mainly on laboratory animals. Often the application of conclusions to human beings is not possible. Most studies on human beings are, and of course must be, retrospective.

Some drugs may not change body structure but may be *fetotoxic,* causing metabolic changes, electrolyte imbalance, central nervous system or respiratory depression, and (in the case of narcotic addiction or alcoholism) causing withdrawal symptoms in the newborn (Table 19·1).

Sedative, analgesic, and anesthetic drugs affect the central nervous system of the mother and her unborn fetus. The timing of the dose and the level in the mother's blood at the time of delivery are the decisive factors in the amount of infant depression. There are varying reports on optimum time of administration. Recent research indicates that it may be the metabolites of sedative and analgesic drugs given early in labor which have a long-lasting effect on the infant after birth, and the depressant effects of drugs given 2 to 3 h prior to delivery which may depress the respiratory centers, causing apnea and difficulty with resuscitation at birth. There remains a very narrow margin of safety. Effects, of course, increase with increasing dosages (1).

Knowledge gained about the long-lasting effects of heavy maternal sedation during labor will perhaps change the current practices of administering analgesics in labor. Studies are being conducted to determine in an unbiased way the immediate and ultimate results of obstetric analgesia and anesthesia on the newborn. Until conclusions are clear, medications to make the mother comfortable should be given as judiciously as possible; they affect the mother for less than a day, but their effect in the infant may last for its lifetime.

After being affected by labor analgesia and anesthesia, infants may have prolonged recovery periods. Sucking and feeding behavior may be slow, and extra mucus may be present, especially during the second period of reactivity. The mother finds it more difficult to feed her infant, who requires more stimulation to suck, and falls asleep easily. This poor feeding behavior may disrupt the initial intimacy between mother and infant and have a cumulative and lasting effect on the development of the mother-child relationship.

An early study by Stechler (2) indicated that depressant medications in labor (meperidine, alphaprodine, pentobarbital, and promethazine) resulted in significant differences in infant ability to "pay attention" to visual stimuli at 2 and 4 days of life. Recently Brackbill et al. found that meperidine medication during labor had a long-term effect on the "coping ability" of the infant, which lasted through one month of age.

The greater the environmental demands on the infant, and the more complex the action required of him to cope with these demands, the greater the difference in quality of performance among infants in terms of their perinatal premedication history (3).

With the concern over the large number of children in our society with learning disabilities and behavior disturbances, a great deal of attention is being focused on these studies of infant response to medication at birth.

administration of medications

Drugs are administered to the newborn through intravenous, intramuscular, or oral routes, and by instillation. Medications may be instilled into the eyes or occasionally into the ears. With eye medications, care must be taken to place the medication in the conjunctival sac, *not* directly on the pupil. Silver nitrate, the most commonly used eye drug, illustrates this point (see "Silver Nitrate," further on).

Oral medications are administered with a plastic disposable dropper or a rubber-tipped dropper, or are placed in a nipple so that the infant can suck the medication. Oral medications are usually given prior to the feeding while the infant is awake and eager to

table 19.1

POSSIBLE EFFECTS OF MATERNAL DRUG INGESTION ON THE FETUS

MEDICATION TAKEN BY MOTHER	POSSIBLE EFFECTS ON FETUS AND NEWBORN
Anticoagulants:	
Heparin	No untoward effect, quickly metabolized
Coumarins	Fetal hemorrhage, intrauterine death, or long-lasting anticoagulant effect in newborn
Antidiabetic agents:	
Insulin	No proved untoward effect unless severe insulin shock occurs
Oral agents:	
Chlorpropamide	Increased risk of fetal death
Tolbutamide	Neonatal hypoglycemia
	Teratogenic effect (?)
Antihistamines:	
Dimenhydrinate (Dramamine)	No evidence of untoward effect
Cyclizine (Marezine)	
Meclizine (Bonine)	Some suspicion of untoward effect (?)
Diuretics:	
Thiazides	Neonatal thrombocytopenia
	Neonatal electrolyte imbalance
Narcotics:	
Morphine	Respiratory depression, apnea
Meperidine (Demerol)	Hypothermia, slow response to mother
Alphaprodine (Nisentil)	Slow feeding in early neonatal period
Heroin, methadone	Withdrawal symptoms from 24 h up to 6 to 8 weeks
Narcotic antagonists:	
Nalorphine (Nalline)	May depress respirations
Levallorphan (Lorfan)	
Sedatives:	
Phenobarbital	Reduces bilirubin level in neonate
Secobarbital	Large doses cause apnea and depression
Pentobarbital	and depress EEG. All sedatives cause decreased responsiveness in early neonatal period
Thalidomide	Congenital anomalies proved
Ethyl alcohol	Withdrawal symptoms if mother is a chronic alcoholic
Steroids:	
Androgenic steroids:	
Testosterone:	Masculinization of female fetus in early months of development
Progestins (and some synthetic estrogens)	
Diethylstilbestrol	Vaginal carcinoma after puberty in some instances
Corticosteroids:	
ACTH, hydrocortisone	Cleft palate, cleft lip(?)

table 19·1 (continued)

Tranquilizers:	
Chlorpromazine (Thorazine)	Do not depress the fetus or newborn.
Promethazine (Phenergan)	Heavy doses may cause alteration
Hydroxyzine (Atarax, Vistaril)	of infant behavior for several months
Meprobamate (Miltown)	(withdrawal)
Benzodiazepines (Librium, Valium)	
Vitamins:	
Vitamin K analogues	Hyperbilirubinemia, kernicterus
Vitamin D_2 (irradiated ergosterol)	Large doses may cause congenital
	cardiac anomalies

suck. Medication is not generally mixed with the formula unless it is administered by nasogastric or gavage tube, as the taste of the milk may be changed. Since such small doses are ordered, medication must be measured by a calibrated dropper or a tuberculin syringe. When medications are administered by dropper, place the dropper tip at the back of the tongue to stimulate the sucking reflex. Hold the baby in the usual feeding position to promote swallowing without aspiration (Fig. 19·1).

Intramuscular administration is usually into the *vastus lateralis,* the major muscle of the quadriceps femoris (Fig. 19·2). Gluteal muscles are not sufficiently developed to be used for injections. Injections into this area could impinge on the sciatic nerve, either directly or by the irritation and swelling resulting from the medication. Since nerve damage sometimes occurs, even when injections are carefully given in the vastus lateralis muscle, it is best to use the oral route whenever possible.

When giving intramuscular injections, the procedure is changed in minor ways from that used for adults. After checking the order and drug, determine the best way to measure the amount (usually a tuberculin syringe is used) and draw up the medication. Check the infant's arm band against the medication card. Palpate the area to determine the injection site (either midanterolateral or upper anterolateral is acceptable). Restrain the leg, and grasp the muscle tissue with one hand, in-

serting the needle with the other. Nurses need not *thrust* the needle into the muscle, since newborn skin is very tender and the needle readily inserted. Aspirate, and then inject very slowly. If injection is made too rapidly, the medication enters the surrounding tissue under pressure and causes more swelling and irritation than with slow injection. Each medication is then charted and the infant observed for the effect.

Intravenous administration may be ordered when the infant cannot retain fluids given orally, when high doses of antibiotics are needed, or when electrolyte or glucose imbalance is present.

A sick infant can become dehydrated very rapidly because of a rapid metabolic rate, immature kidneys that do not efficiently concentrate urine, and a large skin surface in

fig. 19·1 Feeding infant with medication by dropper.

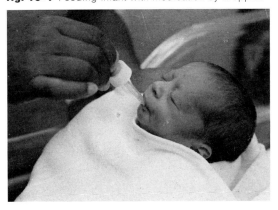

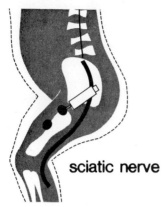

sciatic nerve

fig. 19·2 Intramuscular injection sites for newborn and preterm infants. (*From E. J. Dickason, and A. Ritz, Normal Premature Infant, McGraw-Hill Book Company, New York, 1970.*)

comparison with body weight. The principles of intravenous therapy outlined in Chap. 30 for premature infants are readily applicable for full-term infants as well.

types of medications in use

At the present time several drugs are used prophylactically for most newborns. The high incidence of gonorrhea in the population and the tragic effect of blindness resulting from neonatal gonorrheal infection have led to prophylactic treatment of all newborn infants in the delivery room. Newborn infants often have a lowered level of vitamin K until they are well established on oral feedings; therefore, vitamin K is routinely ordered on the birth day.

VITAMIN K

The newborn's ability to use vitamin K is dependent upon his gestational age; an increased prothrombin time will be present the first 3 to 7 days of life in the term infant and will persist 10 to 14 days in the preterm infant (4). A fluid preparation of vitamin K_1 is administered in a 0.5- to 1.0-mg dose by intramuscular injection into the vastus lateralis

muscle. If any surgical procedure is to be done in the early days of life, it is of utmost importance that the infant have received the injection and that the prothrombin time be tested before the procedure (Fig. 19·3).

SILVER NITRATE AND PENICILLIN

A variety of medications is available to prevent gonoccocal infection of the newborn (*gonococcal conjunctivitis,* sometimes termed *gonococcal ophthalmia neonatorum*). Some states have legislated the drug to be used, others are more flexible and allow a choice of drug. Silver nitrate 1 percent is still recommended by the Committee on Drugs of the American Academy of Pediatrics. One or two drops are placed in the conjunctival sac and then flushed out with sterile physiologic saline solution. Silver nitrate can discolor the skin and is rather irritating to the mucosa; therefore the rinse should be thorough. Infants often react to silver nitrate with slightly reddened and swollen eyelids. Explanation can be made to the concerned mother. Waiting to instill the eye drops until the mother and father have had a chance to see and hold the infant in the delivery area is important, since later the infant will not open its eyes easily if there is a reaction to the medication.

Penicillin ophthalmic ointment (100,000 units/Gm) is also used for eye prophylaxis. It is less irritating to the conjunctiva, but it may be more unsightly, since the ointment remains in the eye and around the eyelashes. The new mother may be alarmed by this apparent exudate unless she receives an explanation. Again, waiting for the parents' first look at the baby before instilling the ointment is important.

SEDATIVES AND TRANQUILIZERS

Some infants are born to addicted mothers. The severity of withdrawal for the infant will depend to a large extent on the dose the mother was taking and the duration of ex-

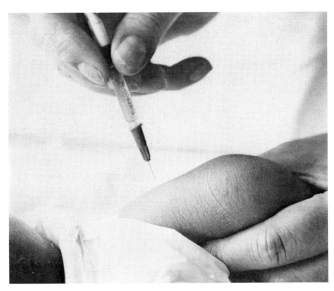

fig. 19·3 Vitamin K injection into midanterior thigh. (*Photo by Ruth Helmich.*)

posure of the fetus. The time of the mother's last dose and the age and condition of the infant also affect the recovery period. The infant usually will appear normal at birth and gradually develop the symptoms of tremors, irritability, "distressed, shrill cry," poor feeding, and perhaps vomiting and diarrhea. Convulsions are rare with treatment. Swaddling the infant and providing warmth and support through this period with fluids and medication allow most infants to withdraw successfully.

Phenobarbital Phenobarbital elixir (2 to 3 mg/kg q6h) may be chosen to depress the central nervous system and calm the newborn. One of the side effects of phenobarbital has been demonstrated to be the lowering of the bilirubin level. Phenobarbital dose is adjusted according to the infant's condition and response, of course. Treatment is maintained for 2 to 3 weeks, during which time the dosage is gradually lowered.

Paregoric Camphorated opium tincture U.S.P. (paregoric) contains a 4 percent tincture of opium. It is usually ordered by drops per kilogram (1 to 2 drops/kg every 4 to 6 h). After symptoms have been controlled, the

dose is gradually reduced by 10 percent per day. Treatment may have to be continued for several weeks. If the infant is sent home before being completely withdrawn, the mother or caretaker should be thoroughly instructed in the method of administration and be given a syringe or calibrated dropper to use so that the dose will be accurately measured.

Chlorpromazine (Thorazine) Thorazine (0.75 mg/kg q6h) is administered intramuscularly until fluids are retained, and then orally. Thorazine is most often used in difficult cases when the above two methods are not able to control symptoms. As a tranquilizer, it acts to reduce agitation and central nervous system irritability.

NARCOTIC ANTAGONISTS

Narcotics used during labor, or present in the mother's circulation prior to delivery in cases of narcotic addiction, can cause *narcosis* in the newborn. Severely narcotized infants at birth are in respiratory difficulty and experience apnea and asphyxia. The interference with the respiratory center function results in biochemical asphyxia with hypoxia, hypercapnia, and a lower pH.

Antagonists to opioid drugs are *Nalline, Lorfan,* and *Narcan.* In some instances these drugs are administered to the mother before birth, and in rare instances are given directly to the infant. Care must be taken to be sure that the cause of respiratory depression is a narcotic, since Nalline may have a powerful respiratory depressant effect if used alone.

> *Nalorphine* (Nalline) is used to overcome depression from morphine and morphine-like drugs. Given to the mother before delivery, it can prevent respiratory depression in the infant. It is not effective against barbiturate- or general anesthetic–based depression. Dosage for the mother is in the range of 3 to 10 mg IV prior to delivery, and for the newborn, 0.2 mg via the umbilical vein or by the intramuscular route.
>
> *Levallorphan* (Lorfan) is used to counteract depression caused by narcotics. Lorfan may be administered to the mother prior to delivery (1 mg IV 5 to 10 min before delivery) or 0.05 mg to the newborn via umbilical vein or intramuscularly. Occasionally when a potent drug such as Nisentil is used for analgesia, Lorfan is administered subcutaneously with Nisentil.
>
> *Naloxone* (Narcan) may be given in doses of 0.4 mg IV, IM, or subcutaneously to the mother in labor to counteract the depressive effect of narcotics. Although it has been used for a few newborns without adverse effects, the evidence for its use is inconclusive, and it is recommended that Narcan not be used for the infant.

ANTIBIOTICS

Antibiotics are ordered by doses calculated per kilogram of body weight. Some of the antibiotics thought to be safe for the newborn are discussed below.

> *Kanamycin* (Kantrex), oral or intramuscular injection (15 mg/kg/day divided into two doses at 12-h intervals), is useful for short-term administration for the newborn. Kanamycin is especially effective in treating infant diarrhea caused by *Escherichia coli,* and in *Klebsiella-* and *Proteus*-induced infections. It is not recommended for long-term therapy because of its potential nephrotoxic and ototoxic action. It is not used with gram-negative *Pseudomonas* infections.
>
> *Neomycin* (50 to 100 mg/kg/day divided into four to six doses) as an oral preparation is useful in the treatment of gastrointestinal disorders caused by *E. coli.* Its effectiveness is limited to the gastrointestinal tract; parenteral administration is not advised.
>
> *Mycostatin* (Nystatin), oral suspension (200,000 units/day in four divided doses), is used for its antifungal activity against *Candida (Monilia) albicans,* the cause of thrush in the newborn. Its absorption from the gastrointestinal tract is limited—thus its specific use for gastrointestinal infections. Adverse reactions are negligible unless very large doses are used.
>
> *Penicillin G* (100,000 to 200,000 units/kg/day, IM or IV, in two divided doses) is used for a variety of infections caused by gram-positive organisms, especially hemolytic *Streptococcus, Staphylococcus,* and *Pneumococcus.* Procaine penicillin is never used with young infants.
>
> *Ampicillin* (Polycillin) (IM or IV, 200 mg/kg/day in four divided doses) is used for a variety of gram-positive and gram-negative organisms. Its bactericidal activity makes it useful in treating many infections in the newborn.
>
> *Cephalothin* (Keflin) (IM, 50 to 100 mg/kg/

day in four to six doses) and *Cephalexin* (Keflex) (25 to 50 mg/kg/day orally) are broad-spectrum antibiotics in current use. Research on the effects of these drugs in the neonate is still incomplete.

The best therapy is preventive, so that drugs will not have to be used routinely for the newborn. When drugs are necessary, precautions in dosage and administration by the nurse are as important as the selection of a nontoxic drug by the physician.

references

1. Y. Brackbill, J. Kane, R. L. Manniello, and D. Abramson: "Obstetric Premedication and Infant Outcome," *American Journal of Obstetrics and Gynecology,* **118**(3):383, 1974.
2. G. Stechler, "Newborn Attention as Affected by Medication during Labor," *Science,* **144**:315, 1964.
3. Brackbill et al., op. cit., p. 382.
4. Marshall H. Klaus and Avroy Fanaroff, *Care of the High-risk Neonate,* W. B. Saunders Company, Philadelphia, 1973, p. 273.

bibliography

Adamssons, K., and I. Joelsson: "The Effects of Pharmacologic Agents on the Fetus and Newborn," *American Journal of Obstetrics and Gynecology,* **96**:437, 1966.

Behrman, R. E., and D. E. Fisher: "Phenobarbital for Neonatal Jaundice," *Journal of Pediatrics,* **76**:945, 1970.

Borgstedt, A. D., and M. G. Rosen: "Medication during Labor Correlated with Behavior and EEG of the Newborn," *American Journal of Diseases of Children,* **115**:21, 1968.

Cohen, S. N., and T. K. Olson, Jr.: "Drugs That Depress the Newborn," *Pediatric Clinics of North America,* **17**:835, 1970.

Davies, P. R.: "Bacterial Infection in the Fetus and Newborn," *Archives of Diseases in Childhood,* **46**:245, 1971.

Green, H. Gordon: "Infants of Alcoholic Mothers," *American Journal of Obstetrics and Gynecology,* **118**(5):713, 1974.

Lenz, W. : "How Can the Teratogenic Action of a Factor Be Established in Man?" *American Journal of Diseases of Children,* **112**:99, 1966.

Stone, M. L., L. J. Salerno, M. Green, and C. Zelson: "Narcotic Addiction in Pregnancy," *American Journal of Obstetrics and Gynecology,* **109**:716, 1971.

Sutherland, J. M., and I. J. Light: "The Effects of Drugs on the Developing Fetus," *Pediatric Clinics of North America,* **12**:781, 1965.

Wilson, James G.: "Environmental Effects on Development and Teratology," chap. 5 in N. Assali (ed.), *Pathophysiology of Gestation: Fetal-Placental Disorders,* vol. 2, Academic Press, Inc., New York, 1972.

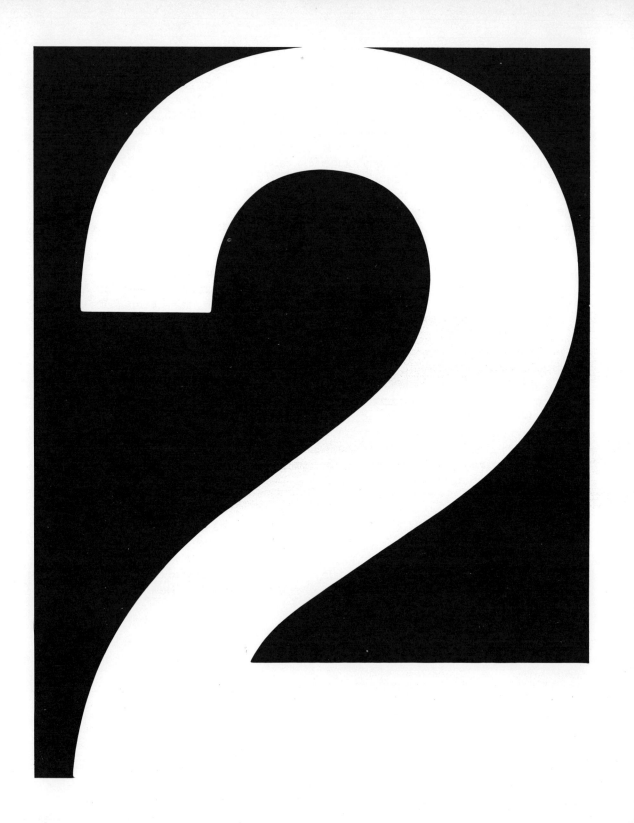

the high-risk mother and infant

A high-risk pregnancy is one that does not progress within the usual pattern. Problems may stem from medical, psychologic, obstetric, and socioeconomic causes, or a combination of these causes. A high-risk pregnancy is a gestation that may produce an abortion or a stillbirth, or which may result in a stressed, malformed, or premature infant. These complicated pregnancies, on the other hand, may result in a normal infant but present a real stress to the mother's health and well-being.

The term "reproductive wastage" aptly describes a pregnancy which is ended by death or disability of the fetus. Causes of difficulty in the pregnancy include diseases existing prior to the pregnancy which impinge on the health of the mother and fetus, complications caused by the pregnancy, and complications occurring during the delivery and newborn periods.

A high-risk pregnancy may result in the conception being lost by spontaneous abortion before the age of viability. About 15 percent of all conceptions are lost in this way. Many of the reasons for spontaneous abortion are unknown, but the known maternal factors include poor nutrition, anemia, borderline fertility, and maternal chronic disease. About 30 percent of the aborted conceptions are lost because of poor implantation or because of a malformed, poorly developing embryo. Fortunately the body will often spontaneously reject a malformed conceptus, thus reducing the numbers of infants born with serious birth defects.

After the age of viability the rate for an abnormal outcome is higher than one would expect; 3 to 5 percent of all these surviving pregnancies end in stillbirth or neonatal death. Part of the reason for this rate is that the high-risk pregnancy may result in an infant born too early, before its development is completed. Such an infant is handicapped by immaturity in every body system. Immaturity and low birth weight are no longer synonymous, although about two-thirds of the low-birth-weight infants (under 2500 Gm) are also immature in development. Other infants, though immature in development, may be born with an adequate body weight (over 2500 Gm). About one-third of the low-birth-weight infants are fully developed but have poor fetal weight gain because of intrauterine stress or malnourishment. Whatever the case, if all low-birth-weight infants are included in a single group, they account for about 64 percent of all deaths in the first year of life, even though low-birth-weight infants make up only about 10 percent of all infants born.

The handicaps and long-term effects produced by intrauterine stress or malnourishment are being widely studied. If the infant is subjected to a reduced nutritional or oxygen supply, inevitable effects occur that prevent optimal development. Only in the last few decades have the results of reduced oxygen levels during the perinatal period been fully recognized (1). The injury to the fetal brain may be severe (resulting in cerebral palsy or mental retardation) or less severe but just as significant (resulting in minimal brain dysfunction which causes learning disabilities or disturbed behavior). Both retrospective and prospective studies are in progress to determine the full implications of perinatal asphyxia. For instance, in one study of a group of children who had suffered perinatal asphyxiation 16 years before, it was found that these children now had similar behavior patterns when compared with controls, but that under stress they showed significantly more behavior disturbances.

It is becoming clear that in dealing with the high-risk pregnancy we must be as concerned for the long-term outcome for the infant as we are for the immediate comfort and safety of the mother. For instance, medication to reduce the discomfort of labor is of immediate benefit to the laboring woman, but its ultimate value must be measured against the years of difficulty for the child should it become hypoxic and its functions depressed during the process of birth. Because of the many factors which we now know lead to future disability in children, a sense of responsibility for the future well-being of all children needs to permeate the thinking of those handling obstetric management and nursing support of the high-risk pregnancy.

morbidity and mortality rates

The term *morbidity* comes from the word *morbid*, meaning "abnormal," "pathologic," or "sick." The morbidity rate is the rate of occurrence of a particular disease expressed in a ratio with a given nonsick population. In making statistical statements it is important to define the given population in each situation.

infant mortality

The *infant mortality rates* include all deaths from the day of birth through the end of eleventh month (the first birthday). From the brief listing in Table I it can be seen that most infants who die do so within the *neonatal pe-riod*, that period which extends from birth through the first 28 days of life. (To obtain the death rate for the period from one month through eleven months, subtract the neonatal from the infant mortality rate.) The *perinatal death rate* includes all deaths from the period of viability (the beginning of the twentieth week in utero) through the first 28 days of life and is quoted as a ratio per 1000 births. Neonatal and infant death rates are quoted as a ratio per 1000 *live* births. Thus in order to read the rates of survival, or the rates of death, in a given year one must know the number of births for that year.

maternal mortality and morbidity

Maternal mortality refers to the death of a woman while pregnant or within 90 days after the end of the pregnancy, no matter how it was terminated. The overall United States maternal mortality rate is an average of all groups and is reported as per 100,000 live births.

Causes of death are currently listed as sepsis, toxemia, hemorrhage, ectopic pregnancy, abortion, and other complications. Table II gives the figures for 1967–1968. Since that time, the advent of legalized abortion in several states has reduced the numbers of maternal deaths due to abortion. In the last decade deaths due to toxemia have dropped by 50 percent, whereas deaths due to infection have remained at the same rate of occurrence. Increased understanding of how to diagnose and treat ectopic pregnancy and hemorrhage has reduced the deaths due to these causes by about 50 percent.

When the average death rate is broken down into "white and nonwhite," a huge discrepancy becomes apparent (see Table III). The rate of death among nonwhite mothers in our society (three to four times higher than for white mothers) is a scandal most directly attributable to the effects of poverty. This is underscored by the fact that the rates even out if mothers are divided along socioeco-

table I

INFANT AND NEONATAL DEATH RATES*

	1950	1960	1970	1972
Births	3,632,000	4,258,000	3,718,000	3,256,000
Infant death rate	29.2	26.0	19.8	18.2
Neonatal death rate	20.5	18.7	14.9	13.7

*Rates per 1000 live births.

table II

CAUSES OF MATERNAL MORTALITY IN THE UNITED STATES, 1967–1968

	WHITE	NONWHITE	TOTAL
Sepsis	3.4	7.2	4.0
Toxemia	3.0	13.5	4.8
Hemorrhage	2.7	7.3	3.5
Ectopic pregnancy	1.0	7.4	2.1
Abortion	2.3	13.4	4.2
All causes	18.1	66.6	26.3

Source: *Statistical Bulletin*, vol. 53, Metropolitan Life Assurance Company, New York, June, 1972.

table III

MATERNAL MORTALITY RATES*

	1950	1957	1960	1967	1970	1972
Overall rate	83.3	39.2	37.1	28.0	27.4	24.7 (780 women)
White	61.1	26.0	26.0	19.5	NA	NA
Nonwhite	221.6	108.0	97.9	69.5	NA	NA

*Rate per 100,000 live births.
Note: NA, not available.
Source: Division of Vital Statistics, National Center for Health Statistics, Washington.

table IV

MATERNAL MORTALITY IN THE UNITED STATES BY REGION, 1967–1968

	WHITE	NONWHITE	TOTAL
United States	18.1	66.6	26.3
New England	11.3	41.1	13.0
Middle Atlantic	17.6	84.0	28.0
East North Central	17.8	71.7	25.1
West North Central	13.7	49.9	16.4
South Atlantic	16.0	63.2	29.6
East South Central	24.2	89.8	42.5
West South Central	24.9	58.3	32.1
Mountain	23.6	57.6	26.7
Pacific	17.7	37.8	20.5

Source: Division of Vital Statistics, National Center for Health Statistics, Washington.

CHARACTERISTICS AND CONDITIONS OF PREGNANCY
WHITE

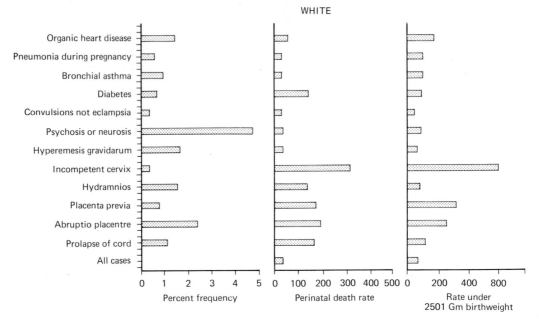

CHARACTERISTICS AND CONDITIONS OF PREGNANCY
NEGRO

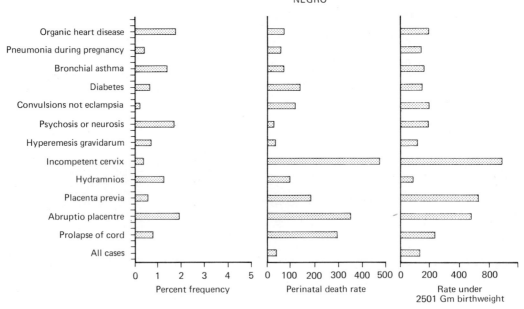

fig. 1 Birthweight and perinatal mortality associated with maternal problems during pregnancy. (*From Kenneth R. Niswander and Myron Gordon,* The Women and Their Pregnancies, *The Collaborative Study of the National Institute of Neurological Disease and Stroke, W. B. Saunders Company, Philadelphia,* 1972.)

nomic lines rather than racial lines. The problem of high-risk pregnancy can be further illustrated by the regional statistics found in Table IV. Areas of the country with a higher mortality rate have more rural or urban poor mothers, both white and nonwhite.

maternal morbidity

Maternal morbidity during the pregnancy period, excluding deaths from abortion, ectopic pregnancy, and toxemia, can be seen on a comparative basis in Fig. I. The figures are slightly lower than the national average because the mothers in this perinatal study (2) received adequate prenatal care.

Most studies come to the conclusion that the overall risk of a complicated pregnancy is influenced by the prior health and socioeconomic level of the mother. Despite the many advances of the last decade, women in our country may be at a disadvantage when it comes to preventive obstetric care. The location, expense, waiting, and travel time prevent poor women who work during the day or who have overwhelming family responsibilities from seeking prenatal care. Medical practitioners and obstetricians are concentrated in the private care sectors, leaving a number of clinics only minimally staffed, or others partially staffed with foreign medical personnel who may have communication difficulties with patients.

We must recognize that poverty creates a cycle that is most difficult to break. Schneider states:

The socioeconomic factors making for high risk pregnancy reduce themselves in practice to one: poverty. In theory, a number of independent factors might be singled out, but in actuality, they manifest themselves as a vast Gordian knot of overcrowding, poor nutrition, fatigue, dirt, maternal stature, poor education, and the need to work even during a difficult pregnancy. . . . (3)

In urban areas where recent immigrants to the city struggle with overwhelming adjustments, a visit to the clinic may be too frightening a process to undertake voluntarily. The woman waits until there is no alternative and problems already exist. In rural areas, poverty, fear, and prejudice are as debilitating as they are in the city. Also, distances are more of a factor to consider in seeking care, for most poor women will not go for preventive care if the clinic is too far from their homes.

When we quote statistics showing nonwhite mothers with a more than double mortality and morbidity rate, and a much higher infant mortality rate in our society, Schneider's statement should be burned into our minds: "The repeatedly noted higher risk among black women is not due to any genetic or racial factor but to the fact that so many of them are poor" (4). That statement can be applied to any group of poor women who show an increased rate of trouble during their pregnancies.

There are signs of hope that some resolution of these problems is taking place.

The pages to follow will discuss the factors precipitating problems in pregnancy and detail the medical and nursing care of the mother and her infant.

references

1. Y. Brackbill, J. Kane, R. L. Manniello, and D. Abramson: "Obstetric Premedication and Infant Outcome," *American Journal of Obstetrics and Gynecology,* **118**(3):377, 1974.
2. Kenneth R. Niswander and Myron Gordon, *The Women and Their Pregnancies,* The Collaborative Perinatal Study of the National Institute of Neurological Diseases and Stroke, W. B. Saunders Company, Philadelphia, 1972.
3. Jan Schneider, "The High-risk Pregnancy," *Hospital Practice,* October, 1971, p. 133.
4. Ibid., p. 135.

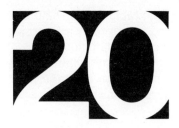

infectious diseases during pregnancy and the puerperium

Herbert S. Heineman

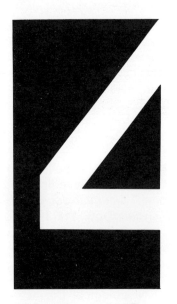

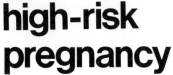

high-risk pregnancy

During pregnancy, the types of infection acquired and their method of acquisition are essentially the same as during the non-pregnant state. Etiologically, therefore, infection during pregnancy is mere coincidence. The need to consider this coincidence as a subject at all arises in part from the alterations in physiology which may modify the woman's response to infection, but even in this respect, as far as the mother is concerned, such modifications are only quantitative. Of much greater concern is the fetus, for whom maternal infection may have far-reaching, possibly fatal, consequences.

Puerperal infections, on the other hand, are strictly complications of childbirth. In the true sense of the term, they may be regarded as wound infections. As such, they are significant, sometimes fatal, for the mother but of no consequence to the infant.

When infection occurs during pregnancy, questions naturally arise about the safety of both mother and child. It is reassuring to know, therefore, that the majority of infections may be treated in the usual manner without harm to either. Little thought needs to be given, for example, to the common respiratory and intestinal infections which most women may experience at least some time during a 9-month pregnancy. In some cases, such minor upsets lead to excessive disability when added to the burden of pregnancy. It is difficult to determine, however, whether the physiologic or metabolic alterations of pregnancy have anything to do with this phenomenon or whether fatigue, muscle strain, and health consciousness merely lower the threshold for symptoms. From a practical point of view, since infected cuts, colds, and viral gastroenteritis are virtually unavoidable in any case, it is probably in the best interest of the patient to permit normal human contact and activities.

Life-threatening infections, such as meningitis, pneumonia, or septicemia, may result in abortion or stillbirth. In these cases, however, damage to the fetus is merely an extension of the extreme metabolic or circulatory insult suffered by the mother; in the less severe cases, the pregnancy may proceed normally to term following control of the infection.

This chapter is concerned chiefly with those infections that bear a unique relationship to pregnancy. The relationship may take one of two forms: (1) the pregnant woman is particularly susceptible to the infection, copes with it less well, or more readily suffers complications than her nonpregnant counterpart; (2) development of the fetus, or the pregnancy itself, is threatened out of proportion to the severity of the maternal illness. In the management of infections, furthermore, consideration must be given to the effect of antimicrobial drugs on the fetus.

infections related to increased susceptibility during pregnancy

INFECTIONS AND HEART DISEASE

The mere presence of heart disease does not prevent successful pregnancy. The limiting factor is the ability of the damaged heart to cope with the added circulatory demands of the last trimester. Three infections present particular hazards in terms of heart failure; streptococcal pharyngitis, bacterial endocarditis, and influenza.

Streptococcal Pharyngitis Streptococcal sore throat must be prevented in patients with rheumatic heart disease, for it may be followed by a recurrence of rheumatic fever, with possible heart failure or additional damage to compromised valves. Fortunately, prevention is available in the form of penicillin or other antibacterial agents; their effectiveness is limited only by the regularity with which they are taken. Monthly injections of long-acting penicillin counteract the problem of forgetfulness; many physicians prefer this regimen over any other.

Bacterial Endocarditis Bacterial endocarditis occurs in patients with rheumatic and many forms of congenital heart disease in which the inner lining (endocardium), including the heart valves, is already damaged either by previous inflammation (rheumatic fever) or by misdirected blood flow (congenital abnormalities). Bacterial infection occurring on these scarred surfaces, especially the valves, may inflict enough damage to cause acute heart failure. Severe kidney damage, cerebral embolism due to fragments of bacterial growths, and other complications may occur, necessitating termination of the pregnancy. Bacteria that cause this infection frequently enter the bloodstream from the gums, especially if the periodontal tissues are diseased. Penicillin in fairly high doses is therefore recommended at the time of dental treatments. Unfortunately, though, bacterial endocarditis is not totally preventable.

Influenza For the great majority of people, influenza at worst causes temporary incapacity, with eventual complete recovery. For the person with heart disease, however, even when the influenza is so slight as to cause only minimal restriction of activity, it poses a real danger of progression to pneumonia; this viral pneumonia is much more serious, with a considerably higher mortality rate, than the common bacterial (pneumococcal) pneumonias. The combination of pregnancy and heart disease predisposes a woman more to this complication than does either factor alone. A woman thus predisposed should be protected by immunization as early as possible in the influenza season. Influenza immunization, which involves the injection of killed virus, is harmless to the fetus and can therefore be safely performed during pregnancy.

OTHER INFECTIONS

Poliomyelitis Poliomyelitis is, fortunately, more of historic than of current interest, although it is by no means extinct in the United States. One of the interesting observations in past outbreaks was the susceptibility of pregnant women to the severest paralytic form. Susceptibility probably resulted both from the pregnant state and from the more intimate exposure of these women to young children, who frequently were carriers of the virus. The only protection is immunization, which should be completed in early childhood but can be accomplished at any age and also during pregnancy.

Tuberculosis Pulmonary tuberculosis may relapse during pregnancy, leading to the reopening of healed cavities and the shedding of tubercle bacilli *(Mycobacterium tuberculosis)* in the sputum. Extrapulmonary foci may also be reactivated. In addition to deterioration in the mother's health, consideration must be given to the danger in which the newborn infant is placed. Infection in utero is very rare in this form of tuberculosis, so that the infant is normal at birth. However, he is also highly vulnerable to infection by airborne bacteria, and if the mother is coughing up tuberculosis-positive sputum close to the newborn's face, infection of the neonate can be anticipated.

Good prenatal care should, therefore, include a tuberculin skin test early in pregnancy. If positive, it should be followed by a chest x-ray and such additional studies as are clinically indicated. If active tuberculosis is diagnosed at this time, it can usually be brought under control with appropriate therapy before term, so that the mother can care for her infant in the normal manner. If the infection is not controlled, drastic measures are necessary to protect the infant, including total separation from the mother until her sputum is negative for tubercle bacilli.

Urinary Infection Even in nonpregnant women, the urinary tract is host to more bacterial infections than any other organ system. Most commonly, infection takes the form of *asymptomatic bacteriuria* or cystitis, the latter characterized by burning and the frequent urge to void. Acute pyelonephritis, which is accompanied by shaking chills, high fever, other constitutional symptoms, and pain and tenderness in the area of the kidneys, is the most severe but fortunately quite uncommon form of urinary infection. Pregnancy and the puerperium, however, are associated with an increased incidence of acute pyelonephritis. The altered physiology and anatomic relationships in the abdomen of the pregnant woman undoubtedly help account for this fact, but the actual mechanisms are not fully understood. For practical purposes, it has been found that many potential pyelonephritis victims can be identified early in pregnancy by examination of their urine. The syndrome *asymptomatic bacteriuria in pregnancy* has assumed great importance among obstetricians, since one-quarter to one-third of women affected, if not treated, have been found to develop overt symptoms. Fortunately, this development can be largely prevented by antibiotic treatment during the asymptomatic phase. Culture of the urine (which must be properly collected, under professional supervision, in order to prevent contamination) is, therefore, one of the important components of good prenatal care.

In the majority of women with no history of prior urinary infection, the responsible organism is *Escherichia coli,* which is susceptible to most broad-spectrum antibiotics. If there has been previous infection with antibiotic therapy, less common and more resistant organisms, such as *Klebsiella, Proteus,* and enterococci, may be found. Therapy must then be more carefully selected and the chances for success are diminished.

Vaginitis Of the various kinds of vaginitis, that due to *Candida (Monilia) albicans* is most characteristically linked to pregnancy. It is a benign but uncomfortable fungal infection of the vaginal mucous membrane characterized by intense itching, redness, and frequently a creamy discharge. Although it occurs commonly without apparent predisposing cause, pregnancy (and the pseudopregnant state induced by oral contraceptives) is associated with a higher incidence and greater resistance to treatment. Symptoms respond fairly readily to topical therapy—e.g., use of vaginal tablets containing nystatin—but relapse is common; definitive cure usually follows the end of pregnancy.

Vaginitis due to *Trichomonas vaginalis* is also common during pregnancy. However, pregnancy is not etiologically related to this infection and provides no obstacle to successful therapy; currently, metronidazole is the drug of choice.

infections in pregnancy that affect the fetus

The chief characteristic of the group of infections that affect the fetus during pregnancy is their severity in the fetus—often leading to death or irreversible developmental defects—compared with their benign manifestations in the mother. Their essential features are summarized in Table 20·1.

BRUCELLOSIS

Brucellosis is worth mentioning in a negative sense. *Brucella abortus,* one of the common etiologic agents of brucellosis, characteristically causes abortion when it occurs in cattle. In human beings, however, abortion is not a common feature; the usual presentation of brucellosis is subacute illness with fever, loss of appetite and weight, fatigue, and occasionally symptoms referable to a particular organ.

CYTOMEGALOVIRUS INFECTION (CYTOMEGALIC INCLUSION DISEASE)

Cytomegalovirus is one of a group of viruses that are capable of traversing the placenta and infecting the fetus in utero. The severe congenital malformations first drew attention to this agent because infection acquired after birth is rarely serious and cannot be recognized without special laboratory studies. Most commonly, acquired cytomegalovirus infection is a rather mild febrile illness in childhood, unaccompanied by specific physical findings even though the virus is disseminated throughout the body. In the great majority of affected children, the illness runs its course without diagnosis. If, however, hematologic tests are performed, *lymphocytosis* with many atypical cells may be found, leading to a mistaken diagnosis of infectious mononucleosis (see also "Toxoplasmosis," below). Antibodies are formed, which prevent dissemination of the virus should subsequent reexposure occur. A woman who has escaped infection during childhood may acquire the virus for the first time during pregnancy. She will then undergo a characteristically mild illness, recovering without any damage to herself but with possible extreme damage to, or even lethal effects on, the fetus.

The most vulnerable organ in the young fetus is the brain, which may remain underdeveloped, leading to microcephaly and mental retardation. Jaundice, enlargement of the liver and spleen, purpura, hernias, and other complications may occur.

No preventive measures are available, either in the form of a vaccine or in early treatment of the mother. Since acquired infec-

table 20·1

MATERNAL INFECTIONS POSING A THREAT TO THE FETUS

INFECTION	EASE OF RECOGNITION IN MOTHER[a]	CRITICAL MONTHS OF PREGNANCY	MOST COMMON MANIFESTATIONS IN NEWBORN [b]	PREVENTION	THERAPY
Cytomegalovirus	vs	Unknown	Microcephaly; cerebral calcification; jaundice	None available	None available
Gonorrhea	(C)B	9	Ophthalmitis; septicemia	Antepartum treatment of mother	Antibiotics
Herpes simplex	(C)vs	9	Disseminated infection	Cesarean section[c]	Chemotherapy[d]
Listeriosis	Bs	8–9	Septicemia; meningitis	Antepartum treatment of mother	Antibiotics
Malaria	CMs	Unknown	Fever; nonspecific signs	Antepartum treatment of mother	Chemotherapy
Rubella	CvS	1–3	Cardiac defects; cataracts; deafness	Immunization of mother before pregnancy	None available
Smallpox; vaccination	Cvs	Unknown	Disseminated infection	Vaccinia immune globulin	None available
Syphilis	(C)S	5–9	Bone and tooth deformities; progressive nervous system damage	Antepartum treatment of mother	Antibiotics
Toxoplasmosis	(C)S	4–6[e]	Microcephaly; cerebral calcification; chorioretinitis	Unknown	None available[f]
Tuberculosis	CB	Postpartum	Tuberculous pneumonia; meningitis; disseminated infection	Antepartum treatment of mother; separation from mother after birth	Chemotherapy

[a] C, clinical; B, bacteriologic; V, virologic; S, serologic; M, microscopic. Small letters indicate that tests are specialized and not routinely available. Parentheses indicate that typical features are more often absent than present.

[b] Only characteristic manifestations are listed; many others may be present.

[c] Value not definitely established.

[d] Iododeoxyuridine and cytarabine; insufficient data available for evaluation.

[e] Best available information.

[f] Irreversible damage present at birth.

tion is so difficult to recognize, elimination of this source of congenital anomalies appears to be a formidable task at present. It would be reasonable and feasible to investigate all febrile illnesses during pregnancy at least with a blood count. If atypical lymphocytosis is found, further studies for cytomegalovirus infection would be indicated.

GONORRHEA

Though birth defects due to fetal maldevelopment have not been reported, maternal infection with *Neisseria gonorrhoeae* may endanger the fetus in two ways. *Ophthalmia neonatorum,* or conjunctivitis of the newborn, is believed to result from inoculation of one or both eyes during passage through an infected birth canal. Improperly treated, the infection may result in corneal perforation, destruction of the eye, and blindness. The universal use of topical prophylaxis (generally silver nitrate drops or antibiotic ointments) in the eyes of infants born in American hospitals has reduced the incidence of this infection. More recently, evidence has been presented that gonococcal infection may occur in utero during maternal septicemia; the infant may then be born with neonatal sepsis or pneumonitis.

At least three obstacles prevent total control of neonatal gonococcal infection. The first is the sheer number of women infected, which is constantly increasing. Second is the lack of acquired immunity following infection, making it possible to become infected repeatedly. Third, more than 80 percent of women with active gonorrhea have no symptoms and therefore do not attract attention to the possibility of this diagnosis. Proper handling of this problem requires routine culture of the cervix during the last month of pregnancy. Because of the intensified care of pregnant women at this time, obtaining a cervical culture should be an easy matter, but the obstetrician must be aware of the special growth requirements of gonococci and use appropriate culture technique. (Public health departments cooperate very willingly in this endeavor.) Treatment can then be instituted, usually with penicillin, and danger to the newborn can be minimized.

HEPATITIS

Because of the occasional occurrence of hepatitis in the newborn infant, a possible relationship has been sought with infectious hepatitis in the mother. No relationship, however, has ever been proved. With the recent discovery of hepatitis-associated antigen (Australia antigen), it has been possible to use laboratory techniques to look for transplacental transfer of a possible etiologic agent in hepatitis; this research has been mostly negative. Hepatitis, therefore, seems to have no significance beyond its effect on the mother herself.

HERPES SIMPLEX

Two strains of herpes simplex virus commonly infect human beings. The genital strain (type 2) causes *herpes progenitalis,* a recurrent vesicular eruption of the genitalia that can be venereally transmitted. In its typical form, it is fairly easily recognized by the clinician. Using special laboratory diagnostic techniques, however, it has been determined that the infection occurs also in atypical and even asymptomatic forms; just how often is unknown, but it may safely be assumed that, like gonorrhea, genital herpes is much more common than would be suspected on the basis of symptoms alone. Congenital malformations have not been reported, but it is suspected by some that spontaneous abortion may occur with excessive frequency if the mother contracts genital herpes in the first half of pregnancy. The best known threat to the fetus occurs as a result of maternal herpes active at the time of delivery. The infant may be infected at birth, and the virus spreads throughout his body to produce a frequently fatal disease characterized by necrotizing lesions in lungs, liver, brain, and other organs, and a vesicular skin eruption (resembling chickenpox). In the belief that infection is acquired during passage through the birth canal, some obstetricians advocate cesarean section if active herpetic infection can be diagnosed at term. However, the additional possibility of in utero infection via the placenta has not yet been excluded, and prevention of neonatal herpes by abdominal delivery has not been conclusively proved.

LISTERIOSIS

Listeriosis occurs in several forms. An adult occasionally develops a severe disease associated with septicemia or meningitis. More often, however, infection is mild and escapes identification. Infection in this form, manifested as a cold, fever, or malaise days to weeks before term in the pregnant woman, may transmit the bacterium, *Listeria monocytogenes,* to the fetus. Depending on the stage of pregnancy and the severity of the infection, the result may be abortion, stillbirth, or neonatal sepsis. The last of these is best known. An older term, *granulomatosis infantiseptica,* describes the tissue pathology in newborn infants dying of listeria sepsis. Meningitis may also occur in newborns. If promptly recognized, these infections can be treated successfully with penicillin or other antibiotics.

MALARIA

Malaria, a parasitic infection, is quite uncommon in American women, although intercontinental travel sometimes leads to exposure in endemic areas. A less obvious danger confronts the mainline drug user who shares a needle with others, for she may acquire malaria by direct transmission from an asymptomatic carrier. Infection thus acquired seldom poses great danger to the mother in the absence of other debilitating conditions because the species of malarial parasites usually involved (*Plasmodium malariae* and *P. vivax*) cause relatively benign infection; the diagnosis may not be suspected, however, because the woman has never visited an endemic area. In many cases, mothers who have borne malarious infants have had no symptoms at all during pregnancy but have been long-term carriers, thus further obscuring the diagnosis. Fever, irritability, and other nonspecific signs may then appear, often without any clue to the true diagnosis because the periodic fever pattern typical of adult infection may not be present in the infant. The diagnosis of malaria is worth considering in any infant with fever of unknown

origin if the mother has ever been in an endemic area or has taken illicit drugs intravenously.

MUMPS

The majority of women are immune to mumps by the time they reach maturity, either through natural infection or through immunization. A substantial minority, however, escape both and may have their first exposure when a young child (commonly preschool age) brings home the infection to his pregnant mother. It has been proposed, on the basis of a small group of children studied, that endocardial fibroelastosis, a serious congenital cardiac condition in which the inner lining of the heart is thickened and stiffened, is the result of intrauterine mumps virus infection. This correlation is not proved, however, and mumps is not considered sufficient cause for interrupting pregnancy. On the other hand, the Advisory Committee on Immunization Practices of the U.S. Public Health Service does not recommend immunization with live mumps vaccine during pregnancy. Pending further knowledge of possible consequences, no routine preventive measures are taken against mumps in pregnancy.

MYCOPLASMA

The mycoplasmas are a group of microorganisms resembling bacteria but lacking their characteristic shape and cell wall. The best known is *Mycoplasma pneumoniae,* the cause of what was formerly called "primary atypical pneumonia." Other species, *Mycoplasma hominis* and so-called T-mycoplasmas, are frequent inhabitants of the female genital tract. Their full pathogenic potential has not yet been elucidated. It has been suggested that they may be responsible for some cases of spontaneous abortion, stillbirth, prematurity, and low birth weight, and that the risk of these complications may be reduced by treatment during pregnancy with a tetracycline, to which the organisms are susceptible. However, tetracyclines are very undesirable antibiotics in the pregnant woman, and in the absence of more definitive indication, their use for mycoplasma prophylaxis is not recommended. No fetal maldevelopments have been attributed to mycoplasmas.

RUBELLA

German measles, or rubella, has achieved notoriety as the prototype of *teratogenic* infections (i.e., infections causing embryonic developmental defects) (Table 20·2). Infection acquired after birth is almost universally benign, but rubella, unlike a number of other maternal infections dangerous to the fetus (such as cytomegalovirus infection, listeriosis, and toxoplasmosis), produces a characteristic syndrome of rash and swollen lymphs glands which readily attracts attention. It is this property that first led to recognition of the association between rubella and congenital deafness, cataracts, and heart disease. The more recent development of serologic tests has made it possible to confirm the diagnosis or rule it out in cases of other illness with similar clinical findings.

table 20·2

PROBABILITY OF RUBELLA-ASSOCIATED CONGENITAL ABNORMALITY ACCORDING TO TIME OF MATERNAL INFECTION*

GESTATIONAL MONTH	CONGENITAL ABNORMALITY, %†
1	50–60
2	25–35
3	7–15
4	5
5–9	‡

*Based on various reports.

†Percentages of live births; additional losses through spontaneous abortion not included.

‡No significant risk due to rubella.

Equally important, a woman can be tested before or during pregnancy for susceptibility to rubella. A positive test (titer greater than 1:10) indicates immunity and the virtual absence of any danger to the fetus from this infection. A negative test (titer less than 1:10), on the other hand, if discovered during the childbearing age but in the nonpregnant state, is a strong indication for immunization. Early in pregnancy, immunization cannot be carried out for fear of infecting the fetus with the live vaccine; women discovered at this stage to be nonimmune must be observed for compatible symptoms and, in such circumstances, retested for developing antibody titers, which would prove that rubella had occurred and that the fetus had been exposed to the virus in utero.

The management of pregnancy complicated by rubella depends on a number of factors. Underlying the choice of alternatives is the central fact that there is no known way to protect the fetus once infection of the mother has occurred, nor, indeed, any way to reduce the chance of infection in a susceptible woman if she has been exposed. (Gamma globulin has been shown to be worthless for this purpose.) Thus the decision involves (1) determining whether maternal infection has occurred, which can be done reliably in each case by serologic tests; (2) determining whether the fetus has been damaged, which cannot be done on an individual basis but requires an estimate of probability. The estimate is based on the stage of pregnancy at which infection occurs. Table 20-2 shows current estimates of the frequency of fetal maldevelopment related to the time of infection. The high probability of severe congenital defects following first- and second-month infection has led to consideration of therapeutic abortion for these mothers. Purely medical judgment has to be tempered by appropriate legal, moral, and religious considerations that vary from case to case. Universal immunization of girls before puberty holds the best hope for future control of congenital rubella. A woman who is discovered while pregnant to be nonimmune and who shows no serologic evidence of infection during pregnancy, should be immunized as soon as practical after delivery to avoid future difficulties.

SMALLPOX

Smallpox is so rare in the United States now as to deserve only passing mention. However, *vaccination* is an important consideration, because the live virus (vaccinia) used has been known to cross the placenta and lead to disseminated infection in the fetus, which may then be stillborn. The abandonment of routine vaccination in infancy could enhance the problem because primary vaccination, which is much more likely to be associated with complications than is revaccination, is also more likely to be delayed until adulthood. The chief indications for vaccination now are travel to endemic areas and work in hospitals and laboratories. Since vaccination is contraindicated in pregnancy, a pregnant woman without immunity must weigh very carefully her risk of exposure before undertaking either of these activities.

SYPHILIS

The causative organism of syphilis, *Treponema pallidum,* can cross the placenta and infect the fetus, with disastrous results. Congenital syphilis can range in severity from stillbirth, at one extreme, to a positive serologic test unaccompanied by clinical findings, at the other. Between these extremes are various forms of damage. Some, such as skeletal and dental malformations, may be evident in infancy or early childhood, while others, such as general paresis (dementia), may not develop until adolescence. Special

conditions are required for placental passage to occur: (1) Treponemes must be circulating in the bloodstream, which is characteristic of primary and secondary syphilis but rarely occurs more than 2 to 4 years after maternal infection first took place. (2) The pregnancy must be beyond the fifth month, because up to that time the placenta affords an effective barrier. The latter feature permits prevention of congenital syphilis by treatment of infected mothers during the first half of pregnancy, usually with penicillin. Identification of such women is achieved by a simple serologic test, which is routinely performed in any good prenatal care program.

Although therapy for syphilis is well standardized, its effect is not immediately apparent. Only a steady diminution in titer of antibodies, or their total disappearance, can be accepted as evidence of cure, and this takes many months to determine. In addition, if the maternal titer is sufficiently high, placental transfer of antibody will occur and the infant will be born *seropositive*. Providing the mother has received standard treatment during pregnancy, the infant should not be treated unless his titer persists unchanged for 3 months or actually increases; a positive serologic test resulting from transplacental passage of maternal antibodies reverts to negative in 3 to 6 months. Conversely, an infant born seronegative to a seropositive mother should be retested in 3 months; infection could have occurred shortly before birth, with antibodies first becoming detectable several weeks later.

TOXOPLASMOSIS

Toxoplasma gondii is a protozoan parasite of mammals. The closest source of acquisition by human beings has not been identified, although incompletely cooked meat and contamination by cat feces have occasionally been implicated. Regardless of how it is acquired, human infection is much more common than realized, as evidenced by serologic tests. These tests, although well standardized and not difficult to do, are seldom performed unless an infant with characteristic abnormalities is born or, in the case of older children and adults, a characteristic retinal lesion is discovered. Only in these two instances is the infection readily suspected by the clinician. In fact, toxoplasmosis is usually clinically unrecognizable, being manifested as pneumonia, skin rash, myocarditis, meningoencephalitis, or, most commonly of all, fever and lymphadenopathy resembling infectious mononucleosis. Atypical lymphocytosis may further confuse the diagnosis (see also "Cytomegalovirus Infection," above), but the specific heterophil antibody test is negative. Most infections undoubtedly go undiagnosed, and if one occurs during pregnancy, especially in the second trimester, the protozoon may reach the fetus and cause a syndrome characterized by destructive inflammation of the retina (chorioretinitis), maldevelopment of the brain (microcephaly or hydrocephalus), and cerebral calcifications; other organs, particularly liver and spleen, may be involved also. Much remains to be learned regarding prevention of congenital toxoplasmosis. For one thing, since maternal toxoplasmosis is not readily diagnosed (unlike, for example, rubella), the statistical probability of fetal infection is unknown. Secondly, although treatment for acute toxoplasmosis is available, the main drug used (pyrimethamine) itself may be *teratogenic* and is therefore not appropriate for use in pregnancy; thus, the treatment may be more dangerous than the disease. No vaccine is available.

TUBERCULOSIS

The chief danger to the infant from tuberculosis occurs after birth. Infection in utero or at the time of delivery is not an important consideration.

antimicrobial drugs in pregnancy

All antimicrobial agents have the potential for entering fetal tissues via the placenta. Whether the fetus suffers ill effects depends both on the drug and on the stage of pregnancy at which it is given.

Practically all that is known about adverse effects has been learned in retrospect, i.e., through the study of damaged infants whose mothers received drugs that were not known to be harmful during pregnancy. The safety of other drugs has been established in the same haphazard way. Unfortunately, this is the only way. While fully informed volunteers are routinely used to determine the safety of new drugs in their own bodies, it is quite a different matter for a mother to volunteer her unborn child to show that a new drug does not produce a crippling congenital defect. Information derived from animal experiments (which are always conducted before human volunteers are subjected to new drugs) have limited relevance to human beings, because the experimental dosages often are not comparable to those used in human therapy and because there are unpredictable species differences in pharmacology. New drugs are therefore marketed with the warning that safety during pregnancy has not been established. When the life of a pregnant woman depends on the use of a new drug, a calculated risk is justified, and from accumulated experiences of this sort effects on the fetus eventually become known.

Following is a summary of relevant information about the more commonly used, older antimicrobial agents.

1. Aminoglycosides (streptomycin, kanamycin, gentamicin). Chief side effect is

ototoxicity. Prolonged use in pregnancy has resulted in impaired hearing in the infant. Danger is probably slight in short treatment courses.

2. Cephalosporins. Safety is not strictly established. However, their popularity and extensive use promises to yield sufficient information for practical purposes.

3. Chloramphenicol. Beyond the well-publicized myelotoxic effects, there is no known danger unique to the pregnant state or the intrauterine fetus. However, the metabolic process for detoxifying the drug is not fully developed in the newborn, who may retain excessive blood levels and develop the so-called "gray syndrome" (cyanosis and circulatory collapse) (see also "Sulfonamides," below). It is wise not to give the drug so close to delivery that the baby might be born before the mother has completely excreted it.

4. Erythromycin. Safety is not strictly established, but years of use have not revealed any problems related to pregnancy.

5. Isoniazid. Safety is not strictly established, but years of use have not revealed any problems related to pregnancy.

6. Methenamine compounds (methenamine mandelate, hippurate). Safety is not strictly established, but years of use have not revealed any problems related to pregnancy.

7. Nalidixic acid. This drug is considered safe during the second and third trimesters. Caution is advised in the first trimester because of insufficient controlled data.

8. Nitrofurantoin. Safety is not strictly established, but years of use have not revealed any problems related to pregnancy.

9. Para-aminosalicylic acid. Safety is not strictly established, but years of use have not revealed any problems related to pregnancy.

10. Penicillins. Penicillin G and penicillin V are considered safe. For the newer, semi-synthetic penicillins, safety is not established, but their popularity and extensive use promise to yield sufficient information for practical purposes.

11. Polymyxins (polymyxin B, colistimethate). Safety is not established.

12. Sulfonamides. These drugs are considered safe for mother and intrauterine fetus. The newborn, however, is unable to handle sulfonamides and may become jaundiced (see also "Chloramphenicol," above). It is wise not to give the drug so close to delivery that the baby might be born before the mother has completely excreted it; long-acting sulfonamides should be avoided altogether.

13. Tetracyclines. These drugs are unsafe for both mother and fetus. Pregnant women have developed fatal fatty degeneration of the liver and pancreas, usually when treated with very high doses. Dysplasia of the teeth occurs in the child because of the affinity of tetracyclines for calcifying tissues; although not apparent until months after birth, these deformities can be traced back to pregnancy.

immunization during pregnancy

Because of the variety of agents used to produce immunity to infection, their effects on the fetus must be considered individually. Table 20·3 shows the most commonly used immunizing substances and their relative safety during pregnancy.

infections during the puerperium

Labor is a traumatic event. Wounds are regularly inflicted on the uterus, cervix, and vagina. The urethra may be contused, and the anus may be lacerated. It is surprising that infection occurs as infrequently as it does,

table 20·3

SAFETY OF IMMUNIZATION DURING PREGNANCY*

IMMUNIZING AGENT	USE IN PREGNANCY
Toxoids	
Diphtheria	Safe
Tetanus	Safe
Killed viruses	
Influenza	Safe
Rabies	Safe
Live, attenuated viruses	
Measles	Not recommended†
Mumps	Not recommended†
Poliomyelitis	Safe
Rubella	Unsafe
Vaccinia (for smallpox)	Unsafe‡
Yellow fever	Not recommended†
Killed bacteria§	
Cholera	Safe
Plague	Safe
Typhoid	Safe
Gamma globulin¶	
Human	Safe
Equine	Safe

*Based on recommendations of the Public Health Service Advisory Committee on Immunization Practices, 1972.

†Based on theoretic grounds. No solid information available.

‡In emergency (proved exposure), may be used together with vaccinia immune globulin.

§All these agents are used only under special circumstances.

¶Used mostly in emergencies following exposure. Provides only temporary protection against severer forms of hepatitis, measles, rabies, and vaccinia. May also suppress rubella in mother, but without protection to the fetus.

although it is well known that excessive trauma or hemorrhage during labor increases susceptibility.

BACTERIOLOGY

A variety of bacteria may be isolated in puerperal infections. Some are frequently associated with distinct syndromes, so that the clinical picture may suggest the bacterial cause. However, the overlap is too great to justify choice of antimicrobial therapy on this basis alone. Laboratory diagnosis is essential, because the antimicrobial susceptibilities of the different bacteria is quite unpredictable. Since the nurse frequently assists in, and may actually be responsible for, obtaining culture material, it is important that he or she understand the bases of meaningful microbiologic diagnosis. The most important principle is that the information obtained from a clinical specimen can be useful only in so far as the specimen, *at the time of examination in the laboratory,* reflects conditions in the patient. The following guidelines should be remembered:

1. Skin and mucous membranes are *always* colonized by bacteria. A wound culture must therefore be taken from *deep* within the wound—if possible, after sterilizing the surface.

2. A Gram's stain helps in interpretation of culture data, frequently gives additional information, and can be reported within minutes of submission to the laboratory. A smear should therefore be made at the bedside when culturing a wound and submitted for staining along with the culture specimen; a telephone report may be very helpful.

3. A culture specimen consists of *live* material. It changes constantly, in that some bacteria may proliferate, proportions may change, contaminants may assume predominance, and some pathogenic species may die out completely within a short time. Unless the specimen is processed soon after it leaves the patient, the results may not reflect the true state of affairs. In other words, it should be rushed to the laboratory. (One reason for preferring a bedside smear over one made in the laboratory is that further delay has no effect on a dried smear.)

4. Anaerobic bacteria are frequently implicated in pelvic infections. Their tolerance of oxygen is sometimes so poor that sealed specimen tubes with prereduced

atmospheres have been specially prepared and are commercially available for use in anaerobic infections. Whether or not such methods are used, liaison with the microbiology laboratory is important if anaerobic organisms are to be recovered.

5. Blood cultures are important sources of information in puerperal fevers. The proper time to culture the blood is the moment someone suspects that bacteremia may be present. The oft-repeated recommendation to culture the blood when the temperature is rising (which may require waiting for it to fall first) is based on fallacious reasoning. During septic fever, temperature fluctuations are determined by the hypothalamus, not by the intermittent entry of bacteria into the blood. Two blood cultures from different veins 1 h apart, regardless of the temperature during that hour, are sufficient; thereafter, empiric antibiotic therapy may be started if the clinical condition does not permit waiting for culture and sensitivity results.

CLINICAL SYNDROMES

Puerperal Fever Obstetricians are not alarmed at low-grade fever [up to 38°C (100.4°F)] on the first postpartum day, ascribing it to absorption of pyrogen from damaged tissues or to beginning breast engorgement. Needless to say, fever of this type may occasionally persist longer than one day. For practical purposes, however, higher, or more prolonged fever is usually taken as a sign of infection. In the past, infections arising during this period have been collectively termed "childbed fever" or "puerperal fever." Advances in understanding of anatomic and microbiologic varieties of postpartum infections have rendered these terms obsolete, and a satisfactory diagnosis nowadays must include a reference to anatomic location as well as to bacteriologic agent. Depending on these factors, a number of different infections can be recognized.

Episiotomy Wound Infection This infection involves the skin and underlying soft tissue of the posterior portion of the vulva. Staphylococci or enteric gram-negative bacilli are commonly involved. The process tends to localize but may lead to disruption of the wound. Local drainage is usually curative, with antibiotics playing an auxiliary role.

Pelvic Cellulitis (Parametritis) In this situation, the loose connective tissue supporting the internal genitalia, including the broad ligament of the uterus, are invaded by extension from the cervix or, less commonly, the uterus. Although not usually serious, the infection may produce considerable discomfort, local tenderness, and fever. The process may be slow to resolve and may leave internal scarring in its wake. Any of the bacteria normally found in the vagina may be responsible, and without microbiologic studies there is no way to make a definitive choice of antibiotics.

Infections of the Uterus The endometrium is the portal of entry for most serious postpartum infections.[1] All have the potential of spreading through the wall of the uterus, to the pelvic peritoneum, and into the local blood vessels. From the latter, dissemination to distant organs may occur, with disastrous consequences.

Endometritis is the first inflammatory reaction that occurs, regardless of the infecting organism. The subsequent course of events is shaped by an interplay of host and parasite in which resistance and virulence both play important parts. The role of excessive trauma and hemorrhage in predisposing the mother to infection has already been pointed out. The role of bacterial virulence is illustrated by three very different syndromes.

[1]For practical purposes, septic abortion is simply a variant of postpartum uterine infection, except for the underlying circumstances.

HEMOLYTIC STREPTOCOCCAL SEPSIS This infection is characterized by the rapid spread of bacteria through soft tissues with relatively little tissue reaction, necrosis, or suppuration. The lymphatic vessels are favorite channels of extension. The infection may be accompanied by extreme constitutional reaction, such as toxic delirium and shock. General peritonitis may occur, and bacteremia may result in metastatic infection.

This is undoubtedly one of the most virulent infections of the puerperium; its early onset (within the first day or two) and rapid progression are clinical clues to its etiology. The responsible organisms are beta-hemolytic streptococci belonging to group A or, less commonly, group B. Group A streptococci were formerly often implicated in epidemics of childbed fever, because they were carried from one patient to another on the hands or in the pharynx of hospital attendants. If the patient is suffering from a streptococal sore throat at the time, she herself may be the source of uterine infection. These epidemiologic considerations do not apply to group B streptococci, which are often normal inhabitants of the vagina, but uterine infections due to them are equally dangerous.

Penicillin G is the antibiotic of choice; in patients with severe penicillin allergy, erythromycin or clindamycin may be used. Tetracycline is not advised because some group A and most group B streptococci are resistant to it.

MIXED AEROBIC-ANAEROBIC INFECTIONS In addition to its normal bacterial flora, various fecal organisms are frequently present in small numbers in the vagina. Against healthy tissues these organisms are harmless, but they may cause considerable trouble when introduced into open wounds. Their relatively low virulence (compared with hemolytic streptococci) is associated with two clinical phenomena: (1) the tendency for two or more species to be present simultaneously, as though one alone were not powerful enough to cause disease; and (2) the tendency for infections to be contained locally rather than to disseminate rapidly. Local tissue reaction usually establishes an effective barrier so that, even if infection penetrates the uterus, it is likely to be confined to the pelvic peritoneum and may be walled off in the form of an abscess. Such infections develop more slowly and are not as threatening as those due to hemolytic streptococci. However, fever and leukocytosis are always present and in some cases may be the only signs of infection. Etiologic organisms include aerobes (such as *Escherichia, Klebsiella,* and *Proteus* species) and anaerobes (such as *Peptostreptococcus* and *Bacteroides* species) in various combinations.

Infections of this type, especially those involving anaerobes, are often associated with pelvic thrombophlebitis. Under these circumstances bacteria will gain access to the bloodstream, and septic pulmonary embolism is an important and possible serious complication. The effect of such embolism may be pneumonia, lung abscess, or acute right ventricular failure.

Surgery is usually required for drainage of pelvic abscesses, which characteristically do not respond to even the best antibiotic regimens. Anticoagulation has been known to reduce fever which persisted in the face of other remedies; in these cases, thrombophlebitis was evidently an important part of the pathologic process. Ligation of thrombosed veins may be necessary to control recurrent pulmonary embolism.

The choice of antibiotics is difficult for several reasons: (1) both the identity and the antibiotic susceptibilities of the bacteria are unpredictable; (2) the anaerobes are difficult to culture and their antibiotic susceptibilities are difficult to determine; and (3) the fact that the pathogens are also members of the normal perineal flora raises doubts as to which wound isolates are truly significant. (Organisms cultured from the blood are always considered significant.) Recommendations change from time to time. At this writing, a combination of gentamicin (for the gram-negative aerobes), ampicillin (for enterococci), and clindamycin (for the anaerobes) is acceptable pending a reliable bacteriologic diagnosis.

CLOSTRIDIAL MYOMETRITIS Uterine infections due to *Clostridium perfringens* have special characteristics because of the unique properties of the organism. Normally a harmless inhabitant of the intestine and occasionally the vagina, its introduction into devitalized tissue turns it into a life-threatening menace. The conditions for its invasiveness have often been met in unprofessional attempts at abortion, which combined tissue mutilation with unclean techniques; however, any unusually traumatic labor may likewise set the stage.

Under these circumstances, the organisms produce a series of powerful toxins which cause tissue necrosis or gangrene; this permits further invasion, and a vicious circle is set up that, all too often, requires hysterectomy for control. The exudate from such infections usually contains a good deal of gas, and gas shadows may be visible on a pelvic x-ray. The term "gas gangrene" has been given to clostridial infections of this severe type, although the gas itself is incidental, being a product of bacterial metabolism and without known toxicity.

The most serious complication results from the entry of large numbers of clostridia into the circulation. The effects may be similar to hemolytic streptococcal septicemia (see above) with high fever, delirium, and shock. In addition, there may be massive intravascular hemolysis, with more than half the red blood cells being destroyed in a few hours. The hemoglobin released into the plasma is useless as an oxygen carrier and is, further, toxic to the kidneys. Complete renal shut-down may occur, with total cessation of urine formation. Metabolism of free hemoglobin in the liver may lead to deep jaundice. Tell-tale laboratory signs are gross red discoloration of the urine and plasma; the latter is visible on examination of sedimented blood in a tube.

Large doses of antibiotics (preferably penicillin) are essential in management. Gas gangrene antitoxin may also be given, although its value is not firmly established. The outcome, however, depends at least as heavily on supportive therapy, which includes measures to counteract shock, transfusion of red blood cells, and appropriate surgery; days to weeks of dialysis may follow the crisis, until the kidneys regain their function.

Mastitis and Breast Abscess Infection of the breast is a complication of lactation and nursing. Entry of bacteria is facilitated by cracking or fissuring of the nipples, and it is plausible that tissue resistance is lowered by the pressure associated with vascular engorgement. As noted earlier, before lactation actually begins, breast engorgement itself may be associated with fever. Infection, however, is a much later event, so that there is little cause for confusion.

Symptoms vary from mild local pain and tenderness to a severe constitutional reaction with fever and leukocytosis. If not appropriately treated, what starts as diffuse cellulitis may localize in an abscess, which then requires open drainage or needle aspiration of pus.

These infections are almost always due to gram-positive cocci, usually coagulase-positive staphylococci. In selecting an antibiotic, it is well to remember that most staphylococci are resistant to penicillin and, frequently, also to other antibiotics. The agent of choice is one of the semisynthetic anti-staphylococcal penicillins, such as oxacillin, cloxacillin, dicloxacillin, or nafcillin. Ampicillin should never be used, because against staphylococci it is no more effective than penicillin G. For penicillin-allergic patients, clindamycin is recommended. Nursing is generally discontinued on the affected side until the lesion has healed, a breast pump being used to withdraw the milk in the interim.

bibliography

INFECTIONS DURING PREGNANCY

Reviews

Barrett-Connor, E.: "Infections and Pregnancy: A Review," *Southern Medical Journal,* **62**:275–284, 1969.

Medearis, D. N.: "Viral Infections during Pregnancy and Abnormal Human Development," *American Journal of Obstetrics and Gynecology,* **90**:1140–1180, 1964.

Cytomegalovirus

Birnbaum, G., J. I. Lynch, A. M. Margileth, W. M. Lonergan, and J. L. Sever: "Cytomegalovirus Infections in Newborn Infants," *Journal of Pediatrics,* **75**:789–795, 1969.

Hanshaw, J. B.: "Congenital Cytomegalovirus Infection: A Fifteen-year Perspective," *Journal of Infectious Diseases,* **123**:555–560, 1971.

Gonorrhea

Barsam, P. C.: "Specific Prophylaxis of Gonorrheal Ophthalmia Neonatorum," *New England Journal of Medicine,* **274**:731–734, 1966.

Charles, A. G., S. Cohen, M. B. Kass, and R. Richman: "Asymptomatic Gonorrhea in Prenatal Patients," *American Journal of Obstetrics and Gynecology,* **108**:595–599, 1970.

Herpes Simplex

Nahmias, A. J., W. E. Josey, Z. M. Naib, M. G. Freeman, R. J. Fernandez, and J. H. Wheeler: "Perinatal Risk Associated with Maternal Genital Herpes Simplex Virus Infection," *American Journal of Obstetrics and Gynecology,* **110**:825–837, 1971.

Influenza

Widelock, D., L. Csizmas, and S. Klein: "Influenza, Pregnancy, and Fetal Outcome," *Public Health Reports,* **78**:1–11, 1963.

Listeriosis

Gray, M. L., H. P. R. Seeliger, and J. Potal: "Perinatal Infections Due to *Listeria monocytogenes.* Do These Affect Subsequent Pregnancies?" *Clinical Pediatrics,* **2**:614–623, 1963.

Ray, C. G., and R. J. Wedgwood: "Neonatal Listeriosis, Six Case Reports and a Review of the Literature," *Pediatrics,* **34**:378–392, 1964.

Malaria

McQuay, R. M., S. Silberman, P. Mudrik, and L. E. Keith: "Congenital Malaria in Chicago. A Case Report and a Review of Published Reports (U.S.A.)," *American Journal of Tropical Medicine and Hygiene,* **16**:258–266, 1967.

Mycoplasma

McCormack, W. M., P. Braun, Y.-H. Lee, J. O. Klein, and E. H. Kass: "The Genital Mycoplasms," *New England Journal of Medicine,* **288**:78–89, 1973.

Rubella

Plotkin, S. A., F. A. Oski, E. M. Hartnett, A. R. Hervada, S. Friedman, and J. Gowing: "Some Recently Recognized Manifestations of the Rubella Syndrome," *Journal of Pediatrics,* **67**:182–191, 1965.

Rudolph, A. J., M. D. Yow, A. Phillips, M. M.

Desmond, R. J. Blattner, and J. L. Melnick: "Transplacental Rubella Infection in Newly Born Infants," *Journal of the American Medical Association,* **191**:843–845, 1965.

Sallomi, S. J.: "Rubella in Pregnancy. A Review of Prospective Studies from the Literature," *Obstetrics and Gynecology,* **27**:252–256, 1966.

Syphilis

Curtis, A. C., and O. S. Philpott: "Prenatal Syphilis," *Medical Clinics of North America,* **48**:707–720, 1964.

Toxoplasmosis

Couvreur, J., and G. Desmonts: "Congenital and Maternal Toxoplasmosis. Review of 300 Congenital Cases," *Developmental Medicine and Child Neurology,* **4**:519–530, 1962.

Feldman, H. A., and L. T. Miller: "Congenital Human Toxoplasmosis," *Annals of New York Academy of Science,* **64**:180–184, 1956.

Tuberculosis

Avery, M. E., and J. Wolfsdorf: "Diagnosis and Treatment: Infants of Tuberculous Mothers," *Pediatrics,* **42**:519–522, 1968.

Committee on Drugs, American Academy of Pediatrics: "Infants of Tuberculous Mothers: Further Thoughts," *Pediatrics,* **42**:393, 1968.

Urinary Infection

Heineman, H. S.: Urinary Infection in Pregnancy, in J. H. Moyer and C. D. Swartz (eds.), "Symposium on the Management of Pyelonephritis," *Modern Treatment,* **7**:349, 1970.

Immunization

Collected Recommendations of the Public Health Service Advisory Committee on Immunization Practices. Morbidity and Mortality, vol. 21, no. 25 (suppl.), Center for Disease Control, Atlanta, Ga., June 24, 1972.

INFECTIONS DURING THE PUERPERIUM

Collins, C. G.: "Suppurative Pelvic Thrombophlebitis," *American Journal of Obstetrics and Gynecology,* **108**:681–687, 1970.

Goplerud, C. P., and C. A. White: "Postpartum Infections," *Obstetrics and Gynecology,* **25**:227–231, 1965.

Hellman, L. M., and J. A. Pritchard (eds.): *Williams' Obstetrics,* 14th ed., chaps. 34, 35, Appleton-Century-Crofts, Inc., New York, 1971.

Rendle-Short, C.: "*Clostridium welchii* Infection of the Uterus Complicating Delivery," Journal of Obstetrics and Gynaecology of the British Empire, **49**:581, 1942.

Roser, D. M.: "Breast Engorgement and Postpartum Infections," *Obstetrics and Gynecology,* **27**:73–77, 1966.

Rotheram, E. B., and S. F. Schick: "Nonclostridial Anaerobic Bacteria in Septic Abortion," *American Journal of Medicine,* **46**:80–89, 1969.

White, C. A.: "β-Hemolytic Streptococcus Infections in Postpartum Patients," *Obstetrics and Gynecology,* **41**:27–32, 1973.

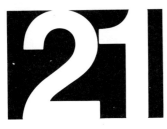

hematologic problems in pregnancy

Evert A. Bruckner

The state of pregnancy results in normal alterations of many functions of the body. When discussing hematologic changes it is important to emphasize that pregnancy is a *physiologic* state, as distinct from a *pathologic* state. Some variation in "expected normal values" is now recognized during varying stages of pregnancy. What is accepted as "physiologically normal" is subject to a specific context of interpretation.

When considering those processes which are abnormal or pathologic which are associated with pregnancy, it is important to clarify whether these pathologic processes are due to or are aggravated by the pregnancy state, or whether they preceded the state of pregnancy and are not directly affected by it.

physiologic changes in the hematopoietic system

BLOOD VOLUME

A major increase in the total blood volume is a prominent feature of the physiologic changes of pregnancy. The plasma volume may increase by 40 percent, and the red cell mass by 15 to 25 percent. The blood thus becomes more dilute and the hemoglobin and hematocrit values may show apparent anemia. This state is termed the *hemodilution of pregnancy*. The phrase "physiologic anemia of pregnancy" is still sometimes found in the literature to describe this change, but is misleading and is thus not the preferred term. The degree of these changes varies considerably among women, but will usually be lower than the normal range of 12 to 14 Gm hemoglobin and 35 to 45 percent hematocrit in nonpregnant women. The hemoglobin level in pregnancy may fall to the range of 10.5 to 12.0 Gm, and the hematocrit level to 30 to 33 percent.

LEUKOCYTES

The leukocyte count increases during the last several months of pregnancy, with a count of 10,000 to 15,000 not being unusual. During and just after parturition there is a further increase in the leukocyte count, frequently to the range of 20,000 to 25,000. The count usually returns to normal within a week after delivery in the absence of other complications.

COAGULATION FACTORS

Blood platelets show little change during pregnancy, with the platelet count, structure, and function typically remaining within the normal range. After delivery a transient rise in count to 500,000 to 600,000 may be observed. An increase in the levels of several of the serum clotting factors is usual during pregnancy.

pathologic changes in the hematopoietic system

Anemia, by far the most common hematologic problem of pregnancy, may be considered in one of three general categories:

1. Inadequate production of erythrocytes (hypoproliferative or maturational anemia)
2. Premature destruction of erythrocytes (hemolytic anemia)
3. Blood loss from the vascular system (hemorrhage)

HYPOPROLIFERATIVE AND MATURATIONAL ANEMIAS

Inadequate blood production to maintain a normal hemoglobin level may result from a variety of distinct causes, including lack of "blood-cell building blocks" (e.g., iron, folic acid, vitamin B_{12}), lack of hormonal stimulus for erythrocyte production, or damage to the bone marrow structure or to the hematopoietic stem cells in the marrow. In more complicated cases examination of the bone marrow is frequently very helpful in determining the cause of a block in erythrocyte production. The morphologic or structural appearance of the developing erythrocyte precursors in the marrow may provide important information as to whether the probable defect is lack of iron, folic acid, or vitamin B_{12}, or whether it is bone marrow damage.

Iron-deficiency anemia Iron deficiency is the most common cause of anemia in both pregnant and nonpregnant women. Anemia may be caused by a decrease in erythrocyte production due to a decrease in hemoglobin production, or it may be caused by a combination of acute blood loss (e.g., at delivery) and an inadequate bone marrow response in replacing erythrocytes, due to lack of iron. Iron deficiency is more common in women than men. The total store of iron is less in women, and the physiologic requirement in females is greater, because of the blood loss during menstruation or delivery, and iron loss to the fetus during pregnancy and lactation (see Fig. 21·1).

The daily requirement of iron in a physiologic steady state averages 1 to 2 mg. The additional requirement of about 400 mg iron

for pregnancy itself and 150 mg for the placenta would require nearly two more milligrams in additional *daily* iron absorption for the mother to remain in iron balance. For the pregnant woman, this usually necessitates iron supplementation, since this amount is not available for absorption from usual dietary sources. Oral iron preparations are usually well tolerated and provide adequate supplementation if taken in the proper manner for absorption and utilization. Iron is absorbed best if taken on a relatively empty stomach (e.g., 30 min before meals). Side effects such as mild nausea, indigestion, and other gastrointestinal symptoms may be decreased or prevented if the dosage is small at first (e.g., 1 tablet daily) and then is increased progressively until a full dosage is attained in 10 to 14 days. When introduced in this manner iron tablets are usually well tolerated. Intramuscular iron administration is not often required if oral supplements are taken in adequate amount and in correct manner. This route of administration should be reserved for those relatively few women who either cannot tolerate oral iron, will not take oral supplements, or for various reasons do not adequately absorb it.

The technique of intramuscular administration is very important. The nurse must learn the exact technique for administering this medication (Chap. 18). It is also very important that she spend enough time with the mother to ensure that she is obtaining an adequate diet and iron and vitamin supplements.

The marrow will respond to iron lack by "economizing," with a resultant moderate decrease in the number of erythrocytes it produces and the development of mild anemia. As the iron-deficiency state becomes more severe, additional "economizing" includes the production of smaller erythrocytes (microcytes) and later the production of pale erythrocytes with a lower concentration of hemoglobin in each one (hypochromic cells).

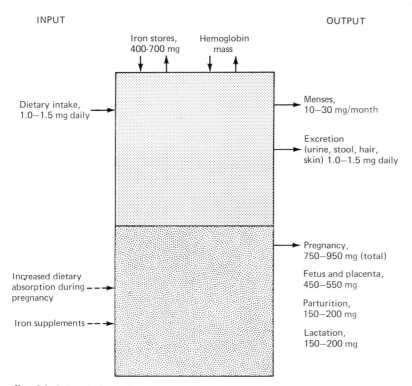

INPUT

OUTPUT

Iron stores,
400-700 mg

Hemoglobin
mass

Dietary intake,
1.0—1.5 mg daily

Menses,
10—30 mg/month

Excretion
(urine, stool, hair,
skin) 1.0—1.5 mg daily

Pregnancy,
750—950 mg (total)

Fetus and placenta,
450—550 mg

Increased dietary
absorption during – –
pregnancy

Iron supplements – –

Parturition,
150—200 mg

Lactation,
150—200 mg

fig. 21·1 Iron balance in women.

Folate-deficiency anemia DNA (deoxyribonucleic acid) is a key part of cell nuclei and chromosomes and is basic to cellular life. Folic acid and vitamin B_{12} are necessary for the synthesis of nucleic acid, and thus for the synthesis of DNA. The more cell division and growth, the greater the amount of DNA required. The more DNA is utilized, the greater is the requirement for folic acid and vitamin B_{12}. The fetus has the capacity of selectively absorbing folate and vitamin B_{12} (as well as other factors necessary for its development, including iron) and will therefore absorb these substances at the expense of the mother. Thus if the available supply of these substances is inadequate for the needs of both the mother and the fetus, the available amount will go primarily to the fetus.

The folate stores in human beings are relatively small and are fairly readily depleted by either increased utilization or decreased intake. A deficiency may result from poor intake, poor absorption from the intestine, liver damage, or frequent pregnancies which may not allow adequate time for replenishing the body folate stores. Since body stores of vitamin B_{12} are somewhat larger than those of folic acid and its sources from the diet are more varied, depletion is considerably less common.

Lack of folate or vitamin B_{12} results in failure of blood cells to divide and mature properly. The cell nucleus matures more slowly than the cytoplasm, and thus the growth patterns of these two cell components become out of phase with each other. Bone marrow showing these changes typical of deficiency of either folate or vitamin B_{12} is described as *megaloblastic.*

In addition to exhibiting slower maturation in the presence of folate deficiency, the erythrocyte precursors typically may skip one of the several mitotic divisions which they would ordinarily make, and thus may remain larger than normal at the end of the cycle. These erythrocytes are called *macrocytes.*

Other causes of folic acid deficiency and resultant macrocytic anemia include certain anticonvulsant drugs and tapeworm infestation of the intestine. The ingestion of estrogenic hormones, as in contraceptive preparations, has also been associated with lower serum folate levels, but the clinical significance of this information is not yet clear. In many of the tropical and subtropical areas anemia associated with megaloblastic marrow is very common and worsens considerably during pregnancy. Its causes are usually multiple, with nutritional deficiencies, including iron, being of major importance. Chronic malaria is an additional factor in some of these cases.

Folate deficiency is fairly common, and is largely preventable by folate supplements. Approximately 50 percent of pregnant women show some evidence of deficiency before the end of gestation. Therefore many hematologists now recommend that a daily oral folate supplement be given, particularly during the last trimester, when folate demands are greatest. Although it has been suggested by some workers that folate deficiency may be a contributing factor to certain obstetric complications such as abruptio placenta and abortion, this remains unproved.

Thalassemia The two previous categories of hypoproliferative anemia dealt with a deficiency of a specific building block or constituent for hemoglobin production. Iron deficiency effectively decreases the production of hemoglobin by decreasing heme production, whereas folate deficiency decreases the production of DNA and slows the development of the nucleus. A third type of hypoproliferative anemia exists which has a distinctively different mechanism and effect. Thalassemia is characterized by a *hypochromic microcytic* anemia, usually associat-

ed with an abnormality of erythrocyte shape. Thalassemia shares with iron deficiency the characteristic of inadequate hemoglobin production. However, at this point a key difference emerges: in iron deficiency the inadequate hemoglobin production is a result of decreased *heme* synthesis, whereas, in thalassemia, anemia results from inadequate *globin* production plus an excessive breakdown of the defective erythrocytes which are produced. Thalassemia is thus both a hypoproliferative anemia and a hemolytic state.

Thalassemia is genetically determined and may occur in either the homozygous or heterozygous state. In homozygous thalassemia (also called *thalassemia major*, Mediterranean anemia, or Cooley's anemia), the anemia is severe and very little normal adult hemoglobin is present. This severe hemolytic anemia is associated with an enlarged spleen, decreased resistance to infection, and other complications. These patients usually do not live beyond adolescence, and pregnancy is rarely encountered in girls with thalassemia major.

The heterozygous form of the disease is called *thalassemia minor.* In general it is not nearly as serious, and there is a wide variation in the symptoms that are experienced. Some patients have very minimal anemia; in others there may be frequent episodes of rapidly worsening anemia, often produced by various types of stresses, including pregnancy. Further complications arise when thalassemia coexists with other hemoglobinopathies such as hemoglobin S (i.e., sickle thalassemia).

The thalassemia syndromes primarily affect populations originating in countries bordering the Mediterranean Sea and in Southeast Asia, but are not strictly limited to these geographic boundaries.

HEMOLYTIC ANEMIA

Hemolytic anemia results from the premature or excessive destruction of erythrocytes, associated with an inability of the bone marrow to replace these cells rapidly enough to maintain a normal hemoglobin and hematocrit level. This group of anemias may be categorized as *intrinsic,* in which an inherent defect in the erythrocyte is the basis for premature cell destruction, or *extrinsic* in which extracorpuscular factors (i.e., factors outside the erythrocyte) are primarily responsible for hemolysis. Although there are many potential causes of anemia, we shall focus on two groups of *intrinsic* erythrocyte defects which account for the great majority of cases of hemolytic anemia: those with abnormal hemoglobin structures and/or production (hemoglobinopathies), and those in which an enzyme deficiency results in an alteration of erythrocyte metabolism (enzymopathies).

The hemoglobinopathies consist of those disorders in which the percentage of normal adult hemoglobin (hemoglobin A) in the red cell is decreased. This can result either from an inability to produce adequate globin to form hemoglobin A, as in thalassemia, or from a condition in which the hemoglobin A has been replaced by an abnormal hemoglobin, as in sickle-cell disease.

A few comments about the structure of hemoglobin may facilitate an understanding of some of the causes of anemia associated with the hemoglobinopathies. The hemoglobin molecule is made up of an iron-containing component called *heme* and two pairs of polypeptide chains called *alpha* (α) and *beta* (β). These chains are attached to heme group, which in turn has the property of reversibly combining with oxygen. The polypeptide chains are made up of 574 amino acids joined in linkage. If a single amino acid is substituted in either of these chains, an abnormal hemoglobin will result. Substitutions of amino acids, with resultant production of abnormal hemoglobin, may occur on either the alpha or beta chain. More than 100 abnormal hemoglobins have been discovered thus far, but the most common and clinically most important is hemoglobin S, or

sickle hemoglobin. This is produced by the substitution of the amino acid valine for glutamic acid in the beta chain of the molecule. In thalassemia, on the other hand, either the alpha polypeptide chain or the beta chain may be affected, with decreased synthesis of the polypeptide chain involved. Depending on which chain is involved, the condition is called *alpha thalassemia* or *beta thalassemia.*

Hemoglobin   S—Sickle-Cell   Disease Sickle-cell disease has an autosomal dominant pattern of inheritance and thus is transmitted equally by males and females. The heterozygous form (designated S-A) is called *sickle-cell trait;* the homozygous form (designated S-S) is called *sickle-cell disease.* In sickle-cell disease most of the hemoglobin in the affected individuals is hemoglobin S, with the remainder usually being hemoglobin F, a fetal form of hemoglobin. The reduced, or deoxygenated, form of hemoglobin S has poor solubility (approximately one-fortieth the solubility of that of hemoglobin A). At the lower range of oxygen tensions it crystallizes out of solution and assumes a characteristic crescentic, or "sickle," shape, with a resultant increase in the viscosity or thickness of the blood. This may result in a "sludging effect" on the blood and a decrease in the blood flow in the very small blood vessels of the tissues, particularly in the spleen, bones, kidneys, lungs, and gastrointestinal tract. Painful sickle-cell crises may be triggered by this chain of events (Fig. 21·2).

INCIDENCE The incidence of sickle-cell anemia in the black population of the United States is 0.3 to 1.2 percent. The sickle-cell trait is present in 8 to 10 percent of the American black population. In tropical Africa the incidence of this gene is considerably higher overall, with considerable variation from one population group to another, with some having an incidence as high as 45 percent (1). Large-scale screening programs to detect unrecognized hemoglobinopathies, particularly hemoglobin S, have been advo-

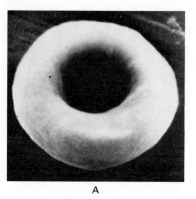
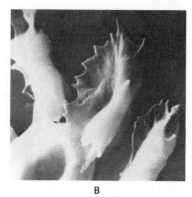
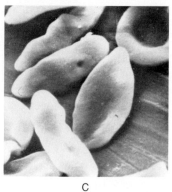

A B C

fig. 21·2 Process of sickling and unsickling of red cells. A Stereoscan electron micrograph of a normally oxygenated red cell showing classic biconcave disk with central cavity and slight surface irregularity. B When deoxygenated, cells take on the typical holly-leaf sickle shape. If reoxygenated, the cells unsickle. The process may go on to an irreversible state (C). C In the oxygenated state *irreversibly* sickled cells have a characteristic oval or cigar shape with a smooth membrane. If deoxygenated and then reoxygenated again, cells return to this shape. (*From "Sickling Damages Red-cell Membrane,"* Medical World News, *Jan.* 26, 1973; *courtesy of Drs. Lessin, Jensen, and Klug.*)

cated, and numerous projects for this purpose are now operative. These studies understandably have generated much discussion pro and con, with a number of difficult questions having been raised concerning the implications of these data. For example, to what extent might the theoretic or practical value of knowing that one is heterozygous—or homozygous—for hemoglobin S be offset by possible social penalities of various kinds (e.g., relating to employment, obtaining medical and other types of insurance, etc.)? These are difficult questions and will require searching and imaginative interdisciplinary study and action, combined with a broad-spectrum approach to education of the public-at-large regarding these issues.

SICKLING CRISIS Crises of sickle-cell disease are of two general types, which frequently coexist. In a *painful crisis,* pain in the back, abdomen, or long bones is frequent, but virtually all the organ systems may be involved in one way or another. Pulmonary infarction, hematuria, and cerebrovascular accidents also may occur. Bone crises have repeatedly been reported as complications of late pregnancy and the puerperium. In a

hemolytic crisis anemia typically develops with great rapidity, which, when superimposed on the already existent moderately severe anemia which is characteristic of sickle-cell disease in the stable state, may result in additional complications such as congestive heart failure, angina, and myocardial infarction. Fever and jaundice are commonly present during hemolytic crises.

MANAGEMENT The management and treatment of the pregnant patient with sickle-cell disease is difficult. Infections, particularly recurrent urinary tract infections, are common and are treated with appropriate antibiotics. Folate deficiency, common in sickle-cell patients, may become much more severe in pregnancy, and the administration of oral folic acid supplements, 1 to 2 mg daily, is helpful. Sickle crises are treated with hydration and analgesia. Blood transfusions for sickle-cell crises occurring during pregnancy have been advocated by some hematologists. Exchange transfusions are probably preferable when blood transfusions are considered necessary. These consist of removing a quantity of blood from the patient and replacing it with normal (i.e., non-hemoglobin

S) blood, thereby increasing the proportion of non-hemoglobin S blood and decreasing the concentration of the hemoglobin S cells, which are predisposed to clumping and hemolysis.

The use of urea or cyanate has been advocated in the treatment of sickle-cell crises. However, their routine use in the treatment of sickle crises is not indicated. Severe, life-threatening dehydration may develop rapidly if the patient's condition is not constantly monitored and if intravenous fluids are not rapidly replaced. Considerable question remains regarding the effectiveness of these agents in preventing sickle crises or in alleviating their effects. At present these agents must therefore still be considered as investigational therapeutic tools. A further contraindication to their routine use in the pregnant woman with sickle-cell disease is the current lack of data on possible effects which these agents could have on the fetus.

MORBIDITY AND MORTALITY Both a high fetal wastage and increased perinatal maternal mortality occur in patients with sickle-cell anemia. Complications are frequent and varied, including an increased incidence of toxemia, infectious complications, increased severity of anemia, painful crises in the bones, and premature labor. Up to one-fourth to one-half of all known pregnancies in women with sickle-cell anemia terminate in neonatal death, abortion, or stillbirth, compared with a fetal wastage of about 15 percent in black patients without sickle-cell disease (2).

Sickle-cell trait Sickle-cell trait is a relatively benign condition, and there is little evidence indicative of any serious complications of pregnancy associated with sickle hemoglobin trait. Urinary tract infections are present with increased frequency in pregnant patients with sickle-cell trait. Hematuria is also relatively common in persons with sickle-cell trait.

Hemoglobin C Hemoglobin C is a relatively common abnormal hemoglobin having an incidence second only to hemoglobin S in the black American population. Approximately 2 percent of American Negroes carry the gene of hemoglobin C, which is approximately one-fourth the incidence of hemoglobin S. Hemoglobin S and hemoglobin C may coexist, with resultant hemoglobin S-C disease. Homozygous hemoglobin C disease (S-C disease) is relatively well tolerated, with only mild to moderate anemia. However, during pregnancy and the puerperium both morbidity and mortality are increased, and pregnancy in a woman with hemoglobin S-C disease is nearly as hazardous as in a woman with sickle-cell disease. Maternal mortality averages about 7 percent, with fetal wastage being considerably higher, averaging about 35 percent (2–5). Because of the frequency and potential seriousness of complications, as well as increased danger of maternal death, avoidance of pregnancy is to be encouraged; contraception or sterilization should be considered. On the basis of these facts a case can be made for an early therapeutic abortion in the event of pregnancy. Strong differences of opinion related to both philosophic and moral presuppositions as well as to the manner in which the available data are interpreted, exist regarding these issues.

GENETIC COUNSELING

In order that they may understand the risks entailed and associated potential problems in any offspring, genetic counseling is of considerable importance to patients with hemoglobinopathies. If the identities of any hemoglobinopathies present in the prospective parents are known, a prediction of probability of occurrence of the entity in question in offspring can be made. For example in an autosomal dominant condition, if one parent is homozygous (e.g., has sickle-cell disease) and the other is heterozygous (e.g., has sickle-cell trait), half their children may be expected to have the disease and the other half the trait. If both parents are homozygotes, all their children would also be expected to be homozygous for the entity in question. Data of this type may be of great assistance to prospective parents in understanding possible risks to any offspring they may have. This has a number of practical implications, including the practice of birth control and other aspects of family planning.

ERYTHROCYTE ENZYME DEFICIENCIES (ENZYMOPATHIES)

Another form of congenital hemolytic anemia is that caused by abnormalities in erythrocyte metabolism resulting in defective energy production within the cell and a subsequent shortening of the erythrocyte life-span. Enzyme deficiencies are the most common example. A large number of erythrocyte enzyme deficiencies have been discovered; glucose 6-phosphate dehydrogenase (G-6-PD) is the most frequently found. Pyruvate kinase (PK) deficiency is less common but is not rare. Both these enzyme defects may either cause a chronic hemolytic process or trigger an acute hemolytic reaction. Various types of stress may trigger such a hemolytic reaction, including oxidative drugs (in the case of G-6-PD) and various other metabolic stresses (infection, fever, pregnancy). Many variants of G-6-PD are known, and the distribution of their deficiency varies widely among different population groups. One common variant is found in approximately 11 percent of American black males, but is much less frequent in black females. Another variant is found in about 50 percent of certain Jewish populations (6). A G-6-PD screening test is indicated in those cases where a hemolytic process is suspected, or where the family history suggests an enzyme deficiency. It is important to identify this enzyme deficiency in order to try to avoid the precipitation of an acute hemolytic crisis by the introduction of medications or other chemicals which may trigger it.

BLOOD LOSS ANEMIA

Acute blood loss of a degree sufficient to produce a decrease in blood volume and red cell mass may result in anemia. Anemia associated with chronic blood loss is due to iron deficiency in most cases, assuming that the bone marrow otherwise has its normal response capacity and is not being inhibited or suppressed by other factors. Iron-deficiency anemia has previously been discussed in this chapter. For discussion of causes and treatment see Chap. 22.

diseases of the leukocytic cell series

NONNEOPLASTIC PROLIFERATIVE STATES

Proliferative disorders of the leukocytic cell series may be either of malignant or nonmalignant type. Examples of nonmalignant or self-limited processes include infectious mononucleosis, lymphadenopathy due to various infections (measles, toxoplasmosis, streptococcal infections, etc.), and allergic reactions. The complications related to these processes are due to the primary process itself, and the proliferative changes in the bone marrow and lymph nodes are merely reflections of this primary process. These changes in the blood, nodes, and bone marrow have no known direct detrimental effect on pregnancy.

LEUKEMIA AND LYMPHOMAS

Examples of a malignant form of neoplastic proliferation of the white cell series include leukemia in its various forms and various types of lymphoma. Leukemia is infrequently encountered in pregnancy. Since chronic myelogenous leukemia has its greatest incidence between the ages of thirty-five and fifty years, i.e., during later reproductive years, it would be expected to be the most common type of chronic leukemia to accompany pregnancy. This is the case. Chronic lymphocytic leukemia has its peak incidence at a somewhat later age and is rarely found in association with pregnancy. Currently available data would suggest that the course of chronic leukemia is not significantly changed by pregnancy. Fetal wastage is considerably increased because of stillbirth and prematurity, but, on the basis of limited data available, maternal mortality does not appear to be markedly increased. Transmission of leukemia from mother to child during pregnancy is not a significant risk.

Pregnancy is an uncommon occurrence in Hodgkin's disease, even though the incidence of this disease is relatively high in the reproductive age group. The available data do not provide convincing support for the common view that pregnancy, per se, has a deleterious direct effect on the course of Hodgkin's disease. However, pregnancy may alter the approach to therapy in a given case, and thus indirectly alter the course of the disease. A history of treated Hodgkin's disease is not in itself a strong basis for terminating pregnancy. Circumstances in which this may be considered or advised include (1) a history of previous radiation to the pelvis, with the associated possibility of fetal abnormality due to radiation effect on the ovaries, (2) the occurrence of pregnancy during the course of an ongoing chemotherapeutic program, or (3) the occurrence of pregnancy in the presence of active or progressive clinical disease.

In the event of recurrence of Hodgkin's disease in sites distant from the uterus, if radiation therapy is deemed the therapy of choice it can be carried out despite pregnancy. Available data provide no evidence of increased fetal wastage in association with radiation therapy to distant sites.

problems of the coagulation system

Coagulation of the blood is a complex phenomenon involving many interrelated factors which are of varying importance in their role in the overall process. The coagulation system exhibits a somewhat precarious balance between excessive coagulation (and thrombosis) and deficient or defective clotting (and hemorrhage). When we speak of "the coagulation system" or "the hemostatic mechanism" it is important to bear in mind that the phenomenon referred to involves *both* the factors that participate in the clotting of blood and those that are involved in the breakdown or lysis of the blood clot. These factors include clotting substances in plasma and tissue fluids, blood platelets, and the function of the blood vessel wall.

THROMBOPLASTIN

One of the key factors in initiating the coagulation sequence which results in a blood clot is thromboplastin. When this material is introduced into the circulation the coagulation system is activated. Thromboplastin is present in most types of body tissue to some degree, but certain tissues contain a relatively high concentration of this substance. Damaged tissues may release thromboplastin into the circulation. For example, abruptio placenta or a retained dead fetus may activate the coagulation sequence by this mechanism. Abruptio placenta is probably the commonest cause of coagulation defect in pregnancy. Shock, gram-negative sepsis, and surgery are examples of other circumstances which may predispose to derangement of the blood clotting mechanism and result in thrombosis or hemorrhage. Of specific importance in obstetrics is the fact that amniotic fluid also contains a significant concentration of thromboplastin which, if introduced into the circulation in amniotic fluid embolism, may likewise trigger clinically inappropriate coagulation.

Illustrative Example: Disseminated Intravascular Coagulation (DIC) Disseminated intravascular coagulation is uncommon in the pregnant or parturient woman, but it is perhaps the best known of the coagulation problems related to pregnancy and parturition. It well illustrates the interaction of multiple factors active in the coagulation process, and will therefore be considered here in more detail than its frequency of occurrence would otherwise indicate. DIC is that condition in which the coagulation sequence is activated in a clinically inappropriate manner, with a resultant series of events which may result in either hemorrhage or thrombosis (or both). This term is being used here in a fairly general or inclusive sense. Other terms which are sometimes used to describe various aspects of this clinical entity include *consumptive coagulopathy* and *defibrination syndrome.*

THE ROLE OF THROMBIN One step in the coagulation process which is key to an understanding of many of the clinical characteristics of DIC is the generation of thrombin from its precursor substance prothrombin, in the presence of certain other necessary clotting factors. Thrombin is an extremely active substance which catalyzes several other reactions related to the clotting-bleeding process. It activates other clotting factors (factors V, VII, and XII), exerts a direct effect on platelets, and splits the molecule of fibrinogen, which is one of the clotting factor proteins produced by the liver. The effect of thrombin on the platelets causes them to clump together, and they are subsequently removed from the circulation by the reticuloendothelial system. Thrombocytopenia may develop as a result of this increased platelet aggregation and destruction, and a "vicious cycle" may be established, with increased utilization of clotting factors (including fibrinogen), decrease in platelet supply, further activation of the coagulation system, and increased thrombin generation, which causes further platelet clumping and their removal from the circulation, and the cycle is thus perpetuated.

MANAGEMENT OF DIC Although DIC of a clinically significant degree is uncommon, self-limiting episodes of increased activity of the coagulation system (including fibrinolysis, that part of the coagulation system which relates to the dissolving or breakdown of the blood clot) are not rare, particularly following certain types of surgery. These episodes usually clear up spontaneously within a few hours, with little or no clinical expression, and do not initiate the "vicious cycle" mentioned above. In those situations where the pathologic state is transient or can be effectively dealt with (e.g., abruptio placenta or removal of a dead retained fetus), treatment for the DIC may not be indicated or required. If, however, a serious bleeding/clotting process results from a condition that cannot be corrected, response to treatment is frequently poor. Administration of platelet transfusions, fresh plasma, and fibrinogen may occasionally be helpful. Heparin therapy has been advocated by some hematologists in an attempt to decrease consumption of clotting factors in DIC. Others, however, avoid its use in this condition because its effectiveness is, at best, very unpredictable and the dangers of its use are considerable.

Platelet Disorders Pregnancy is not a proved etiologic factor in disorders of platelet function or production. It may uncommonly be an intermediary factor in the development of thrombocytopenia due to folate deficiency. A preexisting folate deficiency may be worsened in a pregnant woman because of the folate demands of the developing fetus. Thrombocytopenia may result from the severe folate deficiency thus produced. Pregnant women are subject to the same risks, but not to increased risks of development of an idiosyncratic response to medications or the development of so-called idiopathic (immune) thrombocytopenic purpura (ITP). ITP is an immunologic disorder in which a circulating humoral factor (antibody?) accelerates the destruction of platelets because of changes in the platelet surface, probably related to an antigen-antibody reaction. Children born to mothers with ITP frequently have thrombocytopenia, but it usually clears up spontaneously without clinically significant problems in the infant. Newborn infants may rarely develop transient thrombocytopenia because of the production of antibodies against platelet antigens in their mothers who received platelet transfusions during their pregnancy.

summary

Hematologic problems in pregnancy are usually a reflection of (1) continued or increased expression of a hematologic problem which was present prior to pregnancy, such as a hemoglobinopathy or enzymopathy, (2) increased stresses or metabolic requirements directly associated with the pregnancy, such as anemia due to iron or folate deficiency, or (3) changes in the blood clotting mechanism, such as the development of disseminated intravascular coagulation due to the introduction of thromboplastin into the bloodstream in certain pathologic conditions. This chapter has dealt with several representative problems and questions in these and related categories. It is important to pinpoint as precisely as possible, and as early in the pregnancy as possible, the presence or potential development of hematologic problems so that appropriate corrective or preventive measures may be taken.

references

1. J. V. Neel, "Genetics of Human Hemoglobin Differences, Problems, and Perspectives," *Annals of Human Genetics,* **21**:1, 1956.
2. R. P. Perkins, "Inherited Disorders of Hemoglobin Synthesis and Pregnancy," *American Journal of Obstetrics and Gynecology,* **111**:120, 1971.
3. E. O. Horger, III, "Hemoglobin C Disease during Pregnancy," *Obstetrics and Gynecology,* **39**:873, 1972.
4. M. G. Freeman and G. J. Ruth: "SS Disease, and CC Disease; Obstetric Considerations and Treatment," *Clinical Obstetrics and Gynecology,* **12**:134, 1969.
5. J. P. Hendrickse, K. A. Harrison, E. J. Watson-Williams, L. Luyzatto, and L. N. Ayabor: "Pregnancy in Abnormal Hemoglobin CC, S-Thalassemia, SF, CF, Double Heterozygotes," *Journal of Obstetrics and Gynaecology of the British Commonwealth,* **49**:410, 1972.
6. Ernest Beutler, in W. W. Williams, E. Beutler, A. Erslev, and W. Rundles (eds.), *Hematology,* McGraw-Hill Book Company, New York, 1972, p. 392.

bibliography

Barnes, Cyril, *Medical Disorders in Obstetric Practice,* Blackwell Publishers, London, 1970.
Hematologic Disorders in Pregnancy, vol. 2, Clinics in Haematology, W. B. Saunders Company, Philadelphia, 1973.
Harris, John W., and Robert W. Kellermeyer: *The Red Cell,* Harvard University Press, Cambridge, Mass., 1970.
Williams, William J., et al.: *Hematology,* McGraw-Hill Book Company, New York, 1972.

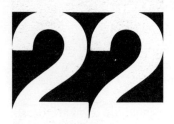

problems causing bleeding in pregnancy

Elizabeth J. Dickason

The medical causes of disturbance in the hematologic system have been discussed in Chap. 21. Pregnancy itself may precipitate many types of bleeding because during pregnancy the blood supply to the uterus increases enormously. The myometrium is supplied mainly from the uterine and ovarian arteries, and as these arteries enter the uterine muscle, they coil and loop to allow for the stretching process of pregnancy (Fig. 22·1). Their pathways into the myometrium at every level of the uterus, from cervix to fundus, allow the uterine muscle to act as an elastic web to control blood flow—constricting vessels which pass through it as the uterus contracts, allowing normal flow as the uterus relaxes.

The normal characteristic action of the uterine muscle is to contract and relax in a rhythmic pattern; early in pregnancy, mild irregular contractions can be observed. Later in pregnancy these increase enough in frequency and intensity to be confused with true labor. As true labor begins, these rhythmic contractions are essential to the blood flow and muscle relaxation that maintain adequate oxygenation of fetus, of the placenta, and of the myometrium itself.

For hemostasis of any bleeding originating in the vessels of the uterus, the myometrium must function as the primary vasoconstricting agent. This unusual action of the uterus in regulating blood flow relates to three basic obstetric problems, the first two of which will be considered in this chapter:

1. Hemostasis in cases such as ectopic pregnancy where the placental blood supply is not under the control of uterine contracture
2. Pre- and postpartal hemorrhage when the causes relate to uterine dysfunction
3. Hypertonic contractions that reduce blood to the placenta and thus oxygen to the fetus during labor

hemorrhage

Any tearing or separation of the placenta will precipitate bleeding through the arterial openings into the placental bed. After delivery of the placenta, relaxation or interference with normal contracture of the myometrium allows a rapid flow of blood into the uterine cavity. The volume of blood that can be lost from the uterus is a reflection of the abundant supply (500 ml/min, at term, flows through the placental area). Thus, bleeding from the placental site can be so severe as to imbalance the supply of oxygen and nutrients to both mother and fetus alike.

HYPOVOLEMIC SHOCK

Hemorrhage which suddenly lowers blood volume causes symptoms of *hypovolemia*. Rapid loss of blood of the equivalent of more than 1 percent of body weight or more than 10 percent of blood volume causes *hypovolemic shock*. [One milliliter of blood is considered equivalent to 1 Gm of body weight. Therefore, in a woman weighing 50 kg (110 lb) or 50,000 Gm, 1 percent of body weight equals approximately 500 ml (1).]

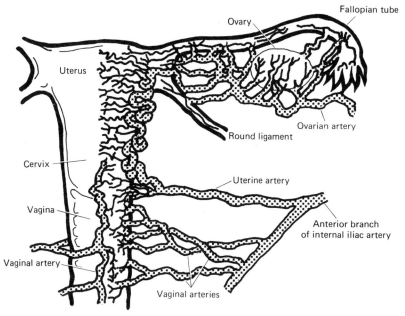

fig. 22·1 Blood supply to the uterus.

The state of shock is a result of inadequate tissue perfusion, leading to deprivation of all nutrients to vital tissues, especially glucose and oxygen, and to a buildup in these tissues of waste products.

Although a variety of body responses occurs as a result of hypovolemia, intricate processes for hemostasis and reflex vasoconstriction also begin (Fig. 22·2). To support the body's own efforts to restore volume, medical intervention to repair the cause of bleeding must take place immediately in cases of obstetric hemorrhage. Treatment follows three main avenues:

Replacement of fluid to restore adequate blood volume

Repair or removal of the causes of bleeding

Support of the patient during the process of treatment

The main medical and nursing support and observations that are carried out during hypovolemic shock in obstetrics are outlined in Table 22·1. More detailed instruction in each area of treatment will be available to you in medical-surgical nursing. A recognition of the urgency and seriousness of bleeding in obstetrics will alert you, the nurse, to the need for prevention, keen observation, and swift treatment of hemorrhage.

ectopic pregnancy

Ectopic implantation always leads to bleeding within the first trimester. An embryo and placenta located outside the normal implantation area cannot grow for more then 10 or 12 weeks without showing the classic signs of pressure and bleeding. The rate of occurrence varies from group to group and appears to be especially influenced by a low health level of the mother and low economic level. For instance, an extremely high rate has been found in Saigon: a rate of 1 in 40 pregnancies perhaps reflected the wartime conditions and lack of care there. The rate in inner city areas of the United States is from 1

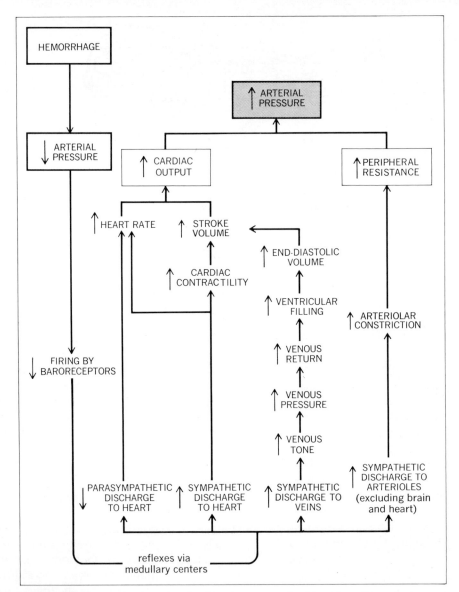

fig. 22·2 Reflex mechanisms to raise blood pressure after blood loss. (*From A. J. Vander, Sherman, and D. Luciano, Human Physiology, McGraw-Hill Book Company, New York, 1970.*)

in 80 to 1 in 120, whereas in areas of higher income levels the rate may be as low as 1 in 500 or 1 in 800. Thus an average figure for the United States of 1 in 200 pregnancies is somewhat misleading (2).

Cell growth will proceed at the same phe-nomenal rate of speed whether the blastocyst implants in the fallopian tube, ovary, cervix, interstitial area of the fundus, or peritoneal cavity (Fig. 22·3). The rapidly developing embryo with its placental tissue will usually begin showing specific pressure effects by

table 22·1

SUMMARY OF TREATMENT AND OBSERVATIONS BASED ON PHYSIOLOGIC RESPONSES DURING HYPOVOLEMIC SHOCK

PHYSIOLOGIC RESPONSES	PATIENT'S SYMPTOMS	MEDICAL/NURSING OBSERVATION	SUPPORTIVE TREATMENT
Cardiac and circulatory status: Decreased venous pressure Decreased cardiac output Tachycardia, lowered pulse pressure	Feels her rapid heartbeat Feels weak and shaky May feel dizzy	Record heart sounds using apical/radial measure	Restore blood volume Draw blood for type and cross-match, hemoglobin and hematocrit, clotting time Be sure blood specimens are taken to laboratory at once Start intravenous fluids, Ringer's lactate, dextrose and saline, large-bore intracatheter. Later, blood will be administered M.D. will begin central venous pressure
		Record frequent indirect blood pressure readings	
		Monitor central venous pressure and record	Keep patient warm
Reduced arterial pressure with peripheral vasoconstriction (blood to vital organs)	Feels cold; peripheral tissues are pale, nails blanch slowly	Check skin color, turgor, moisture, and temperature	
Adrenal medulla is stimulated to produce epinephrine-norepinephrine to add to vasoconstriction	Feels restless, fearful, anxious	Record patient's expressed or observed reactions	Reassure patient, stay with her
Respiratory status: Tachypnea Respiratory center in medulla stimulated by hypoxia	Complains of air hunger; says "room feels stuffy," or "I can't get my breath"	Note rate, rhythm, depth, and changes in respirations	Administer oxygen prn by mask (do not put a pregnant woman in Trendelenburg position as that hinders her respirations) Have patient in side-lying position before delivery
Gastrointestinal status: Fluid shift begins from interstinal spaces and intestinal tract to vascular compartment (takes several hours to compensate) Parasympathetic activity decreases; reduced motility and secretions in GI tract	Sensation of thirst increases	Drop in hematocrit can be observed after shift	Draw blood for serial hemoglobin and hematocrit readings If patient is alert, provide fluids by mouth unless she is to return to operating room or have anesthesia
Kidney status: Conservation of fluids and salts stimulated by vasoconstriction of renal arterioles. (Kidney needs 70 mmHg pressure for effectively filtrating blood and producing urine.)	May have no sensation to void	Oliguria progressing to anuria (lower limit of normal 30 ml/h) Record hourly urine output Record specific gravity on each specimen	Insert foley catheter Measure specific gravity

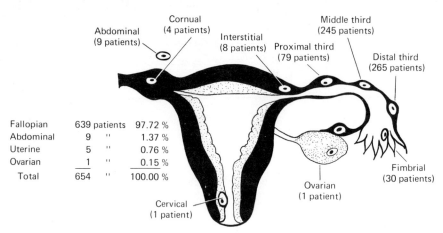

Fallopian	639 patients	97.72 %
Abdominal	9 "	1.37 %
Uterine	5 "	0.76 %
Ovarian	1 "	0.15 %
Total	654 "	100.00 %

fig. 22·3 Ectopic pregnancy: implantation sites. (*From J. L. Breen, "A 21 Year Survey of 654 Ectopic Pregnancies," American Journal of Obstetrics and Gynecology,* **106**:1004, 1970.)

10 weeks of gestation without excessive bleeding. Wherever the trophoblast cells burrow into the implantation site, the effect is the same. Placental implantation stimulates an increase in blood supply, forms maternal pools of blood (lacunae), and produces a spongy vascular area which will bleed profusely should it somehow later become detached from its site.

Breen (3) found in his survey of 654 patients with ectopic pregnancy that 97.7 percent were in the tube. This number corresponds to the incidence in other studies. The other 2.3 percent were distributed, as shown in Fig. 22·3, at interstitial, cornual, cervical, ovarian, and abdominal sites, and are so rare that discussion here will center on tubal implantation.

TUBAL PREGNANCY

Since the tube is 8 to 14 cm in length and 0.5 to 1 cm in diameter, its size cannot support an embryo for long. Normally, the inner mucosal lining of the tube goes through cyclic changes similar to the changes in the endometrium, without the shedding of cells and blood that make up the menstrual flow. Cilia are present to sweep the ovum along the tube; they are assisted by rhythmic contractions that produce the effect of a slow current moving toward the uterus. The fluids produced by the tube appear to be essential for the support of the ovum as it is transported.

Causes Although the exact reasons for many tubal implantations can not be discovered, delayed movement down the tube appears to be the major cause. The most common hindrances to movement are inflammatory changes and scar tissue. Infection can cause both these changes. *Salpingitis* (tubal infection) may be a sequel to endometritis after surgery, childbirth, or abortion, or may be caused by venereal disease. Scar tissue or adhesions may also be a sequel to abdominal surgery, e.g., for appendicitis, ovarian cyst, or cesarean section.

The health or function of the fallopian tube may be affected by lowered progesterone or estrogen levels and by endometriosis, both factors in infertility problems. Occasionally, an ovum may migrate from one ovary to the opposite fallopian tube. This unusual trip has been diagnosed when surgery is done to remove the tubal pregnancy, only to find the corpus luteum located in the opposite ovary

(4). The delay caused by the time for migration of this ovum to the opposite fallopian tube caused implantation to occur in that tube.

When tubal or any type of ectopic pregnancy is confirmed, the treatment is usually surgical removal of the conception. By thetime the pregnancy has developed 10 or 12 weeks, the damage to the tubal tissue is so extensive that it usually cannot be left in place. As an exception to this, if the diagnosis is made early enough, the physician may be able to remove the gestation and repair the tube so that it maintains its function. The procedure is called a *tuboplasty* (5). The surgery may be of an emergency nature, within an hour of admission, or may be delayed if the diagnosis is difficult to make. In any case, the danger of hemorrhage is the primary concern.

Recurrence Since the pathologic condition that caused the tubal implantation is usually bilateral, the woman has a much greater chance of a second tubal pregnancy or of subsequent sterility.

Diagnosis When an ectopic pregnancy is suspected, a careful history of symptoms is taken (Table 22·2). The common indications are amenorrhea, with varying degrees of spotting or heavier bleeding, anemia, syncope, general pregnancy symptoms, and abdominal pain beginning approximately 10 to 12 weeks after the last menstrual period.

To confirm the diagnosis, the physician may, after a vaginal examination, perform a *culdocentesis,* or aspiration of fluid from the cul-de-sac of Douglas (Fig. 22·5). The procedure is done with the patient in a lithotomy position and does not require anesthesia. A needle is inserted into the wall of the vagina just behind the cervix. In cases of slow leaking from an enlarging placental site in the tube, dark unclotted blood can be aspirated from the cul-de-sac where it has collected.

If a culdocentesis is inconclusive, and the diagnosis is still to be determined, a *culdo-scopy* may be the physician's next choice. A small probe with a fiberoptic light is inserted into the cul-de-sac for direct visualization of the tubes. Other physicians prefer a *laparoscopy,* i.e., insertion of a similar probe through the abdominal wall for visualization of the tubes. Both procedures require preparation of the patient, consent, and at least local anesthesia.

These procedures may be carried out on an emergency basis or may be delayed until diagnosis is first sought by nonsurgical means, such as ultrasound evaluation or the culdocentesis. If an emergency *laparotomy* is decided upon to remove the products of conception from the tube, the usual preoperative orders are as follows:

1. Give nothing by mouth.
2. Put Foley catheter in place for straight drainage.
3. Type and cross-match for 2 to 4 units of blood.
4. Determine hemoglobin and hematocrit levels.
5. Perform abdominal shave [or perineal shave, depending on hospital policy].

fig. 22·4 Ectopic pregnancy: sites of referred pain. (*From J. L. Breen, "A 21 Year Survey of 654 Ectopic Pregnancies," American Journal of Obstetrics and Gynecology,* **106**:1004, 1970.)

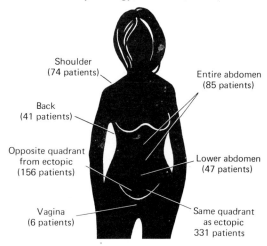

Shoulder (74 patients)

Entire abdomen (85 patients)

Back (41 patients)

Opposite quadrant from ectopic (156 patients)

Lower abdomen (47 patients)

Vagina (6 patients)

Same quadrant as ectopic 331 patients

table 22·2

SYMPTOMS NOTED WITH TUBAL IMPLANTATION

SYMPTOMS	COMMENTS
Various types and degrees of bleeding:	
Painless, periodic vaginal spotting may resemble a light menstrual period	Patient may not notify doctor
	Bleeding may be caused by breakdown of decidual tissue after death of embryo in tube
Hidden bleeding into peritoneum ("a slow leak") causes symptoms of lower abdominal pressure (dark unclotted blood collects in cul-de-sac)	Caused by slow separation of placenta
Sudden massive bleeding associated with rupture of the tubal site causes mother to go into hypovolemic shock	Bleeding is usually preceded by pain
Anemia:	
Fatigue; pale mucous membranes (out of proportion to observed blood loss)	Hemoglobin/hematocrit levels fall slowly, especially with hidden slow bleeding
Abdominal pain of various types:	
Feeling of fullness in lower part of abdomen or backache and mild abdominal aching	3 to 5 weeks after missing the first period, symptoms begin, gradually increasing in intensity
May be referred pain and occur at time of usual menstrual period	(See Fig. 22·4 for sites of referred pain)
May be exquisite pain on vaginal examination when cervix is moved	Vaginal examination often brings first clue to what is wrong
Intense "tearing" pain may occur at time of rupture of tube	May still masquerade as appendicitis
Syncope:	
Light-headedness and fainting have been observed in 35 to 50% of ectopic pregnancies. Termed the "bathroom sign," as fainting often occurs while straining to defecate	Response to feeling of fullness and pressure in rectal area Cause: pressure of growing embryo or collection of blood in cul-de-sac, pressure on nerves of the perineal area
Early symptoms of pregnancy:	
There will be breast tenderness, nausea, and for about 50% a positive pregnancy test, uterus enlarged to about an 8-week size	As long as corpus luteum is functioning, effects of pregnancy hormones will be experienced

6. Have intravenous equipment in place, with large-bore intracatheter.
7. Premedicate only after consent is obtained.

Nursing Care Nursing care is based on the main problem of preventing life-threatening hemorrhage. The patient is maintained on complete bed rest while the diagnosis is confirmed by tests. Sedation may be administered if the patient is not bleeding acutely. The amount of vaginal bleeding is recorded at specific intervals on a *flow chart*. (A flow chart is an output record of vaginal bleeding as seen on vaginal or bed pad. A record of the estimated amount is made every time the pad is changed.)

Vital signs are recorded frequently. It is important to note that unless there is accompanying infection, the temperature is usually normal. Of course, when extensive bleeding has occurred, the patient will show signs of hypovolemic shock (Table 22·1). Prepara-

tions are made for each treatment and for surgery.

Recovery Period The recovery period should theoretically follow that of a tubal ligation. However, since most patients have lost a considerable amount of blood and have had the trauma of losing the pregnancy under these conditions, the recovery period may be more complex. These patients are liable to postoperative distension and to infection because of prior anemia and trauma; a few have postoperative depression. Supportive, anticipatory nursing care can help to reduce complications for the patient.

cystic degeneration of the chorion

The hydatidiform mole, a molar pregnancy, is a rare but potentially dangerous change in the normal placenta. The rate of occurrence in the United States is about 1 in 2000 pregnancies. The chorionic syncytium grows erratically, forming fluid-filled vesicles that are best described as grapelike clusters. (Fig. 22·6). The growth of these vesicles causes the uterus to enlarge much more rapidly than in a normal pregnancy. Strangely, there may also be accompanying hypertensive symptoms similar to those of preeclampsia, but occurring much earlier. Abnormally increasing uterine size and hypertension are accompanied by uterine bleeding, beginning as spotting and progressing slowly to a more serious amount.

Striking changes in laboratory findings indicate a hydatid change in the placenta. The levels of human chorionic gonadotropin (HCG) rise rapidly, since the excessive growth takes place in the chorion. Other laboratory findings in the presence of molar pregnancy are lower estriol levels, lower pregnanediol levels, and lower 17-ketosteroid levels than in a normal pregnancy of the same gestational age (6).

fig. 22·5 Cul-de-sac of Douglas: behind cervix, in front of rectum.

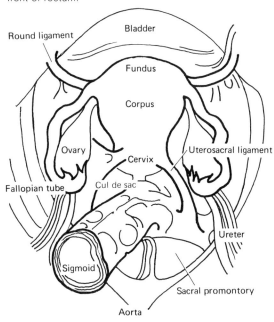

Round ligament
Bladder
Fundus
Corpus
Ovary
Cervix
Uterosacral ligament
Fallopian tube
Cul de sac
Ureter
Sigmoid
Sacral promontory
Aorta

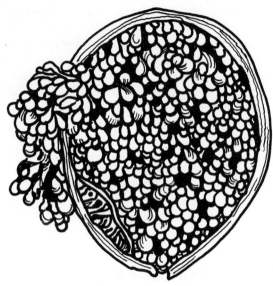

fig. 22·6 Hydatidiform mole. Grapelike clusters fill the uterine cavity.

TREATMENT

The treatment is to empty the uterus of all tissue by careful dilation and curettage, or if the pregnancy is too far advanced, by hysterotomy. After treatment, frequent urine tests are made to check on levels of human chorionic gonadotropin (HCG). Levels should have fallen to the normal nonpregnant rate by the end of 2 months after treatment.

MALIGNANT CHANGES

This follow-up is important because, in a few *very rare* instances, molar pregnancy progresses to one of two malignant changes: to locally *invasive mole,* sometimes called *chorioadenoma destructens,* or to *choriocarcinoma.* Choriocarcinoma is the most malignant form; without treatment, it is invariably fatal. Treatment consists of intravenous therapy with antimetabolite drugs such as methotrexate and actinomycin-D. Early treatment at the first sign of a rising HCG level has led to a cure rate as high as 98 percent (6).

There is a possibility that the changes will be undiscovered if the woman aborts the gestation early and completely. In one study 40 percent of the tissue from spontaneous abortion showed some degeneration of the chorion (7). In another study 70 percent of the actual cases of choriocarcinoma were in patients who had had spontaneous abortions (8). In these cases, symptoms causing the woman to seek medical attention would stem from already existing metastatic disease.

abortion

An abortion is a termination of pregnancy before the fetus is able to survive. An *early* abortion takes place before the sixteenth week of gestation; a *late* abortion occurs during and after the sixteenth week. To be classed as the product of an abortion or as *previable,* the fetus must weigh less than 500 Gm and have a crown to rump length of less than 16.5 cm (9). Should the fetus weigh more than 500 Gm and be born without any signs of life, it is registered as an immature (viable) fetus and a *stillbirth.* If there are any signs of life, such as respiratory or muscle movements or heartbeat, the birth should be listed as liveborn fetus, and as a *neonatal death* if it does not survive.

The age of viability has now been set at the beginning of the twentieth week of gestation, even though very few of the 20- to 27-week-old infants are able to survive. With modern techniques of neonatal intensive care, these infants between 500 and 1000 Gm have a small but significant chance of survival and thus are counted as potentially viable infants.

The word *abortion* can be defined as stopping short of the full growth, or not completing the pregnancy. The word is always modified by an adjective to be specific. Terms describing types of abortion may be classified into two groups:

Spontaneous, or involuntary	Induced, or voluntary
Threatened	Legal
Inevitable	Therapeutic
Complete	Elective
Incomplete	Illegal
Habitual	Criminal
Missed or retained	Self-induced

SPONTANEOUS ABORTION

Seventy-five percent of all spontaneous abortions take place between 8 and 12 weeks of gestation. Many women have experienced early abortions without realizing that they were actually pregnant. Spotting at the first period, then extra bleeding and cramping at the next, may be the only indications of the pregnancy loss; even by 8 weeks the embryo is so small that a woman may pass all the tissue easily. Since an estimated 15 percent of all gestations end in spontaneous abortion, almost every gravida will have experienced an involuntary loss of a pregnancy at some time in her reproductive period.

Causes Causes of spontaneous abortion have been classified by Assali (10) as embryonic and fetal causes (50 to 60 percent), maternal causes (15 percent), and a combination or unknown (20 to 30 percent).

Embryonic or fetal causes include chromosomal and germ plasm defects and placental abnormalities. What is termed a "blighted ovum" is abnormal development or implantation that is inconsistent with growth. Most of the early abortions show embryonic defects. Some women who have lost a pregnancy early find comfort in the fact that early abortion may be the body's way of protecting against an abnormal pregnancy.

Maternal causes tend to be involved in late abortions. These include various infections (Chap. 20), poor nutrition, and, rarely, trauma. Rh incompatibility may be so severe as to prevent the pregnancy from continuing past the first trimester. Systemic diseases that are not well controlled may cause abortion; examples of these are diabetes, sickle-cell anemia, or hypertensive cardiovascular disease. Endocrine imbalance may cause low sex steroid levels which prevent maintenance of the pregnancy without replacement therapy by hormones. Thyroid imbalance, if poorly controlled, often leads to abortion.

Threatened abortion The warning signals of a threatened abortion are those of varying degrees of bleeding, cramping, and abdominal aching. On vaginal examination the physician finds no cervical dilation in process. The lack of dilation distinguishes a threatened abortion from an inevitable abortion. A closed cervix allows hope that treatment with bed rest, sedation, abstinence from coitus, and therapy with uterine relaxants and hormones can avert the progression to an inevitable abortion.

TREATMENT Since the cause is rarely known early enough to use preventive therapy, treatment is symptomatic. Bed rest and sedation may calm the patient. If tests for progesterone and human chorionic gonadotropin reveal low levels, replacement with progesterone may be started. Sometimes thyroid supplements help to maintain a pregnancy. If an abortion is threatening because of psychogenic causes, calm listening and counseling may be helpful. In every case, intercourse will be contraindicated until the pregnancy seems to be well established.

Inevitable abortion Since no therapy really works after true dilation begins, the term *inevitable* is used to describe the inability of therapy to reverse the process of cervical dilation or to save the fetus.

COMPLETE ABORTION The cervix dilates to 4 to 5 cm, and all parts of the placenta and embryo are passed out of the uterus. The recovery period is one of normal involution. Many women do not receive medical care but go through the complete abortion at home.

INCOMPLETE ABORTION After cervical dilation, bleeding, and cramping, fragments of the embryo and placenta are passed. The retained portions of the placenta cause excessive bleeding. In this case the woman must be admitted for evacuation of the uterine contents.

Incomplete abortion may be due to a poorly performed criminal abortion and may be accompanied by injury to the cervix or uterine wall and infection as well. Careful questioning may elicit an admission from the woman that she sought illegal termination of pregnancy. In a New York City hospital, admissions for incomplete abortions were reduced by 50 percent the year after the liberalized abortion law was passed (11).

HABITUAL ABORTION A woman who has lost three or more consecutive pregnancies is called a habitual aborter. The cause may be maternal infertility, chronic disease, or blood group incompatibility. The chief cause is cervical insufficiency, due to prior birth trauma or induced abortion trauma to the cervix, or to intrinsic anatomic problems. The process follows a specific pattern: the cervix begins dilating after 16 weeks, the membranes bulge out of the external os, and the uterus begins the contractions which will lead to delivery of a tiny fetus.

Unless insufficiency, or *cervical incompetence,* is diagnosed and treated, the mother may lose a series of pregnancies between 16 and 26 weeks in gestation. The treatment is to use a *cerclage* procedure, or the placement of a nonabsorbable suture around the cervix to hold it closed. The procedure may be done before conception; if it is done after conception, special precautions must be taken to maintain the pregnancy after the cervical manipulation. Postoperatively, the patient is placed in a Trendelenburg position for 48 h to relieve the pressure of the fetus on the cervix. Sedation and complete bed rest for 48 h are usually ordered. Special checking will be done for vaginal bleeding, contractions, and the fetal heartbeat. Of course, before delivery is possible, this suture must be removed.

Missed Abortion After a pregnancy has been noted, there may in a few cases be a regression of symptoms—or a lack of progression—leading the examiner to suspect a missed abortion. In the previable period, the retention of a conceptus four or more weeks after intrauterine death is called a *missed abortion* or a *retained abortion.* The placental function may continue for some time after fetal death, thus causing confusing pregnancy screening tests. However, it is the nature of things that fetal growth and activity follow a rapidly changing schedule. Absence of the usual weekly changes is a strong indication of fetal death.

Once a missed abortion is recognized, the physician will plan to empty the uterus with suction, or with dilation and curettage, using oxytocin infusion to control bleeding. Late abortion will be treated with oxytocin infusion to soften the cervix. Should this be ineffective, he may try using an intraamniotic injection of saline solution.

Stillbirth Death after the age of viability, still called a miscarriage by lay people, is termed an intrauterine fetal death (IUFD) or, after the delivery, a *stillbirth.* Signs and symptoms of an IUFD follow those of a missed abortion, with the additional changes that are appropriate to the length of time in weeks that the pregnancy had lasted. There are a diminishing of amniotic fluid, a regression of the breast changes, and a reversal of the other physiologic changes of pregnancy. Fetal movements have been felt since 18 weeks and should reach a maximum in the last trimester, decreasing slightly the few weeks before delivery. The mother who has become accustomed to feeling every movement and frequent change of position of the child will state that she feels "empty" when fetal death occurs (12).

Tests for fetal life are the same as those for pregnancy. Especially useful are estriol levels and fetal electrocardiograms. An x-ray view of the fetus some time after fetal death shows overlapping of the skull bones and a generally flaccid posture. If radiopaque dye were introduced into the amniotic fluid, the absence of swallowing (see Chap. 27) would indicate fetal death.

VOLUNTARY INTERRUPTION OF PREGNANCY

The changing laws regarding voluntary abortion reflect the social turmoil of the society. The Supreme Court ruling of January 1973 removed all restrictions on an elective abortion in the first 12 weeks of gestation. The decision was made on the grounds of protecting the woman's right to privacy, leaving the abortion decision to her and her physician. The decision called for clear state restrictions on abortion between 13 and 29 weeks of gestation and asked state prohibition of abortion after 30 weeks. The formulation of each state's regulations as a result of this ruling will take time. All states will probably require that elective abortion be performed by a physician in a hospital or approved clinic. This regulation will at least reduce the number of illegally performed, unsafe abortions that have been done in this country. The rate of *criminal* abortion will drop markedly, and with it the high maternal morbidity from hemorrhage, infection, and trauma. Illegal abortions, minimally estimated at 500,000 per year, caused untold psychologic and physical damage to women desperate enough to seek a termination of pregnancy outside the legal avenues.

In one New York City hospital (13), during 1970–1972 as a result of the elective abortion increase, the incidence of out-of-wedlock births had dropped 11.8 percent, mortality rate was 28 percent lower, and illegal and septic abortions had almost disappeared.

Prior to the Supreme Court ruling, *therapeutic* abortions could be obtained by women for certain medical or psychologic reasons. A panel of physicians, including a pyschiatrist, had to agree to the reasons, a long process that was often expensive in time and consultations. Where there were moderate restrictions abortion could be obtained if one of the following reasons was involved: threatened life or health of the mother, humanitarian-socioeconomic reasons, fetal deformity, or felonious intercourse (incest or rape). Only 15 states were so liberal in their interpretation of therapeutic needs for abortion. After 1970, New York and Hawaii had no restrictions.

Now as information about family planning and abortion become more widely understood and available, the hope is that women, in learning about their own bodies and life situations, will choose the contraceptive method that best suits their life-style.

Abortion should not be used as a method of contraception, but only as a last resort after contraceptive failure. Our efforts as professional nurses involved in health education can go toward helping a woman to prevent future conception when pregnancy is so unwelcome as to cause her to seek to terminate one that has already begun. Nurses who have gained a degree of empathy with a woman going through the turmoil of unwanted pregnancy can begin to comprehend the aspects of her choice. Making a decision when one is in the center of the choice is far different from making it when one is merely observing or debating issues intellectually.

That the choice of abortion constitutes a life crisis situation is clearly stated by Mace (14):

One thing is clear: you must do something, or rather you must decide what to do. Pregnancies do sometimes end of their own accord, but you can't count on that. You need a policy, a plan, and you need it without delay. Every day that passes, the

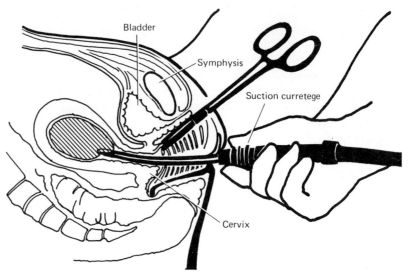

Bladder

Symphysis

Suction curretege

Cervix

fig. 22·7 Suction abortion.

developing life within you grows bigger, more active, more mature. Nine months seems a long time, but it can pass very quickly.

Pregnancy itself is a crisis event for a woman; when it is an unwelcome event the crisis is intensified. Nurses are called upon to use every skill in supporting the mother through the period of the abortion and recovery.

Dilation and Suction Evacuation Suction evacuation of uterine contents is the method of choice for an early termination of pregnancy *before* 12 weeks (Fig. 22·7). The cervix must be dilated wide enough to allow the passage of instruments. Dilation is the most difficult part of the procedure for it must proceed slowly and may be met with considerable resistance, especially in a nullipara. To overcome this problem many physicians are turning to the use of *Laminaria*, a form of seaweed that is hygroscopic (i.e., it swells when wet). Small laminaria sticks can be placed into the cervical os and left in place overnight. Their slow increase in size does painlessly what the physician would have to do under anesthesia. The next day the

patient returns for suction or curettage with a cervical dilatation of 2 to 3 cm. Laminaria are widely used in Japan and only recently have been tried in this country.

Either suction evacuation or curettage can be done under paracervical anesthesia on an outpatient basis when the duration of gestation is less than 11 weeks. Abortion should be done under general anesthesia with admission to the hospital when any question arises about gestational age, or when any medical problems are present. Whichever method is chosen, several precautions are necessary.

1. A complete history should be taken and a complete physical examination made.
2. Ample time should be given for counseling in order for the patient to be clear in her own mind about the decision. (See references by Keller and Shainess.)
3. The statement of the patient's consent should be clearly explained to and understood by her before she signs it.
4. Blood tests must be made. A complete blood count is done, and a tube for type and cross-match should be held in case a transfusion becomes necessary.

5. The patient is instructed to come for her appointment having fasted, i.e., with an empty stomach.
6. She is to be accompanied by a friend who can go home with her after the operation is over.

After the procedure, the patient rests until able to go home. Instructions are as follows: Report any untoward symptoms of bleeding in excess (soaking pad, passing clots), fever, or pain. Do not use tampons or douche or have sexual intercourse until 2 weeks have passed and the physician has checked recovery. If the patient is unreliable about contraception, some physicians will insert an IUD just after an abortion procedure (with consent, of course).

The prevailing mood for a woman who has chosen to terminate a pregnancy is one of relief. There still may follow a period of grieving, and the counselor can prepare the woman for such an event. The importance of good counseling cannot be overemphasized; it is critical to the complete success of the elective abortion process.

Hypertonic Saline Induction After gestational age has been determined as *over 14 weeks* (to allow for sufficient amniotic fluid), a saline induction can be used to terminate pregnancy or to begin labor when there has been an intrauterine fetal death (see Fig. 22·8).

The preparation for the procedure includes taking a hematocrit reading and determining blood type and Rh (RhoGAM is given if the woman is Rh- and Coombs-negative). The patient voids just before the procedure. The abdomen is washed with antiseptic solution and draped. The procedure follows that of amniocentesis (see Chap. 27), but the needle is placed in the miduterus. Local anesthetic is used to anesthetize the skin and area of descent of the needle. A 4- to 5-in needle is used to enter the amniotic fluid; free flow of fluid indicates correct placement. A Teflon catheter is then inserted through the needle. Amniotic fluid is aspirated and replaced with 20 percent saline solution to a total of 200 ml. At the end of the instillation, 1 million units of aqueous penicillin is instilled and the catheter withdrawn.

SIDE EFFECTS A flushed face, thirst, headache, tachycardia, and numbness and tingling in the extremities indicate inadvertent injection into the vascular system. *Hypernatremia* results and must be treated at once with a rapid infusion of 5 percent dextrose and water, plus oral water intake.

Pain in the abdomen indicates incorrect injection into the peritoneum. In some cases, membranes rupture during the procedure and some of the hypertonic saline solution leaks out through the fallopian tubes into the abdominal cavity.

Bladder injection is indicated by a burning sensation and urgency. The bladder must be irrigated at once with physiologic saline solution to dilute the hypertonic fluid and prevent sloughing of the bladder mucosa. Fever may occur as a result of chorioamnionitis, but

fig. 22·8 Saline abortion: how it seems to happen. (*From Marius N. Trinique, Medical World News.*)

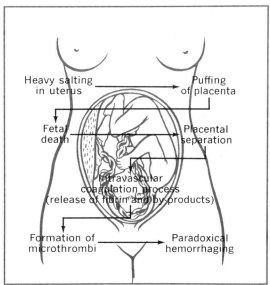

patients appear to respond effectively to antibiotic therapy. Finally, hemorrhage from retained placenta occurs at a rate of about 1:100.

All these are reasons why a saline induction should never be treated as a minor procedure. Staff should be prepared for any eventuality, and clear instructions should be given to the patient to report any untoward symptoms. Most units discharge patients after the procedure, instructing them to return when labor begins.

Labor will ensue within an average of 1 to 3 days (for about 80 percent of women). Other women deliver earlier or have delayed abortions. Usually the cervix dilates rapidly once the process begins, and many women pass the products of conception at home. Thus, patients need a great deal of support and teaching.

Some services use a tape recording, to which the patient listens during the procedure, and in addition provide her with written instructions. An important point to emphasize to the patient is that she will go through a labor process, albeit shortened, and will experience uterine contractions and discomfort. When labor takes place in the hospital, the nurse is the one who monitors the patient's condition and supports her during the process. All the points of postdelivery care are valid for postabortion patients.

placenta previa

On occasion the blastocyst implants in the lower uterine segment. Because the decidua there is less nourishing and the blood supply less adequate, the placenta spreads out over a larger surface and may cover the internal os, *completely*, *partially*, or *marginally*. A fourth type, the *low-lying placenta*, does not impinge on the internal os until the cervix is well dilated during labor (Fig. 22·9). Placenta previa occurs in about 1 percent of all pregnancies and is more common in older gravidas and in those with a multiple pregnancy.

Because low implantation does not favor fetal growth, many of these pregnancies are lost by spontaneous abortion in the first trimester. If the pregnancy is sustained, warning hemorrhages usually do not then occur until the second half of pregnancy. Bleeding is due to the slowly effacing cervix pulling away from the overlying placenta. Hemorrhage may be so severe as to necessitate interruption of the pregnancy to save the life of the mother, with the result of an immature or nonviable infant.

The mother who has been looking forward to this baby will suffer grief at its loss as acutely as the mother who loses her baby at term. Support during the critical decision to terminate the pregnancy is important, because the mother may blame herself for being the cause of the bleeding. She can be reassured that the low-lying placenta is an accident of implantation and is unpredictable, unavoidable, and not usually repeatable.

DIAGNOSIS

The only observable sign of placenta previa is the evidence of degrees of *painless* bleeding; the woman may notice persistent spotting, or she may wake to find a large amount of blood in her bed. Thus, *any* bleeding in pregnancy must be reported to the physician at once. On examination of the woman, the physician is careful not to manipulate the cervix as that might cause further bleeding. However, a gentle speculum examination is necessary to rule out other causes: cervical polyps, infection, cervical erosion, or capillary fragility with blood vessel disruption after sexual intercourse.

To clarify the diagnosis further, isotopic placentography may be performed (Chap. 27). Soft-tissue x-rays may help to locate the placenta when it is preventing engagement of the fetal head. Ultrasonography is also a

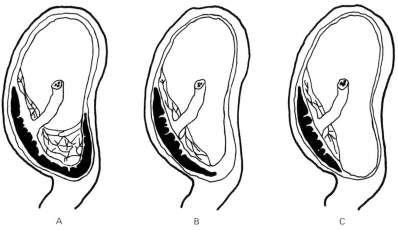

fig. 22·9 Types of placenta previa. A Total; B partial; C low implantation.

useful diagnostic tool for locating the site of the placenta.

TREATMENT

Bed rest until bleeding stops has allowed many pregnancies to mature a few more weeks. Each day in the uterus gives the fetus a better chance of survival. To encourage bed rest, the physician may order sedation (see Chap. 25 for premature labor therapy). Nursing care is planned around keeping the mother quietly in bed, and observing the amount of bleeding. A flow chart is kept to record the amount of bleeding at 4-h intervals. If the bleeding is serious, vital signs are taken more frequently than every 4 h. Unsuccessful tries may raise unnecessary anxiety in the mother; therefore it is preferable to use an amplified fetoscope to obtain the fetal heart rate, as the fetus may be immature and the heart rate hard to hear.

Daily laboratory tests will be ordered to keep track of hemoglobin and hematocrit levels. Blood type and cross-match are determined in order to have at least 2 pt of blood available at all times. Except for the initial gentle speculum examination, vaginal examinations usually are not done, since any manipulation of the cervix may cause an increase in bleeding. The one exception is the "double set-up," in which the patient is examined in the delivery room only after preparations have been made for an immediate vaginal delivery or an emergency cesarean section, should excessive bleeding be precipitated by the examination itself.

Vaginal delivery is possible only when the placenta is marginal or low-lying and the fetal head is well engaged. In this case, the fetal head acts as a ball valve, or tamponade pressing on the edge of the placenta, thus preventing further bleeding during the process of descent.

POSTPARTUM CARE

In placenta previa the placenta site is very vascular, larger than usual, and *friable,* or easily torn. When the placenta has been located in the lower uterine segment, which is thinner and passive during labor, there may have been small tears during delivery that would result in considerably more bleeding during the immediate recovery period. Therefore, any woman who shows signs of placenta previa is watched very carefully for excessive bleeding after delivery.

premature separation of the placenta

In 2 percent of all pregnancies, some degree of placental separation occurs before delivery (15). Another term used to describe placental separation is *abruptio placentae,* a term that reflects the suddenness of the occurrence. The severity of separation has been classified by grades (16):

Grade 0   No clinical symptoms but examination of placenta after delivery shows from one cotyledon to one-third separation of placenta

Grade 1   External hemorrhage only
Mild uterine contracture
More than one-third of placenta, less than two-thirds

Grade 2   External and internal hemorrhage
Uterine contracture, "uterus de bois" (woodlike)
Up to two-thirds separation of placenta

Grade 3   Internal hemorrhage
Severe separation and uterine contracture
Maternal shock and clotting defect
Intrauterine death

Although the causative factors are not clear in every case, 40 to 50 percent of all premature separations are accompanied by maternal hypertension. A multipara has a higher risk of premature separation, as will a woman with folic acid deficiency. Also, abruptio placentae is more likely to occur in a woman who has already experienced one such episode. The mechanism of separation is thought to be associated with vascular changes causing a reduction of blood flow to the uterus. If this reduction is severe enough, vessel necrosis and placental infarcts may occur. As an *infarct,* or area of dead tissue, enlarges, it splits away from the decidua, and hemorrhage from the site begins (Fig. 22·10).

DIAGNOSIS

Premature separation usually produces symptoms suddenly just before or during labor, although the underlying process may have gone on for some time prior to labor. Continuing abdominal pain accompanied by severe bleeding and a change in the character of the uterine contractions are signs that can be easily noted. However, variations in severity of symptoms and grades of separation cause some confusion with placenta previa. With concealed bleeding, or *internal hemorrhage,* the uterus will become rigid and very painful. If touched by the attendant the patient will complain of exquisite uterine tenderness, an unusual sign during labor. The cause of this rigid, hard contracture of the muscle is that blood has been trapped between the decidua and the placenta. The maternal arterial pressure forces more blood into the space, further separating the placenta and disturbing any clots that may have formed; thus the blood may be forced by mounting pressure to *extravasate* into the uterine muscle, forming what looks like a big bruise, leaving the muscle painful, swollen, and unable to relax. The description of the uterus as woodlike, "uterus de bois," is an accurate one for grades 2 and 3.

External, or visible, bleeding occurring with placental separation indicates that the *edge* of the placenta has broken away, allowing the blood to leave the uterus without building up the intense internal pressure that causes so much pain. With grades 0 and 1, the contractions may become erratic but the intense pain of concealed bleeding may be absent.

Fetal survival depends on the ability of the remaining intact placenta to provide oxygen exchange. Fetal death is certain with grade 3 and may occur with grade 2.

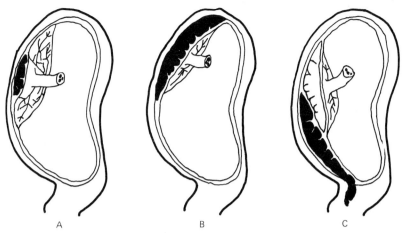

fig 22·10 Types of abruptio placentae. A Partial separation (concealed bleeding); B complete separation (concealed bleeding); C partial separation (apparent hemorrhage).

TREATMENT

Treatment depends primarily on the severity of symptoms and the stage of labor when they occur. The only way to stop the bleeding is for the obstetrician to effect delivery and remove the placenta so that the uterus can contract enough to clamp off arteries leading to the placental site. In case of an extremely bruised uterus with extensive extravasation, uterine contraction may be impossible and a hysterectomy may be required to stop bleeding.

When a great deal of bleeding has occurred, blood coagulation defects cause difficulty in hemostasis (Chap. 21). Thus in every delivery accompanied by moderate to severe premature separation, tests for fibrinogen levels and clotting time will be made. Human plasma fibrinogen is available in every delivery room for emergency replacement.

OUTCOME

Maternal mortality is less than 1 percent when treatment is available, yet fetal mortality from fetal anoxia and immaturity remains at about 40 to 50 percent. Those women who experience abrupt separation when they are some distance from a hospital are usually the ones who succumb to the effects of rapid, uncontrollable bleeding. As a result, statistics from rural areas of the United States may show a higher mortality rate than those from urban areas, where medical care is usually more readily available.

early hemorrhage after delivery

After the placenta has separated, the placental site is a raw wound having numerous arteriole and venule openings that spill out blood if no hemostasis takes place. Normally, strong myometrial contractions pinch off the blood supply and blood clots form. If the uterus stays firmly contracted, all is well and blood loss is minimal. If for some reason it relaxes, the blood flow begins again, pushing out the newly formed clots. Because uterine *atony* is the main cause of early postpartum hemorrhage (i.e., in the first 24 h) frequent checking on the degree of uterine contraction is an important part of nursing care.

During immediate recovery, oxytocin given

intravenously or intramuscularly will actively support normal uterine contracture. When oxytocin is not available or is not given, the infant can be put to breast so that its sucking action can stimulate pitocin release from the posterior pituitary.

The danger period is often the few hours after the intravenous administration of oxytocin is discontinued, or after the medication is diminishing in effect. The likelihood of uterine atony is increased if the newly delivered woman had:

1. A long exhausting labor
2. Uterine inertia during labor
3. A traumatic delivery
4. An overdistended uterus, polyhydramnios, twins, etc.
5. Prior bleeding from abruptio placentae, with extravasation
6. Placenta previa with a large placenta site in the lower uterine segment
7. Fibroids preventing symmetric contraction of the uterus
8. A generally poor condition when she came to delivery, with anemia, preeclampsia, or extreme fatigue

A completely preventable cause of bleeding is that due to overdistension of the bladder. The distended bladder, attached to the tissues of the uterus, pulls it up and pushes it to the right or left of midline, thus preventing contracture. Without the mother herself being aware of bladder distension (see Chap. 10 for reasons), extensive bleeding may occur. If the fundus is to the side and above the umbilicus during early recovery, it will contain many clots. After massage, very firm pressure on the fundus will then expel the clots out into the vagina and then into the bedpan. The amount must be measured, with an estimation of the amount of urine mixed with the blood. Of course, prior emptying of the bladder before massage will allow the uterus to contract properly. In many cases

pain, tension, and anxiety will inhibit voiding. After all techniques to assist the patient have been tried, catheterization may be needed before hemostasis can be obtained.

LACERATIONS

Oxytocin cannot stop bleeding if there are undetected lacerations of the uterine wall, cervix, vaginal wall, or perineum. Lacerations (Chap. 26) are the second most common cause of early bleeding and will show signs of a steady trickle of arterial blood. The mother may show signs of shock without much observable bleeding if the lacerations are deep within the birth passage or in the uterus. The immediate treatment is to return her to the delivery room to repair the laceration, all the while working to restore blood volume.

RETAINED PLACENTAL FRAGMENTS

The third major cause of bleeding after delivery is retention of fragments of the placenta or tissues of the amniotic sac. Good obstetric care includes checking the placenta to see that it has been delivered intact.

If the bleeding is caused by placental fragments, the patient is returned to the delivery table. With light anesthesia, the obstetrician curettes the uterus with his gloved hand wrapped in a sterile gauze sponge, or he uses gentle exploration of the uterus with instruments.

HEMATOMA

A hematoma, or bleeding into the tissues, produces symptoms of swelling, exquisite pain at the site, and often shock symptoms out of proportion to the loss of blood that is evident. Hidden bleeding into the broad ligament, rectal or vaginal wall, or the labia may be the cause of these acute symptoms. Immediate treatment involves a return to the delivery room for examination, clamping, and suturing of the bleeding site. The collected blood in the tissues may be removed as much as possible to reduce the painful pressure.

Severe pain is *always* unusual after a normal delivery. Analgesia such as Darvon compound usually is adequate for postdelivery discomfort. Therefore, a patient complaining of severe pain should always be examined at once for the condition of the perineal area, the bladder, and the uterus.

BLEEDING AND CLOTTING PROBLEMS

On very rare occasions a woman demonstrates a hemorrhagic disorder after delivery (see Chap. 21). The question in treatment is whether the missing factor in the blood coagulation process can be replaced. This situation may become an emergency, especially if the condition was unknown before delivery or developed as a complication such as disseminated intravascular coagulation (DIC). In some situations human plasma fibrinogen is the crucial factor in saving the mother. Vials of this substance are always kept in every delivery area.

Manual Compression If bleeding continues and all factors have been explored, oxytocics have been given, and fluids and blood are being replaced intravenously, the uterus will be compressed manually by the physician. Before or after internal manual compression, *external compression* can be applied by the nurse by grasping the fundus of the uterus firmly with the palm of one hand and pushing down just above the symphysis pubis with the other palm, so that the uterus is compressed between the palms. Massaging the fundus will cause reflex contracture of the muscle, but too much stimulus, too long, will eventually cause exhaustion of the muscle. When bleeding still does not stop, the uterus

may be packed to provide a tamponade. The last resort, a lifesaving measure in severe uterine hemorrhage, is for the obstetrician to do a hysterectomy or to tie off the main arteries leading to the uterus.

late postpartum hemorrhage

One or two weeks after delivery, fresh bleeding is usually the result of retained placental fragments or infection. Rarely, a fibroid tumor of the uterus will delay involution and may cause some extra bleeding. When infection of the endometrium, *endometritis,* is present, *subinvolution,* or poor reduction of the placental site, occurs. This leads to a recurrence of bleeding when the patient is home after having apparently been progressing normally before discharge. Any patient with delayed hemorrhage will be readmitted to the hospital for curettage, oxytocin infusion, blood transfusion, and antibiotic therapy if infection is present.

references

1. Ralph C. Benson, *Handbook of Obstetrics and Gynecology,* 4th ed., Lange Medical Publications, Los Altos, Calif., 1971, p. 182.
2. Thomas F. Halpin, "Ectopic Pregnancy," *American Journal of Obstetrics and Gynecology,* **106**(2):234, 1970.
3. James L. Breen, "A 21 Year Survey of 654 Ectopic Pregnancies," *American Journal of Obstetrics and Gynecology,* **106**(7):1017, 1970.
4. Halpin, op. cit., p. 236.
5. William B. Stromme, "Conservative Surgery for Ectopic Pregnancy," *Obstetrics and Gynecology,* **41**(2):215, 1973.
6. C. B. Hammond and R. T. Parker, "Diagnosis and Treatment of Trophoblastic

Disease," *Obstetrics and Gynecology,* **35**(1):134, 1970.

7. Hammond and Parker, op. cit., p. 138.
8. Nicholas S. Assali and Charles R. Brinkman, *The Pathophysiology of Gestation: Maternal Disorders,* vol. I, Academic Press, Inc., New York, 1972, p. 194.
9. Kenneth R. Niswander and Myron Gordon, *The Women and Their Pregnancies,* The Collaborative Perinatal Study of the National Institute of Neurological Diseases and Stroke, W. B. Saunders Company, Philadelphia, 1972, p. 92.
10. Assali and Brinkman, op. cit., p. 192.
11. Joseph J. Rovinsky, "The Impact of a Permissive Abortion Statute on Community Health Care," *Obstetrics and Gynecology,* **41**(5):781, 1973.
12. Joan Marie Johnson, "Stillbirth—A Personal Experience," *American Journal of Nursing,* **72**(9):1595, 1972.
13. Rovinsky, op. cit., p. 787.
14. David R. Mace, *Abortion: The Agonizing Decision,* Abingdon Press, New York, 1972, p. 13-14.
15. Niswander and Gordon, op. cit., p. 409.
16. Assali and Brinkman, op. cit., p. 223.

bibliography

Diddle, A. W.: "Postpartum Hemorrhage," *Hospital Medicine,* **4**(6):91–104, 1968.

Friedman, Emanuel A., and Marlene R. Sachtleben: "High Risk Labor," *Journal of Reproductive Medicine,* **7**(2):52, 1971.

Greenhill, J. P., and Emanuel A. Friedman: *Biological Principles and Modern Practice of Obstetrics,* W. B. Saunders Company, Philadelphia, 1974.

Hall, Robert E.: *A Doctor's Guide to Having an Abortion,* Signet Books, New York, 1971.

Hammond, Charles B., L. G. Borchet, L. Tyrey, W. T. Creasman, and R. T. Parker: "Treatment of Metastatic Trophoblastic Disease: Good and Poor Prognosis," *American Journal of Obstetrics and Gynecology,* **115**(4):451, 1973.

Harting, Donald, and Helen J. Hunter: "Abortion Techniques and Services: A Review and Critique," *American Journal of Public Health,* **61**:2101, 1971.

Keller, Christa, and Pamela Copland: "Counseling the Abortion Patient Is More than Talk," *American Journal of Nursing,* **82**:102–106, 1972.

Lebfeldt, Hans: "The Psychology of Contraceptive Failure," *Medical Aspects of Human Sexuality,* May, 1971.

Lewis, John L., Jr.: "High Risk Pregnancy: Hydatidiform Mole and Choriocarcinoma," *Journal of Reproductive Medicine,* **7**(2):57, 1971.

Mace, David R.: *Abortion: The Agonizing Decision,* Abingdon Press, New York, 1972.

Nelson, Bristol H., and James E. Huston: "Placenta Previa: A Possible Solution to the Associated High Fetal Mortality Rate," *Journal of Reproductive Medicine,* **7**(4):188, 1971.

Neubardt, Selig and Harold Schulman: *Techniques of Abortion,* Little, Brown and Company, Boston, 1972.

Pritchard, Jack A., R. Mason, M. Corley, and S. Pritchard: "The Genesis of Severe Placental Abruption," *American Journal of Obstetrics and Gynecology,* **108**:22, 1970.

Quinlivan, W. L. G., and J. A. Brock: "Blood Volume Changes and Blood Loss Associated with Labor," *American Journal of Obstetrics and Gynecology,* **106**:843–849, 1970.

Roberts, James M., and Russel K. Laros: "Hemorrhagic and Endotoxic Shock: A Pathophysiologic Approach to Diagnosis and Management," *American Journal of Obstetrics and Gynecology,* **110**:8, 1971.

Scott, James R.: "Vaginal Bleeding in the

Mid-trimester of Pregnancy," *American Journal of Obstetrics and Gynecology,* **113**(3):329, 1972.

Shainess, Natalie: "Abortion, Social, Psychiatric and Psychoanalytic Perspectives," *New York State Journal of Medicine,* **68**:23, 1968 (Reprint C 34).

Silverman, B. B., R. T. O'Neill, and G. T. Fields: "Delayed Postpartum Hemorrhage: a Reappraisal," *Obstetrics and Gynecology,* **36**:32, 1970.

Tanner, M. Leonide, Carolyn B. Stamler, Eleanor Klein, and Beverly Lee: "Attitudes of Personnel: Determinants of or Deterrents to Good Patient Care," *Clinical Obstetrics and Gynecology,* **14**:4, 1971.

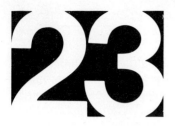

cardiovascular problems in pregnancy

Elizabeth J. Dickason

Cardiovascular changes during pregnancy are quite distinct and would be considered a disease state in a nonpregnant adult. Each of the adjustments that take place has a purpose, and each affects the symptoms experienced by the woman as well as affecting the healthy outcome of the pregnancy. Many of the changes are caused by progesterone in cooperation with estrogen and placental lactogen. Understanding cardiovascular problems in pregnancy requires a knowledge of these normal changes.

normal cardiovascular changes during pregnancy

If the circulatory system is thought of as a very long elastic tube of varying diameters which is already full of fluid, the fact that pressure must be applied at one end to move the fluid is understandable. The amount of pressure, measured as blood pressure, and the rate of flow depend on many factors. Figure 23·1 identifies these factors.

CARDIAC OUTPUT

Cardiac output (the volume of blood the left ventricle pumps into the aorta per minute)

and *stroke volume* (the amount of blood sent into the aorta with each systole) can both be measured and are used to determine how effectively the heart is working. During pregnancy an increase of about 30 percent in cardiac output appears as early as the tenth week. Nonpregnant women average an output of 4.5 l/min. The change in pregnancy of 1.5 l/min raises the volume to a total of 6 l/min in the last two trimesters.

The nonpregnant heart rate averages 70 beats/min. An overall increase of about 15 beats/min helps to accomplish the extra work and push through this extra volume, until after delivery when the rate slowly returns to normal.

CHANGES IN BLOOD VOLUME

Blood pressure will usually rise in cases of *hypervolemia,* or increased blood volume, and always will drop in cases of *hypovolemia.* In pregnancy, however, although the blood volume rises 30 percent (1500 to 1800 ml over the normal nonpregnant average of 4000 ml), this large increase in volume does not seem to cause a basic elevation of blood pressure. Most of the fluid is accommodated in the growing placenta, uterus, body tissues, and breasts. The body also adjusts to the increased volume by shunting blood through the placental circulation. In fact, about 500 ml a minute travels through the placenta, which, acting as an arteriovenous shunt, bypasses the usual capillary bed. This shunting effect actually causes a *decrease* in blood pressure during the first two trimesters of pregnancy.

Blood volume increases early in pregnancy and then is maintained at about the same peak level until just before delivery, when there is a slight decrease. After delivery there is a sudden rise in blood volume as 300 ml of blood is suddenly forced into the circulation with the removal of the placenta (1). The blood pressure may rise 10 to 20 mmHg during the immediate recovery period, and then will decrease slowly until the blood volume

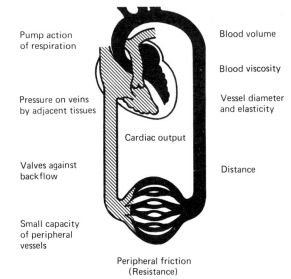

Pump action of respiration

Blood volume

Blood viscosity

Pressure on veins by adjacent tissues

Vessel diameter and elasticity

Cardiac output

Valves against backflow

Distance

Small capacity of peripheral vessels

Peripheral friction (Resistance)

fig. 23·1 Factors influencing circulation. (From E. L. Coodley, "Anatomy of Circulation"; reproduced with permission of the copyright owner, *Consultant, The Journal of Medical Consultation.*)

returns to normal by 4 to 6 weeks postpartum.

An increase of 1200 to 1500 ml of *plasma* makes up most of the increase in blood volume. The *hematocrit* level, or the ratio of red blood cells to plasma, may drop from the normal ratio of 35 to 45 percent to about 30 to 35 percent because the volume of red cells increases only by about 250 to 400 ml. This results in a state of *hemodilution*. The oxygen-carrying capacity of the hemoglobin is unchanged, and the physiologic change is considered normal.

Tissue tension increases as *total body water* rises all during pregnancy to 20 percent above normal, accounting for some of the weight gain and mild dependent edema of pregnancy. In the postpartal period, diuresis occurs in the second through fifth days, ridding the body of most of this excess water (Fig. 23·2).

VISCOSITY OF BLOOD

The viscosity of the blood affects the flow rate, the resistance to flow, and the pressure needed to pump the blood from the heart. Obviously, the thicker or more viscous the fluid, the slower it flows and the more pressure is needed to move it. Blood is about five times more viscous than water. When there is a state of dehydration with reduction in plasma volume and a rise in hematocrit, or *hemoconcentration,* the blood becomes more viscous. If there is fluid retention in the vascular system, with a slight reduction in hematocrit, the blood becomes less viscous.

QUALITY OF VESSELS

The flow rate varies with the lumen of the tube: in a wider tube the blood will flow faster, in a narrower one it will flow slower. Any disease of the vessels, such as arteriosclerosis, affects the diameter of the lumen and the elasticity of the vessels. Mechanisms of vasoconstriction and vasodilation affect the lumen of the vessels and thus the flow rate and blood pressure.

Some capillaries in the circulatory system are so small that red blood cells go through in single file, even squeezing through by changing shape. Flow slows down in these small capillaries to about 1 mm/s, quite a change from the speed of flow in the large superior vena cava, which is about 200 mm/s, and in the aorta, which is about 300 to 500

fig. 23·2 Distribution of increased cardiac output in pregnancy. (*From F. E. Hytten, and I. Leitch, The Physiology of Human Pregnancy, Blackwell Scientific Publications, Ltd., Oxford, 1971.*)

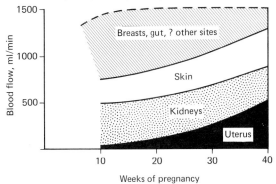

Breasts, gut, ? other sites

Skin

Kidneys

Uterus

Blood flow, ml/min

Weeks of pregnancy

mm/s! The average round trip takes 25 s (2). Circulation time is usually measured from arm to tongue, using a liquid injected intravenously which causes a burning sensation when it reaches the tongue. The nonpregnant rate is 15 to 16 s; during pregnancy the rate averages 12 to 14 s.

DISTANCE OF FLOW

Blood pressure is affected by the distance the blood has to travel; pressure is highest in the large arteries and lowest in the vena cava. One estimate is that the adult system covers 70,000 miles through all the capillary beds of the body (2). Figure 23·3 shows the relationship between the rate of flow and blood pressure. Age makes a difference: blood pressure rises as the infant matures to adulthood and the heart must pump through a longer circuit. The normal blood pressure for a twenty-year-old primigravida at the beginning of pregnancy is about 120/80. By the twelfth week this has dropped to 114/65 because of the circulation bypass through the placenta and the vasodilator effect of increased progesterone.

PERIPHERAL RESISTANCE

Peripheral resistance, or the forces causing friction as fluid and cells pass through the vessels, is a major factor in the amount of pressure needed to move fluid through the circulatory system.

> Total peripheral resistance . . . the measure of the totality of all the factors which affect the blood flow: effective viscosity of blood, the lengths of the vessels, their cross sectional areas as determined by intrinsic tone, vasomotor nerve impulses, presence of constrictor or dilator substances and extra-vascular pressures provided by tissue tensions (3).

DIRECTION OF FLOW

Finally the direction of flow of fluid affects the pressure needed to move it, Man has adjusted to standing upright, but as a result, blood must flow through the venous system 4 to 5 ft against the force of gravity. Any pressure or process which hinders this flow will cause pooling, or *stasis,* of fluid in the lower portions of the body. In many cases fluid moves into the interstitial spaces as pressure rises in the venules. Body position, posture, constriction of circulation, lack of muscle movement, or pressure of the growing uterus on the muscular veins of the pelvis may hinder fluid flow.

SUPINE HYPOTENSION SYNDROME

An example of obstruction of venous return is the supine hypotensive syndrome, or the *vena cava syndrome.* The large uterus pressing on the inferior vena cava or the iliac and femoral arteries as the woman lies supine causes a pooling of venous blood in the legs, raising the pressure in the femoral vessels and reducing the volume and pressure of blood returning to the right atrium. The result is a dropping blood pressure and stroke volume, profuse diaphoresis, and pallor; if the woman is in labor, fetal bradycardia may be re-

fig. 23·3 Blood pressure and velocity. (*From E. L. Coodley, "Anatomy of Circulation"; reproduced with permission of the copyright owner, Consultant, The Journal of Medical Consultation.*)

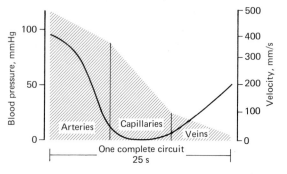

corded. A woman near term, lying supine 3 to 7 min, could experience the effect (4). Most women will, as a reflex, turn to one side unless they are heavily sedated in labor. Some obstetric units, unfortunately, have had the policy of keeping every woman in labor in the back-lying position. A clearly documented syndrome such as supine hypotension must be recognized by the nurse at the bedside as she monitors vital signs (see Chap. 27). Basic treatment is to turn the patient to a side-lying position. Near term, women should be encouraged to assume a side-lying position for sleep and rest.

The vena cava syndrome seems to occur more commonly in the woman with an extra large uterus, as in multiple pregnancy or polyhydramnios. It occurs more often in primigravidas with firm abdominal muscles and taut uterine muscles. Any type of interference with vascular return will predispose the mother to uterine pressure on the vena cava. Severe varicosities, where blood pools in veins in larger than normal amounts, aggravate the condition. During regional anesthesia, loss of neural control affecting venous dilation in the lower extremities may cause the same symptoms (5).

varicose veins

Varicose veins in the lower extremities occur fairly often in pregnancy. Precipitating factors may be some inherent weakness in the wall of the superficial veins, aggravated by obstructed venous return, hypervolemia of pregnancy, obesity, poor muscle tone, and lack of exercise. With care, varicose veins can be minimized and chronic problems prevented.

During pregnancy, treatment is conservative and aimed at reducing any venous obstruction by rest in bed and elevation of the legs several times a day. Ace bandages or firm elastic stockings simulate good muscle tone and prevent stasis of blood in the lower

legs. An increase in the amount of mild exercise will help, as will weight reduction.

To prevent obstructed venous return, instruct the patient to:

Avoid tight constricting clothing
Elevate legs when sitting
Exercise moderately; walk 1 or 2 miles daily
Lie down on her side several times a day to rest
Sleep using a side-lying position in later pregnancy
Use elastic stockings or ace bandages if varicosities exist

Varicosities may also occur in the vulvar, vaginal, inguinal, and rectal veins. Each site is affected by the normal pressure factors during pregnancy. Vulvar varicosities, especially, complicate delivery because they may tear and bleed excessively. During pregnancy, a foam pressure pad held in place by a perineal belt over a sanitary pad may be used to reduce discomfort in the vulva.

HEMORRHOIDS

Rectal varicose veins are called hemorrhoids. From 20 to 50 percent of all pregnant women have some problem with hemorrhoids, beginning early in the first trimester. Hemorrhoids are aggravated by constipation, sitting for long periods, and obstruction of venous flow by the uterus. These rectal varicose veins are painful, itchy, and odorous, as some liquid leaks from the rectum in severe cases. Good perineal hygiene is essential for the pregnant woman with hemorrhoids. Treatment is symptomatic, and the varicosities tend to subside in the postpartal period.

The following are recommended for *treatment of hemorrhoids:*

Medication:
Stool softeners

Gylcerin suppositories
Topical anesthetic spray or ointment
Sitz baths
Witch hazel soaks to anus
Ice bag to perineum
Diet:
High bulk, nonconstipating, with increased fluid intake

thrombophlebitis

SUPERFICIAL VEIN THROMBOPHLEBITIS

Thrombophlebitis is clot formation in the venous system with accompanying moderate to severe inflammation, causing pain, swelling over the site, and some generalized fever. *Superficial vein* thrombophlebitis in the saphenous veins occurs more commonly than deep femoral vein phlebitis, and occurs more often when the woman has preexisting varicose veins. Because the clot tends to be fixed, there is little danger of an *embolus* traveling up to the heart or lungs with superficial thrombophlebitis. With treatment, the symptoms usually subside within 2 weeks.

Women at risk of having this condition should be taught that the early signs of thrombophlebitis are swelling and aching in the legs; they should be reminded to use prophylaxis, i.e., bed rest, elevation of legs, ace bandages or elastic stockings. The highest incidence occurs in the first 4 days of the postpartal period. Early ambulation has reduced the incidence markedly because the muscle activity of walking increases circulation and thus reduces venous stasis. Women discharged early may develop the symptoms at home, and with their attention on the infant, may ignore their own condition until it is full blown. Basic treatment for superficial thrombophlebitis is:

Complete bed rest with *elevation of both legs,* to shunt blood to deep veins and reduce edema

Heat (dry or moist) to assist in improving circulation
Analgesics to manage the pain of swelling and inflammation
Elastic stockings to reduce swelling when condition has improved and patient is out of bed again

In a comprehensive 19-year study by Aaro at the Mayo Clinic (6), thrombophlebitis of some type occurred in 457 out of 32,337 deliveries, or an incidence of 1.4 percent. The majority of these were superficial vein thrombophlebitis and occurred during the postpartum period (85 percent). Observations made during the study were that superficial vein involvement almost always occurred in women who had experienced former episodes or who had varicose veins, whereas deep vein involvement was linked with delivery trauma, bleeding, infection, and operative delivery.

DEEP VEIN THROMBOPHLEBITIS

When a thrombus forms in the deep veins of the leg, the term *phlegmasia alba dolens* has been used to describe the edematous, pale, painful leg. Reflex arteriolar spasm causes severe pain and turns the skin a cyanotic color. There is a deep aching along the line of the vein, plus chills, high fever, and usually an absent popliteal pulse. The onset varies—a few cases begin during the antepartum period, most of them begin within 72 h of birth, with some beginning as late as 22 days after delivery.

Basic treatment parallels that of superficial vein thrombophlebitis, plus use of antibiotics and anticoagulant medication. Heparin, given subcutaneously, is most often used antepartally, as the large molecule does not easily pass the placenta to affect the baby in the uterus. Heparin is quickly metabolized and removed from the system, so that, if necessary, it may be used until a few hours before delivery. When labor begins, heparin is discontinued and vitamin K given to the mother. Later, if necessary, it will be administered to the infant.

SEPTIC PELVIC THROMBOPHLEBITIS

When infection of the endometrium or parametrium follows a traumatic or infected delivery, phlebitis of the femoral, ovarian, uterine, or iliofemoral veins may follow. Signs are tachycardia, chills, spiking fever, and a boggy, very tender uterus. This type of phlebitis is extremely serious, because small emboli and infected particles can easily break off and drift through the venous system to the heart and lungs. Treatment focuses on the infection, as it is usually very severe (see Chap. 20).

pulmonary embolism

The first signs of pulmonary problems are a sharp sticking pain in the chest, shortness of breath, and, in some cases, hemoptysis, or coughing up blood-tinged mucus. Small warning emboli may be thrown off in deep septic phlebitis. The disease may progress very rapidly, with infected particles causing widespread infection or abscesses in the lungs.

In *very rare* instances, a large clot will break off from the deep femoral vein thrombus, travel to the heart, and then to the pulmonary artery, causing sudden death. Signs of such an accident are sudden severe dyspnea and extreme cyanosis.

Pulmonary embolism was the third leading cause of death in reports from New York City in 1967 to 1969 (7). Recently, in England and Wales, pulmonary embolism was second only to abortion as the cause of maternal death. Seventy percent of these deaths occurred in the puerperium (8).

When the patient who is beginning to be active after delivery experiences dyspnea, diaphoresis, or chest pain, the first thought should be of embolism. The patient should be put to bed immediately, a chest x-ray made, sedation and oxygen administered, and anticoagulants given.

amniotic fluid embolism

In high-risk delivery where there may have been tumultuous, hypertonic labor and/or abruptio placentae, amniotic fluid may be drawn up into the venous circulation. Acting as an embolus, the fluid enters the arterioles of the lungs. Since the fluid contains meconium, vernix, lanugo, and fetal cells, these substances will act as foreign bodies in the system. There ensues what appears to be anaphylactic shock, with collapse, hypotension, and uterine hemorrhage. Death follows in most cases within a few minutes. There is no successful means of treating this accident or of preventing it during delivery (9).

heart disease in pregnancy

When heart function has been affected by heart disease, pregnancy may be complicated for the woman and her infant. The three major types of heart disease seen in pregnancy are rheumatic heart disease (RHD), congenital heart anomalies, and heart changes resulting from severe hypertension.

INCIDENCE

The incidence of rheumatic heart disease, though decreasing because rheumatic fever is being treated more successfully, is still 60 to 80 percent of all pregnant patients with cardiac disease. The number of fertile women with congenital heart disease has increased because of better survival to adulthood due to improved care in childhood. Multiparas with hypertension predating pregnancy may have damaged hearts, but newer methods of detecting hypertension and treating it effectively will, it is hoped, reduce heart damage from this cause.

The Combined Maternal Infant Study (10) found an incidence of about 1.7 percent, or 622 cases, of cardiac disease out of 38,823 pregnancies. There was a doubled stillbirth rate and a doubled low-birth-weight incidence among infants of these women.

CLASSIFICATION

The Functional Classification of Heart Disease (11) classifies women with heart disease in groups according to symptoms of dyspnea, palpitations, pain, or cyanosis on different levels of exertion.

Class I	No symptoms on exertion
Class II	Symptoms on ordinary exertion
Class III	Symptoms on limited activity
Class IV	Symptoms at rest

Eighty percent of women with heart problems are in classes I and II and go through pregnancy with minimal trouble. Mothers in classes III and IV are treated as having very high-risk pregnancies and are guarded carefully; extended bed rest and hospitalization during pregnancy are required. The more severe the heart ailment, the higher the incidence of maternal complications and fetal death. In fact, for some women in classes III and IV, therapeutic abortion may be recommended.

SIGNS AND SYMPTOMS

In the examination of a pregnant woman, the doctor will look for signs of heart disease:

Cardiac enlargement seen on chest x-ray
Heart murmur either on diastole or systole
Changes in normal heart *rhythm* or *rate*
Symptoms of *dyspnea, orthopnea,* or *anginal pain*

Congestive heart failure is the big problem to be avoided in cardiac disease. Failure may be precipitated by the normal cardiovascular changes in pregnancy as they stress the weakened heart. Signs of failure are cough, increased dyspnea on exertion, a feeling of being smothered, hemoptysis, tachycardia, and increasing edema (12).

TREATMENT

Treatment of the cardiac patient will be carefully regulated according to her functional ability and diagnosis. Basic problems to avoid in pregnancy are anemia, infection, overweight, fatigue, and emotional stress. The visiting nurse in home visits can determine how the patient is carrying out her diet, rest, and medication orders. Ideally, the mother needs a full-time home aide in order to avoid fatigue, but realistically, many of the women in poorer sections of the country have to manage with heavy social and economic burdens. When high-risk obstetric clinics are alert to social and economic needs of the mothers, some assistance can be arranged. Ideally, too, the pregnant cardiac patient is admitted to the hospital 2 weeks early for evaluation of cardiac and fetal status. Worry about home problems may aggravate her condition; the staff must be alert to this aspect of cardiac care.

As long as the mother's condition is good and tests show that the fetal state is positive, labor may begin naturally. Induction or cesarean section is used only when fetal problems are present. The question of the safety of vaginal delivery as against cesarean section is decided on the basis of obstetric factors. The cardiac strain is much the same in vaginal and abdominal delivery, similar to that of moderate exercise (13). Thus women in classes I and II functionally can go through labor and delivery without great difficulty, whereas those in classes III and IV show increasingly severe symptoms of cardiac strain.

During labor the patient's condition should

be continuously monitored to detect signs of strain. She should be in a semi-Fowler's position and have oxygen by mask available at the bedside. It has been noted that for the cardiac patient, *fear, pain,* and *excitement* are more harmful in terms of elevated pulse, respirations, and blood pressure than is the work of labor. Women who have had childbirth classes are helped by relaxation techniques and an understanding of the labor process. Nurses should work to aid the mother during labor and delivery with her relaxation techniques.

Normal amounts of analgesia are used (with the exception of scopolamine, because of the tachycardia and agitation this drug can precipitate). Caudal anesthesia is ideal for late first stage and second stage, as the stress of bearing down with contractions is eliminated. Hypnosis has been used in a few instances for labor and delivery and seems to be an ideal method. Low-outlet forceps are used to speed the second stage.

Just after delivery, the mother is at risk of having cardiac failure and shock. With the sudden drop in intraabdominal pressure, blood quickly pools in the large abdominal vessels. This, plus the sudden elevation in blood volume as the reservoir of the placenta is eliminated, may imbalance the precarious adjustment of her cardiac function.

Special precautions must be taken to see that the mother does not receive intravenous fluids too rapidly. Oxygen is given by mask as occasion demands, vital signs are taken frequently, and a firm abdominal binder is applied to supply pressure on the deep abdominal veins during the postpartum adjustment period.

In the postpartum period, the need for bed rest is countered by the need for early ambulation to prevent thrombophlebitis in these especially susceptible patients. There are no clear-cut rules for activity (14) except that patients in classes II, III, and IV will be kept in bed until cardiac function has stabilized.

Patients in classes I and II may breast-feed their infants if they wish. Postpartum care at home parallels antepartum care and includes activity based on tolerance, assistance in the home, and careful medical control of symptoms.

hypertension in pregnancy

The pregnant state is delicately balanced and can be disturbed by changes anywhere in the body physiology. Knowledge of cardiovascular dynamics will help to clarify the effect of elevation of blood pressure in pregnancy. Types of hypertension were classified in 1972 by a Committee of the American College of Obstetrics and Gynecology as follows:

I. Preeclampsia-eclampsia
II. Chronic hypertension—of whatever cause
III. Chronic hypertension—with superimposed preeclampsia
IV. Late or "transient" hypertension (15)

It is important to distinguish as much as possible between these classifications, as the treatment, process, and outcome of pregnancy may be quite different with each one. Differentiation may be difficult because the classic presenting symptoms of class I— *hypertension, edema,* and *albuminuria*—may be present in each class.

HYPERTENSION

Seriousness of hypertension in pregnancy is borne out by statistics: one-fifth of maternal deaths and approximately 20,000 perinatal deaths each year are related to hypertensive diseases (16).

Hypertension is defined as a lasting elevation of blood pressure to 140/90 or above *or* a change of 30 systolic points and 15 diastolic above a normal base-line reading. Thus a woman who normally has a blood pressure of

100/70 would be affected by hypertension if her pressure changed to 130/85. All blood pressure is relative to the individual's physiologic state and is affected by many factors. Stress, excitement, and activity which might cause transient elevation must be reduced by rest before an accurate blood pressure reading can be recorded.

The diastolic pressure is more significant than the systolic and should be recorded at the change of sound (Korotkoff's phase 4), since, in pregnancy, the vascular hyperkinetic state may cause a sound to be heard at zero cuff pressure (17). There tends to be great inaccuracy in taking indirect blood pressure readings. Some improvement is made by having the patient's arm relaxed and well positioned, and by using a well-fitting cuff.

The observation has been made that during the first 28 weeks of pregnancy both the systolic and diastolic pressures are slightly decreased from normal nonpregnant averages (15, 17). As the third trimester progresses, increased peripheral resistance and fluid retention cause a slight rise in blood pressure *even in normal* pregnancies. The nurse must get from the chart the base-line prepregnant or first trimester reading in order to recognize pathologic significance in any third trimester elevation.

EDEMA

Seventy-five percent of pregnant women normally experience edema in the lower extremities, especially toward evening. Its development depends on elevated femoral venous pressure, mechanical obstruction produced by the enlarging uterus, and the effects of gravity when the woman is in the upright position. Changing position to the horizontal by resting in bed relieves the collection of fluid in the *interstitial* spaces and causes diuresis to occur. This type of edema is termed *dependent edema*.

In hypertensive states, edema is associated not just with mechanical factors but with salt retention. Fluid may move into the *intracellular* spaces and may be seen "above the waist," or in face, hands, and abdomen, unrelated to body position. This kind of edema, which may indicate a hypertensive problem, is *generalized body edema.* Weight gain may indicate early edema and is the most easily observed sign during the antepartum period. Ten pounds of excess water is stored before *pitting edema* can be demonstrated in the lower legs.

Sodium conservation is a normal physiologic change in pregnancy. During pregnancy, the glomerular filtration rate in each kidney increases 50 percent, from about 500 ml/min to 750 ml/min. If sodium were not reabsorbed by the kidney, the woman would soon be suffering from *hyponatremia*; thus the body appears to be working overtime to retain sodium and prevent hyponatremia. For many years retained sodium was considered the major cause of preeclampsia, and women were put on rigid low-sodium diets. Now it is thought that this regimen can be hazardous to the mother, and dietary salt intake is only modified (18) or not restricted at all.

ALBUMINURIA

The serious pathologic sign in hypertensive states is albuminuria, or proteinuria. Protein is normally screened out by the glomeruli but is passed into the urine in cases of renal disease, renal damage, or moderate to severe hypertensive disease. The degree of proteinuria is determined by a 24-h collection of urine. A level of 100 mg or more per 100 ml, or 5 Gm or more in 24 h, is considered abnormal. When using test tapes on single urine specimens, a reading of 3+ or 4+ is considered a serious amount. Protein in the urine is a late sign of preeclampsia, or it may indicate renal disease. Since extra cervical secretions are common in pregnancy, the protein tests may be distorted unless the nurse obtains a clean-voided midstream urine specimen from the patient.

CLASS I—PREECLAMPSIA-ECLAMPSIA

From the Greek word eklampnis, meaning "shining forth" or "sudden development," comes the word *eclampsia*—the state of convulsions or coma. We use the word *preeclampsia* with the adjectives mild, moderate, or severe to describe the phases of a complex process of disturbed adjustment to pregnancy. The symptoms of this pathologic state are developing hypertension, edema, and proteinuria, usually appearing after the twentieth week of pregnancy. If a convulsion occurs in the severe phase, the woman is considered to have entered the *eclampsia* stage of the syndrome.

For thousands of years this reaction has occurred. The woman was considered to have been poisoned by her baby or by some unknown toxin in her system. Since she returned to normal once the delivery and early recovery period were over, treatment was aimed at getting the baby out of the uterus as quickly as possible.

The term *toxemia* is sometimes used but is obsolete since no toxin is the cause of this syndrome. Now it is thought that the symptoms stem from a complex process which includes:

Increased sodium retention
Widespread arteriospasm
Slow degenerative changes of the placenta
Glomerular endotheliosis

A chain of effects with no known cause, these changes have puzzled researchers for years.

Sodium Retention Sodium retention causes edema from parallel water retention, thus raising the body water above normal level for pregnancy. The warning sign of rapid weight gain is the outward sign of sodium retention. Fluid moves into interstitial and intracellular spaces, and edema shows up in face, fingers, abdomen—"above the waist." In severe preeclampsia the plasma level falls and the hematocrit level rises as fluid leaves the vascular spaces.

Vasospasm Widespread vasospasm affects the kidney, the placental circulation, arterial and venous flow, peripheral resistance, and eye grounds. The results are seen most clearly in the fundus of the eye, where constriction of the retinal arteriolar lumen is one of the earliest signs of preeclampsia. In later phases of preeclampsia, retinal edema may result from *ischemia* (lack of blood supply) because of this vasoconstriction. The visual disturbances experienced in the severe phase of preeclampsia may come from these changes.

Vasospasm appears to be part of the cause of the rising blood pressure. Forcing the same amount of fluid through a smaller arteriolar lumen causes the heart to work harder and with greater pressure.

Placental Changes Vasospasm appears to injure the placenta, causing typical changes seen only in preeclampsia: small, degenerative *infarcts* in the placenta. These injuries may release thromboplastin, which in turn triggers a slow intravascular coagulation process with glomerular fibrin deposits (19).

Glomerular Changes Injury to the glomeruli results in endothelial swelling and fibrin deposits (termed *glomerular endotheliosis*), thus completing the vicious cycle by reducing the effectiveness of the kidney to retain albumin and to excrete sodium and water.

Finally, the degenerating placenta may fail to nourish the fetus adequately, or may be subject to premature separation. Some infants of preeclamptic mothers suffer from the effects of placental insufficiency and are growth-retarded or "small-for-dates" babies. Premature separation of the placenta occurs in 5 to 6 percent of the cases of hypertension in pregnancy (20).

Incidence Patients at risk of preeclampsia

are those who already have hypertension, diabetes, or polyhydramnios, those who have complications of pregnancy such as multiple pregnancy and hydatidiform mole, and those primigravidas at either end of the age range—very young or elderly. The association of preeclampsia with poverty, protein malnutrition, and primiparity is recognized but not fully explainable. The incidence has dropped markedly in the last 20 years—again for no clear reason, except that when recognized early and treated symptomatically, preeclampsia can be controlled before the severe preeclampsia and/or the eclampsia stage is entered.

Prenatal Care Good prenatal care provides screening tests to detect early signs of developing hypertensive problems. Each visit to the doctor includes taking of weight, a urine test for glucose and protein, a blood pressure reading, and a quick check for edema. Signs of preeclampsia usually appear after the twentieth week of gestation. Preexisting hypertension may be discovered before this time, and class III problems may then be picked up about the twentieth week.

Every patient should be taught the warning signals of rapid weight gain (more than 2 lb a week in the last trimester), scanty concentrated urine, visual disturbances, headache, and edema in face, hands, or extremities upon arising from sleep. In the clinic the doctor will follow the trend of blood pressure and urine tests.

Any medications should be explained, so as to reinforce the doctor's orders. The nurse should emphasize the importance of following the rest, diet, and fluid instructions and should telephone any patient who skips her appointment. If necessary, a home visit should be made by the visiting nurse if a patient does not come in after showing signs of preeclampsia.

The usual progression of preeclampsia and its sypmtoms are listed in Table 23·1. The usual treatment is listed in Table 23·2. If the condition is diagnosed early and treated by bed rest, adequate diet, and an increased fluid intake (21), the progression will most often be arrested in the mild phase. In rare instances, severe preeclampsia will develop without the usual warning signals and within a short period convulsions may develop. Sometimes a woman who has not had prenatal supervision enters the eclamptic state at home. She has had symptoms but has not reported them or sought care. For example:

A sixteen-year-old, obese girl kept her pregnancy a secret from her parents. She was admitted to the emergency room in a convulsive state. Her parents thought she had become an epileptic. The baby was delivered soon after admission, precipitously, stillborn, and of about 32 weeks' gestation. Blood pressure on admission while patient was in postseizure coma was 160/100. There was no prenatal care.

Nursing Care The patient will be hospitalized if any symptoms of moderate preeclampsia occur. Nursing care is based on the therapy of providing complete rest. Rest in the side-lying position is the most effective way to reduce blood pressure and promote diuresis. An explanation of the therapy of bed rest can help the patient to understand and cooperate:

"You are in bed here for two reasons—your heart is pumping blood at a high pressure and you have gained a lot of weight, mainly water in the tissues. Your treatment is to stay resting in bed on your side and to drink up to 3 quarts of water a day. Staying in bed puts your body in a relaxed horizontal position, so that the heart doesn't have to push blood uphill against gravity. Resting helps to lower your blood pressure. When you lie on your back the uterus may press on some of the veins connected to the kidneys, so you must remember to lie on either side. The side-lying position allows free circulation to your kidneys, so that more urine is made. The more you void, the less water stays in your tissues—so you lose weight."

A young patient may have difficulty cooperating after the first few days as she may not feel ill. Books, magazines, or a radio-TV may be provided for diversion.

Laboratory Tests Very few tests are specific in checking on the state of preeclampsia. The following are done as screening tests or to check on the progress of preeclampsia:

Excretion in the urine of *vanillylmandelic acid (VMA),* a metabolite of the catecholamines epinephrine and norepinephrine, is measured as a screening test to see whether excessive amounts of these adrenal hormones are being excreted. Excessive excretion occurs, for instance, in the presence of an adrenal tumor. These hormones have a marked effect on blood pressure (22).

Estriols in the blood and urine tell something about the fetal state. If estriol levels are falling below the normal pattern (Fig. 27·9), the fetus may be in danger of intrauterine death.

Blood uric acid shows higher levels in severe preeclampsia. Levels of 5 mg/100 ml or more are significant. Uric acid levels will not be elevated in patients with preexisting class II hypertension.

Medications A variety of doses and sequences will be ordered, because there is not total agreement on the methods of treating preeclampsia.

- Sedative: Usually phenobarbital, 30 to 60 mg tid or q6h to calm and sedate the patient. Phenobarbital is an effective central nervous system sedative and may prevent convulsions.
- Antihypertensive: Only when preexisting hypertension exists or the diastolic pressure rises above 100 to 110, hydralazine may be given in titrated doses until the desired blood pressure level is reached (23). Such therapy requires continuous monitoring of blood pressure.
- Diuretic: Diuretics are used in some areas of the country but are not the best choice of therapy since they do nothing about

the *cause* of the edema, and may *deplete* the body of sodium and potassium. Some doctors order a short test of hydrochlorothiazide, in cases of severe edema.

Anticonvulsant: Magnesium sulfate is a specific anticonvulsant for preeclampsia. In most pharmacology texts it is listed only as a laxative (Epsom salts). Its action intravenously or intramuscularly is to lower blood pressure by causing vasodilation of peripheral blood vessels. By relieving cerebral vasospasm, depressing the central nervous system, and increasing urinary flow, it decreases the possibility of convulsions. The depressive effect lowers respiratory rate and dulls reflexes. The route of excretion is by the kidneys; therefore oliguria may lead to a cumulative effect.

Before each dose of magnesium sulfate, the patient should be checked for signs of cumulative effects:

Respiration less than 10 to 12 per minute
Urinary output below 30 ml/h

Absent or very poor knee jerk reflexes If any of these signs is present, the doctor is informed and the dose may be omitted. As an antidote, an ampul of calcium gluconate or calcium chloride 10 percent is kept, with a 20-ml syringe, at the bedside. (The ions exchange places and the effect of magnesium sulfate is stopped.)

The drug is administered as a 20 percent solution either by IV drip in 250 to 500 ml of dextrose, 5 percent in water,— or by IV push, or as a 50 percent solution intramuscularly. Deep intramuscular injection into the gluteus medius may still be so painful that the doctor may order 1 ml of 1 percent procaine to be added to the solution if the patient has no allergies. To prevent subcutaneous leaking, the drug should be administered by the Z-track technique, using a long-

table 23·1

SIGNS AND SYMPTOMS OF PREECLAMPSIA-ECLAMPSIA

MILD	MODERATE	SEVERE PREECLAMPSIA	ECLAMPSIA
Weight gain—edema More than 1–2 lb/wk. No visible edema	More than 1–2 lb/wk. Some edema above waist in abdomen, fingers, face, and extremities	Excessive weight gain; usually face puffy, rings hard to get off, etc.	Excessive weight gain. Large amount of generalized edema
Hypertension 30/15 rise over baseline reading	Diastolic, 90 or above; 140/90 or above	Systolic, 160 or above; diastolic, 110 or above; class III—may be very high	May be very high or very labile; in rare cases, only a moderate elevation
Feels some lethargy, fatigue	Complains of headaches, lethargy, fatigue	Complains of frontal headache, lasting, unrelieved by analgesics. Cerebral and visual disturbances, ringing in ears, fainting episodes	Grand mal convulsion may occur in sleep; average number, 5–15 (Fig. 23-4)
		May experience amnesia up to 48 h before convulsion. Patient appears alert and functions normally unless heavily sedated	
		Epigastric girdling pain, result of edema/hemorrhage in liver capsule	
Urine—quality/quantity No proteinuria or just a trace	+1, +2 proteinuria	Proteinuria +3, +4, 5 Gm or more in 24-h specimen	Loaded with albumin
Not much change	Scanty concentrated urine	Oliguria—1000 ml or less in 24 h	Severe oliguria; sometimes anuria—400 ml or less in 24 h
Blood changes None seen	Blood estriols may be reduced, reflecting impaired placental-fetal function	Hematocrit elevated because of hemoconcentration; plasma volume lowered; platelets lowered	Same as in severe preeclampsia
		Uric acid above 5 mg/100 ml	
Fundal changes Some retinal arteriolar spasm	More extensive spasm can be seen	Edema—papilledema, ischemia of retina	Papilledema, ischemia
Infant If delivered at this time, usually no problem	Usually no major problems	Infants may be malnourished or "small-for-dates" babies because of placental changes	Precipitate delivery may occur; infant anoxic, stillborn. Premature separation may occur
			Infant may survive if convulsions controlled before delivery

table 23.2
TREATMENT FOR PREECLAMPSIA-ECLAMPSIA

	MILD	MODERATE	SEVERE PREECLAMPSIA	ECLAMPSIA
Home care *(italic)*	Rest in bed as much as possible. Stay home—no shopping, tiring activities, etc.	*Hospitalize* Bed rest in side-lying position, with bathroom privileges	*Hospitalize* Strict bed rest, padded side rails, tongue blade at bedside, close observation. Check levels of consciousness	*Hospitalize* Strict bed rest, padded side rails, padded tongue blade, close observation. Check levels of consciousness
Diet *(italic)*	Moderate salt intake; high protein; limit carbohydrates if overweight	Fluids, 1800 kcal, high protein, moderate salt intake	Clear fluids or IV fluids only	IV fluids only
Intake and output *(italic)*	Record not necessary	Careful output record	Measured intake and output; balance intake against output q4h. Hourly output from Foley catheter	Hourly intake and output Foley catheter
Vital signs *(italic)*	Not necessary. Report any untoward symptoms to doctor	q4h while awake; FHT bid	May be more often than q4h, depending on medication and condition	Frequent, depending on condition and medication. Oxygen by mask prn, tracheostomy set at bedside. Suction at bedside
Medical supervision *(italic)*	See doctor 1–2 times a week	Daily Ophthalmoscope exam	prn Ophthalmoscope exam	prn Ophthalmoscope exam
Tests *(italic)*	Urine for protein	Urine for protein (24 h) Blood uric acid Vanillylmandelic acid(VMA) Serum electrolytes Creatinine Blood uric acid	Same as for moderate preeclampsia Hematocrit, platelets	Same as for severe preeclampsia
Medication *(italic)*	None, or low dose phenobarbital, 30 mg, tid	Phenobarbital, 30–60 mg, q6h Diuretic: short trial to see effect Administer Kay Ciel if patient on diuretics Many doctors feel diuretics contraindicated and dangerous	Phenobarbital, 30–60 mg, q6h Apresoline trial—up to 200 mg daily, carefully titrated if diastolic over 110 Depending on condition: Magnesium sulfate IV 2–4 Gm on admission; then 1 Gm/h or 5 Gm q4h	Some physicians order Dilantin during eclampsia but treatment usually used is: Magnesium sulfate IV 1 Gm/h after initial dose—or 5 Gm q4h If urine 30 ml or more per h, reflexes present, respirations over 10–12 per min

enough needle to accomplish a true intramuscular deposit of fluid.

Severe Preeclampsia-Eclampsia If, in spite of treatment, the trend in blood pressure continues to rise, the patient may enter the phase of severe preeclampsia. She will feel very sick, and with good reason, for she is acutely ill. Equipment must be made readily available and convulsion precautions started, as follows:

Padded side rails on bed
Padded tongue blade (Fig. 23·6) and an airway at bedside
Tracheostomy set at bedside
Oxygen available by mask
Suction equipment at bedside (Fig. 23·5)
Foley catheter (urinary output recorded every 1 to 4 h as ordered)
Nothing by mouth or clear fluids as ordered
Fluids intravenously, using intravenous catheter, well secured
Darkened, quiet room
Vital signs checked every 1 to 4 h as ordered; fetal heart tone (FHT) every 4 h
Close nursing observation

Convulsions are preceded by periods of amnesia, although the patient appears awake and rational. The chief complaint will be severe frontal headache, *unrelieved by analgesics*. The patient may complain of visual disturbances, ringing in the ears, or girdling epigastric pain, caused by edema of the liver capsule. Convulsions may occur during sleep and, contrary to some types of seizures, are not specifically triggered by light or noise (Fig. 23·4). A dark, quiet room is set up to reduce stimuli to the patient's edematous, irritated brain, and to encourage rest. The patient in severe preeclampsia will feel so sick that she will be very passive, and of course she will be heavily sedated (Fig. 23·5). Levels of consciousness should be checked at intervals because she can slip into coma without a convulsion. A rising

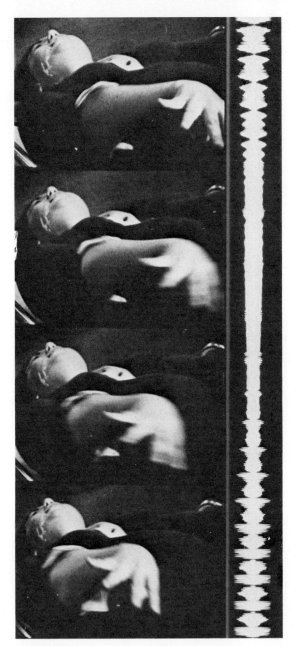

fig. 23·4 The first phase of a convulsion is tonic, rigid muscle contraction. (*From "Modern Obstetrics: Pre-eclampsia-Eclampsia"; courtesy of Ortho Pharmaceutical Corporation.*)

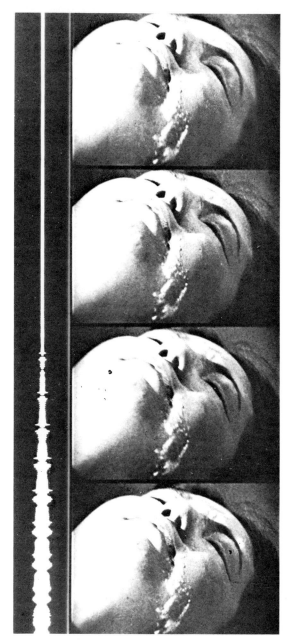

fig. 23·5 Vomiting or excessive mucus may require suctioning. (*From "Modern Obstetrics: Pre-eclampsia-Eclampsia;" Courtesy of Ortho Pharmaceutical Corporation.*)

blood pressure and decreasing urinary output are alarming signs of the rapid progress of the illness.

Care during the convulsion is limited to trying to protect the patient and to providing adequate oxygenation (Fig. 23·6). Oxygen is given by mask. If there is a rapid series of convulsions, a tracheostomy may be needed to provide a clear airway. Anoxia of the mother will affect the infant, but no labor will be induced until the convulsions are controlled for at least 24 h. "Immediate delivery of a convulsing patient doubles her chance of dying" (20). In some instances labor begins during a convulsive period. In those cases labor usually progresses rapidly to a precipitate delivery in bed, often with an abruptio placentae and excessive bleeding.

The seriousness of eclampsia is borne out by the statistics: 6 to 8 percent of all pregnant women develop hypertension; 6 to 8 percent of these hypertensive women develop eclampsia; among these, the maternal death rate has been as high as 10 to 15 percent. Death is due to uncontrolled convulsions, precipitate delivery, bleeding, and in some cases hypofibrinogenemia (24).

Recovery from eclampsia may be very rapid, with the blood pressure returning to moderate levels within 48 h of delivery. However, the danger of convulsions is not over for any preeclamptic or eclamptic patient until 3 or 4 days after delivery. Even without radical changes in blood pressure, convulsions have been known to occur on the delivery table and in the postpartum period. The patient with hypertension is in danger until her pressure is safely near her normal nonpregnant levels.

CLASS II—CHRONIC HYPERTENSION

The second group of hypertensive patients in pregnancy are those who have preexisting chronic hypertension from various causes. Elevation of blood pressure is always a se-

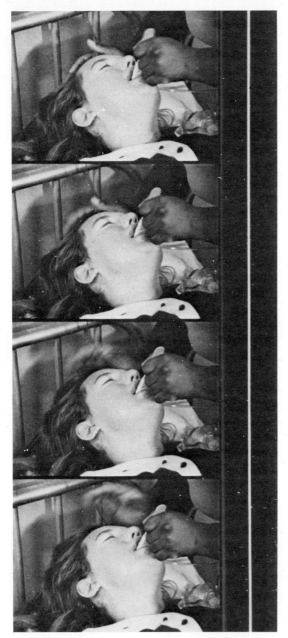

fig. 23·6 Place a padded tongue blade to the side of the mouth between the molars. (*From "Modern Obstetrics: Preeclampsia-Eclampsia;" Courtesy of Ortho Pharmacequtcal Corporation.*)

condary symptom of a primary disease in the body; many diseases cause hypertension. If pregnancy is superimposed on chronic hypertension the patient's symptoms may be aggravated. Close medical attention is needed throughout the gestational period. Severely hypertensive women may be warned not to become pregnant or may be advised to have a therapeutic abortion.

Because of the slight *decrease* in blood pressure during the first two trimesters, there may be an improvement in the symptoms, only to have a return to hypertension in the third trimester. Table 23·3 outlines the symptoms and severity in a pregnant woman of hypertension that was present before pregnancy.

The *cause* of hypertension is treated where possible. There is a high fetal mortality rate in pregnancies with moderately severe hypertension, as well as a much higher risk of the woman's developing preeclampsia. Very often infants are growth-retarded and placentas are smaller than usual. Patients with moderate to severe hypertension are treated as cardiac patients are, with as much bed rest as possible, a controlled diet, and hospitalization during the last trimester.

Since high blood pressure is only a symptom, medication specifically to reduce blood pressure may be used if the diastolic pressure rises above 110 and there is proteinuria. Apresoline (hydralazine) is often prescribed, as it relaxes smooth muscle and may cause renal vasodilation with improved urinary output.

CLASS III—HYPERTENSION WITH SUPERIMPOSED PREECLAMPSIA

About 25 percent of hypertensive pregnant women develop preeclampsia in some form. Of these, those with moderate to severe hypertension existing before pregnancy are in the most danger (refer to Table 23·3). Note the pathologic bodily changes which can be aggravated by the effects of superimposed

table 23.3

CLASSIFICATION OF SEVERITY OF HYPERTENSION IN GRAVID WOMEN

BY DIASTOLIC BLOOD PRESSURE

	1st AND 2d TRIMESTERS	3d TRIMESTER
Mild	80	90
Moderate	100	110
Severe	120	130

BY OTHER CLINICAL CRITERIA

	CARDIAC	FUNDOSCOPY*	RENAL
Mild	Normal cardiac size. Normal electrocardiogram	Normal/minimal (KW I)	Normal renal function 30–50% increment in pregnancy
Moderate	Cardiac enlargement may be evident. ECG evidence of left ventricular hypertrophy. Few symptoms	Spastic or sclerotic changes (KW I, II)	Renal function decreased to approximately that of normal nonpregnant women, i.e., 500 ml/min. Filtration fraction may be increased
Severe	Cardiac enlargement usually evident. ECG evidence of hypertrophy and ischemia. Some symptoms (i.e., headache, palpitations)	Above and occasional hemorrhages and exudates (KW III)	Decreased renal function Increased filtration fraction
Accelerated and malignant	Above symptoms of cardiac failure, ischemic pains, and/or encephalopathy	Frank hemorrhages and exudates, papilledema (KW IV, malignant phase)	Rapidly decreasing renal function, hematuria, proteinuria

*KW = Keith Wagener classification.

Source: Reproduced by permission from Philip J. Feitleson and Marshall D. Lindheimer, "Management of Hypertensive Gravidas," *Journal of Reproductive Medicine,* **8**(3):1972.

preeclampsia. The disease develops earlier in pregnancy and moves to a crisis more rapidly than in normotensive women. Severe renal failure, an increased incidence of abruptio placentae, and more stillbirths are found in this group of women. Finally, preeclampsia tends to recur with each subsequent pregnancy when the woman is already hypertensive.

The signs of preeclampsia in these women are a rise in diastolic blood pressure of 15 mmHg over the usual reading, and any of the classic symptoms of headache, fatigue, edema, oliguria, and proteinuria. Hospitalization is the only safe way to care for this class of hypertensive patients.

CLASS IV—TRANSIENT HYPERTENSION IN PREGNANCY

Transient hypertension occurring *only* in pregnancy parallels *preclinical* or *gestational diabetes* in its prognosis. It has been predicted that women who develop hypertension without preeclampsia in pregnancy. will develop essential hypertension later in life (15, 17). Blood pressure returns to normal soon after delivery. There are no other untoward symptoms. Once the diagnosis of transient hypertension is made, treatment is symptomatic: adequate rest in bed in a side-lying position, and an adequate, controlled diet. No salt restriction is made, nor are diuretics given.

CASE STUDY
Apr. 12
A sixteen-year-old, white primigravida at first visit to the prenatal clinic has a blood pressure of 130/80; pulse, 88; respirations, 18. Height, 5 ft 7 in. Weight, 168 lb. Estimated gestational age—32 weeks.

Counseled, sent home on a restricted-carbohydrate, high-protein, moderate-salt diet. Instructed to rest in bed several times a day and to return in 2 weeks. Instructed to call doctor for any signs of edema, headache, dizziness, visual disturbances.

Apr. 26
Kept appointment, complained of headache. Bp, 144/98; weight, 181 lb. 1+ pitting edema. Admitted to antepartum unit.

Orders: Strict bed rest, side-lying position
Record of liquid intake and urinary output
Preeclampsia check; bp, q4h while awake; FHT, bid; weight, qd.
Regular diet, force fluids
Urinalysis, qd for sugar, albumin, and specific gravity
Urine test for VMA, SMA 12, estriols
Blood for uric acid, CBC, hematocrit
Medications: Hygroton, 50 mg po qd × 2
Phenobarbital, 60 mg po q6h

Apr. 28
Bed rest and diuretic have caused 8-lb weight loss. 36 h after admission, 1 A.M., labor began. Patient very anxious about labor. Bp, 180/100. Seen by resident, who on basis of diastolic reading, ordered:

Magnesium sulfate, 2 Gm IV and 8 Gm IM stat.
7:30 A.M. At 7:30 A.M. in good labor; bp, 140/100; temperature, 36.7°C; pulse, 110; respirations, 24
8:30 A.M. FHT, 140. Membranes ruptured at 8:30; FHT to 180 for 20 min. Patient very wild and restless; Demerol, 50 mg, and Phenergan, 25 mg, administered
9:00 A.M. Blood pressure dropped from 140/100 to 120/90 to 100/80; turned to side, quieted; pressure rose slowly to 140/114
12:00 P.M. Delivered by low forceps, 5 lb 3 oz, healthy baby, Apgar score 8–9
1:00 P.M. Bp, 160/110
1:30 P.M. Bp, 140/90
Returned to ward. Orders: Continue preeclampsia check, record intake and output, administer phenobarbital, 60 mg tid.
May 2
The patient had an uneventful recovery and was discharged on the sixth postpartum day, with a blood pressure of 124/75; weight, 155 lb.

references

1. Ralph C. Benson, *Handbook of Obstetrics and Gynecology*, 4th ed., Lange Medical Publications, Los Altos, Calif., 1971, p. 198.
2. Eugene L. Coodley, "Anatomy of Circulation," *Consultant*, May, 1972, p. 103.
3. Joseph J. Rovinsky, "Blood Volume and

the Hemodynamics of Pregnancy," chap. 6 in Elliot E. Phillip (ed.), *Scientific Foundations of Obstetrics and Gynecology*, F. A. Davis Company, Philadelphia, 1970, pp. 335, 336.

4. Douglas M. Haynes, *Medical Complications during Pregnancy*, McGraw-Hill Book Company, New York, 1969, p. 75.
5. Nicholas S. Assali and Charles R. Brinkman, *Pathophysiology of Gestation: Maternal Disorders*, vol. I, Academic Press, Inc., New York, 1972.
6. Leonard A. Aaro, and John L. Jeurgens, "Thrombophlebitis Associated with Pregnancy," *American Journal of Obstetrics and Gynecology*, **109**(8):1128, 1971.
7. Joseph J. Rovinsky, Correlated Seminar on Thromboembolic Disease in Pregnancy—ACOG Meeting, New York, 1970.
8. D. J. Daniel, "Estrogens and Puerperal Thromboembolism," *American Heart Journal*, **78**:720, 1969.
9. Louis M. Hellman, and Jack Pritchard, *Williams' Obstetrics*, 14th ed., Appleton-Century-Crofts, Inc., New York, 1971.
10. Kenneth R. Niswander and Myron Gordon (eds.), *The Women and Their Pregnancies*, The Collaborative Perinatal Study of the National Institute of Neurological Diseases and Stroke, W. B. Saunders Company, Philadelphia, 1972, p. 226.
11. Ibid., p. 227.
12. Haynes, op. cit., p. 35.
13. Jerome W. Niswonger and Charles F. Langmade, "Cardiovascular Changes in Vaginal Deliveries and Cesarian Section," *American Journal of Obstetrics and Gynecology*, **107**(3):337, 1970.
14. Benson, op. cit., p. 304.
15. Philip J. Feitleson and Marshall D. Lindheimer, "Management of the Hypertensive Gravida," *Journal of Reproductive Medicine*, **8**(3):111, 1972.
16. Hellman, and Pritchard, op. cit., p. 685.
17. Ian MacGillivray, "Blood Pressure in Pregnancy," chap. 2 in Elliot E. Phillip (ed.), *Scientific Foundations of Obstetrics and Gynecology*, F. A. Davis Company, Philadelphia, 1970, p. 293.
18. Edward N. Ehrlich, and Marshall D. Lindheimer, "Sodium Metabolism, Aldosterone, and the Hypertensive Disorders of Pregnancy," *Journal of Reproductive Medicine*, **8**(3):106, 1972.
19. Norman M. Simon and Frank A. Krumlovsky, "The Pathophysiology of Hypertension in Pregnancy," *Journal of Reproductive Medicine*, **8**(3):102, 1972.
20. Haynes, op. cit., p. 161.
21. Leon C. Chesley, J. E. Annitto, and R. A. Cosgrove, "Long-term Follow Up Study of Eclamptic Women," *American Journal of Obstetrics and Gynecology*, **101**:886, 1968.
22. Ruth M. French, *The Nurse's Guide to Diagnostic Procedures*, 2d ed., McGraw-Hill Book Company, New York, 1967, p. 35.
23. Feitleson and Lindheimer, op. cit., p. 114.
24. Lester T. Hibbard, "Maternal Mortality Due to Acute Toxemia," *Obstetrics and Gynecology*, **42**(2):263, 1973.

bibliography

Benson, Ralph C.: *Handbook of Obstetrics and Gynecology*, 4th ed., Lange Medical Publications, Los Altos, Calif., 1971.

Flowers, Charles E.: "Magnesium Sulfate in Obstetrics," *American Journal of Obstetrics and Gynecology*, **96**:763–776, 1965.

Haynes, E. M.: *Medical Complications during Pregnancy*, McGraw-Hill Book Company, New York, 1969.

Hytten, Frank E., and Isabella Leitch: *The Physiology of Human Pregnancy*, Blackwell Scientific Publications, Ltd., Oxford, 1971.

Jovanovic, Dusan: "The Pathology of Pregnancy and Labor in Adolescent Patients,"

Journal of Reproductive Medicine, **9**(2):61, 1972.

Rovinsky, Joseph J., and Alan F. Guttmacher (eds.): *Medical, Surgical and Gynecologic Complications of Pregnancy,* 2d ed., The Williams & Wilkins Company , Baltimore, 1965.

Standards for Hospital Services, American College of Obstetrics and Gynecology, Chicago, 1969.

Vander, Aurthur J., James H. Sherman, and Dorothy S. Luciano: *Human Physiology,* McGraw-Hill Book Company, New York, 1970.

Weekes, L. R.: "Thromboembolic Disease in Pregnancy," *American Journal of Obstetrics and Gynecology,* **107**:649, 1970.

Zuspan, F. P.: "Symposium on Toxemia of Pregnancy," *Clinical Obstetrics and Gynecology,* December, 1966, pp. 859–990.

———: "The High-risk Pregnancy—A Series: Acute Hypertension in Pregnancy," *Contemporary OB/GYN,* **1**(3):27, 1973.

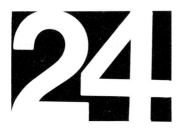

metabolic problems during pregnancy

Hilda Koehler

vomiting

In Chap. 4 you read about typical "morning sickness," or nausea of early pregnancy. When constant and excessive vomiting continues to the sixteenth week of pregnancy, resulting in 5 percent or more loss of body weight, it is termed *hyperemesis gravidarum*. If it continues without treatment, ketosis, ketonuria, neurologic disturbances, liver damage, and renal damage result, and finally death. In the past many women died of this condition; now therapy is started before death threatens.

Although no one knows the cause of hyperemesis gravidarum, the following have been offered as contributing reasons:

1. High levels of chorionic gonadotropin (HCG)
2. Decreased secretion of free hydrochloric acid simultaneously with reduced gastric motility
3. Psychologic intensification of physiologic factors

The peak of vomiting, coinciding with the peak level of chorionic gonadotropin in the blood, is at the tenth week (see Fig. 4·2). Because of the higher levels of HCG in those conditions, pernicious vomiting is more common when there is a multiple pregnancy or hydatidiform mole. Since gastric secretion and motility are decreased and the stomach is displaced upward and to the left early, this seems a reasonable factor in causing vomiting.

Conflicts surrounding the prospect of motherhood—such as fear of the responsibilities, worry about the threat to body image posed by the changing figure, dread of losing independence, or difficulty in thinking of oneself as a mother rather than a daughter—may provide the type of stress that produces vomiting as a reaction.

DIAGNOSIS

Since the woman is unable to retain anything ingested, she may lose an enormous amount of weight, to the point of emaciation. Resulting dehydration may lead to hemoconcentration; carbohydrate depletion will result in ketosis. Existence of acetoacetic acid and acetone in the blood and urine confirms the diagnosis.

TREATMENT

Hospitalization for correction of electrolyte balance and dehydration with intravenous infusions, until oral intake can be resumed, is usually necessary. Vitamin supplements (particularly the B complex group, because of its action on the nervous system) are frequently added to the intravenous infusions. Sedation in injectable or suppository form is usually ordered; the most common drugs are phenobarbital and/or prochlorperazine. Psychologic counseling is instituted, either formally, by a psychiatrist or social worker, or more informally by the attending physician and nurses. Once oral feedings are possible, frequent small meals are given.

NURSING RESPONSIBILITIES

The sympathetic but deliberately firm care given by nursing staff contributes immensely to the recuperation of patients with hyperemesis. By maintaining a calm, compassionate atmosphere, projecting confidence in the certain effectiveness of treatment, and accepting vomiting episodes matter-of-factly, the nurse will truly provide reassurance. Be sure to be careful that the woman is served only foods that are palatable to her, and that they are attractively arranged in very small portions. Hot foods must be hot and cold foods cold; lukewarm foods are intolerable.

PROGNOSIS

Complete recovery can be expected. In the rare cases in which treatment fails, interruption of the pregnancy will be necessary.

PREVENTION

Leppert (1) suggest that if young people receive education promoting healthy attitudes toward adult sexual roles, with emphasis on prevention of disturbed relationships—mother/daughter, parent/child—the incidence of hyperemesis will decrease. Meanwhile, the obstetric health team must become more skillful and consistent in providing family-centered care which supports couples in assuming their new parenthood roles.

obesity

Approximately 60 million Americans are overweight (2). There is always a number of pregnant women who are obese and whose bodies are thereby taxed by two simultaneous stresses. The following facts about the overweight pregnant patient illustrate the handicap they are under:

1. Chronic hypertension is more common.
2. Babies tend to be larger—8 lb or more.
3. Latent diabetes becomes overt during pregnancy.
4. Uterine dysfunction is more common, because of:

 a. The oversized fetus
 b. Compromised pelvic capacity
5. Perinatal mortality is four times greater than for women of normal size (3)

Present practice discourages weight loss during pregnancy. But with care and motivation some overweight women can maintain their prepregnant weight and keep wellnourished and healthy, properly nourishing the fetus.

thyroid disorders

Iodine uptake and thyroxine secretion are controlled in the body by the thyroid-stimulating hormone. Iodine trapped in the thyroid gland is essential for the synthesis of thyroid hormone; if the synthesis into the hormone does not take place, a goiter will develop. Large amounts of iodine can be used to inhibit the hypertrophied thyroid gland by inhibiting the release of the thyroid-stimulating hormone from the pituitary.

HYPERTHYROIDISM (GRAVES' DISEASE)

Hyperthyroidism occurs in 0.5 to 1:100 pregnancies (4). It is related to increased frequency of premature delivery, postpartum hemorrhage, and possibly preeclampsia, but it does not cause abortions or fetal anomalies (5). Pregnancy itself contains some of the ingredients of mild hyperthyroidism: the thyroid gland enlarges, women tend to be bothered by heat, their pulse is faster, they are more moody, and, of course, they have no menses. Overtreatment of the mother with hyperthyroid drugs may result in fetal hypothyroidism and deficient development, especially of the central nervous system (6). Radioactive iodine is not usually used because it would pass freely across the placenta, concentrating in the baby and causing damage to the baby's thyroid and gonads(7).

Treatment In severe cases, the internal medicine specialist and the obstetrician collaborate in caring for the hyperthyroid gravida. Drugs are prescribed to suppress the activity of the thyroid (Lugol's solution, thiouracil, with or without thyroxine), so as to improve the mother's condition without compromising that of the fetus. In the second trimester, a subtotal thyroidectomy may be performed, if indicated, by an experienced surgeon.

Prognosis The mother will recover completely. The baby's thyroid function should be monitored carefully so that if it has been suppressed the baby can receive prompt treatment.

The only thyroid disease unique to pregnancy is hyperthyroidism accompanying hydatidiform mole, which is due to placental secretion of thyroid stimulator. Removing the mole effects the cure (8).

HYPOTHYROIDISM (MYXEDEMA)

Conception and hypothyroidism are usually incompatible (9). However, should a hypothyroid woman become pregnant, early diagnosis is mandatory, because abortion, premature delivery, preeclampsia, and congenital anomalies (most notably cretinism and/or mental retardation) are common. Since the baby's thyroid develops independently of the mother's, however, a normal infant may be born to a hypothyroid mother. Nonetheless, since thyroid disease has a familial tendency, there is a slightly greater expectation of thyroid disturbance in the fetus if the mother is hypothyroid (10).

Treatment Sodium L-thyroxine is prescribed in gradually increasing doses until symptoms disappear.

Prognosis The mother's condition will be stabilized by the thyroid hormone. [In untreated patients, a characteristic exquisite sensitivity to anesthetic agents can be a hazard to the mother (11).] The infant can be expected to be normal when the mother receives proper treatment; however, with delayed or insufficient treatment permanent mental or physical retardation is likely.

diabetes

Diabetes mellitus, from the Greek *diabētēs,* meaning "siphon," and the Latin *mellitus,* "honey-sweet," is the inability to metabolize glucose properly. It is inherited through recessive genes, with 75·percent of the population free of diabetes, 20 percent not diabetic but able to transmit the gene, and 5 percent who are diabetic although not necessarily symptomatic, and who can and do transfer the disease to offspring (12). It is not race-related. In women, symptoms of diabetes occur more frequently during menopause or in their fifties.

Before the discovery of insulin in 1921, diabetic women rarely became pregnant. Infertility and sterility were probably related to loss of ovarian function secondary to malfunction of the anterior pituitary gland, and severe dietary restriction to control the diabetes reduced the nutritional elements necessary for reproduction (13). Of the diabetics achieving pregnancy, 25 percent died; and 60 percent of the babies died (14). Currently the incidence of diabetes is 1:100 to 200 pregnancies. Since the gravid state frequently unmasks unsymptomatic (latent) diabetes, many cases of diabetes are discovered for the first time during pregnancy.

Diabetes is manifested by an increased amount of glucose in the blood and subsequently in the urine. Abnormality is dependent upon actual or relative deficiency of insulin, resulting from functional disturbance of the islets of Langerhans in the pancreas. (Insulin is necessary for metabolism of glucose into glycogen.) Glucose is not metabolized, and it accumulates in the blood. Since the cells cannot use this form of carbohydrate for energy, they metabolize fat instead; thus the result is that the person loses weight. The kidneys attempt to excrete the excess glucose, and the liver is unable to store glycogen properly.

The following are *signs and symptoms of diabetes*:

Polyuria (excess urination)
Polydipsia (excess thirst/fluid intake)
Polyphagia (excess hunger/food intake)
Neuritis (there may be pain in fingers and toes)
Skin disturbances, e.g., pruritus and slow healing
Weight loss
Weakness, fatigue, drowsiness
Visual disturbances

Because of the metabolism of fats, the liver produces an oversupply of ketone bodies; these combine with sodium, tending to make the blood more acid. If untreated, polyuria causes dehydration, with loss of valuable water-soluble minerals. Shifts of electrolytes from cells to body fluids result in the following:

Hemoconcentration and dehydration (elevated hematocrit)
Loss of base and chlorides, reduction of carbon dioxide—combining power, and thus, a shift of pH to the acid side
Fall in blood pressure, circulatory collapse
Labored breathing (Kussmaul respirations)
Depressed renal activity, retention of non-protein nitrogen
Subnormal temperature

Sugar in the urine during pregnancy may be from three main causes: lactose (milk sugar), transient glycosuria (benign), or diabetes. Investigation is needed to determine the cause.

The following conditions should *prompt suspicion of diabetes*:

A family history of diabetes, particularly in parent(s) or twin
History of large babies (weight above 9 lb)
History of increasing birth weights with each child
Unexplained perinatal mortality
Unexplained congenital anomalies
Maternal obesity
Glycosuria during current pregnancy
Hydramnios
History of repeated abortions
History of repeated infections

The most commonly used, because it is the most specific, White's classification for diabetes during pregnancy is that outlined below:

Class A: Slightly abnormal glucose tolerance test; dietary control sufficient; no insulin required
Class B: Onset after age twenty; duration less than 10 years; no vascular disease
Class C: Onset between ages ten and twenty; duration 10 to 19 years; minimal or no vascular disease (retinal arteriosclerosis or calcification of leg vessels only)
Class D: Onset before ten; duration more than 20 years; vascular disease demonstrated by retinitis, transitory albuminuria, or transitory hypertension
Class E: Calcification of pelvic arteries evident on x-ray
Class F: Kidney involvement

TREATMENT

Close collaboration among internist, obstetrician, and pediatrician is mandatory in the care of the pregnant diabetic and her fetus, during pregnancy and through the puerperium and neonatal period. A thorough history is basic. When a known diabetic suspects that she is pregnant, she is most wise to get immediate medical attention, to minimize the chances of risk. Oral hypoglycemics should not be used during pregnancy, because the effects on fetal differentiation and development are unknown (17); however, it is not unusual for a diabetic to present herself to the obstetrician already 8 to 10 weeks pregnant, and having maintained herself on oral agents!

Management of diabetes and pregnancy

table 24·1

INTERACTION OF DIABETES AND PREGNANCY

DIABETES CHANGES PREGNANCY	PREGNANCY CHANGES DIABETES
Oversized babies (metabolic acceleration: true skeletal growth, fat, water retention)	Subclinical (latent) diabetes may become clinical (overt, gestational) diabetes

Fetal death after 36 weeks likely (due to acidosis or placental dysfunction)	Renal glucose threshold is increased:
	  a. Glucose tolerance test is changed
	  b. 2-h postprandial level is elevated

Fetal anomalies more common (3% are lethal)	

Infertility and spontaneous abortion rate higher	Glucose tolerance is changed:
	  a. Elevated needs for insulin, but sometimes
	  b. Lowered needs for insulin if fetal pancreas functions to provide mother's need

Higher incidence of hypertension	
Higher incidence of preeclampsia (one-third to one-half of patients are affected)	Status of diabetes changes because of differing metabolic needs throughout pregnancy
Placenta ages more rapidly	
Abruptio placentae more common; hemorrhage more common	Metabolic complications (hyperemesis, nausea) difficult to treat
Premature labor more common	Work of labor depletes glycogen stores; ketosis may result
Hydramnios more common (10 times more common in the diabetic)	Anabolic activity changes to catabolic activity after delivery, upsetting diet and insulin needs
Higher incidence of infection	High estrogen levels may affect glucose tolerance of liver

DIABETES AFFECTS THE NEONATE

Hyaline membrane disease more common because of prematurity, cesarean section delivery, disordered metabolic state, increased risk of intrauterine asphyxia

Hypoglycemia (below 30 mg/100 ml) can return to normal within 8 h after birth; symptoms are tremors, apnea, cyanosis, seizures, lethargy, poor sucking reflex

Hypocalcemia and hypomagnesemia may be present

Elevated bilirubin, potassium, and phosphate levels (15, 16)

May have congenital anomalies, cardiac enlargement, lighter-weight brain

Poorer temperature control. Red skin, fat, puffy cheeks, returns to normal by 1 mo.

aims at careful evaluation and classification of the condition of the diabetic woman before or early in pregnancy, meticulous and constant supervision and intervention throughout pregnancy, labor, and the puerperium, early termination of pregnancy, and careful pediatric care of the newborn. Prevention of acidosis, toxemia, infections, and intrauterine death are ongoing goals. Usually the obstetrician and internist take turns seeing the patient every 2 weeks until the twenty-eighth week; then she will be seen weekly or more often, depending on her intelligence and cooperation and the severity of the disease (Table 24·1).

To determine dietary and insulin management, the following tests are made at frequent intervals during pregnancy: fasting blood sugar level (70 to 120 mg/100 ml is the normal range in most facilities); 2-h postprandial blood sugar level; urinalyses for glucose, ketone bodies, and albumin; and blood urea nitrogen. Periodic eye examinations by an ophthalmologist are recommended; cardiovascular and renal function tests may be needed.

DIETARY MANAGEMENT[1]

The aim of dietary management for the pregnant diabetic woman is to stabilize her blood glucose level. The carbohydrate, protein, and fat content of her food intake should be relatively constant from day to day, since these nutrients contribute to blood sugar levels.

There are two methods of dietary management for the diabetic patient. The liberal dietary management is known as the "free diet." The more conservative method is the use of the diabetic exchange system, developed by the American Dietetic Association, the American Diabetic Association, and the U.S. Public Health Service.

The patient on the free diet is taught to eat an adequate diet and to avoid sugar and concentrated sweets. It is based on a more tolerant view toward glycosuria. The patient does not measure the amount of food she eats, but is taught to eat foods in the basic four food groups. During pregnancy, she should eat foods as outlined in Chap. 4.

If meticulous dietary management is desired, the physician will prescribe a diet for the patient, giving the desired level of carbohydrate, protein, and fat. The diabetic exchange system is based on the grouping of foods according to their similarity in carbohydrate, protein, as well as in fat content. Foods that do not need to be measured are coffee, tea, clear broth, bouillon, lemon, unsweetened gelatin, vinegar, spices, and seasonings. Foods which are not allowed are sugar, syrups, and other concentrated sweets.

An example of a diabetic diet suitable for a woman in her second and third trimesters is the 2200-kcal diet containing 220 Gm carbohydrates, 95 Gm protein, and 105 Gm fat. This diet allows the following daily food plan:

FOOD EXCHANGES	AMOUNT
Milk, whole	4 cups
Vegetable, group A	As desired
Vegetable, group B	1
Fruit	3
Bread	9
Meat	6
Fat	7

Meal Plans:

Breakfast
1 fruit exchange
1 meat exchange

Lunch
2 meat exchanges
3 bread exchanges

DIABETIC EXCHANGES

EXCHANGE	PORTION SIZE	CARBOHYDRATE, Gm	PROTEIN, Gm	FAT, Gm	kcal
Milk, whole	8 oz	12	8	10	170
Vegetables, group A	As desired				
Vegetables, group B	½ cup	7	2		36
Fruit	Varies	10			40
Bread	1 slice or varies	15	2		68
Meat	1 oz or varies		7	5	73
Fat	1 tsp			5	45

[1]Written by Beatrice Lau Kee.

2 bread exchanges
1 fat exchange
1 cup milk

Vegetable A
2 fat exchanges
1 fruit exchange
1 cup milk

Dinner
3 meat exchanges
2 bread exchanges
Vegetable A
1 vegetable B
2 fat exchanges
1 fruit exchange
1 cup milk

Snack
1 cup milk
2 bread exchanges
2 fat exchanges

Sample Menus:

Breakfast
Orange juice ½ cup
1 egg
1 slice bread
1 tsp butter or
   margarine
1 cup milk

Lunch
2 oz tuna fish
2 slices bread
2 tsp mayonnaise
Celery sticks
Apple
2 graham crackers
1 cup milk

Dinner
Meat loaf, 3 oz
½ cup mashed potato
Green beans
Carrots ½ cup
1 slice bread
2 tsp butter or
   margarine
½ cup fruit cup
1 cup milk

Snack
1 cup milk
2 slices bread
2 Tbsp cream
   cheese

Additional information about diabetic diets may be obtained from

The American Diabetes Association
1 East 45 Street
New York, New York 10017
or
The American Dietetic Association
620 North Michigan Avenue
Chicago, Illinois 60611

The local health department is another resource for patients who are put on diabetic diets by their physicians.

INSULIN REQUIREMENTS

Insulin requirements vary considerably. Some diabetic gravidas need none; unpredictable variations call for constant surveillance. In general, insulin requirements become greater, peaking · at about the seventh month. Ordinarily satisfactory regulation can be attained by administering one of the long-acting preparations. Complications, notably hyperemesis gravidarum, infections, gastrointestinal upset, toxemia, or the stress of labor, require a shift to regular insulin to secure more accurate regulation (18) (Table 24·2).

During the first trimester nausea and vomiting may lead to acidosis and must be treated after examination rather than over the telephone. During the second trimester, infections, especially of the urinary tract, are most likely to be a problem. Pyelonephritis must be prevented. In the third trimester, signs of sugar intolerance and toxemia are potential hazards. Deciding on the best time for delivery of the baby is considered the biggest challenge; hospitalization at about 35 weeks as an aid in making this determination is the usual practice. The following tests are performed: determination of size and age of the baby by palpation; x-ray for presence of distal femoral epiphysis and/or edematous fetus (halo sign); sonogram; urinary estriol determination (Fig. 24·1); and/or amniocentesis for determination of creatinine and pulmonary lipid levels. Because a diabetic fetus tends to be large, the possibility of maternal dystocia is greater, the placenta ages more rapidly, and the infant tends to have a higher mortality rate if left until term, most obstetricians consider the thirty-seventh week optimum delivery time. Seventy percent will have a cesarean section, with a 90 percent fetal survival (19).

table 24·2

CHARACTERISTICS OF VARIOUS TYPES OF INSULIN

TYPE	INDICATIONS	PEAK ACTION, NO. OF HOURS AFTER ADMINISTRATION	DURATION, h
Regular	Emergencies Acidosis Acute infections and chronic infections Surgery, delivery Very young children Supplement to other insulins	1	5–7
Protamine zinc	If more than 30 units insulin required daily	14–20	36
NPH	If more than 30 units insulin required daily	10–16	24–28
Lente	If more than 30 units insulin required daily	10–16	24–28
Semilente	To speed action	4–6	12–16
Ultralente	To prolong action	18–28	36+

NURSING RESPONSIBILITIES

With the rest of the health team, the nurse seeks to assist the expectant diabetic mother to understand the complications that might arise, manifestations of her disease, its treatment, and its prognosis (20). Central to the nurse's teaching is stress of the following:

1. The importance of early prenatal care in pregnancy and of keeping all appointments.
2. Reviewing the role of the diet, both for good nutrition and for diabetic control.
3. Reviewing or teaching examination of urine for sugar and acetone. The woman should test a fresh specimen, which will mean emptying her bladder, waiting ½ h, voiding again, and testing the second specimen. (Toward the end of pregnancy, it may be necessary to use a method specific for glucose, as some methods do not differentiate between lactose and glucose.)
4. Recognizing the signs and symptoms of hypo- and hyperglycemia (Table 24·2).

5. The necessity of reporting any infections or illness to the physician.
6. Reviewing care of teeth, skin, feet, personal hygiene.

fig. 24·1 Patterns of estriol excretion in four categories of diabetic patients. Category 1: fetal death occurred when estriol remained below 4 mg for 24 h. Category 2: mother needed an early cesarean section when estriol level fell rapidly; infant survived. Category 3: section scheduled for thirty-seventh week; infant survived. Category 4: labor ended pregnancy naturally, with infant survival. (*From John W. Green, "Assessing Maternal Estriol Excretion,"* Contemporary OB/GYN, **2**(3):63. 1973.)

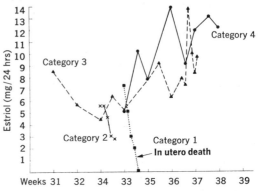

table 24·3

SIGNS AND SYMPTOMS OF DIABETIC COMA AND INSULIN SHOCK

	DIABETIC COMA (HYPERGLYCEMIA)	INSULIN SHOCK (HYPOGLYCEMIA)
Signs:		
Onset	Slow	Rapid
Skin	Dry	Sweating
Reflexes	Normal or absent	Positive Babinski's reflex
Eyeballs	Soft	Normal
Color	Florid face	Pallor
Urine	Sugar	Negative for sugar
Breath	Acetone odor	Normal
Breathing	Kussmaul (deep, labored)	Shallow
Pulse	Rapid	Normal
Symptoms	Thirst	Inward nervousness
	Nausea/vomiting	Hunger
	Headache	Weakness
	Abdominal pain	Paresthesia
	Dim vision	Blurred vision
	Dyspnea	Stupor, convulsions
	Constipation	Psychopathic behavior

7. Reviewing exercises and rest needs. (Overfatigue decreases carbohydrate tolerance.)
8. If insulin is needed, teaching or reviewing its administration. (The nurse must know the information in Table 24·2 in order to anticipate insulin reaction.)
9. How to collect 24-h urine specimens for estriol determination, glucose testing.
10. Importance of wearing identification as a diabetic.
11. Referral to other health personnel and agencies as indicated.

After delivery, diabetes is most difficult to control. Wide and sudden changes in blood sugar level occur because of endocrine and metabolic disruption associated with the termination of pregnancy, slight postpartum infection, change of blood glucose to lactose for breast milk, and perhaps the withdrawal of the availability of fetal insulin. After the second day, placental lactogen is gone and the nursing staff must be alert to the possibility of insulin shock.

For nursing care of the neonate, see Chap. 28.

PROGNOSIS

Maternal mortality of less than 2:1000 is expected with adequate modern therapy. Eye and kidney disorders are usually increased during gestation (21). The baby's prognosis depends on the severity of the diabetes, complications (either medical or obstetric), and prematurity, as well as on method of delivery (vaginal delivery is preferred). Infant mortality rate is currently between 10 and 15 percent, and anomalies occur in about 5 percent of cases (22).

kidney disease

From early in pregnancy through the puerperium the renal collecting structures become dilated to produce the so-called physiologic hydronephrosis of pregnancy (23). Hormone activity accounts for ureteral hypomotility and ureteral muscle changes, resulting in a greater volume of urine staying in the pelvis and ureters. Later in gestation, either the supine or the upright position can cause partial ureteral obstruction (24), since the enlarged uterus may entrap the ureters at the pelvic brim (Fig. 24·2). During pregnancy, many changes affect the excretion of salt, water, and total fluid balance maintained by the kidney. Normally 6 to 8 l water is retained, both within and outside the cells (25) (Fig. 23·2). Various hormones concerned with electrolyte filtration (aldosterone, renin substrate, progesterone, and estrogen) increase, modifying the kidney's ability to excrete, especially its ability to excrete sodium (Fig. 24·3).

Ideally, the woman with a known renal disorder should consult her physician before attempting to conceive (26). Among the back-ground renal conditions that may be complicated by pregnancy are chronic glomerulonephritis, nephrotic syndrome, solitary kidney, polycystic kidney, and, of course, class F diabetes (27). Significant proteinuria will invariably accompany these conditions, leading the physician to investigate.

CHRONIC GLOMERULONEPHRITIS

Ranging in severity from tolerable impairment of kidney function to severe disability, this condition used to be incompatible with pregnancy but now is considered manageable in a cooperative patient. Usually a sequel to a severe systemic disease, most notably streptococcal glomerulophritis, chronic glomerulonephritis results in proteinuria and/or persistent urinary sediment. In pregnancy it produces palpitation, visual disturbances, headache, fatigue, dizziness, nausea, vomiting, edema, hypertension, and eventually some degree of cardiovascular disease and renal insufficiency (28). Anemia is usually severe enough to require transfusion (29).

Treatment Treatment is based on laboratory and clinical findings, which must be closely monitored. Generally therapy includes a high-protein diet, sodium restriction, administration of antihypertensive agents, and, with cardiac insufficiency, digitalis and perhaps diuretics. Preeclampsia necessitates hospitalization. Azotemia (nitrogen in the blood), hyperkalemia (high potassium content in the blood), and continuing blood pressure rise indicate the need to interrupt the pregnancy.

Prognosis The mother's condition is basically unchanged following pregnancy. The primary risk is to the fetus, although without hypertension or renal failure 90 percent fetal salvage can be expected (30). Even with the best of management, however, there is a risk of spontaneous abortion, premature labor, or intrauterine death. Induction of labor must not

fig. 24·2 Intravenous pyelogram demonstrates ureteral dilatation of pregnancy. Note: right ureter is sharply cut off at pelvic brim (single arrow). (*By permission of Dr. Marshall Lindheimer and Dr. Adrian Katz, "Managing the Patient with Renal Disease,"* Comtemporary OB/GYN, **3**(1)49, 1974. *Photo Courtesy of Dr. Peter Dure-Smith.*)

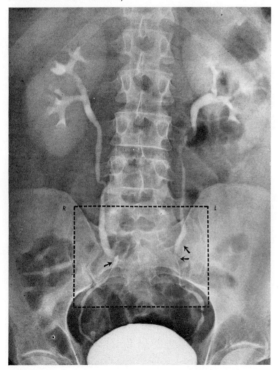

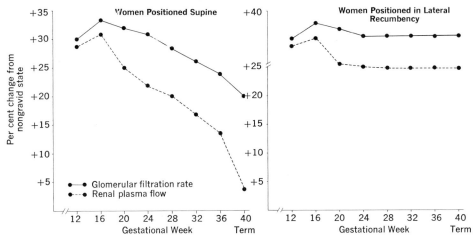

Renal Hemodynamics in Pregnancy

fig. 24·3 Renal hemodynamics in pregnancy. Differences in glomerular filtration rate and renal plasma flow in supine and lateral positions. Increases occur early in pregnancy and are sustained to term if women maintain lateral recumbency position. (*By permission of Dr. Marshall Lindheimer and Dr. Adrian Katz, "Managing the Patient with Renal Disease,"* Contemporary OB/GYN, **3**(1)49, 1974.)

be delayed beyond the end of the thirty-seventh week, and the neonate should be placed under intensive care immediately (31).

NEPHROTIC SYNDROME

If the nephrotic syndrome appears during pregnancy, the findings may be thought to indicate preeclampsia: edema, massive protein in the urine, low blood protein, and lipemia, with or without hypertension. Renal biopsy is required for definitive diagnosis (32). Usually the kidney functions sufficiently to allow the pregnancy to continue; interruption is indicated in the presence of severe malfunction, hypertension, or uremia. Thromboembolism (due to elevated fibrinogen or depressed antithrombin level) and infection as a consequence of low gamma globulin level must also be anticipated (33).

Treatment Nephrotic syndrome is treated according to symptoms and the other conditions accompanying it. Bed rest in the lateral recumbent position, high-protein/restricted-sodium diet, and diuretics are commonly ordered. Steroids are contraindicated during the first 2 months of gestation. Infections must be vigorously treated (34).

Prognosis Depending on the cause, recovery may take place or the disease may progress to renal failure and death; pregnancy itself seems to have no serious effect on the course of the disease (35).

SOLITARY KIDNEY

Usually when a person has only one kidney it enlarges to compensate for the extra demands put upon it; pregnancy does not seem to cause any special problems. The duration of the solitary-kidney condition, the present ability of that kidney to function, and the cause of the condition must all be taken into account.

Treatment Monthly urine cultures are the minimum for scrupulous monitoring against infection. Provided that no infection or hypertension intervenes, pregnancy progresses to term.

Prognosis Excellent in the absence of the above complications.

POLYCYSTIC DISEASE

Polycystic kidney is mainly a problem of older gravidas (36). If function remains normal, complications are not expected. The severest complication, indicating termination of the pregnancy, is hypertension. Infection, as always, is a threat.

Treatment None unless clinical findings demand medical intervention.

Prognosis Excellent in the absence of complications.

In all patients with known renal disorder, frequent evaluations are in order. If renal function deteriorates at any stage of gestation, reversible causes—such as urinary tract infection, subtle dehydration, and electrolyte imbalance—should be sought. Failure to find such a cause is grounds for recommending termination of the pregnancy (37).

references

1. Phyllis Leppert, "Hyperemesis Gravidarum: A Discussion of a Symptom Complex with a Connecting Bridge to Anorexia Nervosa," *Journal of Nurse-Midwifery,* **17**(4):20, 1973.
2. Daisy Lindner, "The Nurse's Role in a Bariatric Clinic," *RN,* **37**(2):28, 1974.
3. Nicholson J. Eastman and Louis M. Hellman, *Williams' Obstetrics,* 13th ed., Meredith Press, New York, 1966, p. 787.
4. Albert B. Gerbie, "Endocrine Diseases Complicated by Pregnancy," chap. 6 in Douglas M. Haynes (ed.), *Medical Complications during Pregnancy*; McGraw-Hill Book Company, New York, 1969, p. 352.
5. S. Gorham Babson and Ralph C. Benson, *Management of High Risk Pregnancy and Intensive Care of the Neonate,* The C. V. Mosby Company, St. Louis, 1971, p. 51.
6. Ibid.
7. Mary B. Dratman, "Managing Hyperthyroidism in Pregnancy," *OB-GYN Observer,* May, 1971, p. 6.
8. Jerome Hershman, "Some Births Normal Despite Enlarged Thyroid in Gravida," *OB-GYN News,* **8**(23):44, 1973.
9. Dratman, op. cit., p. 6.
10. Ibid.
11. Gerbie, op. cit., p. 356.
12. Sheldon Berger, "Medical Management of the Diabetic," *Hospital Topics,* **49**(12):62, 1971.
13. Eastman and Hellman, op. cit., p. 779.
14. Albert Gerbie, "Obstetrical Management of the Diabetic," *Hospital Topics,* **49**(12):64, 1971.
15. Babson and Benson, op. cit., p. 276.
16. John Boehm, "Neonatal Management of the Infant," *Hospital Topics,* **49**(12):65, 1971.
17. Berger, op. cit., p. 62.
18. Gerbie, "Endocrine Diseases Complicated by Pregnancy," p. 344.
19. Gerbie, "Obstetrical Management of the Diabetic," p. 64.
20. Elizabeth Laugharne and Felicity Duncan, "Gestational Diabetes: When Teaching Is Important," *The Canadian Nurse,* **59**(3):34, 1973.
21. Babson and Benson, op. cit., p. 77.
22. Ibid., p. 78.
23. John B. Nettles, "Renal Complications of Pregnancy," chap. 9 in Douglas M. Haynes (ed.), *Medical Complications during Pregnancy,* Meredith Press, New York, 1969, p. 444.
24. Marshall D. Lindheimer and Adrian I. Katz, "Managing the Patient with Re-

nal Disease," *Contemporary OB-GYN,* **3**(1):49, 1974.

25. Ibid., p. 50.
26. Russell Ramón de Alvàrez, "The Kidney in Pregnancy," *Hospital Practice,* May, 1973, p. 133.
27. Ibid.
28. Ibid.
29. Nettles, op. cit., p. 504.
30. Ibid.
31. de Alvàrez, op. cit., p. 134.
32. Ibid.
33. Ibid., p. 135.
34. Ibid.
35. Nettles, op. cit., p. 550.
36. de Alvàrez, op. cit., p. 136.
37. Lindheimer and Katz, op. cit., p. 55.

bibliography

de Alvàrez, Russell: "The Kidney in Pregnancy," *Hospital Practice,* May, 1973, p. 129.

Babson, S. Gorham, and Ralph C. Benson: *Management of High-risk Pregnancy and Intensive Care of the Neonate,* 2d ed., The C. V. Mosby Company, St. Louis, 1971.

Berger, Sheldon: "Medical Management of the Infant," *Hospital Topics,* **49**(12):65, 1971.

Boehm, John: "Neonatal Management of the Infant," *Hospital Topics,* **49**(12):65, 1971.

Burt, Richard L.: "How to Reduce the Hazards of Diabetes in Pregnancy," *Consultant,* June, 1972, p. 37.

Carrington, Elsie R.: "Diabetes in Pregnancy," *Clinical Obstetrics and Gynecology,* **14**(1):28, 1973.

Danowski, T. S.: "Why Milk Glucose Intolerance Can be Significant," *Consultant,* June, 1972, p. 37.

Delaney, James J., and Ptacek, John: "Three Decades of Experience with Diabetic Pregnancies," *American Journal of Obstetrics and Gynecology,* **104**(4):550, 1970.

Dratman, Mary: "Managing Hyperthyroidism in Pregnancy," *OB/GYN Observer,* May, 1971, p. 2.

Eastman, Nicholson J., and Louis M. Hellman: chaps. 27, 29 in *Williams' Obstetrics,* 13th ed., Meredith Press, New York, 1966.

Garnet, James D.: "Pregnancy in Women with Diabetes," *American Journal of Nursing,* **69**(9):1900, 1969.

Gerbie, Albert: "Obstetrical Management of the Diabetic," *Hospital Topics,* **49**(12):65, 1971.

Gottesman, Robert L., and Samuel Refetoff: "Diagnosis and Management of Thyroid Diseases in Pregnancy," *Journal of Reproductive Medicine,* **11**(1):19, 1973.

Haynes, Douglas M. (ed.): chaps. 6 and 9, *Medical Complications during Pregnancy,* McGraw-Hill Book Company, New York, 1969.

Hazlett, B., and Douglas Gare: "The Pregnant Diabetic," *Modern Medicine,* **27**(12):37, 1971.

Kinch, R. A.: "Management of the Diabetic Pregnancy," *Journal of Reproductive Medicine,* **7**(2):40, 1971.

Kucera, J.: "Rate and Type of Congenital Anomalies among Offspring of Diabetic Women," *Journal of Reproductive Medicine,* **7**(2):61, 1971.

Laugharne, Elizabeth, and Felicity Duncan: "Gestational Diabetes: When Teaching Is Important," *The Canadian Nurse,* **69**(3):34, 1973.

Leeper, Robert D.: *Laboratory Texts in Diagnoses of Thyroid Disease,* vol. I, no. 1, Upjohn, Kalamazoo, 1972.

Leppert, Phyllis C.: "Hyperemesis Gravidarum: A Discussion of a Symptom Complex with a Connecting Bridge to Anorexia Nervosa," *Journal of Nurse-Midwifery,* **8**(4):12, 1973.

Lindheimer, Marshall D., and Adrian I. Katz: "Managing the Patient with Renal Disease," *Contemporary OB/GYN,* **3**(1):49, 1974.

————: "Pregnancy and the Kidney," *Journal of Reproductive Medicine,* **11**(1):14, 1973.

Man, Evelyn B., et al.: "Thyroid Function in Human Pregnancy," *American Journal of Obstetrics and Gynecology,* **111**(7):905, 1971.

Merkatz, Irwin R.: "Managing the Renal Transplant Recipient," *Contemporary OB/GYN,* **3**(6):63, 1973.

O'Sullivan, John B., et al.: "Screening Criteria for the High Risk Gestational Diabetic Patient," *American Journal of Obstetrics and Gynecology,* **114**(7):895, 1972.

————: "Gestational Diabetes and Perinatal Mortality Rate," *American Journal of Obstetrics and Gynecology,* **114**(7):901, 1973.

————: "Treatment of Verified Prediabetics in Pregnancy," *Journal of Reproductive Medicine,* **7**(2):21, 1971.

Rivlin, Michel E., et al.: "Value of Estriol Estimations in the Management of Diabetic Pregnancy," *American Journal of Obstetrics and Gynecology,* **104**(6):875, 1970.

Robin, Noel I., et al.: "Thyroid Hormone Relationships between Maternal and Fetal Circulations in Human Pregnancy at Term: A Study in Patients with Normal and Abnormal Thyroid Function," *American Journal of Obstetrics and Gynecology,* **108**(8):1269, 1970.

Schneeberg, Norman G.: "Thyroid Therapy: First Do No Harm," *Consultant,* September, 1971, p. 89.

Souma, John A., et al.: "Comparison of Thyroid Function in Every Trimester of Pregnancy," *American Journal of Obstetrics and Gynecology,* **114**(7):905, 1972.

Tsai, Albert, et al.: "Diabetes and Pregnancy," *Journal of Reproductive Medicine,* **11**(1):23, 1973.

Yen, S. S. C., et al.: "Gestational Diabetogenesis: Quantitative Analyses of Glucose-Insulin Interrelationship between Normal Pregnancy with Gestational Diabetes," *American Journal of Obstetrics and Gynecology,* **111**(6):792, 1971.

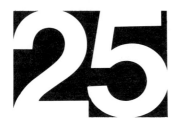

preterm birth, multiple pregnancy, and emergency delivery

Margaret Dean
and
Marretje Jelles Bührer

preterm birth

In current statistics, preterm birth is the chief factor in neonatal morbidity and mortality. Neonatal intensive care facilities have reduced the mortality rates somewhat; however, the prevention of preterm birth will continue to be the major obstetric problem being researched in the 1970s.

The prevention of preterm labor is a problem because of the incomplete understanding of the factors that begin true labor. To prevent labor that starts before the fetus is ready demands a knowledge of how to interrupt the cycle of factors that allow that labor to begin.

MATERNAL FACTORS

What maternal factors seem to precipitate early labor? Very early, after 20 weeks, causes are often related to malfunction of the cervix, such as the incompetent cervix, or to complications such as placenta previa. Abortion, especially that due to poor implantation or lowered fertility, may be related to the same factors that cause labor to start prematurely after the age of viability. Some researchers think that one factor is an alteration of uterine blood supply, since premature contractions occur in connection with heavy smoking, high altitudes, severe hypertension and preeclampsia, and overstretching of uterine muscles by multiple pregnancy or polyhydramnios (1). All these situations have in common a reduction in blood flow to the uterine muscle. See Chap. 8 for other factors in the initiation of labor which are interdependent and complex. Once the process of labor begins, it usually goes through to completion. If it starts before 38 weeks of gestation, or preterm, the outcome is an infant compromised by immaturity.

PREVENTION OF PRETERM LABOR

Labor can be halted only if diagnosed before the cervix has dilated to 4 cm or is 75 to 100 percent effaced (in a primipara) (2). The presence of ruptured membranes usually contraindicates a delay in labor, because the natural barrier against infection has been breached.

At present, therapy involves several pharmacologic agents plus bed rest. Physicians vary in their choice of these agents but agree on the need to diagnose first the existence of true labor.

Three major agents in use are alcohol (ethanol), isoxsuprine hydrochloride (Vasodilan), and its relative, ritodrine hydrochloride (DU-21220). Even with drug availability, sedation and bed rest are sometimes the only choices selected by the obstetrician. Ritodrine is five to ten times more active than isoxsuprine (3) and has fewer side effects. Both the latter are potent vasodilators, acting on smooth muscle. Ethanol works by a different pathway, appearing to block the oxytocin release from the hypothalmus to reduce the number of uterine contractions.

Vasodilators If a vasodilator is chosen, an intravenous infusion is begun and the dose is *titrated* against the patient's response. Expected side effects are hypotension (average decrease of 10 to 15 mmHg blood pressure) and tachycardia (average increase of 30 beats/min). The patient should always be placed on her side, because these drugs, as they relax smooth muscle, will affect the tone of the vena cava and may cause the vena cava syndrome if the patient is supine.

After contractions have been effectively slowed, either drug can be given intramuscularly or orally. Some patients have been carried for more than 2 weeks farther into the pregnancy by means of therapy with ritodrine or isoxsuprine. The patient is instructed that hypotension and tachycardia may recur with the maintenance dose that can be taken at home. She is taught to take her own pulse and to report it at intervals to the physician. She is also instructed to report the recurrence of any painful, regular contractions. For other women, labor begins again and membranes rupture right after the intravenous therapy is discontinued. At this point they move into the active phase of labor which cannot be halted by any known means.

Bed rest Bed rest in the side-lying position continues to be useful in addition to drugs and where drugs are not available. Bed rest is effective because production of epinephrine and norepinephrine is decreased. These adrenal hormones affect uterine activity.

Ethanol The use of intravenous alcohol (ethanol) has been reported by Fuchs (4) and Bienarz (5) to be an effective method of slowing contractions and in some cases of halting labor. The side effects experienced by the patient may be nausea, vomiting, and inebriation. After contractions slow, some physicians maintain the patient on oral doses of whisky until contractions cease (6).

Nursing Care When a patient is admitted to the hospital in preterm labor, the nurse will need to prepare for the possibility of a low-birth-weight infant (Fig. 25·1). Several observations and actions are necessary on admission. After vaginal examination the mother is placed on complete bed rest, on her side. The enema is omitted and further vaginal exams are kept at a minimum. Since future therapy will be based on observations during the first few hours after admission, base-line fetal heart tones and maternal vital signs are taken and labor is monitored. An external labor monitor is applied so that even mild contractions unfelt by the mother can be recorded. During this period of diagnosis, x-ray pelvimetry or ultrasound measurements can aid in determining fetal size. Usually several hours pass before a decision regarding treatment is made because the decision depends upon the predicted size and condition of the infant. The mother will be very apprehensive and need continuing support and clear explanations of the decisions as to the method of treatment.

PREMATURE RUPTURE OF MEMBRANES

One-third of all premature labors appear to be related to premature rupture of membranes (PRM). The cause of early rupture is often unknown, but some of the factors leading to this event are infection of the cervix or vagina, cervical incompetency, multiple

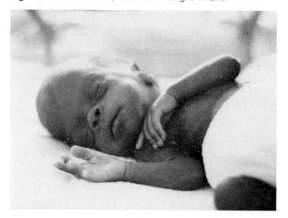

fig. 25·1 Premature, low-birth-weight infant.

pregnancy, hydramnios, malpresentation, and disproportion. Labor begins in about 70 percent of these cases within 12 h (7). Once membranes have ruptured most physicians do not delay labor, for the incidence of infection rises with each hour after the first 24 h.

There is a great risk of infection ascending from the vagina and cervix to the remaining amniotic fluid, membranes, decidua (endometrium), and placenta. The longer the delay before delivery, the more likely will be the possibility of *amnionitis* and *placentitis.*

If infection has already begun before admission, the signs will be an elevation of maternal temperature and a change in odor of the fluid. The membranes and placenta on delivery may appear cloudy. *Nitrazine paper* can indicate the presence of ruptured membranes, as amniotic fluid is more alkaline than vaginal secretions.

The risk of amnionitis is mainly to the fetus, as the mother can usually be effectively treated with antibiotics. Normal respiratory movements in utero serve to pull amniotic fluid into the trachea, but if fetal hypoxia occurs, deep gasping respiratory movements are triggered which move fluid deep into the alveoli. The infant is then born with the likelihood of amnionitis pneumonia, or perinatal aspiration syndrome (PAS). Swallowing movements also occur in utero, and infected fluid can be taken into the gastrointestinal tract, causing gastroenteritis after birth. The more preterm the infant, the worse the threat of infection encountered in the intrauterine environment, and the harder it is for the infant to fight infection, because of his immaturity.

INDUCTION

Under normal circumstances, most women need no stimulus to begin labor. The popularity of "babies by appointment," elective induction, has waned since the advent of fetal monitoring, and most obstetricians now use induction of labor only for those situations in which a problem indicates that the normal body processes need to be augmented. *Induction,* or the use of agents to bring on the onset of labor, and *stimulation,* the use of agents to increase the speed and intensity of labor, both should require a situation that demands artificial intervention in the body timing. The following are the *major indications for induction*:

Placental insufficiency
Premature rupture of fetal membranes
Prolonged pregnancy (+41 weeks)
Preeclampsia
Rh sensitization
Diabetic mother
Hypertensive mother
Fetal death

Since oxytocin was first accepted in 1948, several agents have been studied for their effective physiologic action on the uterine muscle: sparteine sulfate, buccal and subcutaneous oxytocin, and now, intravenous oxytocin and prostaglandins. The first three have been largely discarded; prostaglandins are the subject of intensive studies and promise to be quite satisfactory in optimum doses. Nonpharmacologic methods have been used: exercise, enemas, castor oil, and more recently, amniotomy (rupture of the membranes) and "stripping of the membranes" (digital separation of the membranes from the lower uterine wall). Of these methods, walking stimulates labor once it has begun, an enema in early labor clears the lower intestinal tract and may slightly stimulate contractions, and castor oil makes the woman miserable. Rupturing the membranes before labor begins places the mother at risk of acquiring infection (see above), as does stripping the membranes.

Although there is no completely safe way to change the speed of labor or initiate it, yet with careful observation, regulated dosage, and fetal monitoring, induction and stimulation with oxytocin and perhaps with prostaglandins can be used effectively where indicated.

Under ordinary circumstances, the blocks to uterine contractility are extremely effective. Therefore the readiness of the body for labor has always been a key factor in the success of induction. The Bishop score has been constructed to evaluate readiness. A value is assigned each criterion—0, 1, 2, or 3 points. The higher the number the better is the condition for labor. A score below 9 indicates an unready patient.

	0	3 points
Dilation of the cervix	Closed $\longrightarrow$	5 cm dilated
Effacement of the cervix	Zero $\longrightarrow$	80 percent effaced
Station of the presenting part	−3 $\longrightarrow$	+2
Consistency of the cervix	Firm $\longrightarrow$	soft
Position of the cervix	Posterior, central, or anterior (8)	

The processes during prelabor which normally take several weeks prior to the beginning of regular contractions and dilation must be effected within a few hours during induction. These changes are movement of the head into the pelvic inlet to engagement station, stretching of the lower uterine segment and upper vaginal wall, and softening (ripening) of the cervix. If induction is begun before the cervix is ready, there will be a time lag before true labor begins. An oxytocin infusion may be administered for 8 to 12 h and then discontinued so that the patient can sleep. The next morning marked changes may be seen in the progressive cervical effacement. Contractions during this period are painless and yet have an effect and can be monitored by the external sensor.

If induction is used, the nurse must understand that the patient goes through the same "work of labor" only over a shorter span of time. Thus, the total pressure needed (measured in Montevideo units) (see Fig. 9·2) to dilate the cervix completely and to cause the descent and expulsion of the fetus is the same as for spontaneous labor, but the contractions may be more intense, more frequent, and longer in duration. And here is where the problem of induction lies. As the body responds to oxytocin, the hope is that the contractions will be physiologic, i.e., normally effective. However, the individual sensitivity to oxytocin changes from phase to phase of labor and from woman to woman, so that the dosage must be *titrated,* adjusted by her response to the infusion. It is important to avoid *hypertonus,* or excessively strong, long contractions with inadequate periods of relaxation.

Method of Oxytocin Administration The pharmacologic effect of oxytocin is explored in Chap. 18. Because of its short half-life, it is safest to administer the drug by the intravenous route. One ampul (10 units) diluted in 1000 ml Ringer's lactate solution or dextrose and water yields 10 milliunits/ml of solution. Although different concentrations are ordered, the drug is always administered in terms of *milliunits per minute.* The only way accurately to regulate flow is to use an infusion pump, with the solution being added by a "piggy-back" needle to an infusion containing a solution of 5 percent dextrose in water. In this way, should hypertonus occur, the intravenous flow can be stopped immediately.

Precautions Nurses often react negatively to oxytocin use because they have seen abuses and know the real dangers of fetal distress if labor is not carefully monitored. However, knowledge of the way in which oxytocin changes the normal labor pattern will help to objectify nursing care. There are some important factors to remember.

1. Very few patients can tolerate oxytocin-augmented contractions and remain "in control" in the true Lamaze sense. Therefore, patients usually will need some analgesia.

2. Oxytocin sensitivity varies markedly from person to person, and sensitivity varies from phase to phase of labor. The patient may indicate her progress in labor by a change in her response to oxytocin.

3. The setup, observation, and maintenance of a problem-free infusion fall within nursing measures, but the obstetrician is responsible for beginning the intravenous infusion and for titration of the dosage (which includes remaining with the patient for a sufficient period after each change in rate or dosage to ensure a problem-free administration). The physician must be within call for unexpected problems.

4. An infusion pump is the preferred means of controlling the rate of flow; second best is a microdropper setup. Both are used as a piggy-back addition to a plain infusion.

5. Labor may be substantially shortened and may move toward delivery more rapidly than expected. Therefore close observation is mandatory.

6. Because the labor is speeded up, there will be more pressure on the head (presenting part), less recovery time between contractions, and greater possibility of fetal distress. Therefore, fetal heart tones must be regularly observed. (Hon recommends a minimum of every 10 min in normal labor.) External or internal monitoring of each patient is highly recommended and may become mandatory in the future (Chap. 27).

7. The nurse may shut off the infusion at the first indication of a hypertonic, or *tetanic,* contraction. She must never flush the IV tubing or manipulate a poorly running IV infusion in such a way as to inject larger doses of oxytocin into the vein.

Properly controlled, induction and stimulation remain helpful tools in labor when there are problems with its process and progress. What place these techniques will hold in the future remains to be seen.

multiple pregnancy

A multiple pregnancy carries a much higher risk of perinatal morbidity and mortality, mainly because the incidence of preterm delivery of low-birth-weight infants is much higher than that with single gestations. Infants may be "small for date" or preterm, or both. Medical care is aimed at maintaining the pregnancy as long as possible to give the infants the best chance of survival.

TYPES OF MULTIPLE PREGNANCY

Monovular Twins Monovular twins are the result of a single fertilized ovum (zygote) which has divided exactly in two before implantation. This process of "two-ing," or twinning, may occur from 2 to 7 days after fertilization. The time of division affects whether the two fetuses have separate amnions and chorions, but there will always be a single placenta. Each of the blastocysts develops into an individual with similar intelligence, physical characteristics, and sex. Monovular, or identical, twins are intensely interesting from the psychosocial, biologic aspects, as these two individuals have the same genetic consitution. Twin studies are done often to test the effects of environment as compared with genetic inheritance.

Diovular Twins Diovular, or fraternal, twins stem from two ova, released at the same time, that have been fertilized. They may have placentas fused together or ones that develop absolutely separately. Even if the placentas fuse, each has an individual chorion and amnion. Fraternal twins may look so much alike that they can be thought identical, or

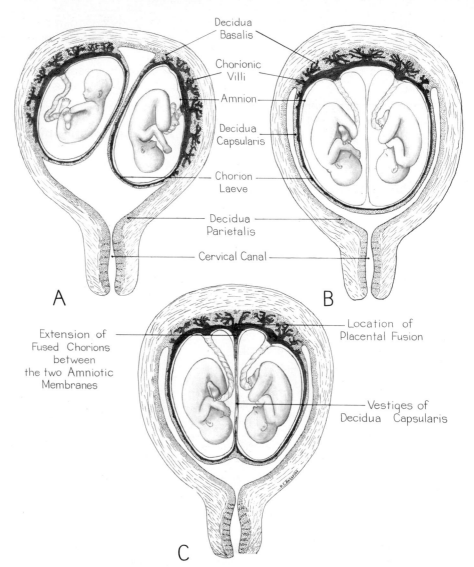

Decidua
Basalis

Chorionic
Villi

Amnion

Decidua
Capsularis

Chorion
Laeve

Decidua
Parietalis

Cervical Canal

A

B

Extension of
Fused Chorions
between
the two Amniotic
Membranes

Location of
Placental Fusion

Vestiges of
Decidua Capsularis

C

fig. 25·2 Schematic diagrams showing: A diovular twins with independent membranes; B monovular twins; C diovular twins implanted close to each other, resulting in fusion of their membranes. (*From: Bradley M. Patten, Human Embryology, 3d ed., McGraw-Hill Book Company, New York, 1968.*)

may be as different in size, coloring, personality, and ability as brothers and sisters in a family can be (Fig. 25·2).

Patton states that "fairly good evidence is available that approximately three-fourths of all twins are fraternal and only about one-fourth are monovular" (9). Twinning chances increase with increasing parity, but so far no hereditary causes have been found to predispose toward monovular twinning. Fraternal twinning appears to be a hereditary tendency for the woman to mature more than one ovum during the ovulatory period (10).

Triplets and Quadruplets Triplets and

quadruplets may be either fraternal or identical, but single-ovum pregnancies are least frequent. There may be mixed groups, with a set of monovular infants and one or two diovular infants.

Quintuplets and Sextuplets It is very rare for single-ova pregnancies to produce so many infants. In most cases, either two or three distinct placentas, or masses of two or three, have fused together. These pregnancies are most often linked to drugs that stimulate the ovary, resulting in hyperovulation.

Siamese Twins One of the odd accidents which can occur only with identical twinning is the failure in some cases to separate completely during early development. The infants are born as *conjoined* or "Siamese" twins. Nursing care of these infants is interestingly outlined by Dicksen (11).

TESTS FOR TWIN TYPE

Blood factors must be identical in monovular twins, as must be the chemical substances such as haptoglobins and gamma globulins. Footprints and fingerprints will be nearly the same. "Ear prints" can assist in identifying identical twins, since ear formations are distinctive from birth onwards. Often an identical twin appears to be a mirror image of the other, for instance with the whorl of hair on the crown of the head on the opposite side. Skin grafts from one identical twin will always be accepted by the other twin.

MULTIPLE PREGNANCY CAUSED BY DRUGS

In recent years, treatment for infertility has led to an increased incidence of multiple gestation. Because of this, the statistics for naturally occurring multiple pregnancies are somewhat changed. Prior to this change, multiple births occurred most frequently in the black population and least often in the

Oriental. Identical twinning occurs at much the same rate in every racial group.

Two major drug therapies are in use for lowered fertility. Clomiphene citrate and menotropins plus human chorionic gonadotropin are very specifically used to stimulate ovulation in a woman who is subfertile.

Clomiphene Citrate (Clomid) Clomid appears to stimulate increased output of pituitary gonadotropins, which in turn affect the growth of the graafian follicle. The drug is very potent and can cause abnormal ovarian enlargement. Side effects are related to the enlargement of the ovary. Vasomotor symptoms, "hot flashes," and blurred vision disappear soon after the drug is discontinued. Dosage is usually 50 mg for 5 days beginning on the fifth day of the cycle. If treatment is unsuccessful with properly timed coitus, no more than two more cycles can be attempted.

Because of the drug's potency, very careful instructions for the patient are important, as well as a discussion with the couple about the chances of having a multiple gestation. That possibility is ten times more common than in spontaneous conception (12). If the drug is inadvertently taken during a very early pregnancy, malformation is possible. Therefore careful basal temperature readings are essential every day after beginning the first 5-day course. The woman is instructed in the method and is asked to report any changes suggestive of pregnancy.

Menotropins (Pergonal) Human menopausal gonadotropin (Pergonal) and human chorionic gonadotropin (HCG) are administered intramuscularly in sequence to obtain ovulation in patients with low fertility. Twenty percent of those taking this drug conceived more than one fetus. Pergonal is a combination of FSH and LH obtained from the urine of postmenopausal women. When administered intramuscularly for 9 to 12 days, it produces ovarian follicle growth only. To cause *ovulation* HCG must be given intramuscularly on day 13 of the menstrual

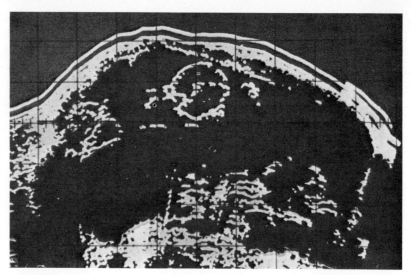

fig. 25·3 Ultrasound scan of quintuplets showing only three heads. (*Courtesy of B. Reaney, M.D., and B. Kaye, M.D., "Delivering the Chicago Quints," Contemporary OB/GYN, March,* 1973.)

cycle. Administration of this therapy requires daily visits to the physician and, after day 14, every other day follow-up until success or failure is evident.

Side effects include ovarian enlargement, causing abdominal distension and pain in some cases. The therapy may be used over a longer period than Clomid.

DIAGNOSIS OF MULTIPLE PREGNANCY

Twins often came as a surprise when confirmation depended only on palpation and auscultation of fetal heart beat. Even now, diagnosis is difficult before 20 or 24 weeks, when the signs become more evident that there is more than one fetus developing. The most accurate methods of diagnosis are fetal electrocardiogram, ultrasound, and x-ray. The twin heartbeat can be recorded as early as the sixteenth week. With x-ray, when more than two babies are present, diagnosis is complicated by overlapping outlines. Still occasionally, at birth time, there is one more baby than predicted (Fig. 25·3)!

PREMATURITY AND LOW BIRTH WEIGHT

The great majority of multiple pregnancies follow a normal course but delivery comes early. The length of gestation from the onset of the last menses to birth is about 22 days less than in a single birth, averaging birth at 37 weeks(13). Birth weight is often a misleading parameter of gestational age, for in many instances, even if there are identical twins, they may differ considerably in weight. Especially in fraternal girl-boy pairs, girls often weigh less than the boy partner at birth. Sometimes one infant has dominated because of better placement of the placenta nourishing it. In some cases, the second twin may be so depleted of nourishment that it does not survive more than a few hours after birth (Fig. 25·4).

PRENATAL CARE

Pregnancy proceeds normally during the first trimester when the embryos are small. The only problem noted for some consists of

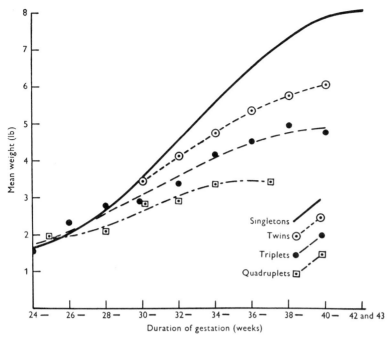

fig. 25·4 Duration of gestation and mean weight for single infants, twins, triplets, and quadruplets. (*From Frederick C. Battaglia et al., "Birth Weight, Gestational Age and Pregnancy with Special Reference to High Birth-Weight–Low Gestational Age Infants,"* Pediatrics, **37**:418, 1966.)

increased nausea and vomiting. As the growth rate increases, however, the major physiologic problems will be due to *pressure* of the overlarge uterus on the surrounding organs, *anemia,* and *fatigue.* There may be an increased incidence of polyhydramnios and preeclampsia for some women. There are increased risks of an early complex delivery. Prenatal care for the mother includes precautions against these problems, and therapy is directed toward maintaining the pregnancy as long as possible.

Pressure Effects The uterus causes pressure on the ureters, bladder, intestines, vena cava and renal veins, and later, on the diaphragm. Increased pressure on the venous circulation may lead to varicose veins of the rectal, saphenous, or vulvar veins. Constipation and digestive problems may be accentuated during the second and third trimester. Pressure on the ureters may favor urinary stasis and chronic infection. Pressure in each case is relieved by a side-lying position whenever the mother rests. Toward the end of the third trimester, she may have to use a semi-Fowler's position for sleep. During the day she may have to wear a well-fitted maternity corset to provide some support for the abdomen.

Anemia Maternal anemia can be prevented by a diet rich in iron and the addition of supplemental iron and folic acid, since the iron requirement is increased for a multiple pregnancy. Complicating intake is the fact that the mother usually can tolerate small meals only, because of increased pressure on the stomach.

Rest Rest for the mother carrying a multiple gestation is the most important single factor in preventing preterm delivery. In a Colorado series (14), perinatal mortality was 6 percent in a bed-rest group compared with 23 percent in a non-bed-rest group. The average weight of each baby in the bed-rest group was 250 Gm more, and the pregnancies averaged about six more days in duration.

Along with bed rest and limited activity, many physicians are now using medication (Vasodilan) to prevent premature labor. Once the cervix begins to efface, the mother is admitted to the hospital in hopes of giving the infants a few more days to mature. She is maintained on complete bed rest and is medicated.

MAJOR PROBLEMS IN MULTIPLE PREGNANCY

Hydramnios Polyhydramnios, the production of an abnormally large amount of amniotic fluid, can precipitate premature labor and may for a period cause the appearance of multiple gestation. Hydramnios is more common in multiple pregnancies and where there are renal or gastrointestinal anomalies in the infant.

Normally, the amnion circulates and reabsorbs about 350 ml of amniotic fluid per hour in later pregnancy. If even a 1- or 2-ml imbalance occurs, the buildup of pressure can be quite dramatic. The uterus enlarges more rapidly than normal in the second half of pregnancy, and the pressure symptoms experienced by the mother may be quite severe. An amniocentesis may be one way of relieving pressure, but there is a definite risk connected to repeated tapping of the amniotic sac. When membranes rupture prior to or during labor, there is a much greater risk of a prolapsed cord.

Preeclampsia The chances of preeclampsia are more common in multiple gestations, but the reasons for this increased incidence are unknown. The regimen of bed rest should help to diminish the incidence of hypertension, edema, and albuminuria in the future.

Hemorrhage Because of the enlarged placental site, the internal os may be completely or partially covered. The warning signs of bleeding prior to labor should be noted carefully. During delivery, a lower uterine or a cervical tear is not uncommon. After delivery the mother may have postpartum hemorrhage because of uterine atony and the large placental site.

Labor With therapy, the mother may approach nearer to term than has been customary in the past. She is observed carefully, and the condition of the cervix checked each week. She is instructed to notify the physician when the contractions begin regularly. Usually, considerable dilatation and effacement of the cervix have already taken place during prelabor, so that it appears that the active phase of labor is shortened.

Problems during labor are those of uterine overdistension, with resultant ineffective contractions, and abnormal presentations of the fetus. It is most important to guard against special hazards to the second twin. Local anesthesia is used because the length of delivery time is unknown and general anesthesia would depress the responses of the second infant. The first infant may have a vertex presentation, but the second twin often is in a transverse or breech position, with the attendant problems of difficult delivery and possible prolapse of the cord.

Delivery room procedures involve notifying the pediatric support staff of the impending delivery. Resuscitation equipment for several infants must be available, and the premature nursery must be ready to receive the infants. Each cord is tagged at the maternal side, and each infant is identified in order of birth. After delivery, the placenta is examined to aid in the diagnosis of zygosity.

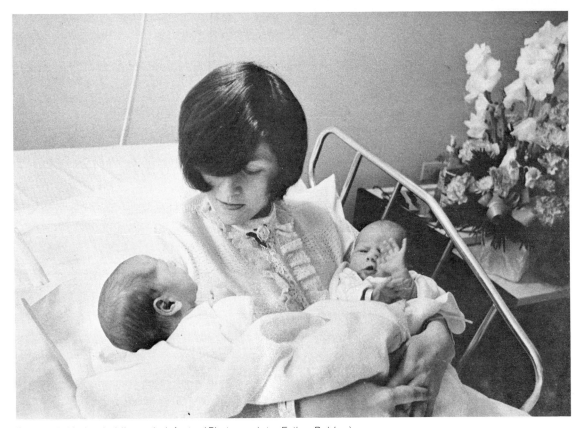

fig. 25·5 Mother holding twin infants. (*Photograph by Esther Bubley.*)

ASSISTING THE MOTHER IN CARE OF HER INFANTS

Mothers who expect the arrival of more than one infant have time to prepare psychologically and economically to receive them. How much of a problem their arrival causes depends on many factors. Fortunately the birth of more than one infant usually rallies the whole family to help. (Fig. 25·5).

There are supportive agencies that can be used by referral from the physician or clinic. Social service assistance, homemaking assistance, and visiting nurses can all be called upon.

Since multiple births usually happen to women who have had children, they already have some skill in child care. Most mothers find that in the first year it makes no difference whether the infants are fraternal or identical. What is important is their birth weight, as well as their gestational age at birth. One infant may be behind the other and, if responses differ, the mother may suffer undue anxiety. Nurses can assist her in recognizing the uniqueness of each infant.

Twins may be so engrossed with each other that they may delay speech until later than a single child. Their growth pattern depends upon their gestational age at birth. The mother should be familiarized with the delay in maturation caused by preterm birth. The differences in growth will emerge fairly soon. A book such as *Infants and Mothers* by

Brazelton will help the mother treat each baby individually.

emergency delivery

A delivery becomes an emergency when it is outside the usual planned, prepared setting. The mechanism of labor remains the same, of course. Four main settings will be considered: home delivery, en route in car or taxi, somewhere in the hospital, and in a disaster situation.

If you were to become involved, what would you do?

The woman who delivers so rapidly is usually a person who has a relatively painless labor, one who does not feel her contractions until the transition stage or until actually bearing down. Often the patient goes to the bathroom because the urge of bearing down is an overwhelming sensation; she then realizes that the delivery is imminent.

Basic medical asepsis can be observed even in an emergency delivery. The home environment is a safe place for a delivery because the mother is used to her own environmental bacteria. (Indirectly, so is the fetus.) The baby is being born through a passage that is not aseptic; because of this, no delivery is really sterile. Once you understand that fact, it is easier to proceed with a home delivery, doing your best with soap and water or whatever is on hand.

If one or more persons are present, the most knowledgeable one handles the delivery while directing the others to seek help by calling the number of the police, ambulance, or fire department. Utilize the family to get equipment and assist with the delivery.

Assess the situation. If the patient is in the bathroom and the baby is ready to be born, lower her to the floor. (It is difficult to deliver a baby while the mother is standing up.) Place several towels under her buttocks to allow some height for delivering the shoulders. If there is time, transfer her to her bed and proceed by placing her crosswise on the bed with her buttocks slightly hanging off the mattress. Instruct her to place her hands under her thighs, to support herself. One can also use a table and the patient can rest her feet on the backs of two chairs. A person's possessions are valuable to her, so to protect the mattress, floor covering, or furnishings, one can use a plastic shower curtain, plastic tablecloth, newspapers, towels and old sheets. A dishpan can be used to catch the flow of amniotic fluid and blood.

While all these preparations are being made, give emotional support to the patient. Comfort her, tell her that she is doing beautifully, and reassure her that everything is going well. In order to win time, ask the cooperation of the mother during a bearing-down contraction to blow instead of push. Short blows, or panting, prevent the mother from bearing down. One less push gives you 3 to 5 min more to prepare. If there is time, wash your hands and wash down the perineum. A wet towel and dishwashing liquid are quick cleansing tools.

THE DELIVERY AT HOME

Once the head crowns, ask the mother not to push but to use the pant-blow respiration pattern. Place one hand fully on the baby's emerging head and give very gentle counterpressure while the head is being born. Sudden popping out of the head should at all times be prevented, since it may cause intracranial hemorrhage. The gentle counterpressure lets the head emerge slowly through the vaginal opening. There is no hurry. When the child's head emerges from the vagina, gently stroke the child's nose downward to expel mucus and amniotic fluid. (This is the way the nose is blown by people unaccustomed to Kleenex or handkerchiefs.) "Milk" the throat by an upward stroking movement on the neck and under the chin. Then place a hand on the nose to get excess mucus out. This method enables the child to have a fairly clear oral and nasal pharynx. Feel for the cord. If there is a loose cord around the neck, slip it over the head. If it is fairly tight, a gentle pull may allow more to come forth and enable you to slip it over the head.

The mechanism of labor at this point is that the child is still enclosed by the vaginal wall with great pressure on the thorax, pressure which is part of the preparation for respiration. Some amniotic fluid will still be bubbling through the trachea because of the squeezing of the chest. Therefore, while you wait, continue milking the nose and stroking the neck and chin.

Take the head in two hands, press it gently downward and ask the mother to push. This will enable you to deliver the anterior shoulder under symphysis pubis. When the beginning of the upper arm appears, lift up the head gently, all the while looking under the baby to see the posterior shoulder emerge. Correct delivering of the shoulders may prevent upper vaginal or perineal lacerations. Remember the vagina is not a straight passage but is almost J-shaped. The head comes down under the symphysis pubis; so must the shoulders. When the shoulders are born, slide a hand along the back and legs and grab the feet, while the other hand supports the neck and head. Release the hand around the neck and rub the back with that hand. Then place the baby, wrapped in a towel, head downward on the mother's abdomen. There's no hurry. If no ambulance service is coming, complete the delivery.

If the delivery takes place with no chance of transport, you may tie the cord. Resist dramatic nonhygienic methods. Through eons of time different means have been used, from a sharp stone to chewing the cord through. The latter method is not recommended because the human mouth contains more organisms than almost any other instrument you could find. Most homes have some sewing notions—wool, heavy cotton thread, string, or button thread. Never use silk or fine thread as it will sever the cord in the tying act. Tie the cord in two places, 3 in from the baby's abdomen, then about 2 in farther up. To cut, you can use a kitchen knife, scissors, or a new razor blade. If fire is available, you can hold the cutting tool over a flame; if alcohol is available, wipe it off well.

If you know that no help is available to complete the delivery, wrap the baby in a baby blanket or a soft old sheet and then a blanket, and proceed to wrap that part of the cord hanging from the vagina in a clean towel or cloth and wait for separation of the placenta. When it separates, ask the mother to push and deliver the placenta. Never pull the cord, for the cord may snap or part of the placenta may come away. The placenta can remain in the uterus for 24 h without injury to the mother. Once separation has occurred, however, postdelivery care is identical to that in the hospital. Keep the patient warm, watch her pulse, check for signs of bleeding or shock, and check the fundus frequently. If the uterus has a tendency to relax, massage it very gently. Other methods include, besides the massage, use of ice cubes wrapped in a cloth, a heavy weight such as a big book placed just above the fundus, and breast stimulation. For breast stimulation, one can either put the child to the breast or use manual stimulation.

Be careful about letting the patient see her blood loss. Estimated blood loss in a normal delivery is anywhere from 250 to 500 ml. Remember that this blood is mixed with a large amount of amniotic fluid. Estimate the amount for a later report.

If the mother is not going to the hospital, she needs fluid replacement. Hot tea with honey, salty broth, or whatever she can drink can be prepared by the family. If transport is available, do not give fluids orally. There may be a need in the hospital for general anesthesia for exploration of the uterus and repair of lacerations.

Infant Care If you have to stimulate breathing, do not *hit* the child or slap the back or buttocks. (One does not hit an unconscious patient to make him breathe.) A gentle slap or flicking on the soles of the feet or rubbing the back is often enough stimuli. Assess quickly the response of the infant to birth. If the infant does not spontaneously cry or breathe, place the child on a flat surface, roll up a towel and place it under the baby's shoulders, extend the head downwards and give mouth-to-mouth resuscitation. Your priority after establishing respiration is maintaining the infant's temperature. Dry the baby, wrap him in whatever is available (something clean and warm), and place the child either in a crib or in the mother's arms.

Preterm Infant Unfortunately, many precipitate deliveries result in preterm infants. Your problems are then multiplied. Gentle handling and a warm environment are especially crucial to the small baby. A good environment for the preterm baby is a small cardboard box within a larger one. In the outer box place warm water bottles and newspapers; use lightweight baby blankets to cover the baby. One can also use a box near an open oven door, with the oven on low heat. The environmental temperature for the preterm infant must be in the low 90° range to prevent cold stress. If no other aid is available, placing the infant next to the mother's skin and wrapping them both will be the safest method of maintaining temperature.

If all is well and no transport is available, you may, when the status of the full-term infant is stabilized, wash it in warm water with mild soap. Since the cord is still wet, you can immerse the baby in the water. After all, water has been his usual environment. The precaution here is to prevent chilling.

DELIVERY EN ROUTE

Delivery in a car or taxi is perhaps the most complicated in terms of setting, lack of equipment, and assistance. If there is enough time, place the patient on the back seat of the car. Place the mother's skirt or pants under her to provide a screen against the much-used seat. Since we are dealing only with the actual delivery, the focus is on protecting the baby. Support the head, ease out the shoulders, and clear the airway. Wrap the baby in anything available, and place it in the mother's arms. If necessary, put the baby next to the mother's skin and then wrap her and the baby in whatever is available. The car should be kept idling to provide heat, but in any event watch the infant for chilling.

At the hospital, a mother who delivers en route will be taken directly to the delivery room, where the cord will be cut. She is then prepared for the removal of the placenta and manual exploration of the uterus, and is examined for cervical and vaginal lacerations. An infusion will be started, and oxytocin will be given, either directly intravenously or added to the infusion. The infant will be routinely taken care of, placed in an observation nursery, and observed for signs of trauma, temperature, intracranial hemorrhage, and infection.

The physician may place both mother and infant on prophylactic antibiotics.

PRECIPITATE DELIVERY IN THE HOSPITAL

A precipitous delivery may also occur in a labor room! The same rules apply as in an emergency delivery. Give the mother emotional support, have her breathe correctly (pant-blow), and ask for her cooperation.

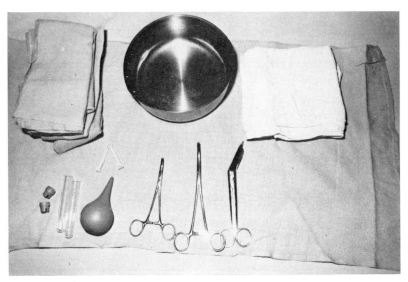

fig. 25·6 Emergency delivery pack.

A portable emergency kit in the labor room contains the following: two Kelly clamps, one plastic cord clamp, one scissor, a bulb syringe, two red-top tubes, a receiving blanket, four towels, 4- by 4-in gauze sponges, and a placenta basin (Fig. 25·6).

After the cord has been cut, the baby and the mother are both transferred to the delivery room where the usual procedures—delivery of the placenta, manual exploration of the uterus, and examination for lacerations—take place. Care to the baby is given as after a normal delivery.

DELIVERY DURING DISASTER

Much has been written about disaster nursing. The type of care that can be provided in disaster conditions depends on whether there has been any prior planning for or warning of disaster. With prior planning, people are prepared to manage an emergency delivery and delivery kits are available. Should you be the *one* doing the planning, and the drug store, dime store, or home is your only resource, remember to provide:

Something for cleansing	alcohol, liquid soap
Something for an airway	ear bulb syringe, meat basting syringe
Something for the cord	strong cotton thread or yarn, razor blade, scissors, or knife
Something for padding or protection	newspapers, brown paper, large plastic bags, old sheets, towels
Something to warm the baby	blanket, towel, clean sheet, shirt, diapers
Something to put the baby in	carton, box
Something to feed the baby	bottles, milk powder, etc., should mother not be able to nurse

In an unpredictable major disaster, rules may be unusable. It is those at the periphery of a disaster who may help in the ways listed above. A woman delivering alone will instinctively try to preserve herself and the child.

If you are a nurse in an area where cultural differences affect childbirth methods, you can follow these differences as much as possible, keeping in mind the essentials. For instance, in many primitive societies, the custom of rubbing soil or cow dung on the cord should be prevented because it causes many infants to die of tetanus within a short time. Preventive medicine with a little common sense can be taught even though people differ in customs.

The rules for emergency situations are well outlined in Mahoney's *Emergency and Disaster Nursing* (see "Bibliography"). Panic will interfere with clear thinking, and since information and experience are the best tools to quell panic, it is usually up to the person with the most medical experience to take charge. When panic is reduced, people will usually work together to deal with crises in quite sensible, remarkable ways.

references

1. Thomas P. Barden, "Premature Labor: Its Management and Therapy," *Journal of Reproductive Medicine,* **9**(3):113, 1972.
2. Robert Landesman, "Premature Labor, Its Management and Therapy," *Journal of Reproductive Medicine,* **9**(3): 95, 1972.
3. Ibid., p. 106.
4. Fritz Fuchs et al., "The Effect of Alcohol on Threatened Premature Labor," *American Journal of Obstetrics and Gynecology,* **99**:627, 1967.
5. Jozef Bienarz, "The Inhibition of Uterine Contractility in Labor," *American Journal of Obstetrics and Gynecology,* **111**:174, 1971.
6. Kenneth R. Niswander and Myron Gordon (eds.): *The Women and Their Pregnancies,* W. B. Saunders Company, Philadelphia, 1972, p. 427.
7. Bradley M. Patton, *Human Embryology,* 3d ed., McGraw-Hill Book Company, New York, 1968, p. 159.
8. E. H. Bishop, "Pelvic Scoring for Elective Induction," *Obstetrics and Gynecology,* **24**:266, 1964.
9. Patton., op. cit., p. 159.
10. Ralph C. Benson, *Handbook of Obstetrics and Gynecology,* 4th ed., Lange Medical Publications, Los Altos, Calif., 1971, p. 216.
11. Wendy S. Dicksen and Dorothy T. Meilieke, "Surgical Separation of Co-joined Twins," *Canadian Nurse,* May, 1973, p. 26.
12. Mary K. Asperheim and Laurel A. Eisenhauer, *The Pharmacologic Basis of Patient Care,* W. B. Saunders Company, Philadelphia, 1973, p. 347.
13. Barden, op. cit., p. 113.
13. James J. Delaney, "Immediate Bedrest in Multiple Gestation Cases," *OBGyn News,* **8**:6, 1973.

bibliography

Preterm Birth

Gunn, Gordon C., D. R. Mishell, and D. G. Morton: "Premature Rupture of the Fetal Membranes," *American Journal of Obstetrics and Gynecology,* **106**(3):469–480, 1970.

Liley, A. W.: "Disorders of Amniotic Fluid," chap. 3 in N. Assali, *Pathophysiology of Gestation: Fetal Disorders,* vol. II, Academic Press, Inc., New York, 1972.

Ostergard, Inc.k,: "The Physiology and Clinical Importance of Amniotic Fluid, A Review," *Obstetrical and Gynecological Survey,* **25**:297, 1970.

Webster, August: "Management of Premature Rupture of the Fetal Membranes," *Obstetrical and Gynecological Survey,* **24**:485, 1969.

Multiple Pregnancy

Allen, G.: *Twin Research: Problems and Prospects,* National Institutes of Health, Washington, pp. 242–269.

Bastzen, Peter J.: "Cycle Regulation with Clomphene Citrate: A Double Blind Study," *American Journal of Obstetrics and Gynecology,* **101**:1032, 1968.

Farooqui, T. O., et al.: "A Review of Twin Pregnancy and Perinatal Mortality," *Obstetrical and Gynecological Survey,* **28**:144, 1973.

Friedman, E. A., W. M. Alpern, and C. G. Allan: "The Multiple Pregnancy," *Journal of the American Medical Association,* **193**:440, 1965.

——— and M. R. Schheben: "The Effect of Uterine Overdistention on Labor: 1. Multiple Pregnancy," *Obstetrics and Gynecology,* **23**:164, 1964.

Gause, Ralph W.: "Multiple Pregnancy, Diagnosis, Delivery and Problems of Development," *Journal of Obstetric and Gynecological Nursing,* **1**(3):22, 1972.

"Multiple Pregnancy," *New England Journal of Medicine,* **288**:1329–1336, 1973.

Pernoll, T. L., and R. W. Carnes: "Electronic Fetal Monitoring of Twin Gestation," *American Journal of Obstetrics and Gynecology,* 115: 582, 1973.

Scheinfeld, Amram: *Twins and Supertwins,* J. B. Lippincott Company, Philadelphia, 1965.

Induction

Christie, G. B., and D. W. Cudmore: "The Oxytocin Challenge Test," *American Journal of Obstetrics and Gynecology,* **118**(3):327, 1974.

Friedman, E. A., and Marlen A. Sachtleben: "Oral Prostaglandin E_2 for Induction of Labor at Term," *Obstetrics and Gynecology,* **43**(2):178, 1974.

Leake, R. D., R. Gunther, and P. Sunshine: "Perinatal Aspiration Syndrome: Its Association with Intrapartum Events and Anesthesia," *American Journal of Obstetrics and Gynecology,* **118**(2):271, 1974.

Suspan, Frederick (ed.): "Induction of Labor: An Invitational Symposium," parts I and II, *Journal of Reproductive Medicine,* **6**(1): 17–34, 1971; **6**(2):17–31, 1971.

Emergency Delivery

Disaster Manual for Nurses, 3d ed., rev., Massachusetts Civil Defense Agency, Framingham, 1966.

Fitzpatrick, Elise, Nicholas J. Eastman, and Sharon Reeder: *Maternity Nursing,* 12th ed., J. B. Lippincott Company, Philadelphia, 1971.

Mahoney, Robert F.: *Emergency and Disaster Nursing,* 2d ed., The Macmillan Company, New York, 1969.

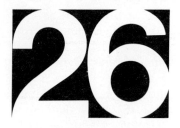

operative delivery

James H. Lee, Jr.

Though the title of this chapter is "Operative Delivery," it seems appropriate, before discussing the common obstetric operations, to consider some of the factors affecting the outcome of labor, particularly insofar as these factors might influence the need for operative intervention in the birth process. In addition, some mention must be made of diagnostic measures of the way that pelvic capacity is determined.

The conditions affecting the outcome of labor are:

1. The effectiveness of uterine contractions
2. The consistency, effacement, and dilatation of the cervix
3. The size and shape of the maternal pelvis in relation to the size, presentation, position, and attitude of the fetus

Other factors affecting the outcome of labor but not in the scope of this chapter might include:

4. Intrapartum infection
5. The general condition of mother and baby

dystocia

The term *dystocia* implies abnormal labor. Once rhythmic contractions of the uterus have begun and associated changes in the cervix—effacement, or thinning, and dilatation—have occurred, we assume that labor has begun and we expect it to continue over a reasonable time span and to terminate with expulsion of the infant. The question of what is a reasonable time span beyond which the length of labor is considered to be abnormal has been a troublesome one, and over the years has arbitrarily been set at anywhere from 18 to 48 h in various centers. Certainly it is the prevailing opinion that there is an increase in perinatal morbidity and mortality associated with prolonged labor.

Our understanding of the clinical course of labor has been greatly enhanced by the work of Friedman, who, by applying graphic analysis techniques to the study of large numbers of labors, has been able to divide labor into three functional stages—*preparatory, dilatational,* and *pelvic*—and to establish the principle clinical features of each stage.

When cervical dilatation is plotted graphically against time, it is apparent that in normal labors a characteristic sigmoid, or S-shaped, curve is produced (Fig. 26·1). Subdivisions of this curve include a *latent phase,* which extends from onset of labor to the upswing of the curve; an *active phase,* which begins with the upswing and proceeds in a nearly straight line until just a rim of cervix remains; and a *deceleration phase,* which ends with complete dilatation of the cervix. The deceleration phase may actually, from a physiologic standpoint, be considered to be part of the second stage of labor, for from this point on descent of the presenting part must occur. Viewed in this way variations from the normal pattern of labor become evident earlier and should lead to prompt reevaluation to diagnose the cause and to provide appropriate management.

The preparatory, or latent, phase of labor ordinarily lasts for several hours and, according to Friedman, should not normally exceed 20 h in nulliparas or 14 h in multiparas.

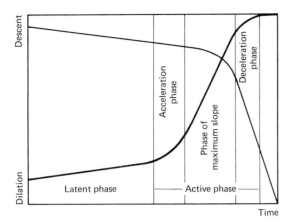

fig. 26.1 Normal labor curve, with functional divisions. (*From E. Friedman, "Normal Labor Curve," Clinical Obstetrics and Gynecology*, **16**(1)176, 1973.)

Unusual prolongation of this phase of labor (Fig. 26·2A) may often be due to the use of excessive amounts of analgesic or sedative drugs too early in labor, to the presence of a thick uneffaced cervix at the start of labor, or more rarely to some form of uterine contractile dysfunction.

Treatment of prolongation of the latent phase may include rest or stimulation. Providing sedation with an adequate dose of a narcotic-analgesic preparation to help the patient sleep will frequently allow her to awaken in active labor after a few hours. Fluid intake must be maintained to prevent dehydration and electrolyte imbalance. If contractions do not stop entirely, indicating "false labor," or if active labor does not follow, labor is stimulated with oxytocin, given in a dilute intravenous infusion of 5 percent glucose in water. The patient's condition must be monitored during oxytocin stimulation, with careful observation of uterine contractions and fetal heart rate.

Disorders of the active phase, or dilatational division, are evidenced by abnormally slow dilatation rates. The normal rates, again according to Friedman, should not be less than 1.2 cm/h in nulliparas or 1.5 cm/h in

multiparas. Two abnormal patterns may be noted in this phase—a prolonged, or protracted, active phase (Fig. 26·2B), and secondary arrest of dilation (Fig. 26·2C). The first, sometimes called *primary dysfunctional labor,* may result from fetal malposition or malpresentation, from cephalopelvic disproportion, or from inefficient uterine contractility—in about that order of frequency. Less commonly, in this phase, excessive sedation or anesthesia may be responsible for the prolongation.

The other abnormality of this division is *secondary arrest of dilation.* This means that some time after active dilation of the cervix has begun, arrest occurs, with no further progress in dilation occurring. This causes concern because of the possibility of cephalopelvic disproportion. The occurrence of either type of pattern indicates the need for prompt evaluation of the patient to determine the cause. Evaluation may require vaginal examination for determining position and presentation of the infant, and for estimating pelvic measurements and capacity. X-ray examinations may be necessary to aid in determining fetal size and position, and for obtaining more accurate pelvic measure-

fig. 26.2 Prolongation of phases of labor. A Prolongation of latent phase; B prolongation of active phase; C secondary arrest of dilation. (*From E. W. Page, C. A. Villee, and D. B. Villee, Human Reproduction: The Core Content of Obstetrics and Gynecology and Perinatal Medicine, W..B. Saunders Company, Philadelphia,* 1972.)

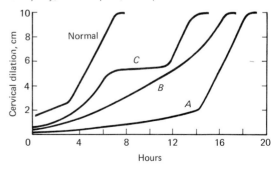

ments (pelvimetry). The use of monitoring equipment (electronic and/or ultrasonic) for aid in evaluating the uterine contractile pattern and the fetal heart response is also helpful and can provide much information.

Prompt diagnosis is important, and will help one to decide whether watchful waiting, rest with narcotic-sedative drugs, oxytocin stimulation, or operative interference is indicated.

The finding of disproportion in patients with either of these protracted active phase patterns would indicate the need for delivery by cesarean section. Patients showing the pattern of secondary arrest of dilatation in whom disproportion can be excluded may often be helped by the administration of oxytocin. On the other hand, those with patterns of primary dysfunctional labor are less apt to be helped by oxytocin stimulation. Continued slow progress of labor can be expected, and thus these women will primarily require support, with attention to their water and electrolyte balance, as well as support for their emotional needs.

What Friedman calls the *pelvic division* of labor is characterized by the final retraction of the cervical rim and by descent of the presenting part through the pelvis to the perineum. In this phase the rate of descent of the presenting part is the basis for estimating progress. The expected rate of descent is at least 1 cm/h in nulliparas and 2 cm/h in multiparas. Rates of descent that are slower than this, or arrest of descent, indicate again the need for careful evaluation for evidence of disproportion, malposition, or malpresentation. Disproportion of any significant degree requires delivery by cesarean section. If disproportion does not exist, labor may be allowed to proceed as long as progress is being made, or delivery may be effected by forceps, if conditions are suitable. Again, if uterine dysfunction seems at fault, the use of oxytocin would be helpful.

pelvimetry

In the foregoing discussion one of the factors that was mentioned repeatedly as affecting the outcome of labor was the presence or absence of *cephalopelvic disproportion.* This term refers to the size and shape of the skeletal pelvis in relation to the size, presentation, position, and attitude of the fetus. Thus maternal and fetal factors are involved.

The maternal factors are the size and shape of the skeletal pelvis. The classification of pelvic shapes most commonly used is that of Caldwell and Moloy, which is based chiefly upon the configuration of the pelvic inlet, although other factors are considered. Since most serious contractions of the pelvis occur at the inlet, this is, perhaps, the most important area to consider. Combination or intermediate forms are perhaps more common than the pure types. The four basic types of pelvis recognized in this classification (Fig. 26·3) are the *gynecoid, android, anthropoid,* and *platypelloid.*

GYNECOID PELVIS

The gynecoid pelvis is the typical female pelvis. The inlet is nearly round, the true pelvis is shallow and roomy, and there is a deep sacral curve. The subpubic arch is amply curved. The walls of the pelvic cavity are straight or may diverge at the outlet. This is the most favorable type of pelvis for normal delivery.

ANDROID PELVIS

The pelvic bones are often of heavier construction. The inlet is rather heart-shaped because of forward protrusion of the sacral promontory and the convergence of the anterior segment. The true pelvis is deep and the side walls converge. The lower end of the sacrum tends to tilt forward, and the subpubic

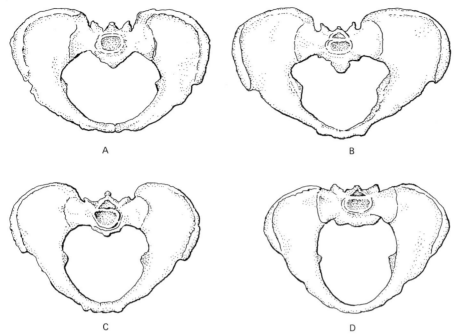

fig. 26·3 Types of pelves: A platypelloid; B android; C gynecoid; D anthropoid. (*Redrawn from Ullery and Castallo, Obstetric Mechanisms and Their Management, F. A. Davis Company, Philadelphia,* 1957, *p.* 39.)

arch is narrowed. This is the worst kind of pelvis from an obstetric standpoint since, even if engagement takes place, the head may be arrested at lower levels by the converging walls.

ANTHROPOID PELVIS

The inlet is oval, with the transverse diameter contracted and the largest diameter anteroposterior. The sacrum is narrow and long. The subpubic angle may or may not be amply curved. Engagement of the fetal head is more likely to occur in the anteroposterior diameter and will undergo little rotation in its descent.

PLATYPELLOID PELVIS

This type of pelvis is anteroposteriorly contracted, with a flattened inlet which is oval in transverse direction. The outlet is usually ample. If the fetal head can pass the inlet, there is usually no problem in delivery.

The size of the pelvis and the determination of its basic shape can be determined approximately by clinical examination (internal pelvimetry). By means of vaginal and rectal examination one can determine the contours of the inside of the pelvis, the thickness and width of the symphysis pubis, the prominence of the ischial spines, the degree of curvature and width of the sacrum, and the distance between the ischial tuberosities.

Determination of the *diagonal conjugate* is a means of estimating the anteroposterior diameter of the pelvic inlet. This is determined by directing the examining fingers back toward the hollow of the sacrum, then directing them upward until the tip of the finger touches the upper margin of the sacral promontory, or until the vaginal inlet prevents the hand from reaching farther. When this occurs the point of contact of the hand with the undermargin of the symphysis pubis is marked, and the distance from that point to the tip of the finger is measured. Subtracting 2 cm from that measurement to allow for the thickness of the pubis gives an approximate measurement of the true anteroposterior diameter of the pelvic inlet.

A more exact method for obtaining pelvic measurements is by means of x-ray pelvimetry. Because of increasing awareness of potential hazards of ionizing radiation to the fetus and the maternal ovaries, x-ray studies are requested less frequently than in the past. However, x-ray pelvimetry can be helpful from a diagnostic standpoint when there is apparent dystocia, when malpresentation is evident or suspected, or when there is a history of previous dystocia or unexplained stillbirth or birth injury. The x-ray studies will be most helpful if done when the patient is in labor, for one can then study the size and position of the fetal head in relation to the pelvis. Dystocia is due frequently to disproportion between the *size* of the head in relation to the maternal pelvis. In addition to actual size, variations in the *attitude* of the head can increase its relative size and retard passage through the pelvis. If the head is well flexed on the neck, as in vertex presentation, the smallest diameters of the head are presented; various degrees of extension of the head cause larger diameters to have to traverse the pelvic inlet. If the pelvic capacity is borderline, this could result in disproportion. *Brow* and *face* presentations are examples of abnormal presentations caused by extension of the head.

ABNORMAL PRESENTATIONS OF HEAD

A *brow presentation* may spontaneously convert to either a vertex or a face presentation. If conversion does not occur, a problem of disproportion is posed because the largest diameter of the fetal head is presented and, unless the head is small or the pelvis quite large, there will not be enough room for the head to descend. A persistent brow presentation that cannot be converted to a vertex or face presentation may thus be an indication for delivery by cesarean section (Fig. 26·4).

A *face presentation* represents the extreme of extension. These are relatively uncommon, occurring about 2 to 3 times per 1000 deliveries. In most instances engagement and descent will occur and the chin will rotate anteriorly to permit delivery by flexion across the perineum. If the chin should rotate posteriorly to the hollow of the sacrum, however, spontaneous delivery is impossible. It will be necessary in this case to rotate the chin anteriorly, either manually or with forceps; if this is not possible, then delivery by cesarean section will be necessary (Fig. 26·5).

Another factor influencing labor and delivery is that of *position* of the fetal head. If, in a vertex presentation, the occiput enters the pelvis and descends in one of the posterior quadrants of the pelvis (occiput posterior position), the process of *internal rotation* will require more time and effort than if it were in an anterior position. This is a factor in some prolonged labors. In the majority of instances

fig. 26·4 Brow presentation. (*Courtesy of Ross Laboratories, Columbus, Ohio, Clinical Education Aid.*)

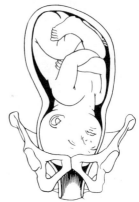

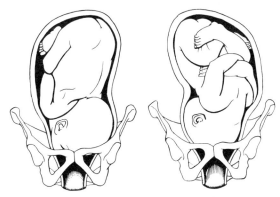

fig. 26·5 Face presentation. (*Courtesy of Ross Laboratories, Columbus, Ohio, Clinical Education Aid.*)

no real problem is encountered in this process and normal delivery occurs. However, if, for some reason (large head, contracted pelvis, ineffectual uterine contractions, etc.), rotation is interfered with, then normal delivery becomes difficult or impossible. The presenting part may start to rotate anteriorly and become wedged in the transverse position (*transverse arrest*), or may rotate posteriorly into the hollow of the sacrum, as was described with the face presentation (*persistent occiput posterior*, if vertex, or *persistent mentum posterior*, if face). This turn of events may then require operative intervention—either rotation with forceps or cesarean section (Fig. 26·6).

The most common, and hence the "normal," presentation is cephalic, i.e., the fetal head is normally the foremost part of the fetus to enter the birth canal. The normal cephalic presentation is the vertex. Abnormal cephalic presentations include the *face* and *brow* which have just been discussed. The other principal abnormal presentations are *breech* and *shoulder* presentations.

Breech Presentation Breech presentations occur in about 4 percent of all deliveries, but the rate varies depending upon the size of the fetus, being much higher in association with premature fetuses. The high

mortality rate of 10 to 20 percent associated with breech presentation is related to the high number of premature fetuses born in this way. Nevertheless, there is still a mortality rate in term fetuses of between 1 and 2 percent, which is 2 to 3 times that of fetuses with cephalic presentation. Other complications associated with breech presentation include a higher incidence of prolapse of the umbilical cord, and a more frequent occurrence of premature rupture of the membranes. The possibility of disproportion causes concern because the fetal head, which is the largest part of the infant, is the last part to pass through the pelvis, producing a next to impossible situation as far as fetal survival is concerned if it proves too large.

There are three varieties of breech presen-

fig. 26·6 Graphic display of cervical dilation-time patterns based on computer-derived data from 10,293 patients studied. The variations in the curves from that occurring in association with occiput anterior fetal positions (heavy line) are apparent. Nearly uniform slowing with occiput posterior (light line) and occiput transverse (heavy broken line), and modified normal pattern with breech presentation (light broken line) are shown. (*Used by permission of Emanuel A. Friedman and Bernard H. Kroll, "Computer Analysis of Labor Progression: V. Effects of Fetal Presentation and Position,* Journal of Reproductive Medicine **8**(3)121, 1972)

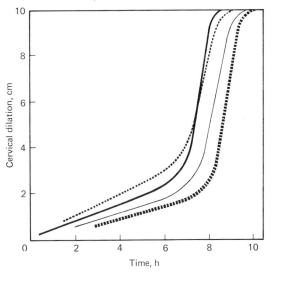

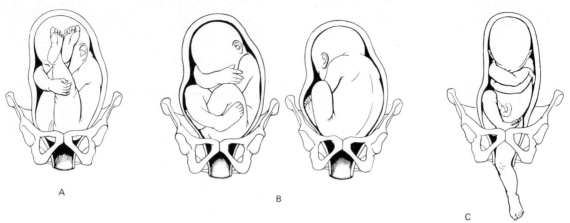

fig. 26·7 Breech presentation. A Frank breech; B complete breech; C incomplete breech (footling). (*Courtesy of Ross Laboratories*, Columbus, Ohio, *Clinical Education Aid.*)

tation, depending upon the position of the legs. In a *frank breech* presentation, the thighs are flexed on the trunk and the legs extended so that the feet are adjacent to the shoulders and rest alongside the head. This is the most frequent type. In a *complete breech* (Fig. 26·7B) the legs are flexed on the thighs and the thighs flexed on the trunk so that the feet and buttocks present. In an *incomplete,* or *footling, breech* the foot, or occasionally the knee, is the leading part (Fig. 26·7A, B, C).

The diagnosis of breech presentation may usually be made by abdominal examination and is indicated by finding the fetal head present in the fundal portion of the uterus. On vaginal examination the hard, smooth dome of the head is not felt, but one can feel the softer, irregular mass of the buttocks, the genitalia, and sometimes the feet.

There is a normal mechanism for the spontaneous delivery of an infant by breech presentation, but because of the increased fetal risk associated with this presentation cesarean section is frequently needed. Perhaps 20 percent of infants presenting as a breech are delivered in this manner. If the fetus is judged to be excessively large (over 8 lb in weight), if the patient is an elderly primigravida, or if

labor is protracted, cesarean section will be considered.

Shoulder Presentation Shoulder presentation associated with *transverse* or *oblique lie* presents a serious problem. This presentation occurs about once in 300 deliveries and is most often associated with multiparity, placenta previa, a contracted pelvis, multiple pregnancy, or bicornuate anomalies of the uterus. Occasionally, if detected before or early in labor, a shoulder presentation may be converted to a cephalic or breech type by *external version*. There is no normal mechanism for delivery in this presentation, and spontaneous delivery can occur only if the child is dead or extremely small. Unless conversion to a cephalic or breech presentation can be accomplished, delivery by cesarean section is indicated (Fig. 26·8).

maternal complications of delivery

It seems pertinent at this point to mention briefly some of the more important or more common complications that are encountered soon after delivery of the infant.

RETAINED OR ADHERENT PLACENTA

The third stage of labor (placental stage) is usually completed within 5 min, but may be prolonged because the placenta is unusually adherent (placenta accreta) or because it is "trapped" by contraction of the lower uterine segment. Perhaps the most common cause of retained placenta is failure to deliver it promptly after separation has occurred. If the placenta has not been delivered within 15 to 20 min, *manual removal* should be done, and this should be done at any time if bleeding is profuse and the placenta cannot be delivered by simple manual expression. In *placenta accreta* the cotyledons invade the uterine muscle; as a result, there is no cleavage plane, and separation of the placenta is impossible unless only a small area is involved. Hysterectomy is usually indicated for this relatively rare condition.

POSTPARTUM HEMORRHAGE

Postpartum hemorrhage is defined as the loss of more than 500 ml blood. The most common cause of immediate postpartum hemorrhage is uterine atony. Less frequent causes are lacerations of the vagina and cervix, and blood loss from the episiotomy incision (see Chap. 22).

Hemorrhage is a leading cause of maternal death, but almost all deaths from hemorrhage are preventable. Prompt recognition and appropriate treatment are necessary.

UTERINE RUPTURE

Uterine rupture is a very serious obstetric complication. Fortunately it does not occur very often on properly conducted obstetric services. Rupture during pregnancy almost always occurs at the site of a scar from a previous operation or injury, such as a myomectomy or a previous cesarean section. Rupture during labor is also most frequently associated with a scar from a previous cesarean section. Other causes include dystocia, particularly from a contracted pelvis, excessive parity, oxytocin stimulation, or injudicious operative deliveries.

The symptoms of rupture during labor are usually unmistakable. At the height of a contraction the patient will complain of a sudden, severe, tearing pain in her abdomen. This is followed by almost immediate cessation of labor. Depending on the amount of blood loss, the patient will show signs of intraperitoneal hemorrhage and shock. As soon as the diagnosis is made, immediate laparotomy is indicated, and blood should be available for transfusion. Occasionally it is possible to repair the laceration in the uterus, but most often hysterectomy will be necessary.

LACERATIONS AND INJURIES

Injuries to the pelvic soft tissues are inevitable because of the overdistension that occurs during the process of labor and delivery. Multiple small tears may occur around the urethra and clitoris and on the inner aspects of the labia minora, if the vaginal introitus is overstretched during delivery. These tears are usually superficial, but may bleed profusely. Bleeding from these superficial tears is readily controlled by suturing. Superficial abrasions of the vaginal mucosa may occur, especially over the ischial spines, and deep tears may extend up the lateral

fig. 26·8 Shoulder presentation. (*Courtesy of Ross Laboratories*, Columbus, Ohio, *Clinical Education Aid.*)

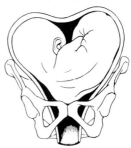

sulci, or folds, of the vagina. These deep lacerations of the vagina may be produced during forceps rotations and difficult extractions, but also may occur during simple forceps deliveries, or even during spontaneous deliveries.

Lacerations of the perineal body occur in many first labors. These injuries are classified according to their extent. *First-degree* lacerations involve only the skin and mucous membrane. A *second-degree* laceration involves the muscles and fascia except for the anal sphincter. *Third-degree* lacerations include division of the anal sphincter; and in *fourth-degree* lacerations the anterior rectal wall is split. Perineal lacerations most commonly result from what is, in effect, disproportion between the fetus and the soft tissues. Lacerations often occur during rapid, or precipitate, delivery.

The problem here is not so much the injury to the perineal body alone, but the deeper injuries accompanying it which are not visible and are not always readily amenable to repair. Lacerations of the perineum result in injury to the urogenital diaphragm and to the levator ani muscles and their fascial coverings. These deeper injuries to the structures which support the pelvic organs—the bladder, rectum, vagina, and uterus—are responsible for the later development of cystocele, rectocele, and uterine prolapse.

Lacerations of the cervix occur frequently during labor, but these are usually shallow and bleed little. More extensive lacerations may be produced by precipitous labor, by the injudicious use of oxytocics, or by attempts to deliver the infant before dilation of the cervix is complete. Bleeding from such lacerations may be profuse.

Careful inspection of the perineum, vulva, vagina, and cervix is necessary following delivery to detect any significant lacerations and injuries; if found, they should be properly repaired.

Extensive damage to the soft tissues of the pelvis can, for the most part, be prevented by good obstetric care.

obstetric operations

GENERAL CONSIDERATIONS

Not all labors and deliveries follow a smooth uncomplicated course; as has been indicated in the foregoing portions of this chapter, problems can arise to complicate delivery and necessitate operative intervention. These problems can often be anticipated, but often they arise unexpectedly during the course of labor and delivery. It is of the utmost importance, therefore, that skilled personnel are available to cope with these problems as they arise, and that the facilities and equipment are adequate.

Obstetric operations must be conducted in a proper setting. The delivery rooms should be fully equipped operating areas with the addition of special instruments and equipment for obstetric use. They must be equipped for normal delivery or for major surgery. Equipment for major anesthesia should be available. In addition, a heated bassinet and resuscitative equipment for the infant are necessary. It is desirable that at least one delivery room should be equipped with an operating table and instruments for the performance of cesarean section. A recovery room for the immediate postpartum observation of patients is also desirable.

EPISIOTOMY

Episiotomy is probably the most frequently performed obstetric operation. The term implies the deliberate incision or cutting of the vulva and perineum. Episiotomy is usually performed when a tear of the perineum appears inevitable during delivery of the infant, most obstetricians preferring a clean cut to a jagged tear. In the natural process of labor, the presenting part of the infant, forced by uterine contractions and voluntary bearing-down efforts of the mother, will gradually stretch and distend the muscles and fasciae of the pelvic floor and the tissues of the vulva as delivery occurs. Unless the tissues are very elastic, damage is bound to result, and the extent of injury cannot really be determined simply by inspection of the visible perineal trauma. It is possible, in fact, for the surface tissues to remain intact while tears in the deeper supporting structures remain hidden from view. As a consequence, most obstetricians feel that the best way to prevent this immediate damage, as well as future disability due to relaxation of the pelvic supporting structures, is to perform an adequate and timely episiotomy. In addition to preventing damage to the pelvic supports, it is also of benefit to the fetus by relieving the pressures on its head that result from its passage through the pelvic floor.

The indications, then, for episiotomy are resistant perineum, a large fetus, or abnormal presentation. Episiotomy is particularly indicated during delivery of a premature infant, to prevent trauma to the head. It should routinely be used in almost all primigravidas and in multiparas whose pelvic supports are well preserved as the result of previous repair. If the episiotomy is performed at the proper time and is adequately repaired, it will amost always be necessary to perform it again at subsequent deliveries.

The two *types* of episiotomy commonly employed are the *median* and the *mediolateral*. The median episiotomy is preferred by many because it is easier to repair and is less uncomfortable during the immediate postpartum period. The main disadvantage is the high incidence of sphincter tears and rectal lacerations that occur. It is performed by making an incision with scissors from the midline of the posterior fourchette through the median raphe of the perineal body as far as the fibers of the external anal sphincter. To make a mediolateral episiotomy, the incision is also started at the fourchette, but the scissor blades are directed at an angle between the anal margin and the ischial tuberosity. The skin, bulbocavernosus muscle, urogenital diaphragm, transverse perineal muscles, fasciae covering the levator ani muscle, and possibly some of its fibers, will be cut with an adequate mediolateral episiotomy.

The type of episiotomy is not as important as its timing and adequacy. The incision should be made when the presenting part is beginning to distend the perineum and remains visible between contractions, but before enough distension has occurred to produce damage to the fasciae and muscles. If the subpubic arch is broad, the perineum of adequate length, and fetal size not excessive, a median episiotomy is suitable. If the subpubic arch is narrowed, the perineum short, or the infant large, a mediolateral episiotomy is preferable.

Blood loss from an episiotomy wound may be significant but can be kept to a minimum by clamping bleeding vessels and applying pressure with a sponge until it can be repaired. Repair generally should not be started until after the placenta has been delivered and the vagina and cervix have been inspected for lacerations. The wound should be repaired carefully in anatomic layers, using sutures of fine catgut (No. 00 or 000 chromic).

Following delivery and repair, the perineal wound should be observed for the development of evidence of hematoma formation or infection. Good perineal hygiene is necessary. To help reduce edema and immediate discomfort an ice bag can be applied to the perineum intermittently for the first 12 h; after that time, heat, provided by sitz baths or a perineal lamp, will help to reduce discomfort.

FORCEPS DELIVERY

The obstetric forceps is an instrument devised to *extract* the fetal head from the birth canal. A secondary function is its use to *rotate* the head to a more favorable position for extraction. It is said to have been responsible for saving more lives than any other instrument or device that has ever been invented.

The use of instruments for delivery goes back to antiquity, but these instruments were used for the destruction and extraction of infants who had died during labor or for whom live birth was impossible because of contracted pelves or abnormal positions or presentations. The use of forceps for the purpose of delivering a live infant began with the invention of the precursor of the modern obstetric forceps by Peter Chamberlen, the Elder, about 1598. The instrument was kept a family secret and was used by four generations of Chamberlens for the next hundred years. By the middle of the eighteenth century the design of the forceps was made public in a book by Edmund Chapman, and since then has been modified almost constantly as more knowledge has been gained concerning the mechanisms of labor. The modern obstetric forceps consists of two halves, designated right or left according to the side of the pelvis to which they are applied. Each half has a handle, a shank, a lock, and a blade. The blade may be solid or open (fenestrated). The blade is curved to fit the fetal head and has another curve in relation to the shank—a pelvic curve—which is adapted to the curve of the axis of the birth canal. The most commonly employed forceps in general use are modifications of two basic types—the Simpson forceps and the Elliot type—each of which has certain advantages and disadvantages. In addition, special types of forceps are used in some situations—the Kielland forceps for rotation and the Piper forceps for delivery of the aftercoming head in breech presentations (Fig. 26·9A, B).

Types of Forceps Delivery Forceps deliveries are classified in various ways. The classification proposed in the *Manual of Standards,* 2d ed., published by the American College of Obstetricians and Gynecologists, is as follows:

1. *Outlet forceps*: The application of forceps when the scalp is or has been visible at the introitus without separating the labia, the skull has reached the pelvic floor, and the sagittal suture is in the anteroposterior diameter of the pelvis.
2. *Midforceps*: The application of forceps when the head is engaged, but the conditions for outlet forceps have not been met. In the context of this term, any forceps delivery requiring artificial rotation, regardless of the station from which extraction is begun, shall be designated a "midforceps" delivery. The term "low midforceps" is disapproved. A record shall be made of the position and station of the head when the delivery is begun. In addition, a description of the various maneuvers and of any difficulties encountered in the application of the forceps and in the extraction of the infant shall be recorded.
3. *High forceps*: The application of forceps at any time prior to full engagement of the head. High forceps delivery is almost never justified.

Indications for use Indications for the use of forceps may be either *fetal* or *maternal.* The usual fetal indications include arrested rotation or posterior rotation of the occiput or chin, failure to make progress in descent, certain abnormal presentations such as face and brow, and fetal distress, as evidenced by slowing of the heart rate and passage of meconium. In addition, the use of forceps is indicated for delivering premature infants to prevent trauma to these more fragile heads. Many obstetricians routinely use forceps for delivery of the aftercoming head in breech presentations.

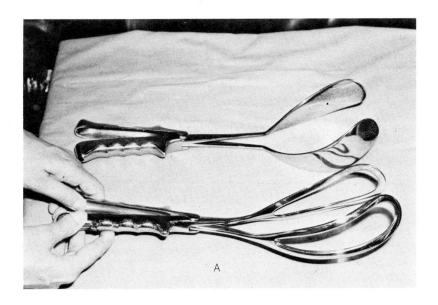

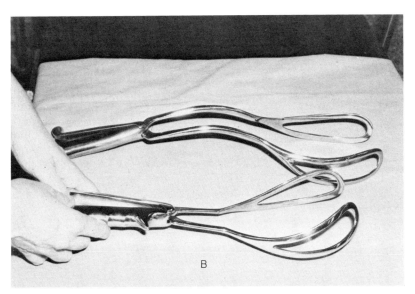

fig. 26·9 Forceps in common usage. A *Top:* Tucker-McLean forceps, with solid, smooth blades. *Bottom:* Elliot forceps. B *Top:* Piper forceps for breech deliveries; note curve of shank. *Bottom:* Simpson forceps.

Maternal factors indicating the use of forceps include uterine inertia, maternal exhaustion, mild or relative degrees of cephalopelvic disproportion, and the presence of systemic diseases making the prolonged expulsive efforts necessary to complete the second stage of labor undesirable. The latter would include such diseases as heart disease, pulmonary tuberculosis or other severe respiratory disease, and hypertension or other cardiovascular disease. The wide use of conduction anesthesia with loss of the bearing-down sensation and interference with voluntary expulsive efforts is a common current indication.

Perhaps most of the forceps operations done today are done *electively,* or *prophylactically.* Many obstetricians today routinely use forceps delivery and episiotomy to prevent trauma to the fetal head, prevent maternal exhaustion, and prevent damage to the supporting tissues of the pelvis. If the criteria for outlet forceps delivery are met, elective forceps deliveries are as safe as spontaneous deliveries, or safer.

Prerequisites for use Certain requirements must be met before forceps are used. If these prerequisites cannot be met, the use of forceps is contraindicated. The *cervix* must be *completely dilated,* otherwise it is very apt to be lacerated. The *head* must be *engaged,* and the operator must know its *position.* There must be no *serious disproportion.* The *membranes* must be *ruptured,* and the *rectum* and *bladder* should be *empty.* The operator must be familiar with the *normal mechanisms* of labor and be *skilled* in the use of *forceps.* The patient should receive some form of *anesthesia* (Fig. 26·10A through H).

Dangers to the mother from difficult or injudiciously applied forceps operations include injury, hemorrhage, and infection. Injuries can occur to the cervix, vagina, rectum, and bladder. Dangers to the child include compression of the brain, fracture of the skull, and injuries to the face and eyes. These risks are minimized by adherence to the requirements listed above. If serious difficulty is anticipated or becomes apparent during the course of forceps delivery, it is much safer for mother and baby for the delivery to be effected by cesarean section.

VACUUM EXTRACTOR

A vacuum extractor has been developed and reintroduced into obstetrics as a replacement for the forceps in vaginal delivery. It consists of a steel cup with an attached suction tube and a metal chain for traction. The cup is applied to the fetal scalp and is held in place by a vacuum produced by a suction pump. By means of the vacuum pressure the scalp is pulled up into the cup, creating an artificial caput succedaneum.

This instrument is used occasionally in some hospitals but has met with limited enthusiasm in this country. It would seem to be of only limited usefulness and to have no advantage over the use of conventional forceps.

cesarean section

One can find references to the operation of cesarean section as far back as mythologic times. This is not surprising, for it is one of the most dramatic of operations. In the sequence of events in the development of the operation we find that, in the beginning, the cesarean operation was performed only upon the dead mother to provide a separate burial for the child, that it later was done upon the dying mother when the child showed signs of life, and finally upon the living mother in the effort to save both baby and mother.

The origin of the operation's name is thought to go back to the eighth century B.C. when Pompilian law decreed that the child should be removed from the womb of any woman who died in late pregnancy. The law continued during the reign of the emperors, or Caesars, and was known as the lex caesarea.

Today, cesarean section is one of the safest of major operations, and many series of over 1000 sections have been reported without a single maternal death. Delivery by cesarean section has an average incidence in this country of 5 percent or greater, depending on the type of community and the philosophy of the physicians. It is performed for indications that have little in common with the severe pelvic contractions and neglected

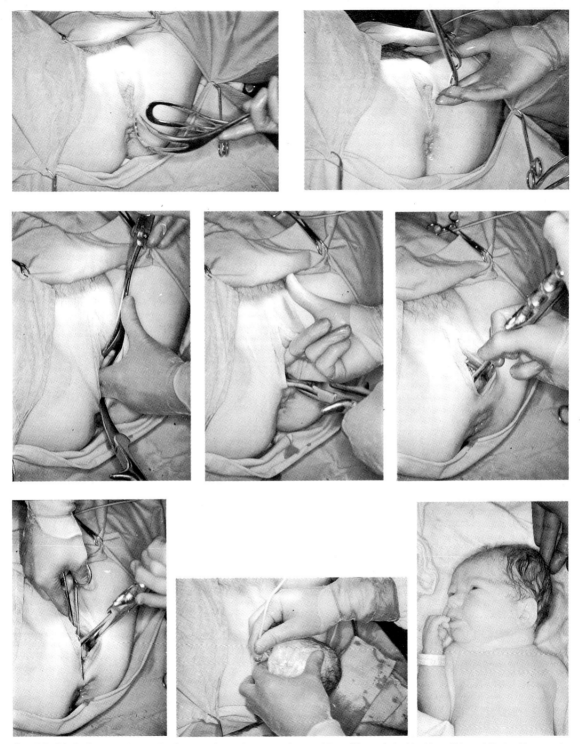

fig. 26·10 Delivery using outlet forceps in occiput anterior position. (*From A. L. Haskins, "Use of Outlet Forceps in Occiput Anterior Position," Modern Medicine,* © *The New York Times Media Company, Inc., Sept.* 4, 1972.)

labors of earlier years, and is used freely when it appears that abdominal delivery offers the most benefit for mother and child.

INDICATIONS

In most hospitals today the most frequent indication is a *previous cesarean section.* Because of the risk of rupture of the uterine scar, most obstetricians adhere to the dictum "once a section, always a section." This risk is not great, but rupture of the uterine scar carries a significant mortality rate. If the reason for the first section was of a temporary nature, some obstetricians are willing to allow labor and vaginal delivery to occur. In such cases · the patient must be watched very closely during labor for evidence of rupture of the scar, blood should be cross-matched, and facilities available for immediate abdominal delivery if rupture should occur.

If repeat operations are excluded, the incidence of primary sections is about 2 to 3 percent. The most frequent indications, in order of frequency, are *disproportion, uterine dysfunction, placenta previa, malposition and malpresentation, toxemia, placenta abruptio, fetal distress, prolapsed cord, diabetes mellitus, previous pelvic surgery* (successful vaginal plastic repair and hysterotomy, etc.).

If delivery by repeat section is planned, it can be done electively and scheduled like any other planned surgical procedure. Ordinarily, delivery will be planned for about a week or 10 days before term (so that the baby will have as much time for intrauterine growth as possible) but before the onset of labor. If there is doubt about the size and maturity of the infant, the performance of *amniocentesis* to obtain a sample of amniotic fluid for analysis may be helpful. Finding creatinine values of 2 mg/100 ml or more, lecithin/sphingomyelin ratios of 2 or over, or fetal fat cells in excess of 20 percent of cells examined, would indicate fetal maturity. The use of ultrasonic techniques for measuring fetal head size as an index of maturity also shows promise of being helpful.

TYPES OF CESAREAN SECTIONS

Several types of abdominal and uterine incisions are used in performing section; the approach and uterine incision used should be those which are safest and best for the individual patient.

Abdominal incision is most frequently the *vertical subumbilical,* or *midline,* incision. Sometimes a paramedian incision may be performed. *Transverse incisions* of the *Pfannenstiel* or *Cherney* type are also used occasionally. In the Pfannenstiel incision the skin and rectus fascia are opened transversely, but the peritoneum is opened vertically. In the Cherney incision the rectus muscles are divided at their attachment to the pubic rami and the peritoneum is opened transversely.

Uterine incisions are made in either the upper segment, or fundus, of the uterus, or in the lower segment. Upper segment incisions are made vertically in the midline. This is known as the *classical* incision. The muscle is incised down to the amniotic sac, and the membranes are stripped from the uterine wall. The incision is then lengthened with bandage scissors, and the membranes are ruptured with suction to aspirate the amniotic fluid. The infant is extracted usually by grasping the feet and extracting it as a breech. The infant's mouth and pharynx are aspirated, the cord is clamped and cut, and the infant is placed in a warm crib. Ideally, a pediatrician should be present to receive the baby and provide immediate care. The placenta is then removed from the uterus, and the uterine wound closed in layers with chromic catgut sutures. The abdominal wound is then closed in routine fashion. The classical incision is used infrequently at the present time, but is still used occasionally in conditions where rapid extraction of the infant is desirable, or by some physicians in the presence of placenta previa.

The *lower segment operation* is used most frequently. After the abdomen has been opened, the vesicouterine fold of peritoneum is incised and the bladder removed by blunt dissection from the lower uterine segment. Either a vertical or curved transverse incision is made in the lower uterine segment; after rupture of the membranes, the infant is extracted, and the uterine wound sutured. The lower segment operation has the advantage that there is often less bleeding from the thinner lower segment, and that after the bladder has been replaced and the vesicouterine peritoneum sutured, the uterine wound is excluded from the peritoneal cavity.

Another type of section is known as an *extraperitoneal section*. Several varieties of this type have been devised. The procedure was developed to approach the lower uterine segment without entering the peritoneal cavity in patients who had actual or potential intrauterine infection. With the development and safety of the lower segment transperitoneal operation and the availability of antibiotics to prevent or control infection, the extraperitoneal operation is seldom used.

In some situations cesarean section is followed by hysterectomy, or removal of the uterus, after the child has been delivered. This operation is known as *cesarean hysterectomy*. It may be performed in patients with uncontrollable hemorrhage, or in the presence of diseases of the uterus such as multiple myomas (fibroid tumors) or carcinoma in situ of the cervix, or because of placenta accreta. In some clinics cesarean hysterectomy is performed as a means of permanent sterilization in preference to tubal ligation.

PREOPERATIVE PREPARATION

If the cesarean section is being performed electively, the preparations are the same as for any abdominal operation, plus arranging for receiving and caring for the baby.

On admission, a complete physical examination is performed and routine laboratory studies are made, including blood count and urinalysis. Blood should be typed and crossmatched and be made available for use during operation. The patient is prepared by shaving the abdomen and perineum. Food and fluids are withheld during the night before surgery, and an enema to empty the bowel is given in the morning. An indwelling catheter is placed in the bladder before the patient goes to the operating room so that the bladder may be kept empty during the procedure.

In the operating room the skin preparation and draping are the same as for any abdominal operation. Equipment for resuscitation and care of the infant must be available, including the customary identification bracelets. If the section is being done as an emergency procedure, all the above preparations must be made more rapidly.

POSTOPERATIVE CARE

Postoperative care consists of postoperative as well as postpartum care. The uterus must be watched carefully for evidence of atony, which is most apt to be a problem after section performed for prolonged labor or for late pregnancy bleeding. Vital signs, including pulse and blood pressure, should be recorded frequently for the first several hours. Fluids are given parenterally for the first 24 h after delivery but may be given orally the day following surgery if bowel sounds are present and there is no distension. By the second day the patient may be ready to take solid food. The catheter is usually removed after 24 h or so. The patient is usually out of bed within 24 h.

ROLE OF THE NURSE

During labor the role of the nurse includes providing support and reassurance to the patient, explaining the procedures, and providing assistance to the physician in the preparation and administration of medications. In addition, she must monitor closely the patient's vital signs, fetal heart rate, and uterine contractions. In some hospitals she may, after special training, be permitted to do sterile vaginal examinations and take additional responsibility for following the patient's progress in labor.

When the patient is in the delivery room or operating room, unless the nurse is scrubbed and actually assisting in the performance of the delivery or operative procedure, her role again is that of lending support and reassurance to the patient. In addition, she must ensure that facilities and equipment are ready for the reception of the infant and its resuscitation, if necessary, and provide needed medications, supplies, and instruments to the operating team.

During the critical time immediately following delivery, whether it was a vaginal delivery or cesarean section, monitoring of the patient is of vital importance. Careful observation and recording of vital signs, urinary output, firmness of the uterus, the presence or absence of excessive bleeding, hematoma formation, etc., are major and primary responsibilities of the nurse attending the patient. During this period, again, the provision of encouragement, reassurance, and emotional support to the patient will pay large dividends.

All these nursing functions during labor and delivery will be better performed if the nurse has acquired a solid understanding of normal obstetrics, of the potential problems that can occur, and of the accepted measures for dealing with these problems if they should arise.

bibliography

Bamptom, Betsy A., and Joan M. Mancini: "The Cesarian Section Patient Is a New Mother, Too," *Journal of Obstetrical and Gynecological Nursing,* **2**(4):58, 1973.

Diddle, A. W., J. R. Semmer, and J. F. Slowey: "Cesarian Section: A Changing Philosophy," *Postgraduate Medicine,* **53**:3, 1973.

Friedman, Emanuel A.: "The Functional Divisions of Labor," *American Journal of Obstetrics and Gynecology,* **109**:274–280, 1971.

————: "Patterns of Labor as Indicators of Risk," *Clinical Obstetrics and Gynecology,* **16**:172–183, 1973.

Laufe, Leonard E.: *Obstetric Forceps,* Paul B. Hoeber, Inc., New York, 1968.

Page, E. W., C. A. Villee, and D. B. Villee: chaps. 14 and 16 in *Human Reproduction, The Core Content of Obstetrics, Gynecology and Perinatal Medicine,* W. B. Saunders Company, Philadelphia, 1972.

Reid, D. E., K. J. Ryan, and K. Benirschke: *Principles and Management of Human Reproduction,* W. B. Saunders Company, Philadelphia, 1972.

Speert, Harold: *Inconographia Gyniatrica, A Pictorial History of Obstetrics and Gynecology,* F. A. Davis Company, Philadelphia, 1973.

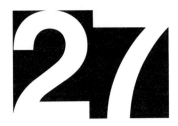

fetal medicine

Elizabeth J. Dickason

The study of the growing fetus, termed *fetology,* is becoming a major area of interest in medicine. New techniques of monitoring and interpreting growth patterns have led to discovery of facts about the fetus unknown even a few years ago. Now it is possible to determine gestational age, condition, problems, defects, and even the sex of the infant.

Because a very large number of infants are lost or handicapped before birth, it is important to work toward reducing the morbidity and mortality rates. Many defects cannot as yet be prevented, but modern techniques allow early diagnosis where the possibility of problems might exist. Early diagnosis is recommended when one or both parents have chromosomal abnormalities or carry genetically sex-linked diseases. Women over forty are usually counseled to have early testing because of the greater risk of bearing a child with Down's syndrome. When one child is affected with a genetic defect, the family is considered to be more likely to have a second child so affected.

Since genetic counseling is time-consuming and expensive, parents should be informed about the costs and the time involved. If the woman is pregnant already, diagnosis should be made early enough to give the parents the option of choosing a therapeutic abortion. Conversely, early discovery of some metabolic defects may allow

for treatment through dietary changes during pregnancy. Complete information on genetic counseling can be obtained from The National Foundation-March of Dimes.[1]

methods of studying the fetus

AMNIOCENTESIS

Amniotic fluid is the best mirror of fetal condition before labor begins. It contains cast-off cells from the respiratory, genitourinary, and gastrointestinal tracts and the skin. Some of these cells can be cultured, i.e., grown in a medium over a period of 10 days to 2 weeks. Cell division occurs, and growth can be stopped at just the right point to obtain a clear microscopic view of the chromosomes. These are photographed under a high-power microscope, arranged in pairs, and studied for abnormalities. This karyotype is useful in determining the infant's sex and the presence of autosomal trisomies, translocations, or mosaicisms (see Chap. 2).

Biochemical studies of enzymes of these growing cells can inform the physician of genetically transmitted metabolic diseases; i.e., inborn errors of metabolism (IEM). Currently, about 40 of these metabolic disorders can be detected before birth.

Amniocentesis for suspected genetic problems is done ideally at the sixteenth week of pregnancy. Before this time there appears to be too little amniotic fluid. Scheduling it at the sixteenth week allows time for the 2 to 6 weeks needed for karyotyping and biochemical studies. There remains time for the parents and the genetic counselor to discuss the alternatives open to them. If a therapeutic abortion is chosen, it should be done before the end of the twentieth week of pregnancy. Abortion may be recommended in cases of translocation and sex-linked metabolic disorders.

[1] 1275 Mamaroneck Rd., White Plains, N.Y.

Signs of Fetal Maturity Amniocentesis later in pregnancy is most often done to determine the condition of the fetus or the degree of fetal maturity. Repeated amniocentesis may be done in cases of isoimmunization as the condition of the infant in jeopardy is followed carefully. If indicated, plans have to be made either for early delivery or for intrauterine transfusion (see Chap. 29).

The fluid obtain by amniocentesis is studied for bilirubin, creatinine, color, turbidity, cell content, and in some cases, hormonal content. The gestational age of the infant can be predicted by four parameters:

1. In normal infants, bilirubin disappears from the fluid by 38 weeks' gestation. There is a predictable curve, which can be analyzed. If the fluid shows no bilirubin, the infant is usually mature enough to survive outside the uterus.
2. Creatinine increases with age after 32 weeks gestation. This rising curve is correlated with a value of 1.5 mg/100 ml as always indicating an infant weighing 2500 Gm or more.
3. Staining the cells found in the amniotic fluid with Nile blue sulfate causes "fat cells" to turn orange. If 10 percent or more of the cells found in the specimen are orange-stained, the infant is usually more than 36 weeks gestation and more than 2500 Gm in weight (1).
4. Lecithin/sphingomyelin ratio. Lecithin and sphingomyelin are surface-active phospholipids found in the amniotic fluid. They reflect the maturity of the fetal lung. By evaluating the concentration of these substances, and the ratio between them, a determination can be made as to the readiness of the fetus for respiratory independence.

   A ratio of 2:1 L/S shows that the lung is mature enough to function. A ratio of 1:1 indicates immaturity. Ratios in between show variable outcomes. The lower the L/S ratio, the more severe the respiratory distress in infants (2).

Because there is danger in premature delivery, amniocentesis is done to determine fetal age in high-risk pregnancies when the chances of waiting until term for an infant have to be balanced against the handicap of prematurity.

The Technique of Amniocentesis The nurse will assist in the amniocentesis by preparing the patient.

1. Have the patient void to empty her bladder.
2. Position and drape the patient in supine position.
3. Gather equipment for the procedure.

Preparation:

Sterile gloves
Sterile drape
Antiseptic for skin
Razor to shave site

fig. 27·1 Aseptic technique of transabdominal amniocentesis. A short needle with stylet for first insertion through maternal tissue makes it possible to avoid contact of the amniocentesis needle with maternal skin. (*Redrawn, courtesy of Bernard Mandelbaum, M.D.*)

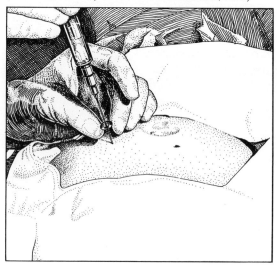

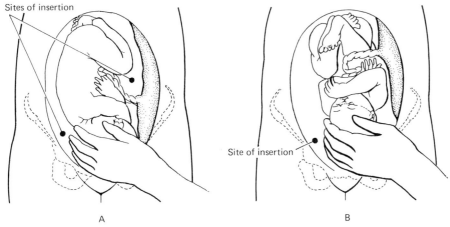

Sites of insertion

Site of insertion

A

B

fig. 27·2 Sites of insertion into amniotic fluid. (*Redrawn, courtesy of Bernard Mandelbaum, M.D.*)

Local anesthetic—lidocaine 1 percent
5-ml syringe with 25-gauge needle

Procedure:

1½-inch 20-gauge needle with stylet—for first insertion
5-in 22-gauge needle with stylet—threaded through 20-gauge needle (Fig. 27·1)
Labeled tubes for fluid specimen (protect from light)
10- and 20-ml syringes

4. Assist the doctor by holding the head of the baby away from the puncture site (Fig. 27·2).
5. Take fetal heart tones before and after procedure.
6. Take mother's vital signs.
7. Observe for untoward effects:

Bleeding   Increased fetal activity
Premature labor   Infection (fever)
Pain   Amnionitis

8. Instruct the mother in follow-up care as prescribed by the physician.

The risks of amniocentesis must be explained to the mother without unduly alarming her. In very rare instances morbidity occurs. The fetus may be punctured and may hemorrhage. Abruptio placentae or amnionitis may also occur. Maternal morbidity—hemorrhage, abdominal pain, or peritonitis—has been reported. Labor may be precipitated; causing abortion or, if later in pregnancy, premature delivery. A consent must be signed after a complete explanation has been given to the patient.

Summary of Uses Amniocentesis is a technique used to:

Diagnose genetically carried diseases
Determine age or sex of the infant
Determine condition of the fetus
Introduce radiopaque liquid for amniography
Induce abortion by salinization
Reduce intrauterine pressure in cases of polyhydramnios
Administer packed red blood cells intraabdominally to the fetus

SOUND

For many years the only methods of evaluating fetal condition were palpation and sound, feeling for size and position, and listening to the fetal heartbeat. The fetal position, the amount of fluid, and the position of the pla-

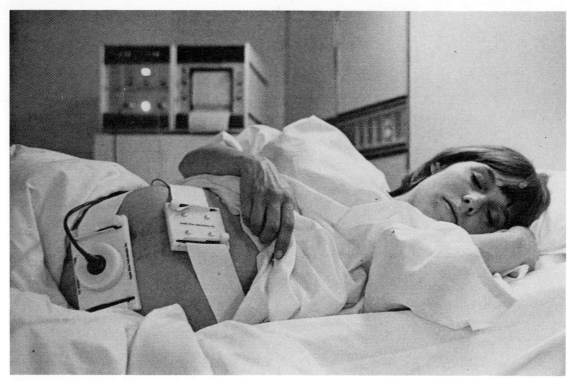

fig. 27·3 Doppler method of ausculation. (*Courtesy of Gould, Inc.*)

centa affect the transmission of sound, as does the quality of the stethoscope. The method of *auscultation* is described in Chap. 4. Auscultation is useful in pregnancy but has been shown to be much less accurate than the newer methods of monitoring the fetus during labor (Fig. 27·3). However, until all labor rooms are equipped with monitors, nurses must still become skilled in listening with a stethoscope to the fetal heart sounds.

Phonocardiography This technique involves the placement of a microphone enclosed in a soft cover over the site of the best fetal heart sounds. When the fetus shifts position, the microphone must be shifted. This microphone may be strapped around the abdomen and left in place during labor. Sounds are amplified and may be recorded to produce a written record. External noise and movements of the patient limit the accuracy of this technique.

Ultrasound Ultrasound is an application of sound waves beamed at very high frequencies, 1 to 20 million cycles per second (normal audible limit is 20,000 cycles per second), into body tissue. It appears to be noninjurious to human tissue within this range. The principle is generally that of sonar. The echoes bouncing back from soft tissues are converted into electrical energy seen as bright spots on an oscilloscope. Just as one can learn to read x-rays, so these characteristic echoes can be read on the oscilloscope. Because ultrasound shows soft-tissue structures without harmful effects of radiation, its use will become very important in obstetrics. In a number of situations where early diagnosis is needed, ultrasound can be of use (Fig. 27·4).

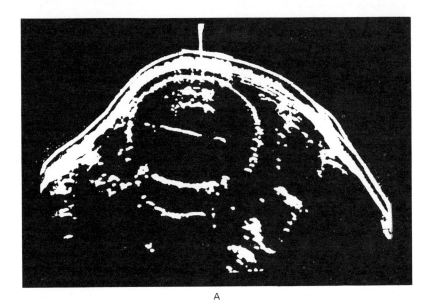

A

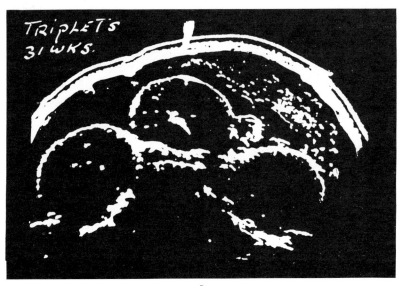

B

fig. 27·4 Ultrasound diagnosis. A Transverse cross-section showing fetal head at 32 weeks. B Triplets at 31 weeks. (*Courtesy of Picker Corporation.*)

Ultrasound is a very accurate method for detecting the ectopic pregnancy. The location of implantation of an embryo can be determined after the eighth week, although the embryo may weigh only a gram and be only 2.8 cm in length. There are almost 40 obstetric situations in which ultrasound can be of use. Among these are:

Placental localization

Detecting abnormal implantation

Detecting abnormalities of fetal development

Determining fetal maturity by accurate measurement of the biparietal diameter of the fetal head

Ultrasound procedure requires 30 to 60 min although the patient is exposed to ultrasound for only a few minutes during this time. The technique is not widely available, but as more physicians are trained in its use, more and more centers will provide ultrasound diagnosis in pregnancy.

X-RAY

Radiation dosage should be carefully controlled in potentially pregnant women. The only safe days for x-rays are the first 10 days after the menstrual period. Otherwise, before a pregnancy is discovered a woman might receive an excessive dose, affecting a highly radiosensitive embryo. The first 3 months of development—the period of *organogenesis*—are the most important. However, as is well known, dosage may be cumulative, and high doses of radiation to the mother have been correlated with an increased incidence of malignant diseases such as leukemia in early childhood. Therefore, x-rays are always used as a last choice in obstetrics, most usually in the last trimester, and then only when other methods are not available (3) (see Fig. 3·14).

Since bony structure can be visualized on x-ray, *pelvimetry,* the measurement of the pelvic size and shape, is one of the uses of x-ray in obstetrics. Fetal position, size, and head diameters in relationship to pelvic size can be determined. Pelvimetry is usually done when the patient is in labor to aid in diagnosis of cephalopelvic disproportion.

In suspected placenta previa, soft-tissue x-rays can show the vague outlines of the placenta in a low-lying position if the head is displaced. One method to aid in visualization of the placenta is the use of contrast material inserted into the bladder or into the amniotic fluid. *Cystography* is the introduction of a radiopaque contrast material, such as 12 percent sodium iodide, into the bladder. This serves to outline the soft tissue of the bladder, helping to delineate the position of the placenta. Plain air can also be used as a contrast material. Lateral and anteroposterior x-rays are then taken.

For *amniography* an amniocentesis is performed, removing 20 to 25 ml fluid. An equal amount of contrast material is introduced into the amniotic sac. The contrast material mixes through the fluid and outlines the fetus. This method is used to detect fetal condition because a healthy fetus swallows amniotic fluid, making it possible to perform a "GI series" in the uterus. The speed with which the contrast material is swallowed can be correlated with normal rates, i.e., 3 to 4 h to outline the small intestine. Absence of swallowing or obstruction of the intestinal tract can be seen in malformed infants. A timed series of x-rays is taken to demonstrate the distribution of the contrast material (2).

ISOTOPIC PLACENTOGRAPHY

Although various radioactive isotopes are being used, a common choice is Cr^{51}, which is injected into an arm vein. After a wait of 10 min for circulation, a counter records the radioactivity over each of nine divided segments of the abdomen. The report returned with the patient will show the placental location expressed as the areas of highest counts of radioactivity. The reason for this is that the placental area receives a larger volume of blood per minute than the rest of the uterus.

FETAL BLOOD TESTING

During labor, after the cervix has dilated and the membranes have ruptured, samples of

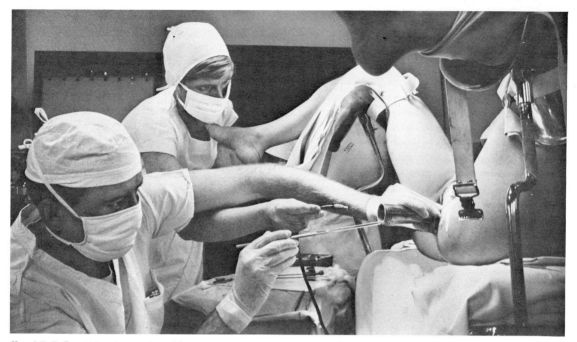

fig. 27·5 Fetal blood sampling. After conical scope is introduced into the vagina with sterile technique, blood sample from fetal scalp is collected in glass capillary tube. (*From* OB/GYN Observer, *November*, 1970.)

fetal capillary blood can be taken from the presenting part—scalp or buttocks. In the technique being used, which was first recorded by Dr. Saling, the fetal scalp is punctured and drops of blood are collected in a long glass capillary tube (Fig. 27·5). By microanalysis of such small amounts of blood it is possible to test the fetal pH, P_{O_2}, P_{CO_2}, glucose, and base deficit values. Hematocrit and hemoglobin can also be determined. There is a good correlation between a series of falling levels of pH and a low Apgar score at birth (4).

Fetal blood testing is carried out in high-risk situations and when fetal distress is noted in the process of labor. Blood testing can only supply periodic information and must be supplemented by heart rate monitoring.

Procedure The mother is positioned in dorsorecumbent or Sims' position and draped. The perineal area is cleansed of all blood,

mucus, and amniotic fluid. Sterile equipment is used:

Gloves, long forceps, cotton swabs, antiseptic
Endoscope for visualizing the cervix
Ethyl chloride spray to cause hyperemia of scalp
Knife blade with long handle
Long heparinized glass capillary tubes
Cotton swabs and swab holders

The time of sampling must be noted as a correlative factor with current fetal and maternal condition. If indicated, blood may be drawn from the mother at the same time to be measured for pH, P_{O_2}, P_{CO_2}, glucose, hematocrit, and hemoglobin.

FETAL ELECTROCARDIOGRAM

An indirect fetal electrocardiogram may be obtained during the prenatal period by means of electrodes placed on the mother's abdomen. The resulting record is a mixture of maternal and fetal cardiograms. This procedure has been especially useful in diagnosing multiple pregnancy or intrauterine death in the antepartal period.

electronic monitoring of labor

To monitor the fetus electronically during labor, the fetal heart rate is obtained either by the direct attachment of an electrode to the presenting part of the fetus or by an ultrasound transducer strapped to the maternal abdomen (Fig. 27·6A, B). Simultaneously intrauterine pressure (uterine contraction pattern) is recorded, either by direct means such as a Teflon fluid-filled catheter passed through the cervix after membranes have ruptured, or indirectly by attaching a pressure-sensitive transducer to the mother's abdomen. The indirect method, i.e., ultrasound detection of fetal heart rate and external transducer, may be used earlier in the course of labor and with intact membranes. Its initiation in the patient in labor is usually a nursing responsibility. The direct method requires more skill and at present is usually a physician's responsibility. Both methods provide a chart showing continuous recordings of fetal heart rate and uterine contractions.

PROCEDURE

The patient is placed in the Sims' position, and the perineum is cleansed. Surgical asepsis is used for the following equipment:

    Gloves, forceps, cotton swabs, antiseptic
    Endoscope for visualizing the cervix
    Special forceps for scalp electrodes
    Teflon catheter with tubing attached to a three-way stopcock
    Introducer for catheter and slide guide for scalp electrodes

    10-ml syringe filled with saline solution to remove air from tubing and catheter

Nonsterile equipment includes tapes to attach leg plate securely (Fig. 27·7A through E).

Learning to interpret fetal monitoring records requires time and practice. Records showing the following features are within a normal pattern:

1. Rate between 100 and 180 beats/min.
2. Good beat-to-beat variation of at least 5 beats/min.
3. Accelerations of the heart rate with uterine contractions.
4. Early decelerations. Moderate slowing of the FHR at the time of contractions. These are uniform in shape, begin with the onset of the contraction, and end with the return of the contraction to the base line. Early decelerations are due to head compression and characteristically appear late in labor, when contractions are intense and frequent.
5. No decelerations during labor.

All the above features in the record correlate very well with a healthy fetus equipped to tolerate the stress of uterine contractions during labor (Fig. 27·8).

ABNORMAL FINDINGS

Abnormal findings in monitoring records are:

1. *Late decelerations* show a pattern of slowing of the FHR beginning during the peak of a uterine contraction and persisting after the contraction is over. Late decelerations are due to fetal anoxia and are serious indications that the fetus is potentially in distress. Any factor which interferes with the arrival of oxygen to the fetus will cause late decelerations. Some examples are partial separation of the placenta, hyperactive uterine contractions without relaxation intervals (usually due to excessive oxytocin dosage), maternal hyperten-

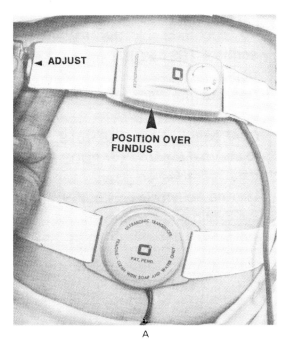

A

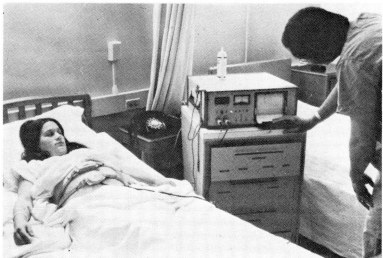

B

fig. 27·6 A Fetal external monitor B External monitor in place. (*With permission of Corometrics Medical Systems, Inc. Copyright,* 1974.)

sion with resultant poor circulation to the uterus, toxemia with poor placental perfusion.

2. *Variable deceleration* is the most common pattern seen in monitored patients. As its name implies, the pattern of slowing bears less relationship to contractions than the more uniform early and late deceleration. The deceleration is more rapid in onset and recovery, and each deceleration dif-

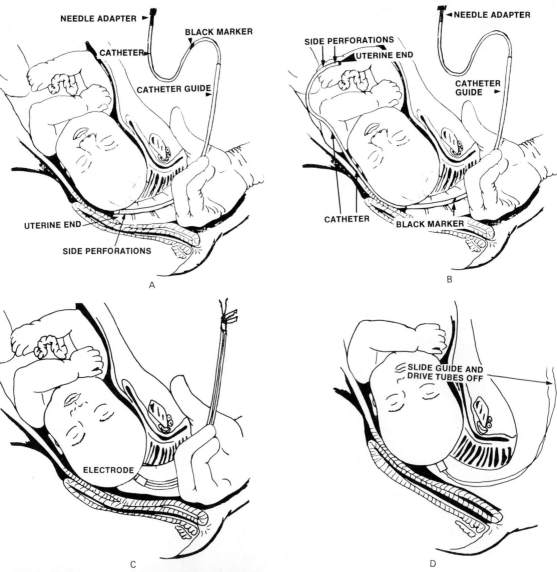

fig. 27·7 Procedure for attaching internal monitor. A and B After membranes are ruptured, the catheter is introduced past fetal head into the uterus. C Spiral electrode attached to scalp; D electrode slide guide removed; E close-up of spiral electrode in slide guide. (*With permission of Corometrics Medical Systems, Inc. Copyright,* 1974.)

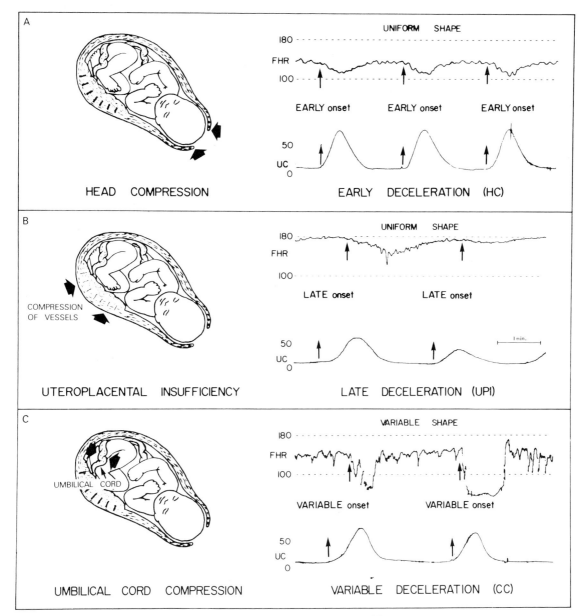

fig. 27·8 Chart of mechanisms of fetal heart rate deceleration patterns. (*From Edward P. Hon,* An Introduction to Fetal Heart Monitoring, *Harty Press, Inc.,* 1968.)

fers from those before and after. It is the most dramatic of the patterns, with dips in rate of 60 beats/min being common. Variable decelerations are due to compression of the umbilical cord. Since the umbilical cord is highly sensitive to compression, variable decelerations do not always mean fetal difficulty. Variation in the pattern (i.e., decelerations that last longer, become greater in amplitude, and are unresponsive to treatment) usually signifies fetal anoxia.

3. *Loss of beat-to-beat variation* in fetal heart rate is a serious sign of fetal anoxia. A straight line on the fetal heart recording is the most serious index of anoxia to the fetal heart itself. The interpretation of such a record must be cautious, because certain drugs administered in labor, such as Scopolamine and Valium, may significantly reduce beat-to-beat variation.

The uterine contraction record is helpful in assessing the quality of labor. It is invaluable in following the course of patients who are receiving oxytocin for the induction or stimulation of labor.

Which patients should be monitored electronically during labor? The condition of any patient in the high-risk category should be monitored during labor. Electronic monitoring answers the question: Can this very important fetus tolerate the stresses imposed by uterine contractions which temporarily reduce blood flow to the fetus? As long as the record is normal, labor can be permitted to continue and a normal baby can be anticipated. An abnormal tracing which cannot be corrected implies a poor tolerance for labor in that fetus, and labor should be terminated; this often is done by cesarean section.

In all patients receiving oxytocin during labor, electronic monitoring should be performed. It allows for the earliest detection of excessive uterine activity and the resultant fetal anoxia secondary to impairment of circulation of blood through the uterus to the placenta.

In normal labor patients, not requiring oxytocin, monitoring will allow for improved observation of the fetal heart (a continuous recording) and the quality of labor. It will detect episodes of umbilical cord compression and usually allow for their correction, permitting optimal circulation to the fetus. Electronic monitoring should prevent the sudden intrapartum death of an apparently normally formed fetus. These deaths may be due to previously unrecognized umbilical cord compression or intolerance to labor contractions and decreased uterine circulation.

fetal distress

Fetal distress may be chronic, occurring all during the course of pregnancy, or acute, usually manifested during labor but also appearing when the mother is deprived of oxygen (e.g., when anesthesia is poorly administered) or with a bleeding complication, such as placenta previa. Since monitoring in labor has been discussed, let us first consider acute distress.

ACUTE FETAL DISTRESS

The classic definition of fetal distress included abnormalities in fetal heart rate, a rate under 120 or over 160 beats/min, and the appearance of meconium in the amniotic fluid. Unfortunately these signs correlate very poorly with the actual condition of the fetus, and the management of labor with only these criteria often results in the emergency delivery of babies who were never in jeopardy and failure to recognize the truly anoxic fetal state.

The proper interpretation of monitoring records has improved our diagnosis of fetal distress. Fetal distress results from the failure of oxygen to be delivered in adequate supply to the fetus. The most obvious interference with the baby's oxygen supply would result from compression of the umbilical cord. Such compression can be caused by prolapse of the cord with pressure by the presenting part against the pelvic wall, tight loops of cord around the fetal neck or trunk, short cords, or true knots in the cord. Cord compression produces *variable decelerations*. If the obstruction to blood flow through the cord increases, the duration of the decelerations will also increase, lasting 20 to 30 s after the contraction is over.

Other causes of inadequate oxygen delivery to the fetus are related to uteroplacental blood flow. Abnormally strong or long uterine contractions will temporarily shut off blood flow to the placenta. A poor "head of pressure" in the blood supply to the uterus which may result from maternal hypotension (e.g., supine hypotensive syndrome or maternal blood loss) will cause fetal anoxia. Uteroplacental insufficiency results in *late decelerations* in the fetal heart rate record. These decelerations may be very subtle at first, and represent a change in the rate of only 5 to 10 beats/min. Any deceleration which persists after a uterine contraction ends must be considered to represent fetal anoxia.

Thus, all late decelerations and progressively severe variable decelerations as well as a loss of beat-to-beat variation in fetal heart rate indicate acute fetal distress.

Treatment of Acute Fetal Distress When signs of fetal distress appear, the following steps should be taken:

1. Change the patient's position to (*a*) relieve pressure on the umbilical cord and (*b*) take the weight of the pregnant uterus off the vena cava, correcting hypotension due to supine hypotensive syndrome. Try both the right and left lateral positions or the Trendelenburg position. This simple maneuver will often correct an abnormal fetal heart rate pattern.
2. Discontinue administration of oxytocin. Uterine contractions may be too long or strong for optimal placental circulation.
3. Administer oxygen 8 to 10 l/min to mother by mask.
4. Examine the patient to rule out umbilical cord prolapse.

If despite these measures an abnormal pattern of fetal heart rate persists, fetal scalp sampling should be performed, if this technique is available. If fetal acidosis, with pH below 7.20, is present, labor must be terminated. If fetal scalp sampling cannot be done, and after 20 min there is no improvement in the pattern, delivery should be performed by the most expeditious method, usually cesarean section.

If the abnormal fetal heart rate pattern is corrected, labor may be allowed to continue. Electronic monitoring has the advantage of displaying the results of therapy to correct fetal anoxia, and allows a more intelligent and scientific decision to be made regarding the management of labor.

In the presence of an abnormal fetal heart rate pattern and a normal fetal scalp pH, fetal scalp sampling must be repeated in 20 to 30 min. If pH remains normal, the fetal condition is considered good enough to allow labor to progress. The reason for this is that fetal scalp sampling is a more reliable index of fetal well-being than fetal heart rate patterns. Electronic monitoring is an excellent screening test to select those babies whose management will be improved by measurement of their acid-base balance. The combined use of both procedures is the ultimate in accurate assessment of fetal condition.

CHRONIC FETAL DISTRESS

Chronic fetal distress arises during the course of pregnancy and results from any condition which interferes with fetal nutrition and oxygenation. It may be present for several months. The common causes of chronic fetal distress are:

1. Maternal diseases such as chronic hypertension, congenital heart disease, diabetes, toxemia of pregnancy, Rh incompatibility, severe anemia.
2. Underdevelopment of the placenta, resulting in a placenta too small to nourish the growing fetus adequately. This results in the "small-for-dates" fetus, which may weigh as little as 2 to 3 lb at full term. The

causes for this condition are not fully understood.

3. Chronic infections of the fetus which interfere with development. Most common of these are rubella, toxoplasmosis, syphilis, tuberculosis.

The condition of the fetus that survives to term in spite of chronic distress, must be carefully monitored in labor, since this stressful interval often produces more damage and even death. Acute fetal distress is a very common complication in labor of these previously jeopardized fetuses.

Diagnosis of Chronic Distress The diagnosis of chronic fetal distress requires a very careful maternal history to discover known factors interfering with fetal growth. Frequent prenatal visits to discover and treat complicating illnesses (e.g., ketosis or infection in a diabetic patient) are mandatory. Clinical and ultrasound determination of fetal growth during the course of pregnancy will often detect the "small-for-dates" baby.

Especially useful is the plasma or urinary estriol determination performed on maternal blood and urine. The fetal adrenal gland produces a steroid which is converted by the placenta to estriol, which can be measured in blood or urine. A rising estriol level from the twenty-eighth week of gestation to term is normal. A flat estriol curve on repeated weekly determinations indicates suboptimal growth. A falling level often precedes intrauterine death by 48 to 72 h. A falling level is an indication for termination of pregnancy, if the fetus is viable (Fig. 27·9).

Unfortunately, at present, recognition of chronic fetal distress, rather than its prevention or treatment, is all that is possible. What is possible, however, is its recognition and the removal of the baby from its hazardous environment in the uterus at the time when the infant is most likely to survive. Very often the fetus suffering from chronic distress will do much better in the nursery than in the uterus. Until that optimal delivery date arrives, most of the fetuses will benefit from maternal bed rest, which will allow maximal uterine circulation.

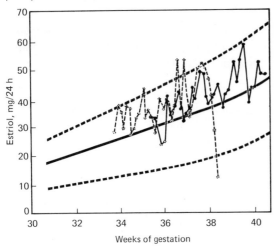

fig. 27·9 Drop in urinary estriol concentration indicates fetal distress late in pregnancy. (*From* Contemporary OB/GYN, **1**(1):15, 1972.)

references

1. Arthur T. Fort, "Prenatal Intrusion into the Amnion," *American Journal of Obstetrics and Gynecology*, **110**:3, 1970.
2. Louis Gluck and Marie V. Kulovich, "Lecithin/Sphingomyelin Ratios in Amniotic Fluid in Normal and Abnormal Pregnancy," *American Journal of Clinical Obstetrics and Gynecology*, **115**:4, 1973.
3. Joseph Sternberg, "Irradiation and Radiocontamination during Pregnancy," *American Journal of Obstetrics and Gynecology*, **108**:3, 1970.
4. Ann M. B. Milic and Karlis Adamsons, "Fetal Blood Sampling," *American Journal of Nursing*, **68**:10, 1968.

bibliography

Clements, J. A., A. C. G. Platzker, D. F. Tierney, et al.: "Assessment of the Rish of RS by a Rapid Test for Surfactant in Amniotic

Fluid," *The New England Journal of Medicine*, **298**:1077,1972.

Daw, Edward: "Fetography," *American Journal of Obstetrics and Gynecology*, **115**:5, 1973.

Dunn, Leo J., and Ajay S. Bhatnagar: "The Use of Lecithin/Sphingomyelin Ratio in the Management of the Problem Obstetric Patient," *American Journal of Obstetrics and Gynecology*, **108**:4,1970.

Grimwade, J. C.: "The Management of Fetal Distress with the Use of Fetal Blood pH," *American Journal of Obstetrics and Gynecology*, **106**:2,1970.

Hon, Edward R.: *An Introduction to Fetal Heart Rate Monitoring*, Harty Press Incorporated, New Haven, Conn., 1969.

Nitowsky, Harold M.: "Prenatal Diagnosis of Genetic Abnormality," *American Journal of Nursing*, **71**:8,1971.

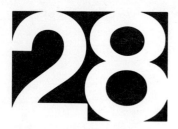

28

the high-risk full-term infant

Marvin L. Blumberg

For 40 weeks, from the time that the ovum is fertilized until the fetus is delivered as an infant and the umbilical cord is severed, this fetus has a parasitic existence inside the mother's uterus, where she nourishes it, breathes for it, and carries off its waste products. Yet, during that time the fetus must gradually mature in its structures and internal functions to utilize properly the nutrients and oxygen furnished to it and to be able to convey away its waste products through the proper organs. Cerebral centers that control proper functioning, enzymes that affect digestion, absorption, and excretion of metabolic by-products, lungs that exchange carbon dioxide for oxygen, and a host of other mechanisms and structures must be mature enough and ready at the instant of birth to take over for the independent existence of the newborn.

Immaturity, dysfunction, or lack of any of the normal control functions may result in temporary or permanent damage to vital structures, especially to the brain. In recent years, medical research in the fields of neonatal physiology, biochemistry, and pharmacology has brought about sufficient expertise to help the prematurely born infant to survive by correcting, treating, or compensating for certain defects and deficiencies. This chapter will discuss the medical problems of the newborn that arise whenever there is difficulty in establishing and maintaining the following functions: respiration, circulation, neurologic function, metabolic function, nutrition, and excretion.

establishing and maintaining respiration

The metabolic functions of all living cells are basically dependent upon an oxidation-reduction cycle. Unicellular animal organisms such as the ameba and the paramecium derive their oxygen from the supply dissolved in the surrounding water in which they live and discharge waste carbon dioxide by the process of osmosis through the cell membrane. As animals became more complex through the evolutionary cycle, an internal mechanism had to be developed within the organism to transport oxygen to all the body cells and to carry off carbon dioxide. Oxygen from air inspired into the pulmonary alveoli osmoses into the surrounding capillaries, where it becomes united in a loose chemical bond with the hemoglobin of the circulating erythrocytes to form *oxyhemoglobin*.

FETAL OXYGENATION

During fetal life, the oxygen enters through the mother's lungs, into her bloodstream to the placenta, where oxygen separates from the materal oxyhemoglobin, passes through the maternal-fetal placental membrane, and is picked up by the fetal erythrocytes. In turn, carbon dioxide in the fetus is transported by the fetal erythrocytes and transferred to the maternal circulation through the placenta.

It must be quite apparent that the concentration of oxygen furnished to the fetus by the mother via the umbilical arteries is lower than the original arterial oxygen blood concentration in her circulation, for she has already used a considerable amount for her own needs. Two mechanisms enable the fetus to function at an average oxygen blood saturation of *40 to 60 percent*, whereas the newborn infant after several hours requires an average oxygen saturation of *85 to 90 percent*.

1. The fetus has a relative *polycythemia*, or increase in red blood cells, ranging from 4.5 to 6.5 million per cubic millimeter, with a hemoglobin content of 17 to 20 Gm/100 ml of blood. The number will drop off gradually in the postnatal period to a norm of 4 to 5 million red blood cells per cubic millimeter and 12 to 14 Gm hemoglobin per 100 ml. This *polycythemia* affords more erythrocytes for transport of the oxygen to the fetal body cells, to compensate for the reduced concentration of oxygen.
2. Fetal hemoglobin has a greater affinity and, therefore, a greater carrying capacity for oxygen, as well as a lower dissociation constant for fetal oxyhemoglobin than for postnatal oxyhemoglobin. The rate and the ease of reduction of fetal oxyhemoglobin are greater, thus furnishing oxygen more readily and more completely to the body cells.

INITIATION OF RESPIRATION

Before 26 weeks of gestation the fetal lung is still very immature. Between 26 and 30 weeks, the lung is still weak and has only a small surface area for the exchange of gases. It is, however, rapidly developing an adequate capillary system. Between 31 and 36 weeks, there is considerable improvement in gas exchange ability and in total lung surface area. By 37 weeks there is enough mature alveoli formation for the lungs to function adequately for a term baby. Prior to 27 weeks of gestation it is virtually impossible to sustain human independent life by any present

means because of the total inability of the existing alveolar functioning surface to oxygenate the blood, no matter how much oxygen is furnished to the infant. After 27 to 28 weeks of gestation, if no other abnormalities or severe dysfunctions exist, pulmonary aeration can be accomplished and life can be sustained.

As the mature fetus is about to be thrust into a postnatal independent existence, the combination of tactile and thermal stimuli upon the infant's skin produces an afferent-efferent reflex which causes him to inspire deeply and to cry. Once established in the normal term baby, respiration will continue spontaneously through a combination of chemical stimulus to the respiratory center of the medulla by blood carbon dioxide level, and other regulatory mechanisms.

The first breath normally requires very high intrathoracic pressures in order to expand the totally collapsed alveoli. After the first expiration, the lungs retain up to 40 percent of the total lung volume as residual air. Subsequently, inspiratory pressures are far lower. Lung inflation can be demonstrated in a simple fashion by blowing up a round toy rubber balloon. It requires more effort to start the first expansion than to continue to expand the balloon with subsequent blowing breaths.

In premature infants, the high inflating pressure of the first inspiration is often required for each following breath as well. This difference from the respiratory process in the mature newborn is due to the developmental immaturity of the lungs, which has left the alveoli incapable of holding residual air on expiration, thereby causing them to collapse with each breath.

The phenomenon which enables an alveolus or a gas bubble of liquid to maintain its round shape and expansion is known as surface tension. In the mature alveolus expansion is maintained by a thin film of fluid, *surfactant*, a phospholipid, which reduces surface tension as the alveolar radius decreases during expiration, thus preventing collapse and retaining residual alveolar volume. Premature infants are unable to synthesize an adequate amount of surfactant, a fact that accounts for the high incidence of respiratory distress syndrome in very premature infants. With each week of fetal growth, more surfactant, and especially more mature surfactant, forms to allow the efficiency of respiration.

RESPIRATORY DISTRESS SYNDROME

Respiratory distress is a broadly descriptive term meaning increased effort of breathing. It may result from a number of causes, often interrelated, such as developmental immaturity, pharmacologic depression, and birth trauma. Respiratory distress syndrome, often referred to as hyaline membrane disease, is the most frequent cause of respiratory difficulty in premature infants.

All infants have some surfactant in their lungs at birth. A sufficient level and a rapid rate of synthesis must be maintained, at least at the start, or else a vicious cycle is set up. Alveolar collapse with each expiration causes *hypoxemia*, or lower oxygen concentration in the blood, which in turn will lead to acidosis. Reflexly, constriction of the pulmonary vasculature and diminished blood flow to the lungs occur with the result of further hypoxemia. Surfactant formation is further inhibited, and *transudation*, or movement of fluid into the alveolar spaces, takes place. Respiratory exchange is progressively blocked and, if untreated, is likely to result in death. Postmortem microscopic examination of the lungs reveals an *eosinophilic*-staining amorphous hyaline membrane lining many of the alveoli. Thus, hyaline membrane is a *result* of respiratory distress syndrome, not the *cause*.

Although this syndrome is most frequent in premature infants, there are conditions predisposing a full-term neonate to this condi-tion, such as delivery by cesarean section, especially from a diabetic mother.

Other Causes of Respiratory Distress Respiratory difficulty may also be due to intrinsic pulmonary factors or to extrinsic problems. Intrinsic disorders include primary *atelectasis*, or failure of a large number of alveoli to expand, *emphysema*, or overexpansion of a lung segment caused by a ball-valve type of obstruction of a bronchiole, *pneumatocele*, or cystic area within the lung, and pneumonia from aspiration of amniotic fluid or of an early oral feeding. These all produce difficulty in breathing because they diminish the gas-exchange ability by direct effect or by indirect compression effect.

Extrinsic disorders produce respiratory distress primarily by compression and displacement of a lung and/or the mediastinal structures. These include *herniation* of abdominal viscera into the thoracic cavity through a congenital defect in the diaphragm, *pneumothorax* (air in the pleural space), and *chylothorax* (free lymphatic fluid in the pleural space).

Congenital *choanal atresia* (Fig. 28·1). or blockage of the nasal passages posteriorly due to a membrane or to a solid bony plate, may produce respiratory distress and suffocation. The affected infant, in trying to breathe through the obstructed passages, becomes

fig. 28·1 Choanal atresia. (Note blockage of the nasal passages posteriorly.)

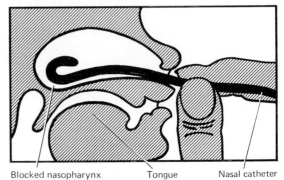

Blocked nasopharynx   Tongue   Nasal catheter

more and more hypoxic and develops all the symptoms of progressive deterioration.

RESPIRATORY DEPRESSION

Respiratory depression in the neonate may produce hypoxia, hypoxemia, and acidosis if it does not subside spontaneously or by the application of stimulant drugs. The two main causes of respiratory depression are (1) heavy recent maternal sedation or narcosis (within about 1 h) that strikes the infant's respiratory center just about the time of delivery, and (2) prolonged cerebral anoxia due to fetal distress during labor or delivery. The *major causes of respiratory distress* are shown in the following outline:

I. Intrinsic problems
   A. Primary atelectasis
   B. Emphysema
   C. Pneumonia
      1. Perinatal aspiration syndrome
      2. Amnionitis pneumonia
II. Congenital anomalies of respiratory tract
   A. Choanal atresia
   B. Tracheoesophageal fistulas
   C. Phrenic nerve paralysis
   D. Vocal cord paralysis
III. Extrinsic problems
   A. Herniation of abdominal viscera
   B. Pneumothorax
   C. Chylothorax
IV. Respiratory depression
   A. Anoxia
   B. Narcosis
V. Immaturity
   A. Exhaustion
   B. Hyaline membrane disease (RDS)

SIGNS AND SYMPTOMS OF RESPIRATORY DISTRESS

The nursery nurses are the front-line professionals in the care of the newborn. It is essential, therefore, that they be familiar with the *signs and symptoms of respiratory distress* in order to alert the physician. These signs are listed in the following outline:

I. Changes in respiratory rate and rhythm
   A. Rising respiratory rate
   B. Tachypnea
   C. Periods of apnea
II. Presence of respiratory sounds
   A. Grunting, expiratory sound (RDS)
   B. Stridor, inspiratory sound, upper airway obstruction
   C. Wheeze—obstruction within thorax
   D. Rales
   E. Feeble cry
III. Use of accessory respiratory muscles
   A. Flaring nostrils
   B. Retractions
      1. Suprasternal
      2. Sternal
      3. Substernal
      4. Intercostal
IV. General condition
   A. Central cyanosis
      1. Circumoral
      2. Head and trunk
   B. Poor muscle tone
   C. Poor reflex responses
   D. Hypothermia

The recognition of early signs is as important as the knowledge of treatment procedures. Persistent *tachypnea*, with a rate over 50 to 60 times per minute, may be an early sign of low blood oxygen level. Obstructive difficulty in the airway, atelectasis, or hyaline membrane disease will cause the infant to have grunting respirations and chest wall retractions. There is drawing in of the intercostal areas between the ribs and the subcostal area beneath the ribs with each inspiration. Because the immature infant has somewhat pliable bones, the whole sternum can be seen to retract. Cyanosis may also be present and is significant if it extends beyond the hands and feet to the face and trunk (central cyanosis).

Grunting has an interesting and important

purpose. As already described, as a result of low surfactant content and poor surface tension, the alveoli of the infant with respiratory distress syndrome tend to collapse completely with each expiration, making each inspiration as labored as the first. In the normal lung, alveoli usually retain as much as 40 percent of the inspired air during expiration, which makes each inspiration unlabored. When an infant grunts, he closes his epiglottis temporarily, thus forcing expiration against pressure and thereby tending to maintain some residual air in the alveoli.

RESUSCITATION OF THE NEWBORN WITH DEPRESSED RESPONSES

The first consideration in supporting respiration must be establishing a clear airway. Pharyngeal secretions must be removed by gentle suction, either by mouth by means of a DeLee catheter with a trap, or by machine with low negative-pressure suction. In the presence of obstructive anomalies of nose, tongue, pharynx, or larynx, it is often necessary to insert a pharyngeal airway to depress and extend the tongue, or even an endotracheal tube, to maintain pulmonary air exchange. When the infant's respiratory effort is too weak or when the lungs cannot expand properly, it may be necessary to assist ventilation. Direct intermittent pressure accomplishes oxygenation at varying concentrations through a firmly but gently applied face mask or through an endotracheal tube (Fig. 28·2). For alternative methods of providing oxygen see Chap. 30.

Use of Oxygen If the airways are clear and if sufficient alveolar surface is available, it is usually unnecessary to supply oxygen at a concentration higher than 35 to 40 percent. (Air at sea level contains 20 percent oxygen by volume.) In severe depression it may be necessary to introduce up to 100 percent for short periods of time. The dangers inherent in exposing the neonate to excessive concen-

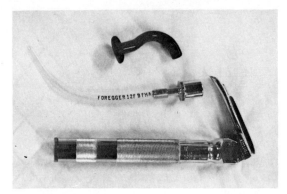

fig. 28·2 Resuscitation of the newborn: equipment for endotracheal intubation. After the larynx has been visualized with the laryngoscope and the fluid, mucus, or other obstruction suctioned out, the endotracheal tube may be left in place while mouth-to-mouth resuscitation or intermittent positive-pressure breathing is carried out. Sometimes a small airway is inserted after the endotracheal tube is removed. Oxygen, humidity, warmth, careful handling, and observation are critical in the follow-up period.

trations of oxygen for any length of time have been well documented. The eyes of the small premature infant are particularly vulnerable to the effects of elevated plasma oxygen concentrations for prolonged periods. Damage to the retina and formation of a membrane within the eye result in a condition known as *retrolental fibroplasia* that can produce permanent blindness.

Another potentially serious effect of overoxygenation is *hyperoxemia*, or too high a blood oxygen level, that may interfere with the enzymatic pathway responsible for the formation of surfactant in the neonate. Any reduction of an adequate amount of mature surfactant may aggravate an already existing situation of respiratory distress.

The third consideration in maintaining oxygen levels is the body temperature. If the environmental temperature drops considerably, the infant's body temperature falls below normal range and his rate of metabolism increases. The increase in metabolism causes an increase in oxygen consumption.

In other words, the infant must increase his oxygen consumption in order to maintain body temperature.

Use of Respiratory Stimulants and Narcotic Antagonists Pharmacologically, respiratory stimulants and narcotic antagonists are not necessarily synonymous. Drugs such as caffeine sodium benzoate and nikethamide (Coramine) stimulate the respiratory center in the floor of the fourth ventricle of the brain and are mainly effective in counteracting the effect of depression by barbiturates. Rarely used for infants, these respiratory stimulants counteract cerebral anoxia of mild to moderate degree. Narcosis and depression may require the more specific antagonist effects of such drugs as nalorphine (Nalline) and levallorphan (Lorfan) (see Chap. 18).

Correcting Acidosis and Hypoglycemia Hypoxemia, if uncorrected, can lead to a build-up of carbon dioxide and a consequent lowering of pH of the blood, causing acidosis and the development of hypoglycemia. The administration of sodium bicarbonate in glucose solution intravenously by way of the umbilical vein or a peripheral vein can prevent these serious chemical imbalances. The concentrations utilized are usually 5 to 10 mEq (4.2 to 8.4 Gm) sodium bicarbonate dissolved in 100 ml of 10 percent glucose solution. The rate of administration of this mixture is usually 65 ml/kg of body weight in 24 h. Using the same solutions at the same rate of administration by way of a nasogastric tube has proved as effective as use of the intravenous route in prevention and treatment of all but severely acidotic neonates, without the risk of infection or thrombosis from intravenous administration (1). With any route, administration must be monitored by blood tests in order to avoid overalkalinization while bringing the pH out of the acidotic range.

If airways are patent, normal chemistries are maintained, and the body structures are mature enough, an infant can be supported through respiratory depression and distress and recover.

Anomalous deformities such as diaphragmatic hernia and pneumatocele, and conditions such as pneumothorax and chylothorax, of course require prompt surgical intervention.

establishing and maintaining circulation

NORMAL FETAL CIRCULATION

The structure of the normal fetal cardiovascular system (Fig. 28·3) is essentially what it will be after birth, with the exception of two main shunts or shortcuts that enable more efficient direction of oxygenated blood, and the presence of the umbilical vessel lifeline from the placenta. Since the fetal lungs are not functional, the pulmonary blood flow is needed only to nourish the lung tissue, not for gaseous exchange. A large amount of the blood that leaves the right ventricle of the heart through the pulmonary artery is, therefore, shunted directly into the aorta and the systemic circulation through the ductus arteriosus between the two vessels. This duct normally closes shortly after birth as the systemic blood pressure builds up (Fig. 28·4).

The second important shunt that exists before birth and closes, at least functionally, after birth is the foramen ovale between the left and right atria of the heart. In fetal life, this allows a portion of the maternally oxygenated blood returning to the fetal right atrium via the vena cava to shunt through to the left atrium, down to the left ventricle, and out to the aorta, thus again bypassing the pulmonary circuit.

At birth the umbilical two arteries and one vein cease their functions of carrying blood for the purpose of gas exchange, nutrition, and waste exchange. Their division is followed by atrophy of their connections from umbilicus to the systemic arteries and veins.

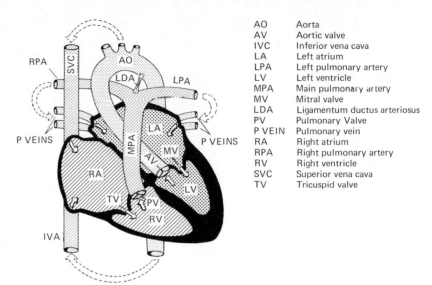

AO	Aorta
AV	Aortic valve
IVC	Inferior vena cava
LA	Left atrium
LPA	Left pulmonary artery
LV	Left ventricle
MPA	Main pulmonary artery
MV	Mitral valve
LDA	Ligamentum ductus arteriosus
PV	Pulmonary Valve
P VEIN	Pulmonary vein
RA	Right atrium
RPA	Right pulmonary artery
RV	Right ventricle
SVC	Superior vena cava
TV	Tricuspid valve

fig. 28·3 Normal heart (adult). (*From Ross Laboratories, Columbus, Ohio, Clinical Education Aid No. 7.*)

fig. 28·4 Patent ductus arteriosus. The patent ductus arteriosus is a vascular connection that, during fetal life, short-circuits the pulmonary vascular bed and directs blood from the pulmonary artery to the aorta. Functional closure of the ductus normally occurs soon after birth. If the ductus remains patent after birth, the direction of blood flow in the ductus is reversed by the higher pressure in the aorta. (*From Ross Laboratories, Columbus, Ohio, Clinical Education Aid No. 7.*)

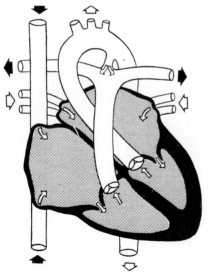

DEVIATIONS FROM NORMAL CIRCULATION

In such a complex mechanism of chambers, conduits, and function, it is a marvel that structural anomalies occur as infrequently as they do. Structural deviations may be manifest in both intracardiac and extracardiac areas. They may vary from defects that are not immediately life-threatening, requiring no early treatment, to severe anomalies that are incompatible with life. If the shunt or communication is large enough or so situated that enough venous or deoxygenated blood is spilled back into the systemic or left-sided vascular system, the infant will be *cyanotic*. Otherwise, the anomaly is described as *acyanotic*. Heart murmurs may or may not be audible, depending on the location and size of the anomaly.

Among the less severe defects are persistent *patent ductus arteriosus* (Fig. 28·4), *coarctation*, or narrowing of a segment of aorta, *stenosis* of the pulmonary artery, *intraventricular septal defect* (Fig. 28·5), *auricular (atrial) septal defect* (Fig. 28·6), or persistence of a patent foramen ovale between the two auricles. Among the more severe anomalies, some incompatibilities can be helped by emergency surgery in the neonate. Later, if the child survives, revision surgery may improve chances for prolonged survival. Among these conditions are transposition of the aorta and pulmonary artery to the reverse ventricles, and total anomalous venous drainage with reversal of the venous return to the auricles. *Cor triloculare*, or three-chambered heart (two auricles and one ventricle), is, of course, impossible to correct surgically at present. The anomalies of heart and great vessel structures known as *tetralogy of Fallot* (Fig. 28·7) and *Eisenmenger's syndrome*, though not incompatible with life, will impair efficient cardiac function as the infant grows.

fig. 28·5 Ventricular septal defect. A ventricular septal defect is an abnormal opening between the right and left ventricle. Ventricular septal defects vary in size and may occur in either the membranous or the muscular portion of the ventricular septum. Because of higher pressure in the left ventricle, a shunting of blood from the left to right ventricle occurs during systole. If pulmonary vascular resistance produces pulmonary hypertension, the shunt of blood is then reversed from the right to the left ventricle, with cyanosis resulting. (*From Ross Laboratories, Columbus, Ohio, Clinical Education Aid No. 7.*)

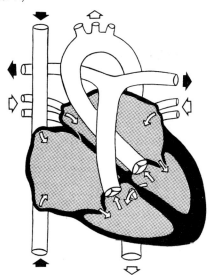

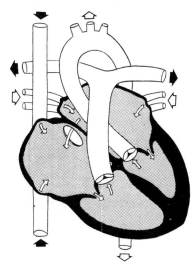

fig. 28·6 Atrial septal defects. An atrial septal defect is an abnormal opening between the right and left atria. Basically, three types of abnormalities result from incorrect development of the atrial septum. An incompetent foramen ovale is the most common defect. The high ostium secundum defect results from abnormal development of the septum secundum. Improper development of the septum primum produces a basal opening known as an ostium primum defect, frequently involving the atrioventricular valves. In general, left-to-right shunting of blood occurs in all atrial septal defects. (*From Ross Laboratories, Colombus, Ohio, Education Aid No. 7.*)

While the cardiac electrical impulse is initiated within the heart itself at the sinoatrial (SA) node, extracardiac neurogenic effects may play a role in regulating heart rate and action by way of the vagus nerve. Central effects on the circulatory center in the medulla of the brain from anoxia, circulating drugs, intracranial pressure from birth trauma, edema, or hemorrhage into the vital centers may indirectly affect the activity of the cardiovascular system.

SIGNS AND SYMPTOMS OF CIRCULATORY ABNORMALITIES

Signs and symptoms of circulatory abnormalities in an infant that should alert the nursery

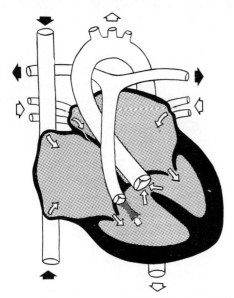

fig. 28·7 Tetralogy of Fallot. This disorder is characterized by the combination of four defects: (1) pulmonary stenosis, (2) ventricular septal defect, (3) overriding aorta, and (4) hypertrophy of right ventricle. It is the most common defect causing cyanosis in patients surviving beyond two years of age. The severity of symptoms depends on the degree of pulmonary stenosis, the size of the ventricular septal defect, and the degree to which the aorta overrides the septal defect. (*From Ross Laboratories, Columbus, Ohio, Clinical Education Aid No. 7.*)

nurse and should be observed and reported by her are similar in some respects to those of respiratory distress. An inefficient heart or anomalous great vessels may manifest signs and symptoms of poor oxygenation of the infant's blood supply in the form of cyanosis. Tachypnea will be due to the body's effort to absorb more oxygen by more rapid breathing. If the strain on an anomalous heart is too great, heart failure may develop. In this case, in addition to signs of air hunger, the infant will be extremely restless and fretful and will be unable to feed because of inability to suck and swallow due to respiratory difficulty.

Some cardiovascular anomalies are asymptomatic in the neonatal period except for the presence of a murmur that can be heard only with a stethoscope on the infant's chest. An experienced nurse can, of course, detect unusual chest sounds when she observes vital signs.

SUPPORTIVE CARE AND TREATMENT

The first line of treatment for a cardiovascular anomaly of the cyanotic type is the use of oxygen at a sufficiently high concentration to alleviate the cyanosis. In the presence of a heart that is beating continuously and consistently too rapidly (i.e., at a ventricular rate over 180 beats/min), it is necessary to slow the heart rate and to increase the force of each beat by administering digoxin or, less commonly, other alkaloids such as Cedilanid, usually intramuscularly. In emergency situations, the drug may be administered intravenously, at least initially.

Emergency surgical procedures are basically designed to channel enough oxygenated blood into the systemic circ'ation to sustain life as efficiently as possible.

As with any infant, normal or not, nutrition and fluid intake must be provided by the most practical method—oral, nasogastric tube, or intravenous routes.

maintaining neurologic function

Basic biologic functions of alimentation, excretion, and mitotic division are performed at the cellular level and are biochemical reactions. The very complexity of higher forms of animal life makes it essential that there be a governing and directing system, in essence a so-called switchboard control, to organize all the specialized functions into a synchronous, reciprocating operation. This sytem is the nervous system, the brain at the center, the spinal cord as the trunk line, and the peripheral nerves beyond.

Anomalies, malformations, and destructive injuries within the nervous system will affect its functions and, therefore, the function of other systems or organs that it controls in variable fashion and degree, depending on the location and extent of the defect.

CAUSES OF NEONATE NEUROLOGIC ABNORMALITIES

The etiology of nervous defects in the neonate is essentially threefold—developmental, infectious, and accidental. Developmental defects may be genetic (usually a recessive trait and usually part of a more general syndrome) or they may be due to *dysgenesis* (faulty development at some stage of early embryonic development). Infections that affect the developing nervous system are mainly viral, and most of the damage occurs in the first trimester of gestation when the brain and spinal cord are evolving. Among the developmental anomalies is *microcephaly*, or totally small cortex. *Hydrocephalus*, or an excessively enlarged head, results when circulation and reabsorption of cerebrospinal fluid are prevented by absence or stenosis of the normally existing channels or foramina by which the ventricles of the brain communicate with the subdural space (Fig. 28·8). A rare anomaly is cerebral agenesis, resulting in what is commonly, and unfortunately, referred to as anencephalic monster—a condition in which the entire brain is absent except for the medullary brainstem with its centers of circulation and respiration control. The entire cranium is open, exposing the rudimentary primitive brain segment.

Certain maternal viral infections occurring especially in the first gestational trimester can be devastating to the developing brain. The principal viral agents are rubella virus and cytomegalovirus. Another type of microorganism, the toxoplasma, can damage the brain even later in gestation (see Chap. 20).

Accidental damage to the brain may be due to anoxia or to hemorrhage. Frequent or appreciable maternal (placental) bleeding during the second or even the third trimester, after the brain has been basically formed, may produce sufficient cerebral anoxia to damage the cerebral cortex. During parturition, damage may result from prolonged deprivation of oxygen to the brain caused by obstruction of the umbilical vessels by knotting or pressure, by premature separation of the placenta (abruptio placentae), a relatively long period before the head is delivered, or possibly even by excessive hypoxic anesthesia to the mother (Chap. 18).

TRAUMATIC EFFECTS

Severe trauma to the infant's head during parturition may cause small cerebral hemorrhages by compression of the skull. Tears in the major cerebral vessels by excessive stretching may be caused by extreme molding of the skull. Small hemorrhages may cause damage indirectly through an anoxic effect on the affected areas, as blood and, thus, oxygen supply are cut off. Major hemorrhages are usually fatal.

Occasionally peripheral nerves are injured by events of delivery. The blade of obstetric forceps may sometimes compress the facial nerve in the area anterior to the ear and below and lateral to the eye, producing a peripheral type of facial paralysis which, in most cases, resolves, since the continuity of the nerve is usually not disrupted. More serious is injury to the brachial plexus where it originates from the spinal cord at the base of the neck and runs to the arm through the axilla. This injury occurs when the head is markedly extended laterally to the opposite side, with the arm extended and the shoulder depressed. The effect of this maneuver is occasionally to *avulse,* or tear away, the plexus of nerves from the spinal cord, an irreparable and irreversible damage. If the lower part of the plexus only is avulsed, the result is Erb's palsy, or partial paralysis of the arm with inability to supinate or elevate it. If the entire

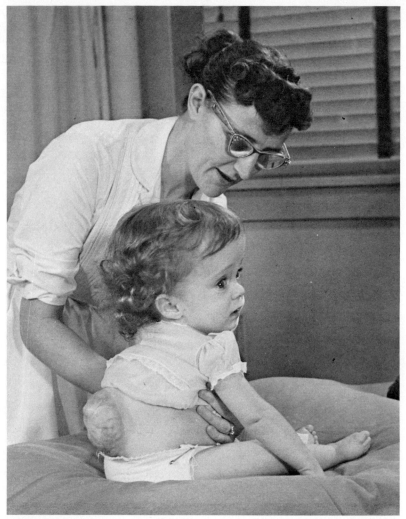

fig. 28·8 Hydrocephalic child with spina bifida. (*Courtesy of The National Foundation-March of Dimes.*)

plexus is avulsed, the result is total flaccid paralysis of the arm, or Klumpke's paralysis. There is usually accompanying damage to the contiguous stellate autonomic ganglion at the level where the brachial plexus emerges from the cord, producing a Horner's syndrome of *ptosis,* or drooping of the eyelid, and *enophthalmos,* or retraction of the eyeball.

CHEMICAL EFFECTS

The brain is sensitive to chemicals or chemical changes in the blood, in addition to the concentrations or partial pressures of oxygen and carbon dioxide. *Hypoglycemia* may occur when the infant's blood sugar level drops too low. Normally the newborn will have and will tolerate glucose levels as low as 40 mg/100 ml for a few hours post partum as he utilizes his sugar reserves from the mother's blood and has not yet begun feedings. In prolonged starvation due to withholding of feedings or to an obstructive or nonabsorptive pathologic condition, *severe hypoglycemia,* or less than 20 mg/100 ml, may result. This state may also result in the infant of a woman with uncontrolled or untreated diabetes. Such a mother, requiring more insulin than her own pancreas is capable of producing, "borrows" insulin from her fetus during gestation. Consequently, the infant may be born with an enlarged pancreas that produces more insulin than he needs. Until he can bring his insulin production and his insulin requirement into equilibrium, his blood glucose level may be depressed low enough to produce generalized twitching, as in a mild motor seizure. Treatment rarely requires more than extra glucose feedings by mouth. Even this may be avoided if the mother's diabetes mellitus is treatment-controlled and if she receives 10 percent glucose solution intravenously during labor and delivery in order to transmit a good level of blood glucose to the infant via the placenta. (See Chap. 30 for a discussion of hypoglycemia in preterm infants.)

Drug Addiction A mother who is addicted to a narcotic such as heroin or morphine, or to methadone as a patient on a methadone maintenance program, will usually impart the addictive state to the newborn as a consequence of transplacental passage of the drugs during gestation. The affected infant will generally exhibit tremors, excessive restlessness and irritability, shrill cry, digestive disturbance, diarrhea, and, in extreme cases, even convulsions. Infants with mild cases may manage withdrawal without sequelae. Others, depending on the severity of the condition, may even die if left untreated. Treatment with phenobarbital may be adequate for mild cases. More severe cases may require chlorpromazine (Thorazine) and, in rare circumstances, may even require an opiate such as camphorated tincture of opium (paregoric).

RESULTS OF NEUROLOGIC DAMAGE

Cerebral anomalies, infections, and some teratogenic drugs early in gestation will virtually always result in some degree of mental deficiency. Sometimes damage from trauma, anoxia, or hemorrhage may be mild enough not to be destructive of brain cells, thereby causing only transient effects. The extent of severe damage depends on the location of the damage. Involvement of the prefrontal or frontal cortex results in impairment of intelligence. Involvement of the motor area of the brain will probably cause neuromuscular *spastic cerebral palsy.* Anoxic damage to the more deeply located basal ganglia that relay and control motor impulses usually leads to *athetoid cerebral palsy,* with its uncoordinated involuntary movements of gross muscle groups.

Cerebral palsy may be defined as a condition of gross neuromuscular defects resulting from widespread damage to the cortex or the basal ganglia of the brain or both during the immature stages of their development after the time that their primitive differentiation is completed, from first-trimester embryo to second-trimester fetus. Damage to the embryonic brain during the first trimester usually results in death or anomaly rather than cerebral palsy. Prenatal cerebral damage after the first trimester accounts for an estimated 20 percent of cases of cerebral palsy. Intrapartum cerebral injury is the main cause of cerebral palsy and is responsible for about 60 percent of cases. Cerebral insults during the first 2 or 3 years of life, before all the nerve centers and nerve tracts have matured, may account for approximately 20 percent of cerebral-palsied children.

SIGNS AND SYMPTOMS OF NEUROLOGIC DEFECTS

Several signs and symptoms should alert the nursery nurse to the existence of neurologic deficits, central, cerebral, or peripheral. Severe depression of the infant's responses, with general poor muscle tone, failure to respond to tactile or mildly painful stimuli such as flicking the soles of the feet, brisk rubbing of the trunk, or pulling a few strands of hair, and a weak brief cry are suggestive evidence of cerebral depressive effects that could be transient, permanent, or even fatal. Cerebral lesions that produce irritation of the brain, such as hemorrhage or anomalies, may cause the infant to cry with a very high-pitched shrill voice almost like the mewing of a cat. Other signs of cerebral irritative lesions are frequent local muscle group tremors or twitching of extremities or face, or even generalized seizure activity of the face, trunk, and extremities.

A flaccid, limp arm is usually indicative of brachial nerve plexus injury. After a forceps delivery, a one-sided facial weakness, drooping of the mouth, and possibly also of the eyelid, are due to facial nerve injury from the forceps application.

SUPPORTIVE CARE AND TREATMENT

Treatment falls into the prophylactic categories of good prenatal care, competent obstetric procedures, and, theoretically, good genetic counseling. Universal vaccination to stop epidemics of rubella must be undertaken. Avoidance of teratologic drugs during pregnancy, the proper usage of sedatives and narcotics during the first stage of labor, and the correct administration of anesthesia during the second stage of labor or during cesarean section, are all important considerations.

Therapy for existing neurologic conditions and effects can be divided into several categories. One is the administration of drugs such as narcotic antagonists, oxygen, and the agents for narcotic withdrawal symptoms. Another is the administration of glucose solution orally or intravenously for hypoglycemic effects. Most other aspects of treatment are long-range and to be applied beyond the neonatal period for mental and neuromuscular deficits.

maintaining genitourinary function

NORMAL URINARY PHYSIOLOGY AND FUNCTION

Though the gonads and the urinary system develop from adjacent embryonic structures and share some portion of an outlet, the two systems function completely independently. The present discussion is concerned primarily with urinary function. The kidneys may be considered to be the most important filtration system in the body for waste elimination. In the normal course of events, the chemical equilibrium of the body is maintained by a balance of function involving renal filtration, pulmonary gaseous exchange, sweating, and intestinal absorption and elimination. The unit of function in the kidney is the glomerulus, through which are excreted by osmosis urea and creatinine, the chief protein metabolic waste products, and excesses of sodium ion, urates, and phosphates to keep the blood electrolytes within normal concentrations. The glomerular filtrate passes into the tubule, where some chemicals are partially resorbed. Eventually the filtrate collects through the *calyces* in the pelvis of the kidney as urine, which then runs into the bladder through the ureters and thence is excreted through the urethra.

PATHOLOGY OF THE URINARY TRACT

In the neonate there is no concern with renal diseases such as glomerulonephritis, collagen disease, and renal chemical malfunc-

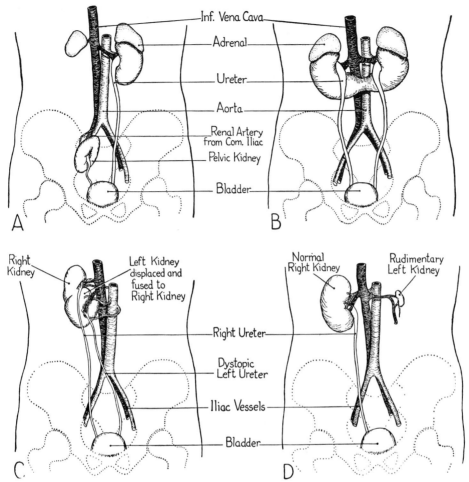

fig. 28·9 Developmental disturbances of the kidneys. (Sketched from museum preparations. A, C, D, in the University of Michigan Anatomical Collection; B, in the Dypuytren Museum, Paris.) A unilateral pelvic kidney; B horseshoe kidney; C dystopic left kidney fused to right kidney; D nearly complete agenesis of left kidney. (*From B. M. Patten,* Human Embryology, *3d ed., McGraw-Hill Book Company, New York, 1968.*)

tion. The pathologic conditions affecting the urinary tract of the newborn are principally congenital anomalies and infection (Fig. 28·9).

Anomalies may involve the kidney, the ureter, the bladder, and even the urethra. Some kidney malformations are *horseshoe kidney* (in which the two kidneys are fused across the midline, forming one horseshoe-shaped organ) and *polycystic kidney* (in which a number of the collecting units fail to empty into the renal pelvis so that they form large cysts of unexcreted urine). *Hydronephrosis,* in which the ureter or bladder outlet is obstructed, causing the entire pelvis and calyces to dilate with urine, and *hydroureter* often coexist. These are not renal anomalies but rather obstructive uropathies. Constriction of the ureter at the ureteropelvic junction, often due to an aberrant blood vessel, narrowing at the ureter junction with the bladder, stricture or posterior urethral valve at the bladder outlet, or even a constricted urethral meatus at the external opening are obstructive uropathies. A severe anomaly is extrophy of the bladder, in which the entire urinary bladder is open onto the lower abdominal surface and the ureters thus are open externally.

Urinary tract infections most often result from bacteria entering the bloodstream of the infant after surface trauma. Ascending infection from the urethra in newborn girls is less common than later in infancy or childhood.

GENITAL ABNORMALITIES

Genital abnormalities may take the form of ambiguous genitalia, making sex determination difficult for the observer. These may be caused by sex chromosomal aberrations, adrenal cortical hyperplasia in the infant, maternal androgenic hormones, and true or pseudohermaphroditism (Fig. 28·10).

Sex chromosomal aberrations may produce a male phenotype (body structure) with a female genotype (sex chromosome pattern) such as Klinefelter's syndrome, or a female phenotype with a male genotype such as Turner's syndrome. Turner's syndrome shows characteristic webbing of the neck and edema of hands and feet in the neonate. Many other types of abberations of sex chromosomes or gonadal dysgenesis may be studied in other texts such as Schaffer and Avery, *Diseases of the Newborn.*

Adrenal cortical hyperplasia produces excess androgenic hormone, which causes clitoral enlargement suggestive of a penis in the newborn girl. Similar masculinization of the female external genitalia may be observed in infants when the pregnant mother had an androgen-producing adrenal tumor or when the pregnant mother was treated for whatever reason with testosterone or other androgenic hormones.

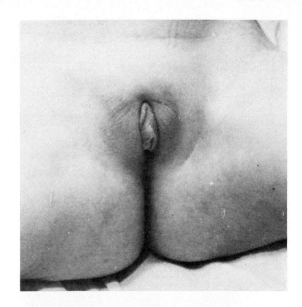

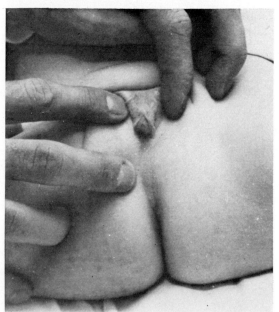

fig. 28·10 Ambiguous genitalia. (*From J. German and J. L. Simpson, "Abnormalities of Human Autosomes: I. Ambiguous Genitalia Associated with a Translocation 46,XY,t(Cq+; Cq−),"* in Birth Defects: Orig. Art. Ser., D. Bergsma (ed.), Part X, The Endocrine System, *published by Williams & Wilkins Co., Baltimore, for The National Foundation–March of Dimes, White Plains, N.Y., vol* VII(6):145, 1971, *with permission of the copyright holder.*)

Hermaphroditism is more commonly pseudo- than true. It is due to faulty embryologic differentiation of the genital precursor tissues. Pseudohermaphroditism may show atypical external genitalia but normal unisexual internal genitalia and a corresponding sex chromosome pattern. The rare true hermaphrodite has characteristics of both sexes, such as both testes and ovaries, and a mosaic sex chromosome pattern of both male and female genotypes.

Two developmental aberrations in the male that are not produced by genetic or hormonal causes are *hypospadias* and *cryptorchidism*. In the former, the penile urethra may lie open for a segment on the undersurface of the penis proximal to the tip of the glans, or it may end in an orifice or meatus proximal to the normal opening at the end of the penis. In cryptorchidism, or undescended testes, one or both testes may remain up in the abdomen or in the inguinal canal. It may be due to a short spermatic cord preventing its descent through the inguinal canal into the scrotum, or to developmental delay that can be rectified later by the administration of injections of anterior pituitary-like (APL) hormone derived from pregnant mares' urine. Correction of severe hypospadias or cryptorchidism unresponsive to hormone therapy is generally relegated to the surgeon.

SIGNS AND SYMPTOMS OF UROLOGIC PROBLEMS

A normal neonate may void urine at the time of delivery or occasionally not for about 24 h. Persistence of *anuria* beyond that time, however, should be reported by the nurse and should become the concern of the physician. A markedly distended abdomen, especially in the lateral flank areas, should be called to the attention of the physician. A palpable mass in those areas should create suspicion of an anomalous kidney, and x-ray studies should be pursued, with injection of radiopaque renal-excreted dye.

External anomalies, such as extrophy of the bladder or grossly abnormal genitalia, of course are readily apparent.

SUPPORTIVE CARE AND TREATMENT

Some anomalies are amenable to surgery and others are not. In the former category, some conditions require emergency surgical intervention that is usually palliative initially and that must be followed later by more definitive procedures. In some, surgery will eventually be necessary but it is not an early lifesaving measure. Horseshoe kidney may conceivably have normal function. In any event, no surgery is indicated. Polycystic kidney cannot be corrected or improved surgically. If it is bilateral, neither kidney can or should be removed. If it is unilateral and asymptomatic, the involved kidney may have to be removed later.

Obstructive uropathy presents a surgical emergency in the newborn. Palliative nephrostomy must be performed in the first days of life by inserting tubes into the renal pelvis through a flank incision to drain the urine continuously out of the kidney in order to prevent irreparable damage to the glomeruli from back pressure. Later, when the infant's condition will permit, surgery will be performed to relieve the cause of the obstruction.

Infection, of course, must be treated vigorously with antibiotics. It is best to identify the invading organism by culture of the blood and urine, in order to ascertain in vitro the most effective antibiotics.

maintaining metabolic function

In a sense, a living organism may be regarded as a chemical factory in which life processes are normally maintained by a balance of anabolic synthesis and catabolic degradation of protoplasm. These chemical reactions are carried out largely through the intermediary action of enzymes, organic compounds that enable reactions to occur without themselves being an integral part of the reaction. Often the chemical reactions involve the alteration of a toxic waste substance by one or more enzymes in a chain reaction, producing a compound that can, in the end, be excreted through the kidneys or the gastrointestinal tract.

ENZYMATIC DEFICIENCIES

This simplistic exposition of metabolism should serve to indicate how readily the delicate balance of normal function can be upset if one enzyme fails to develop or is incomplete in the neonate. A number of such enzyme deficiencies have already been identified, and more are being investigated. The diagnosis is usually made by the detection of higher levels of *metabolites,* i.e., breakdown products, in the urine than would normally be expected. Diagnosis can be further tested by finding abnormally high levels of the metabolites or their chemical relatives in the blood.

Some of the better known syndromes resulting from these deficiencies may be mentioned. Galactosuria reflecting *galactosemia* (galactose in the blood) is due to the lack of an enzyme that normally converts galactose into glucose. Galactosemia, if untreated, can cause mental deficiency. *Phenylketonuria,* so called because of the phenylketone found in the urine, reflects the elevated blood level of phenylalanine, an amnio acid. If uncorrected, PKU will also lead to brain damage and mental retardation. A number of other amino acid enzymatic aberrations fall into the category of *aminoacidurias.*

Another type of enzyme deficiency that is not involved with amino acid metabolism is a condition in which the liver cells fail to produce the enzyme, *glucuronyl transferase,* that normally brings about the chemical reactions

changing unconjugated bilirubin to the conjugated form. Unconjugated bilirubin in high concentrations in the blood may produce *kernicterus,* or toxic brain damage that results in mental deficiency and possible neurologic deficits. Conjugated bilirubin is a form that is presumably nontoxic and can be broken down in the body in order for its chemical components to be reutilized. Clinical examples of congenitally lacking glucuronyl transferase are the Crigler-Najjar syndrome and the Dubin-Johnson syndrome.

Unconjugated biliruin is produced by hemolysis, or the destruction of erythrocytes. Hemolysis may be due to incompatibility of blood types (see Chap. 29) or to congenital anemias such as spherocytic anemia, stomatocytosis, or others. Though these latter rarely produce effects in the neonatal period, occasionally they do. Conjugated bilirubin has already passed through the liver cells and has been chemically altered. It is normally then excreted through the biliary tract into the duodenum. When obstructive problems exist in this system, the conjugated bilirubin is forced back into the bloodstream. Obstruction may be due to *atresia,* or nonpatency, of the common bile duct, intrinsic liver disease such as congenital hepatitis, and blockage of the bile canaliculi by thick, viscous bile, known as *inspissated bile syndrome.*

TREATMENT

No complete treatment exists for any of these metabolic disturbances. The most important step is to recognize the specific deficiency early, e.g., a history of a diabetic mother should alert one to watch for hypoglycemia. In many states, a blood test for phenylalanine level is mandatory before infants are discharged from the nursery. Some hospitals test routinely for galactose in the neonate's urine. Jaundice is a sign that should indicate the performance of appropriate laboratory tests.

In conditions of aminoacidurias, the appearance of elevated blood levels and the presence of the metabolites in the urine are dependent upon protein (milk formula) feedings. The blood test for phenylalanine is not useful until after 2 or 3 days of formula feeding; the phenylketones still may not appear in the urine for 4 to 6 weeks. Physicians and clinics should follow up an initial negative blood test, performed during the neonatal period, with a blood or urine test when the infant is 4 to 6 weeks of age.

When a diagnosis is made, dietary control measures can be started early. Synthetic formula feedings can eliminate the milk sugar (lactose) that is the precursor of galactose, or the protein amino acids, such as phenylalanine and cysteine. These amino acids, however, are essential to normal growth and development in the proper concentrations, although above a certain level in the blood they can be toxic, especially to the brain. Thus, the safe limit for phenylalanine is considered to be 4 mg/100 ml of blood. For this reason, dietary management must include proper amounts of milk to ensure adequate amino acid nutrition while blood samples are titrated to make certain that the levels are within normal bounds. As for galactose, simple glucose can be substituted in the feedings.

Hemolytic disease is treated with exchange transfusions and/or phototherapy, but these measures are only palliative in cases of enzyme deficiency. Obstructive pathologic conditions such as atresia of the bile duct must be corrected surgically. Treatment for hepatitis and inspissated bile syndrome is only supportive.

maintaining nutrition

With the respiratory, circulatory, and nervous systems of the newborn functioning reasonably well, the next important consideration must be the maintaining of nutrition. During intrauterine existence the embryo and fetus required nutrients mainly for growth. In postnatal existence the infant requires nutrients and calories for growth, for body heat, and for muscular activity. Furthermore while antenatally all nutrients were furnished through the umbilical vessels from the mother, postnatally the infant is dependent upon an intact gastrointestinal tract from mouth through anus and upon the ability to suck and to swallow.

NORMAL REQUIREMENTS

Nutritional needs of the independently functioning individual may be considered in several categories. Twenty-four amino acids derived from proteins are known to have nutritional importance. Of these, nine are essential for cell growth and multiplication: histidine, isoleucine, leucine, lysine, methionine, phenylalanine, threonine, tryptophan, and valine. Carbohydrates are simple sugars like glucose and fructose, complex sugars like sucrose and lactose, and starches. The latter two classes of carbohydrates must first be converted to simple sugars which are then used mainly for tissue energy requirements. Proteins and fats can be oxidized for energy or stored by the body. The metabolism and oxidation of all these organic nutrients release heat which can be measured in terms of calories.

In addition to the organic nutrients the organism requires various inorganic elements or electrolytes for proper functioning. These are mainly sodium, potassium, calcium, iron, phosphorus, sulfur, and magnesium, among others. No less important than any requirement already mentioned is sufficient water to dissolve and transport all the nutrients and waste products intracellularly, extracellularly, and intravascularly. Water intake must approximate the amount lost in urine, stool, expired air, and perspiration.

Thus, it is seen that the proper amount of

the proper food must be furnished to the neonate in order to give him a good start in life. Nature has provided every mammalian mother with species-specific milk that has the ideal mixture for her young under normal circumstances. Scientific and technical advances have produced modified cows' milk formulas that approximate human milk and synthetic nonmilk formulas containing a proper balance of nutrient constitutents. The normal term newborn requires about 56 kcal/lb of body weight (117 kcal/kg) per 24 h and about 60 to 90 ml fluid per pound (120 to 180 ml/kg) of body weight per 24 h. The needs of the premature infant run higher, depending on his weight and degree of functional maturity. Thus, his caloric requirements may be 30 to 50 percent higher than those of a normal term infant.

PROBLEMS PREVENTING INTAKE OR ABSORPTION

Problems preventing intake or absorption of food fall into two categories, functional and structural. Functional disturbances may be the result simply of immaturity of the suck and swallow reflexes. They may also be due to the debilitating effects of respiratory distress, systemic infection, or central nervous system damage. Structural problems are essentially congenital deformities in various areas of the gastrointestinal tract (Fig. 28·11A). *Cleft palate* may interfere with sucking (Fig. 28·11B). It is amazing, however, how many infants who have even wide clefts manage to nipple-feed fairly well when they are held upright. Gastrointestinal anomalies below the pharynx are more serious and life-threatening.

Esophageal atresia and *tracheoesophageal fistula,* i.e., a communication between the trachea and the esophagus, may occur in any of five variations. As shown in Fig. 28·12, the commonest, accounting for 87 percent of cases, is the blind pouch proximal es-

ophagus with tracheoesophageal fistula distally. In this condition swallowing of liquids will result in regurgitation, with danger of aspiration into the trachea and beyond. The diagnosis should be suspected by the nurse with the first water feeding when the infant regurgitates or chokes repeatedly after swallowing a small amount.

Intestinal obstruction may be caused by *atresia* anywhere below the stomach. Pyloric stenosis at the stomach outlet does not usually show symptoms until about five to seven weeks of age, when projectile vomiting occurs. Pyloric stenosis occurs mainly in male infants. Atresia may occur in the duodenum, the jejunum, or the ileum at any level and may affect variable lengths of intestine. Functional obstruction may result from congenital adhesion bands constricting the intestinal lumen, intestinal malrotation during embryonic formation, meconium ileus (a failure of intestinal function due to blockage by very thick meconium), and *imperforate anus* (Fig. 28·13). *Omphalocele* is an anomaly in which an abdominal wall defect allows herniation with a membranous covering of a portion of the intestine at the site of the umbilicus. Omphalocele may produce ileus or obstruction.

SUPPORTIVE CARE AND TREATMENT

Treatment must be directed toward correcting any existing obstructive disorder surgically and toward supplying nourishment by one of several routes. Where functional disturbances interfere merely with intake, not with passage of fluids, as in immaturity, sepsis, or cerebral insult, adequate nutrition may be sustained by nasogastric tube feeding. Where chest surgery has been performed to correct tracheoesophageal anomalies, a temporary gastrostomy is performed and a tube sutured into the opening for feedings until the esophageal junction heals. Supple-

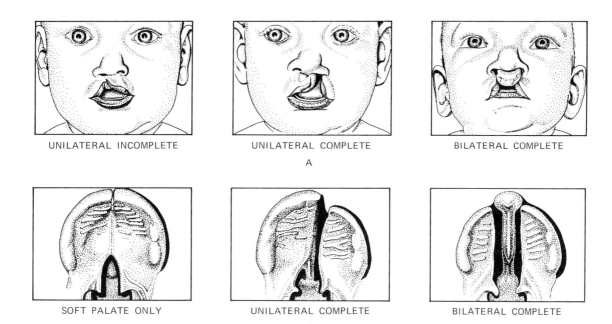

UNILATERAL INCOMPLETE   UNILATERAL COMPLETE   BILATERAL COMPLETE

A

SOFT PALATE ONLY   UNILATERAL COMPLETE   BILATERAL COMPLETE

B

fig. 28·11 A Cleft lip. B Cleft palate. (*From Ross Laboratories, Columbus, Ohio, Education Aid No. 7.*)

mentary intravenous fluids containing glucose and electrolytes or blood transfusions may be indicated.

Infants with obstruction of the colon or with imperforate anus will require a colostomy or a jejunostomy to bypass the distal surgical repair in order to allow healing. These procedures add to the problems of nursing care, for the more liquid stool is quite irritating to the skin surrounding the stoma.

In cases of extensive or protracted intestinal obstruction or dysfunction, adequate nutrition cannot be maintained by peripheral vein infusions. Any solution of adequate amounts of nutrients such as amino acids and hypertonic glucose is too viscous and even sclerosing for small veins with narrow lumens and small blood volume passage. Lately, a technique has been devised known as deep intravenous *hyperalimentation,* by means of which a highly enriched solution equivalent in nutritive value to milk can be furnished to

fig. 28·12 One type of tracheoesophageal fistula, in which the esophagus ends in a blind pouch. The lower esophagus connected with the stomach causes the stomach to be distended with air. (*From B. M. Patten, Human Embryology, 3d ed., McGraw-Hill Book Company, New York,* 1968.)

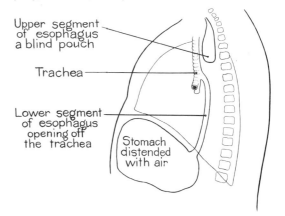

Upper segment of esophagus a blind pouch

Trachea

Lower segment of esophagus opening off the trachea

Stomach distended with air

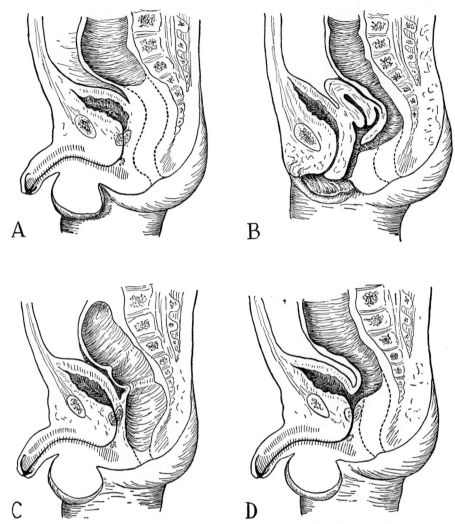

fig. 28·13 Imperforate anus (four types of disorder). (*Redrawn from Corning.*) A Anal atresia combined with obliteration of lower part of rectum; B anal atresia combined with a rectovaginal fistula; C uncomplicated anal atresia; D anal atresia combined with rectovesical fistula and agenesis of the rectum. (*From B. M. Patten,* Human Embryology, *3d ed., McGraw-Hill Book Company, New York,* 1968.)

the infant parenterally. A polyethylene catheter is introduced into the external jugular vein at the side of the neck through a small skin incision. The catheter is threaded down through the superior vena cava to the right atrium of the heart. Thus, the solution is immediately diluted into the rapidly flushing large volume of blood entering the heart

without irritating any vascular walls. The exterior portion of the catheter is tunneled under the skin for several centimeters, from the point of introduction into the jugular vein upward, and brought out through a lateral incision in the scalp. The solution is pumped into the catheter by steady flow by an electric infusion pump with an interposed millipore filter to eliminate any milliparticles of solid matter that could initiate thrombi or otherwise block small blood vessels.

bibliography

American Academy of Pediatrics: "Pediatricians Revise Guidelines on O_2 for Neonates," *American Journal of Nursing,* **71**(5):902, 1971.

Dahm, L. S., and L. S. James: "Newborn Temperature and Calculated Heat Loss in the Delivery Room," *Pediatrics,* **49**:504, 1972.

Filler, Robert M.: "Total Parenteral Feeding of Infants," *Hospital Practice,* June, 1972, p. 79–86.

Gluck, Louis: "Pulmonary Surfactant and Neonatal Respiratory Distress," *Hospital Practice,* **6**(11):45–46, 1971.

Lees, Martin H.: "Cyanosis of the Newborn Infant," *Journal of Pediatrics,* **77**:484–498, 1970.

Martin, L., A. Gilmore, J. Peckham, and J. Baumer: "Nursing Care of the Infant with Esophageal Anomalies," *American Journal of Nursing,* **66**:2463–2469, 1966.

Nelson, Nicholas M.: "On the Etiology of Hyaline Membrane Disease," *Pediatric Clinics of North America,* **17**:4, 1970.

Reynolds, E. O. R.: "Hyaline Membrane Disease," *American Journal of Obstetrics and Gynecology,* **106**:5, 1970.

Schaffer, Alexander J., and Mary Ellen Avery: *Diseases of the Newborn,* 3d ed., W. B. Saunders Company, Philadelphia, 1971.

White, Mary, and William J. Keenan: "The Recognition and Management of Hypoglycemia in the Newborn Infant," *Nursing Clinics of North America,* **6**(1):67–69, 1971.

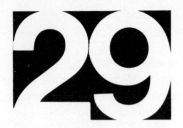

immunologic problems of the newborn

Marvin L. Blumberg

The process of immunization is the mechanism by which the body produces antibodies to neutralize or destroy foreign protein substances known as *antigens.* These antigens may be live microorganisms or inert organic structures such as red blood cells and killed bacterial vaccines. The specific antibody structure remains fixed in the "memory" of the plasma and other cells of the reticulo-endothelial system, so that when the host is again challenged by either the natural disease organisms or a booster dose of vaccine, a rapid rise in level (titer) of the specific antibody will occur. Immunity in response to antigen stimulus is called *active immunity.*

In contrast, if preformed antibodies from another source are injected into the host just before or during an attack of an antigen, the host will have no need to form specific antibodies. The donated antibodies from human serum from another already immunized person or in animal serum (e.g., from a horse) can confer *passive immunity* on the host. The donated antibodies will last in the system about 4 to 6 weeks, after which there is neither protection nor "memory" for recall of antibody formation by future antigen invasions.

ISOIMMUNIZATION

The mechanism of becoming *sensitized* or of forming antibodies against antigens from the same species is termed *iso*immunization. Normally, immunization is essential for survival of the host, but in several cases it is a detrimental process. Where there is the Rh factor incompatibility or ABO incompatibility between parents the infant may be jeopardized. Several other incompatible blood groups exist, but problems with Rh and ABO factors are most commonly seen.

When incompatibility exists between two parents, the infant of these parents will inherit a red blood cell group from the father that may differ from the mother's group. As a result, specific antibodies that can destroy those erythrocytes may be produced in the mother's serum against the antigen of the fetal red cells.

By the same antigen-antibody reaction, a nulliparous Rh-negative woman may be immunized and build up anti-Rh antibodies by receiving a transfusion of Rh-positive blood. The antibody buildup in either the gestation or transfusion situation will not harm the woman herself but will be detrimental to future Rh-positive fetuses.

The placenta is usually a very effective barrier between maternal and fetal circulation, so that an antigen-antibody reaction takes place during or after pregnancy only if there is intermingling of fetal cells into the mother's circulation. Movement may go in the mother's direction when minute breaks occur in the placental interface—in cases of infection of the placenta itself, during trauma at delivery or abortion, or when normal small tears occur in the placenta as it separates naturally during the third stage.

Studies have shown that it takes as little as $1/2$ ml blood containing the antigens to cause a significant antibody response (1). It requires about 72 h for this critical process to be stimulated, an important factor in the application of preventive therapy. Antibody formation may take 6 weeks to 6 months after stimulus. Once there has been an antibody response, however, the maternal antibodies can traverse the barrier to enter the fetal circulation and attack the erythrocytes. With Rh, the stimulus usually occurs after one pregnancy and affects the next pregnancy.

ABO incompatibility

Genetic inheritance of one factor from each parent leads to six possible genotypes in the ABO blood group system.

Homozygous	Heterozygous
OO	AO
AA	BO
BB	AB

Depending on which antigen is in the red cell, the opposite antibody is present in the plasma. For example, if a person has type B, then there will be anti-A antibodies in the plasma (see Table 29·1).

The pathogenesis of ABO incompatibility differs from that operating in Rh incompatibility because the group O mother already possesses a and b agglutinins (i.e., anti-A and anti-B antibodies) which may cross the placental barrier and interact with the A or B antigens in the erythrocytes of the fetus. There appear to be some mechanisms that protect the fetus in such cases which are not as yet clearly understood. Interestingly, when both Rh and ABO incompatibility coexist between mother and infant, the production of anti-A and anti-B antibodies in the mother seems to suppress her production of Rh antibodies.

ABO may account for about two-thirds of the maternal isoimmunization with consequent neonatal disease (2). There are three possible combinations that are incompatible.

Mother	Infant
O	A, B, or AB
A	B
B	A

Problems are most frequent with an O mother and an A infant, less common with the O mother and a B infant, and very rare in the other combinations. The results of ABO incompatibility are usually milder than those of Rh incompatibility. In rare cases where it is a severe disease, it is thought that the mother's "natural" antibody titer has been augmented by the antibodies she has formed in response to the fetal erythrocytes that had entered her circulation during pregnancy to sensitize her further.

Rh incompatibility

The Rh group is made up of several factors of varying strengths. We refer to *positive* factors as to the strongest factors in reaction with a specific antiserum test. In this country we usually refer to the Rh group using the *CDE* typing, but others use the Rh-Hr system. Table 29·2 indicates the equivalents. Factor *D* is the major factor in Rh incompatibility, although in rare instances the infant will be jeopardized by other factor (*c* or *e*) incompatibility.

An Rh-negative person must be homozygous because the Rh-negative cell group is a recessive genetic factor; both the genes involved are lacking the dominant Rh factor

table 29·1
ABO ANTIGEN PLACEMENT

TYPE	ANTIGEN IN RED CELL	ANTIBODIES IN PLASMA
O	None	Anti-A, anti-B
A	A	Anti-B
B	B	Anti-A
AB	A and B	None

table 29.2

CDE TYPING OF Rh GROUP, WITH Rh-hr
EQUIVALENTS

Rh 1	= D	= Rh₀
Rh 2	= C	= rh'
Rh 3	= E	= rh"
Rh 4	= c	= hr'*
Rh 5	= e	= hr"

*At present Hro(d) is not demonstrable but is considered as part of the scheme.

and are therefore "negative." An Rh-positive person may be either homozygous or heterozygous, for the dominant gene overshadows the others in the group. The infant of an Rh-negative mother and a homozygous Rh-positive father will always be heterozygous for positive (Fig. 29·1A). The genetic inheritance laws indicate that if both parents are heterozygous for positive, the infant has a 50 percent chance of being heterozygous positive, a 25 percent chance of being homozygous positive, and a 25 percent chance of being homozygous negative (Fig. 29·1C).

This pattern demonstrates one of the reasons why incompatibility does not always result in problems for the infant. In fact, as long as the Rh-positive fetal cells do not breach the barrier to enter the maternal circulation, nothing untoward will happen (Fig. 29·2).

EFFECTS ON THE FETUS AND NEONATE

Though there are no clinically apparent effects on the mother as a result of isoimmunization, the consequences for the fetus and infant may range from mild to fatal, if untreated. Depending on the level of the mother's antibody titer and the concentration of her antibodies that entered the fetal circulation before birth, the degree and duration of hemolysis of the infant's blood cells may be more or less severe.

Hemolysis is the breakdown of hemoglobin into globin (globulin fraction) and heme.

Heme is then broken down into iron and *bilirubin.* There are five steps in bilirubin metabolism and excretion; slowing or interference at any step raises the blood concentration of bilirubin in an *unconjugated,* indirect, fat-soluble form. To be excreted promptly, bilirubin must be *conjugated* within the liver by an enzymatic reaction with *glucuronyl transferase.* The conjugated form is a water-soluble, direct form, which is excreted mainly through the bile into the intestines; some is reabsorbed and stored for reuse, and some is partially excreted by the kidneys in the form of urine urobilinogen.

The process of metabolism of hemoglobin goes on normally in every person, but the newborn is handicapped at birth by two factors; an immature liver, and an extra load of fetal erythrocytes with a shorter life-span than adult erythrocytes. The blood of a normal full-term infant contains on an average 17.1 ± 1.8 Gm hemoglobin per 100 ml and has a hematocrit value of 52 ± 5 percent. Normally only as much as 1.5 percent of the red cells are in the form of reticulocytes.

jaundice

Jaundice is a symptom of elevated blood levels of unconjugated bilirubin. Since an elevated bilirubin level shows as a yellow color in skin and sclera, it gives a dramatic indication of its presence. In neonates jaundice usually stems from an imbalance of red cell destruction and formation. Fetal hematocrit is high because of lower oxygen levels at the placental exchange site. After birth, inspired air containing more readily available oxygen allows the neonate to reduce the numbers of circulating red cells. The dumping of excess fetal erythrocytes overloads the immature liver (the site of transformation of bilirubin to its excretable form), thus causing bilirubinemia and jaundice.

Jaundice can also be caused by other

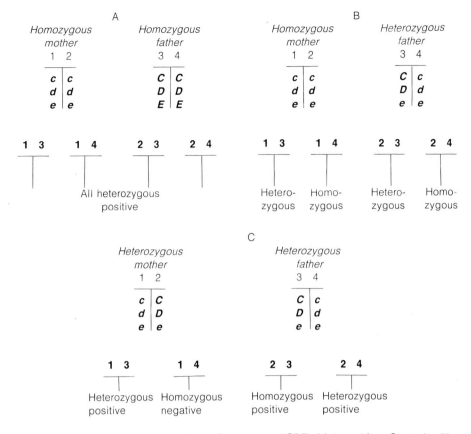

fig. 29·1 Examples of zygosity with the Rh grouping (*CDE*). (*Adapted from* Obstetrics Illustrated.)

factors interrupting the metabolic cycle: newborn infection, congenital malformations, metabolic defects, or maternal drug intake affecting fetal liver function.

PHYSIOLOGIC JAUNDICE

Developmental hyperbilirubinemia is a new term for *physiologic jaundice,* the state of having an elevated bilirubin level because of physiologic immaturity. All newborns (unless postmature) experience some hyperbilirubinemia, with a mean peak at 6 mg/100 ml blood on the third to fourth day of life (2). Since jaundice is evidenced when the level reaches about 5 mg/100 ml by the yellow coloring of

the skin and sclera, about 50 percent of all newborns will *not* demonstrate observable jaundice, although they may have slightly elevated bilirubin levels.

KERNICTERUS

When bilirubin levels rise to 18 mg/100 ml or more, brain damage may occur because of deposit of the fat-soluble, indirect-reacting bilirubin in brain cells. This event, *kernicterus,* is to be avoided because of the permanent damage to the brain cells. Symptoms of kernicterus are lethargy, poor feeding, opisthotonus, and hypertonus. Kernicterus may result in the child having chorioathetoid cere-

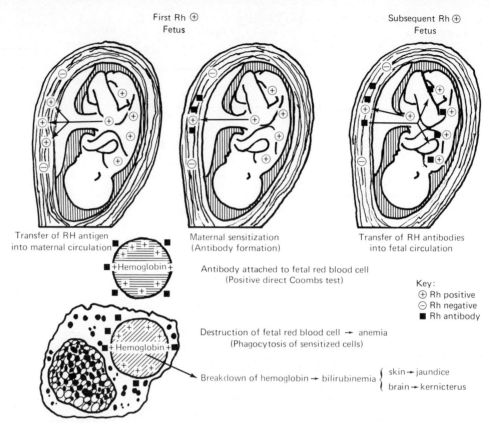

First Rh ⊕
Fetus

Subsequent Rh ⊕
Fetus

Transfer of RH antigen
into maternal circulation

Maternal sensitization
(Antibody formation)

Transfer of RH antibodies
into fetal circulation

+Hemoglobin+

Antibody attached to fetal red blood cell
(Positive direct Coombs test)

Key:
⊕ Rh positive
⊖ Rh negative
■ Rh antibody

+Hemoglobin+

Destruction of fetal red blood cell → anemia
(Phagocytosis of sensitized cells)

Breakdown of hemoglobin → bilirubinemia { skin → jaundice
brain → kernicterus

fig. 29·2 Method of transfer of antigen-antibody. (*Courtesy of Ross Laboratories, Columbus, Ohio, Clinical Education Aid No.* 9.)

bral palsy, deafness, and mental retardation. In lesser degrees it results in minimal brain dysfunction, with clumsiness and learning disabilities.

Between physiologic jaundice with levels under 10 mg/100 ml and kernicterus there lies a range of bilirubin levels that are serious but treatable. Keeping bilirubin levels below 18 to 20 mg/100 ml has fairly consistently prevented kernicterus. However, a compromised, sick infant can be damaged at lower levels. Premature infants are especially vulnerable because of immaturity of body systems. If the baby is anoxic or has acidosis, hypoglycemia, or infection, it is much more vulnerable to kernicterus at lower levels of bilirubinemia (2).

anemia

In severe cases of incompatibility, it is anemia which threatens survival before birth. The maternal antibodies destroy fetal erythrocytes faster than they can be reformed by the hematopoietic organs.

treatment of hemolytic disease

Until the early 1960s the only treatment available for use in serious cases of hemolysis and jaundice was an exchange transfusion. A fetus severely affected with erythrocyte destruction from incompatibility early in gestation was virtually doomed to fetal death and stillbirth or to a very premature birth. Now, in severe cases, when the infant is deemed too small to survive, and is suffering from severe anemia because of red cell destruction, an intrauterine transfusion can be done.

After correct placement of the transfusion cannula by paracentesis through the mother's abdominal wall into the uterus, Rh-negative, type 0 packed red cells are administered into the fetal peritoneal cavity. Amazingly, the red cells can be absorbed intact across the peritoneal wall into the circulation of the infant. Intrauterine transfusions may have to be administered as early as the twenty-first week of gestation and may have to be repeated several times to maintain an adequate hemoglobin and hematocrit level. Although there is a high risk of complications, many cases are on record in which a jeopardized infant has been carried to a safe delivery and become a normally thriving infant (3).

It is possible to predict if the infant will have trouble by testing two factors; the mother's antibody titer (rising titers mean increasing antibody production) and the level of bilirubin excreted into the amniotic fluid by the fetus (rising levels mean increasing hemolysis) (3).

The physician may have to estimate the best time for delivery, balancing immaturity against a rising titer and bilirubin level. Delivery as early as 4 weeks preterm may prevent a considerable amount of hemolysis and hyperbilirubinemia, but the resultant immaturity may handicap the infant in other serious ways in addition to inadequate bilirubin metabolism.

COOMBS' TEST

The most frequently used test to determine antibody presence in fetal or maternal blood, the Coombs' test, uses the serum of rabbits immunized against human globulin. Because the maternal Rh antibodies are globulins, the rabbit immune *antiglobulin* will cause agglu-

tination (direct Coombs' positive) when added to the affected infant's cord blood, the cells of which are coated with maternal antibodies. The direct Coombs' test is often negative in the presence of ABO incompatibility, perhaps because of the lack of sensitivity of A or B antigens in the infant's cells.

The indirect Coombs' test may be used by a different process to measure maternal antibody levels as well. The indirect test uses the mother's serum rather than her red cells to demonstrate whether antibodies are present, either from a prior transfusion of incompatible blood or by isoimmunization during pregnancy. The indirect Coombs' test may be used to test levels of reactivity during pregnancy. A rise in the level or titer indicates that the process is continuing to proceed, more antibodies are forming, and the fetus will be jeopardized. A positive reaction at a titer of 1:8 is acceptable, but anything stronger than that is a sign of maternal sensitization (4). For instance, a titer of 1:64 means that the serum has been diluted 64 times and still gives an agglutination reaction when placed with the antiglobulin.

EXCHANGE TRANSFUSION

When there is a serious degree of jaundice in the first 24 h of life or low levels of hemoglobin because of hemolysis, an exchange transfusion may be the most effective way to rescue the infant. The process involves removing and replacing about 20 ml at a time, by way of an umbilical vein catheter and a three-way stopcock connected to a syringe, a blood container, and the catheter, usually until as much as 500 ml of blood has been exchanged. A low-birth-weight baby might be given less blood.

In order to prevent the clotting of the donor blood in the container, sodium citrate is added to it at the time of collection. Sodium citrate will combine with serum calcium, the factor that would initiate coagulation. When this citrated blood is given to the infant, it tends to deplete his own serum calcium by combining with it. Since low calcium levels can cause tetany with convulsions, and possibly even death, 1 ml of 10 percent calcium gluconate should be injected slowly through the venous catheter after each 100 ml of blood has been exchanged.

The rationale for performing an exchange transfusion is the removal of about 80 percent of the infant's Rh-positive antigenic red cells along with the maternal anti-Rh antibodies, and replacement with Rh-negative nonantigenic red blood cells. The infant's own type (A, B, or O) with Rh-negative blood is used. The donor blood is also cross-matched against the mother's serum to test for serologic compatibility. When ABO incompatibility is severe enough to call for an exchange transfusion, the infant is given type O, Rh-negative blood. In very severe cases of either, there may be enough circulating antibodies that a second or even a third transfusion may be required.

PHOTOTHERAPY

For a long time it was known that when blood was drawn from a patient for bilirubin determination, the specimen had to be shielded from light. Light produced a chemical change, wherein the specimen would yield a false low reading. Then some observers noted that there seemed to be a lower incidence of jaundice among newborns on the sunny side or in the brightly lighted areas of the nursery than among those infants in the less bright areas. It took a while for these observations to be synthesized into a hypothesis that could be tested and proved (5). The findings were that unconjugated, indirect bilirubin could be degraded into a water-soluble compound by exposing the infant to bright, cool, fluorescent light.

The chemical reaction is a photic one, dependent on light intensity at the blue-short-wavelength end of the visible spectrum. During treatment, which lasts about 3 days, the baby's eyes must be shielded from the light. Eye pads covered by a light-proof outer bandage or pad protect the delicate retina from prolonged exposure to bright light. Most nurses remove the baby from the lights and remove the eye shield during feeding times (Fig. 29·3).

Though phototherapy has become widely accepted, there is some lingering doubt about its complete safety. Questions exist about the possible long-range toxicity of bilirubin breakdown products and about the effect of light energy on the chemical elements of the blood and other body cells. Therefore, some limitations and guidelines for the application of phototherapy are important. It is not used prophylactically to prevent physiologic jaundice but is used only after bilirubin levels have risen above 10 mg/100 ml, and the duration of use is only long enough to drop the blood level back down below 10 mg/100 ml. When properly employed, phototherapy is an excellent tool to prevent damaging hyperbilirubinemia.

prevention of isoimmunization

The mechanism of passive immunization forms the rationale for preventing isoimmunization of Rh-negative mothers who bear Rh-positive infants. Rh-negative gamma globulin (RhoGAM) is a serum concentrate containing pooled anti-Rh D antibodies. These antibodies, if injected within 72 h after delivery or abortion, will destroy any Rh-positive fetal cells that may have entered the mother's circulation at the time of delivery. When the mother is given antibodies, she has no need to form her own, with cells then imprinted with "memory" for the next occasion. Just *after* each subsequent pregnancy the mother who is not isoimmunized must be

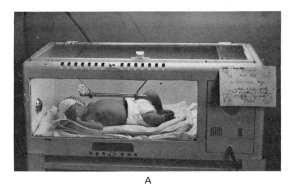
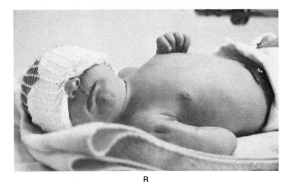

fig. 29·3 A Phototherapy. B Eyes must be bandaged to protect against light. (*Photographs by Ruth Helmich.*)

passively reimmunized. In this way any development of hemolytic disease for the newborn can be completely prevented. Once she becomes sensitized, RhoGAM can no longer be given to her.

So far, no similar procedure exists for preventing ABO incompatibility. There are no amniotic fluid tests or blood tests to distinguish between naturally present a or b agglutinins in an O mother's serum and an augmented titer due to the introduction of fetal A or B erythrocytes into her blood. Nor has there been developed an antiserum for passive immunization if such tests were available. Fortunately, ABO incompatibility is usually less severe and rarely requires exchange transfusion.

Prevention is the key to future elimination of Rh-negative problems. Every woman who is typed as Rh-negative with a homozygous or heterozygous mate should be educated about prevention. Anti-D gamma globulin should be administered to her within 72 h of any delivery, abortion, or stillbirth, to provide protection against active isoimmunization.

references

1. Elmer R. Jennings, "Fetal-Maternal Hemorrhage: Its Detection, Measurement and Significance," *RhoGam Symposium,* New York City, Apr. 17, 1969.
2. Lawrence M. Gartner and Melvin Hollander, "Disorders of Bilirubin Metabolism," chap. 8 in Nicholas Assali (ed.), *Pathophysiology of Gestation: Fetal and Neonatal Disorders,* vol. 3, Academic Press, Inc., New York, 1972, p. 466.
3. John T. Queenan, "Amniocentesis in Rh Disease," *Contemporary OB/GYN,* **1**(2):49, 1973.
4. Louis M. Hellman and Jack A. Pritchard, *Williams' Obstetrics,* Appleton-Century-Crofts, Inc., New York, 1971, p. 1038.
5. Jerold F. Lucey, "Neonatal Jaundice and Phototherapy," *Pediatric Clinic of North America,* **19**(4):827, 1972.

bibliography

Barnett, Henry L. (ed.): *Pediatrics,* 15th ed., Appleton-Century-Crofts, Inc., New York, 1972.

Gill, Thomas J.: "Transfer of Immunity to the Fetus," *Contemporary OB/GYN,* **1**(5):53, 1973.

Mollison, Patrick L.: *Blood Transfusion in Clinical Medicine,* 4th ed., F. A. Davis Company, Philadelphia, 1967.

Nelson, Waldo E. (ed.): *Textbook of Pediat-*

rics, 9th ed., W. B. Saunders Company, Philadelphia, 1969.

Pochedly, Carl: "The Exchange Transfusion, Newer Concepts and Advances in Technic," *Clinical Pediatrics,* **7**:383–388, 1968.

Schaffer, Alexander J., and Mary Ellen Avery: *Diseases of the Newborn,* 3d ed., W. B. Saunders Company, Philadelphia, 1971.

Woody, N. C., and M. J. Brodhey: "Tanning from Phototherapy for Neonatal Jaundice," *Journal of Pediatrics,* **82**:1042, 1973.

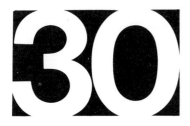

the preterm infant

Arlene Ritz

The death toll among babies born too soon and too small has been appallingly high. Even with intensive research and advances in the medical and nursing care of such infants, they account for approximately 63 percent of the infants that die every year. Not only does preterm birth carry with it a high death rate, but studies have repeatedly confirmed the increased frequency of sequelae such as mental retardation, neurologic diseases, and visual handicaps.

classification

What is now called preterm birth was formerly referred to as premature birth. Recent investigations have clearly demonstrated that the use of the word "prematurity" has been an oversimplification in classifying infants by birth weight. Formerly, a premature infant was defined as one with a birth weight of 2500 grams (5½ lb) or less. The use of birth weight alone is often misleading in diagnosing prematurity. In many cases, the newborn weighing under 2500 Gm is a small but mature neonate without any physiologic underdevelopment. Because of this confusion, both the American Academy of Pediatrics Committee on the Fetus and the Newborn (1) and the Expert Committee of the World Health Organization have recommended that a clear distinction be made between the terms "low birth weight" and "prematurity," as follows:

Low-birth-weight infant—any live-born infant with a weight at birth of 2500 Gm or less.
Premature infant—a live-born infant with a gestation period of less than 37 weeks regardless of weight.

Most recently, the following nomenclature has been used so as clearly to distinguish developmental differences in low-birth-weight infants:

Preterm infant—a live-born infant with a gestational age of less than 37 weeks. These infants may be called premature, and they characteristically suffer from immature development.
Small-for-dates-infants—infants whose birth weights are below average for their gestational age (Fig. 30·1). It is estimated that this group makes up to 30 to 50 percent of all low-birth-weight infants. These infants may be distinguished as follows:

1. Infants of low birth weight having a gestational age of 37 weeks or more. Despite their low weights, these infants are well developed and mature. Familial, genetic, or racial factors account for their small size. For example, in India, a low-birth-weight infant is considered one weighing under 2150 Gm.
2. Infants of low birth weight who are small for gestational age due to intrauterine growth retardation (Fig. 30·2). The difficulties encountered by these infants are generally due to maternal or fetal problems such as multiple births, nutritional deficiencies, placental circulation insufficiency, endocrine disorders, and congenital

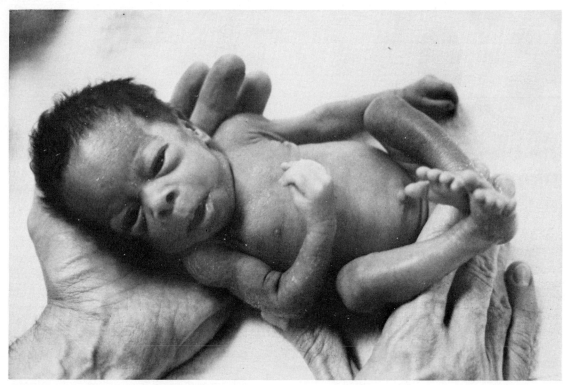

fig. 30·1 Small-for-date infant. Infant weighing 960 Gm at birth in the thirty-sixth week of gestation shows the effect of severe intrauterine malnutrition. (*From Pedro Rosso, "Nutrition and Abnormal Fetal Growth,"* Contemporary OB/GYN, **2**(3):54, 1973.)

anomalies. The morbidity encountered among these infants is generally due not to the immaturity of their body systems but to malformations, malnutrition, or intrauterine problems.

Some infants are doubly handicapped by being both preterm and "small-for-dates." Being disadvantaged by maternal or fetal diseases as well as immaturity, their mortality rate is exceedingly high.

This chapter is limited to the study of the preterm infant whose survival is at considerable risk because of anatomic and physiologic immaturity. However, reflecting the nomenclature used in the vast literature on the subject, in this chapter the word *preterm* is used interchangeably with the words *premature, immature,* and *low birth weight*.

incidence

Using weight as the criterion for prematurity, there is a wide variation in the general incidence throughout the world, which ranges from approximately 4 to 15 percent. Of the 3,256,000 babies born in the United States in 1972, about 10 percent were premature.

A significantly higher premature birth rate exists among nonwhites, reportedly as high as 12 to 15 percent. Many etiologic factors have been implicated in this intolerably high incidence—e.g., poor socioeconomic considerations, inadequate nutrition, heavy phy-

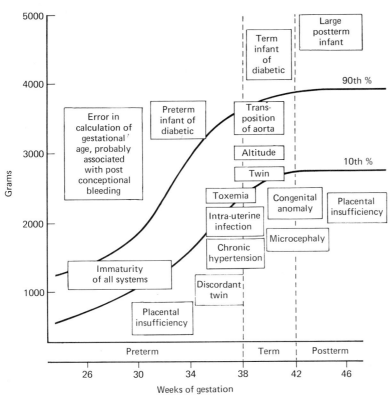

fig. 30·2 Conditions associated with intrauterine growth—related to birth weight and gestational age classification. (*From L. O. Lubchenco, C. Hausman, and Leena Backstrom, "Factors Influencing Fetal Growth," in* Nutricia Symposium: Aspects of Praematurity and Dysmaturity, *H. E. Stenfert Kroese B.V., Leiden,* 1968.)

sical labor, prolonged employment during gestation, and inadequate antepartum care.

mortality

The size and gravity of the problem are reflected in the wastage associated with premature birth. The overall mortality rate of these immature infants reportedly ranges from 20 to 30 percent, which is 30 times that found in mature infants. Studies indicate that approximately 60 to 85 percent of premature neonatal deaths occur in the first 2 days of life. Immaturity accounts for about two-thirds of all infant deaths in the first month of life, and remains the major cause of death throughout infancy. Death is most frequently attributed to immaturity of body systems, intracranial hemorrhage, and infection.

Survival rate is directly proportional to the birth weight. The weight of the fetus increases from 700 Gm at the end of the second trimester to 3500 Gm at full term. It is this prodigious growth in the last trimester which influences the ultimate survival rate. For each 500-Gm group below the 2500 Gm level, the mortality rate increases fourfold (2). Mortality reaches almost 90 to 100 percent in the newborn weighing 1000 Gm (2 lb) or less, although some centers report survival rates of about 20 percent for infants in this category. As the

NEWBORN CLASSIFICATION AND NEONATAL MORTALITY RISK
BY BIRTH WEIGHT AND GESTATIONAL AGE

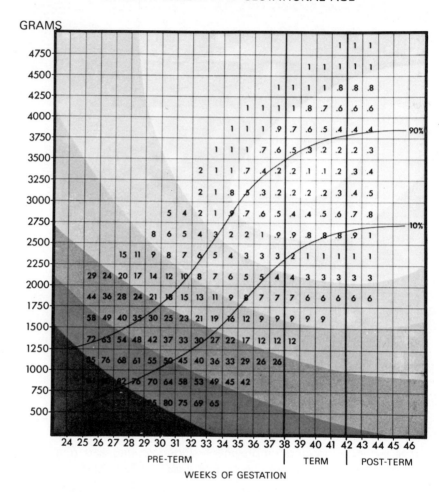

From Lubchenco, Searls, Brazie,
J Pediat, 81:814, 1972

Interpolated data based on mathematical fit from original data
University of Colorado Medical Center newborns, 7/1/58 - 7/1/69

fig. 30·3 Newborn classification and neonatal mortality risk by birthweight and gestational age. (*From L. O. Lubchenco, D. T. Searls, and J. V. Brazie, "Neonatal Mortality Rate: Relationship to Birth Weight and Gestational Age,"* Journal of Pediatrics, **81**:814–822, 1972.)

newborn's weight approaches 2500 Gm, the survival rate approximates that found in full-term babies.

There is ample evidence that gestational age—if correct—is a valid diagnostic criterion for prematurity. The major difficulty in using this parameter is the unreliability of the menstrual history in the average patient.

The nurse can predict the survival possibility of the high-risk infant by looking at the classification chart in Fig. 30·3. Here, weight plus the gestational age is used to predict survival. Investigations indicate that the use of both factors is a more significant determinant of survival than use of either weight or age alone. For example, if an infant is admitted to the nursery weighing 1300 Gm and having an estimated gestational age of 29 weeks, he will have about a 50 percent chance of survival. But if the same infant had a gestational age of 33 weeks, his chance of survival would be as high as 70 percent.

morbidity

In addition to this tragic human loss, there is a dreadful risk of morbidity for the infants who survive. During the neonatal period, the preterm infant is especially liable to cerebral hemorrhage, respiratory problems, anemia, dehydration, infections, failure to thrive, and kernicterus.

In general, the lower the birth weight the greater the incidence of disability in the various aspects of growth and development such as weight, height, and teething. Preterm infants surviving the first year are much more likely to have neurologic and psychologic abnormalities than infants born at term. In a long-term follow-up study on infants weighing under 1500 Gm at birth, Lubchenco and coworkers (3) reported two out of three infants with central nervous system or visual damage, 50 percent with spastic diplegia, and 40 percent with an IQ under 90.

Social and cultural deprivation so frequently found with these children compounds and complicates the neurologic problems. Emotional immaturity is commonly found during childhood, and prognosis in this regard depends upon the degree of parental emotional stability or distortion.

With the significant improvements in the medical and nursing care of premature infants, survival of very low-birth-weight (under 1500 Gm) infants has increased. Follow-up studies on these infants have confirmed the pessimistic view that a large number (ranging from 33 to 70 percent) of survivors inevitably suffer from serious abnormalities. This raises an ethical question. Are such extraordinary efforts towards survival justifiable unless there is promise of lessening the incidence of severe handicaps? Rawlings and co-workers (4) point out that modern methods of care aimed at preventing and treating such critical abnormalities as hypoxia, hypoglycemia, and hyperbilirubinemia should not only result in increased survival, but also lead to a marked lessening of brain damage in the survivors. Their contention is supported in an initial study of infants weighing 1500 Gm or less born at University College Hospital in London between 1966 and 1969. Although this study is limited and incomplete, it offers a new outlook for these infants from the established association of improved survival and increased handicap. Let us hope future studies will confirm this optimism.

characteristics

The physicial appearance of the preterm infant startlingly reflects the deprivation suffered as a result of preterm birth. Figure 30·4 shows a 1300-Gm, thin, fragile infant suffering from a host of problems common to such babies.

The preterm infant's physical characteristics correlate with his gestational age at birth, and classically he presents a majority of the features listed in Table 30·1. The more immature the baby, the more exaggerated will be the external differences from the term infant (Fig. 30·5A through E).

Two main parameters have been used by Dubowitz (5) to assess gestational age. The first is a series of 10 neurologic signs reflecting postures and primitive reflexes, and the second is a series of 11 external characteristics. Figure 30·6 illustrates the neurologic responses with the scores assigned to each, and the procedures for evaluating the postures and reflexes. The external features and their scores are described in Table 30·2. A score of 35 is assigned both to the neurologic signs and to the external criteria, comprising a maximum total score of 70. The graph in Fig. 30·7 correlates this total score with the estimated gestational age. For example, a

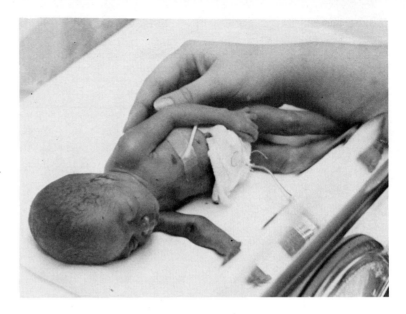

fig. 30·4 A 1300-Gm infant with estimated gestational age of 31 weeks. This small infant has an arterial catheter in the umbilical cord (to provide fluids and to monitor blood gases) and, attached to the skin of the chest, a temperature-sensing device which leads to the incubator and regulates the environmental temperature according to the infant's variations. (*Photograph courtesy of Long Island Jewish–Hillside Medical Center, New York.*)

table 30-1

COMMON CHARACTERISTICS OF THE PRETERM INFANT

SKIN
Thin, delicate, loose, wrinkled
Blood vessels readily seen
Presence of lanugo on face and shoulders
Ecchymosis from trauma or handling at birth
Color reflects baby's condition
First 24 h—smooth, wrinkle-free soles of feet

TRUNK
Broad and long
Very small chest—wide in transverse, but narrow in anterior-posterior plane
Abdomen round, full, and larger than the chest
Absence of breast nodules

GENITALIA
Small
Labia majora are open and gaping, and labia minora and clitoris are prominent
Scrotum small; rugal folds and pigmentation absent; testes may be undescended

NEUROLOGIC STATUS
Minimal activity
Feeble, whining, muted cry
Facial grimacing
Uncoordinated, jerky, asymmetric movements
Gagging, swallowing, and sucking reflexes are weak or absent
Moro reflex is incomplete—throws out arms but does not fist-clench and return arms

FACE
Head round and relatively large
Eyes prominent
Tongue large
Ears soft and flabby; hug scalp; easily pushed into different shapes
Neck short

EXTREMITIES
Short in relation to trunk
Fingernails and toenails are soft and extend to the ends of the digits

MEASUREMENTS
Length—less than 47 cm (18 in)
Head circumference—less than 33 cm (13 in)
Disproportion between circumferences of head and thorax; head usually 3 cm or more larger than the chest

POSITION
Lies flat in frog-leg position with shoulders, elbows, and knees all touching mattress. Head is on one side or the other

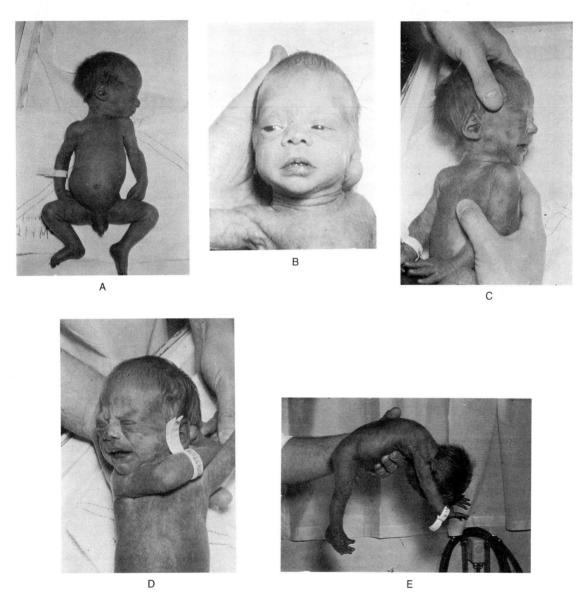

fig. 30·5 Characteristics of the preterm infant. A Preterm infant lying supine; note lack of muscle tone, resulting in froglike position with extremities flat on the bed. B Preterm infant facies; note lack of subcutaneous fat. C Head turned beyond the point of the shoulder. Full-term newborn does not turn head as far as shoulder. D Scarf sign: the arm can be pulled around the neck much farther than the arm of a full-term infant. E Ventral suspension: the preterm infant hangs limply with straight legs and arms when tested for strength of back and neck muscles. (*Photographs, courtesy of Kenneth Holt, M.D., from tape-slide program, "Neurologic Examination of the Newborn."*)

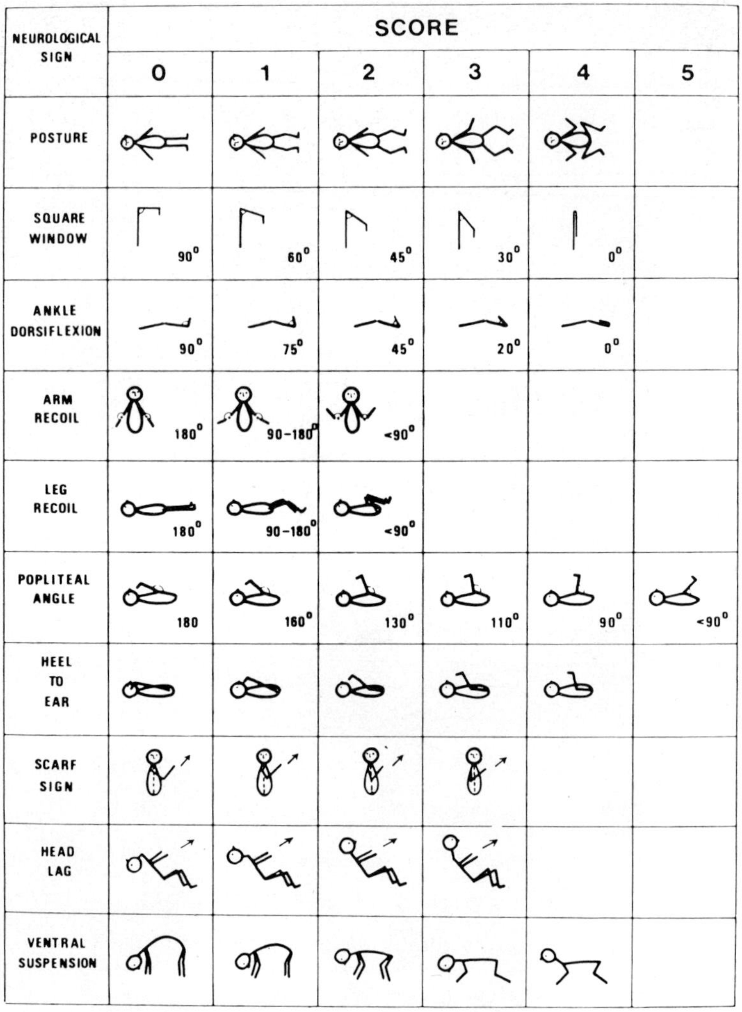

NEUROLOGICAL SIGN	SCORE					
	0	1	2	3	4	5
POSTURE						
SQUARE WINDOW	90°	60°	45°	30°	0°	
ANKLE DORSIFLEXION	90°	75°	45°	20°	0°	
ARM RECOIL	180°	90–180°	<90°			
LEG RECOIL	180°	90–180°	<90°			
POPLITEAL ANGLE	180	160°	130°	110°	90°	<90°
HEEL TO EAR						
SCARF SIGN						
HEAD LAG						
VENTRAL SUSPENSION						

fig. 30·6 Scoring system of neurologic signs for assessment of gestational age. (*From Victor Dubowitz, "Clinical Assessment of Gestational Age in the Newborn Infant,"* Journal of Pediatrics, **77**:1–10, 1970.)

table 30-2
SOME NOTES ON TECHNIQUES OF ASSESSMENT OF NEUROLOGIC CRITERIA

POSTURE: Observed with infant quiet and in supine position, Score zero—arms and legs extended; 1—beginning of flexion of hips and knees, arms extended; 2—stronger flexion of legs, arms extended; 3—arms slightly flexed, legs flexed and abducted; 4—full flexion of arms and legs.

SQUARE WINDOW: The hand is flexed on the forearm between the thumb and index finger of the examiner. Enough pressure is applied to get as full a flexion as possible, and the angle between the hypothenar eminence and the ventral aspect of the forearm is measured and graded according to diagram. (Care is taken not to rotate the infant's wrist while doing this maneuver.)

ANKLE DORSIFLEXION: The foot is dorsiflexed onto the anterior aspect of the leg, with the examiner's thumb on the sole of the foot and other fingers behind the leg. Enough pressure is applied to get as full flexion as possible, and the angle between the dorsum of the foot and the anterior aspect of the leg is measured.

ARM RECOIL: With the infant in the supine position the forearms are first flexed for 5 s, then fully extended by pulling on the hands, and then released. The sign is fully positive if the arms return briskly to full flexion (score 2). If the arms return to incomplete flexion or the response is sluggish, it is graded as score 1. If they remain extended or are followed only by random movements, the score is 0.

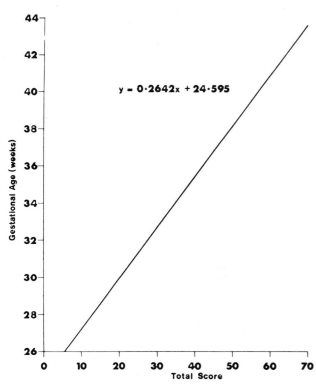

$$y = 0.2642x + 24.595$$

Gestational Age (weeks)

Total Score

fig. 30·7 Graph for reading gestational age. The score from Table 30·3 is added to the score from Fig. 30·6. A line is drawn from the horizontal axis to the diagonal line; then from the intersecting point, a line to the perpendicular axis will indicate the age in weeks. (*From Victor Dubowitz et al., "Clinical Assessment of Gestational Age in the Newborn Infant,"* Journal of Pediatrics, **77**:1–10, 1970.)

table 30·2 CONTINUED

LEG RECOIL: With the infant supine, the hips and knees are fully flexed for 5 s, then extended by traction on the feet, and released. A maximal response is one of full flexion of the hips and knees (score 2). A partial flexion scores 1, and minimal or no movement scores 0.

POPLITEAL ANGLE: With the infant supine and his pelvis flat on the examining couch, the thigh is held in the knee-chest position by the examiner's left index finger and thumb supporting the knee. The leg is then extended by gentle pressure from the examiner's right index finger behind the ankle and the popliteal angle is measured.

HEEL-TO-EAR MANEUVER: With the baby supine, draw the baby's foot as near to the head as it will go without forcing it. Observe the distance between the foot and the head as well as the degree of extension at the knee. Grade according to diagram. Note that the knee is left free and may draw down alongside the abdomen.

SCARF SIGN: With the baby supine, take the infant's hand and try to put it around the neck and as far posteriorly as possible around the opposite shoulder. Assist this maneuver by lifting the elbow across the body. See how far the elbow will go across, and grade according to illustrations. Score zero—elbow reaches opposite axillary line; 1—elbow between midline and opposite axillary line; 2—elbow reaches midline; 3—elbow will not reach midline (Fig. 30·5D).

HEAD LAG: With the baby lying supine, grasp the hands (or the arms if the infant is very small) and pull him slowly toward the sitting position. Observe the position of the head in relation to the trunk, and grade accordingly. In a small infant the head may initially be supported by one hand. Score zero—complete lag; 1—partial head control; 2—able to maintain head in line with body; 3—brings head anterior to body.

VENTRAL SUSPENSION: The infant is suspended in the prone position, with examiner's hand under the infant's chest (one hand in a small infant, two in a large infant). Observe the degree of extension of the back and the amount of flexion of the arms and legs. Also note the relation of the head to the trunk. Grade according to diagrams (Fig. 30·5E). If score differs on the two sides, take the mean.

Source: From Dubowitz et al. (5).

table 30-3
SCORING SYSTEM FOR EXTERNAL CRITERIA

EXTERNAL	SCORE*				
SIGN	0	1	2	3	4
Edema	Obvious edema of hands and feet; pitting over tibia	No obvious edema of hands and feet; pitting over tibia	No edema		
Skin texture	Very thin, gelatinous	Thin and smooth	Smooth; medium thickness. Rash or superficial peeling	Slight thickening	Thick and parchment-like; superficial or deep cracking
Skin color	Dark red	Uniformly pink	Pale pink; variable over body	Pale; only pink over ears, lips, palms, or soles	
Skin opacity (trunk)	Numerous veins and venules clearly seen, especially over abdomen	Veins and tributaries seen	A few large vessels clearly seen over abdomen	A few large vessels seen indistinctly over abdomen	No blood vessels seen
Lanugo (over back)	No lanugo	Abundant; long and thick over lower part of back	Hair thinning	Small amount of lanugo and bald areas	At least half of back devoid of lanugo
Plantar creases	No skin creases	Faint red marks over anterior half of sole	Definite red marks over > anterior half; indentations over < anterior third	Indentations over > anterior third	Definite deep indentations over > anterior third

Nipple formation	Nipple barely visible; no areola	Nipple well defined; areola smooth and flat, diameter < 0.75 cm	Areola stippled, edge not raised, diameter < 0.75 cm	Areola stippled, edge raised diameter < 0.75 cm
Breast size	No breast tissue palpable	Breast tissue on one or both sides, 0.5 cm diameter	Breast tissue both sides; one or both 0.5–1.0 cm	Breast tissue both sides; one or both <1 cm
Ear form	Pinna flat and shapeless, little or no incurving of edge	Incurving of part of edge of pinna	Partial incurving of whole of upper pinna	Well-defined incurving of whole of upper pinna
Ear firmness	Pinna soft, easily folded, no recoil	Pinna soft, easily folded, slow recoil	Cartilage to edge of pinna, but soft in places, ready recoil	Pinna firm, cartilage to edge; instant recoil
Genitals: Male	Neither testis in scrotum	At least one testis high in scrotum	At least one testis right down	
Female (with hips half abducted)	Labia majora widely separated, labia minora protruding	Labia majora completely cover labia minora		

Source: Adapted from Farr and Associates, *Developmental Medicine and Child Neurology*, **8**:507, 1966. Reproduced from Dubowitz (5).

*If score differs on two sides, take the mean.

score of 50 corresponds to a gestational age of 38 weeks; a score of 20 corresponds to 30 gestational weeks.

It is important that the neonatal nurse be familiar with these signs and characteristics. Experience will permit her to complete the whole procedure in approximately 10 min. If possible, the assessment should be made within 24 h after delivery. Using this system, the estimated gestational age is reported to be accurate within 2 weeks.

physiologic handicaps

RESPIRATORY ADJUSTMENTS

Crucial to the baby's survival is the adjustment of his vital physiologic systems to extrauterine life. The immediate difficulty that the preterm infant encounters is maintaining respirations. By the twenty-seventh week of life, an infant's lungs may be able to function to sustain life (see Chap. 28). However, many factors contribute to impair respirations in these infants with a precarious hold on life—instability of the rib cage, weak chest muscles, soft and collapsible bronchi, incomplete development of alveoli and capillary blood supply, small surface area for the exchange of gases, and inadequate production of surfactant. The high incidence of respiratory distress syndrome in preterm infants is related to this last factor. Aspiration resulting from absent or poor gag or cough reflexes may further embarrass respirations. The nurse must be alert for signs of respiratory distress, which are elaborated on later in the chapter.

TEMPERATURE ADJUSTMENT

Maintaining stability of body temperature is extremely difficult for the preterm infant. Because of weak, underdeveloped muscles and inactivity, the baby cannot produce adequate heat. Excessive loss of heat results from the infant's large surface skin area in relation to body weight, and the inadequate supply of fat needed for heat production and insulation.

Since lipid accumulation occurs late in gestation, the preterm infant suffers from insufficient stores of fat in both white and brown adipose tissues. For the mature neonate, white adipose tissue in the subcutaneous areas not only provides energy, but also serves as an insulation against heat loss. Brown adipose tissue, which is unique to the neonate, possesses a greater thermogenic activity than ordinary fat. This mechanism of increased heat production, termed *non-shivering thermogenesis*, is particularly effective during periods of cold stress. Brown fat is located around the heart, kidneys, adrenals, and great vessels, and superficially is deposited around the neck, between the scapula, and behind the sternum. Although starvation reduces the stores of white fat, and cold stress depletes the reserves of brown fat, there is probably some overlap of function. In the normal maturing infant, the progressive replacement of brown with white adipose tissue approximates the development of the ability to shiver.

The preterm infant is incapable of adjusting to environmental changes. His temperature-regulating center in the brain is immature. He cannot shiver in response to cold stress; nor can he perspire, so that his entire body becomes red and flushed when overheated. Problems related to overheating infants have only recently received attention. Perlstein and coworkers (6) reported on the frequent occurrence of apneic spells in premature infants kept in incubators where automatically controlled heating suddenly increased the ambient temperatures.

In order to enable the preterm infant to stabilize his temperature with minimal effort, a controlled environment must be provided through the use of an incubator. Environmental temperature control is intended to maintain the infant's metabolism at the lowest effective rate. Cold stress increases the baby's metabolic rate, necessitating increased oxygen consumption. If thermal stress remains unchecked, glycogen is broken down and the preterm infant's very limited stores are rapidly consumed, resulting in hypoglycemia. This anaerobic breakdown of glycogen also results in an increased production of lactic acid, contributing to metabolic acidosis. *Critical* temperature refers to that temperature below which the infant's metabolic rate and oxygen consumption will increase in an effort to raise body temperature. Should the baby's temperature drop below this critical point, his survival will be impaired by a host of metabolic difficulties, including oxygen deprivation, depletion of glycogen stores, reduced blood glucose level, and metabolic acidosis.

NUTRITIONAL ADJUSTMENT

Preterm infants present many feeding and nutritional problems. The sucking and swallowing reflexes are often absent or weak, necessitating gavage feeding, and contributing to the easy aspiration of fluids. Storage of glycogen is affected by the immaturity of the liver and the small muscle mass. Small, frequent feedings are essential in order to compensate for the very small stomach capacity, and to prevent hypoglycemia. Digestion and absorption are impeded by low gastric acidity, an immature enzyme system, and incomplete absorption of nutrients such as fats and vitamins.

The rapid growth rate of these infants conflicts with the anatomic and physiologic handicaps that interfere with nutrition. Distension often results from sluggish peristaltic activity. Vomiting and regurgitation are frequently encountered as a result of the small stomach capacity and the weak cardiac sphincter in the stomach (Fig. 30·8).

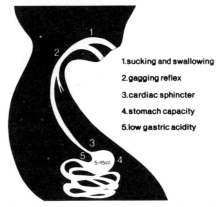

1. sucking and swallowing
2. gagging reflex
3. cardiac sphincter
4. stomach capacity
5. low gastric acidity

fig. 30·8 Anatomic and physiologic handicaps interfere with nutrition in the small infant. (*From E. J. Dickason and A. Ritz,* Care of the Normal Premature Infant, *McGraw-Hill Book Company, New York, 1970.*)

care of the high-risk infant in neonatal intensive care centers

In the last decade a revolution has occurred in the care of babies at high risk. A greater understanding of the pathophysiology of the neonate, along with advances in electronics and biochemistry, has drastically altered the complexity of ideal care. The practices of isolation, minimal handling, delayed feeding, and limited oxygen therapy have yielded to more aggressive approaches.

Neonatal specialists in the fields of medicine and nursing have emerged to care for these babies. The demands made on the nurse caring for these infants are great. She must be extremely knowledgeable in perinatology, intensely committed, able to work under stress, and skilled in executing all activities with great attention to detail. Nursing responsibilities include (1) close observation; (2) physical care of the infant; and (3) the use and management of incubators, oxygen and resuscitative equipment, respirators, monitors, infusion pumps, radiant heaters, and phototherapy lamps. Obviously, providing the highest quality of nursing care requires specialized education and experience. Presently, educational programs are being offered by many neonatal intensive care centers on an in-service basis.

Since there is sufficient evidence to show that mortality rates decrease when infants at high risk are cared for in intensive care units, it is now recommended that infants in need be given this advantage. It is unrealistic to expect all hospitals to have the facilities, equipment, and specially trained personnel to establish this type of service. The ultimate solution is to have special care units operate as regional centers. Many hospitals and communities have moved in this direction, and offer excellent transport services to infants in jeopardy requiring specialized care.

IMMEDIATE CARE IN THE DELIVERY ROOM

The first minutes of life are critical for the preterm infant, and survival and prognosis depend upon the quality of early treatment. It is essential that a physician and nurse adept in the care of prematures be on hand to devote complete attention to the baby. It is the nurse's responsibility to ensure that all equipment needed in caring for the infant is available and in good working condition.

As soon as the infant is delivered, the physician holds the head down and suctions the nostrils and oropharynx with a bulb syringe. Every effort must be made to avoid chilling the baby, since cold stress complicates birth asphyxia and depletes the stores of fat and glycogen. Heat loss occurs from exposure to cool ambient temperature, and from evaporation of amniotic fluid on the baby's skin. The baby should be dried immediately with a warm towel, wrapped in a warm blanket, and placed in a warm incubator. Examination of the infant, eye treatment, and identification can all be done after the infant has been placed in the incubator. Babies subjected to cold stress often have unrecorded temperatures, and develop cya-

nosis and shock. Asphyxia occurs more often in the premature than in the full-term infant, and resuscitation procedures should be performed under a radiant heat lamp.

The nurse should appreciate that the Apgar score not only identifies high-risk infants but also provides a widely understood quantitative evaluation of the infant's condition. This scoring system should be used to evaluate the status of the infant at 1 and 5 min after delivery. The procedure has proved most accurate when performed by an impartial nurse or physician not involved in the delivery.

As soon as possible, the infant should be transported to the intensive care nursery in an incubator equipped with a battery-operated heat source (Fig. 30-9). Hospitals not equipped to offer specialized services should make immediate arrangements for transfer of the infant to an appropriate institution. Until transfer is accomplished, efforts are directed at maintaining the infant's respirations and applying external heat. Modern transport facilities are equipped to provide the infant with heat, oxygen, intravenous infusions, and drug therapy (Fig. 30·10).

ADMISSION TO THE INTENSIVE CARE NURSERY

Since the nursery personnel are generally notified that a patient is in premature labor or that a baby is arriving via transport service, they have the advantage of being prepared for the infant's arrival. A clean incubator must be prepared, heated, and humidified. The incubator is heated to a temperature of between 32.8 to 33.8°C (91 to 93°F), and the relative humidity set at approximately 60 to 85 percent. The incubator temperature is adjusted according to the needs of the baby. The nurse must have all items and equipment needed to care for the infant at hand; i.e., linen, measuring tape, a sling and scale,

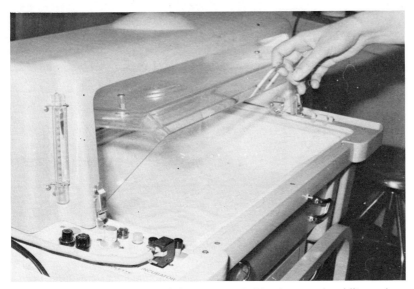

fig. 30·9 Portable incubator with battery-operated heat source, humidity, and oxygen supply to transport infant from delivery room to intensive care nursery. (*Courtesy of Booth Memorial Medical Center, Flushing, N.Y.*)

thermometer and tape to apply the electrode if an automatically controlled machine is used, suction apparatus, resuscitative tray, and intravenous equipment. The supply of oxygen must be checked, and tubing available to deliver it to the incubator.

The major responsibilities of the nurse regarding admission of the infant to the nursery are summarized below.

1. Notify the pediatrician of the infant's arrival.
2. Before removing the infant from the transport carrier, check the oxygen concentration and the baby's temperature.
3. Transfer the infant to the prepared incubator.
4. Verify the identification of the baby with the transport or delivery room nurse. Ensure that:
   a. The infant has been properly tagged and foot-printed.
   b. The birth record is available and complete.
   c. The name of the hospital sending the infant, as well as the name, address, and telephone number of the mother, are available.
   d. Correct identification of the infant is marked on his incubator, chart, etc.
5. Check to see that eye prophylaxsis and vitamin K_1 were administered. (Most hospitals have a policy of administering 1 mg vitamin K_1 to the infant in the delivery room or nursery to prevent hypoprothrombinemia. It is now known that large doses given to the newborn or to the mother at term may result in hyperbilirubinemia and kernicterus.)
6. Weigh the infant in a sling inside the incubator (Fig. 30·11). The scale must be set to compensate for the weight of the empty hammock.
7. If an automatically controlled incubator is used, attach the electrode to the infant's skin (Fig. 30·4).
8. Keep the infant nude so that he may be

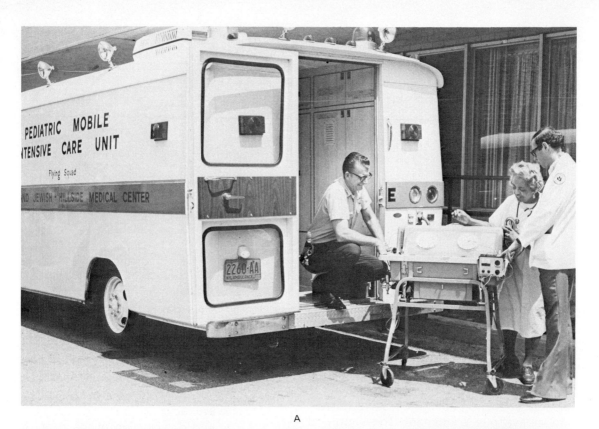

A

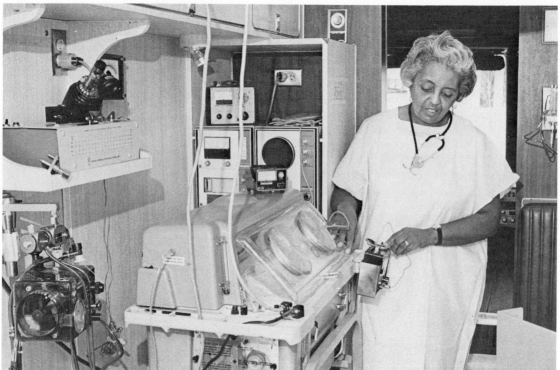

B

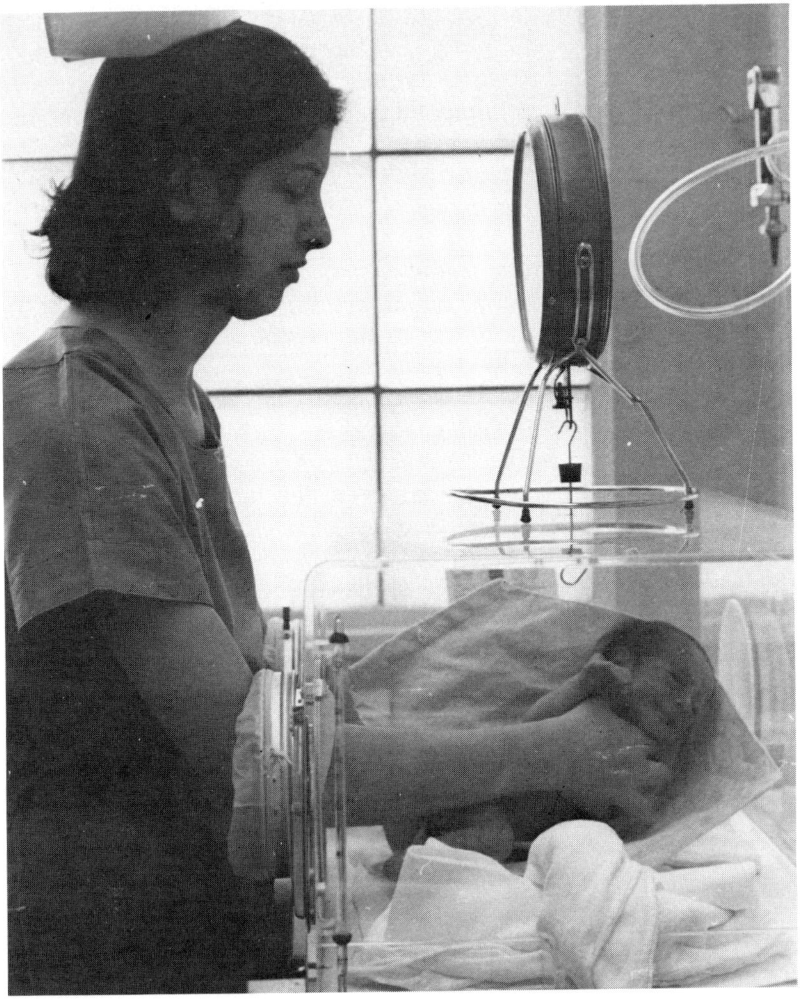

fig. 30·11 Weighing infant in a sling inside the incubator.

carefully observed in regard to the following:

a. Excess secretions which require removal by suctioning

b. Rate and type of respirations, and signs of respiratory distress

c. Color—particularly ashen appearance or pallor, cyanosis, and jaundice

d. Activity and cry

9. Investigate the maternal history for early rupture of the membranes, traumatic delivery, diabetes, infection, sterility of delivery—all of which may serve as clues in identifying an infant in serious jeopardy.

10. Assist the physician with the physical examination. (If no obvious problems were observed in the delivery room, a thorough and careful examination should be delayed until the infant's temperature is stabilized.)

11. If possible, all specialized procedures performed on the infant should be done in the incubator. If the baby must be

fig. 30·10 Transport ambulance equipped with every possible type of assistance for the small infant during the trip from a community hospital to the regional neo- natal intensive care unit. (*Courtesy of the Long Island Jewish–Hillside Medical Center, N.Y., photographed by Herbert Bennett.*)

removed in order to receive treatment, the infant should be cared for on a table warmed by an overhead heater.

12. Record all pertinent information on the baby's chart.

CONTROL OF THE INFANT'S ENVIRONMENT

Temperature Incubators range from those offering only such features as heat and humidity control to sophisticated machines which provide a totally controlled environment for the infant. Small preterm infants generally require incubators constructed to provide a filtered circulation of air, optimal *ambient* (surrounding) temperature, desirable oxygen and humidity concentrations, and an ingress through portholes so that the baby can be cared for in the incubator. Since the baby remains naked in the incubator, very close observation is possible.

Despite the high temperature of air in the incubator, radiant heat loss will occur in the infant if the incubator walls become cold. Therefore, incubators should not be placed near cold windows or in the direct path of cool air. Generally, the nurse can make a judgment in this regard simply by feeling the outside of the incubator walls. Ideally, the temperature of the walls should not be more than 2°C (3.5°F) below the temperature of incubator air, but such precision would require electronic testing.

Incubators are often livesaving instruments for infants whose thermal stability is precarious. The thermal state of the infant is indicated by his temperature, and the machine is either manually or automatically adjusted to regulate the environmental temperature in accordance with the baby's needs.

If the machine is manually controlled, axillary temperature readings are taken. However, the very first reading on admission should be taken rectally to check the patency of the anus. The incubator thermometer reading should be noted before opening the portholes to take the baby's reading. In preterm infants, axillary temperature readings have been found dependable, and the thermometer should be held in place for 1 to 3 min. The infant's axillary temperature readings should be between 36.5 to 37°C (97.8 to 98.6°F). Significant changes in the infant's temperature require that the nurse adjust the incubator temperature by gradually raising or lowering the thermostat. The infant's temperature should be checked every $1/2$ to 1 h until stabilized. It is generally recorded at 3- to 4-h intervals thereafter. The nurse should remember, however, that once the baby's temperature is stabilized, the incubator temperature dial should not be changed. After stabilization, a change in the baby's temperature may be a sign of disease, and this sign could be confused by constant changes in the incubator temperature.

Many incubators are equipped with automatically controlled regulators that respond to a temperature *thermistor probe* which is taped to the baby's skin—generally on the abdomen. The control is set to maintain the skin temperature at the desired level—about 36.1 to 37.2°C (97 to 99°F). Through a control mechanism, the incubator is regulated to increase or reduce heat output in accordance with the predetermined setting. Paper tape is usually placed under the probe to protect the skin, and over it to secure proper placement. If the baby is placed in a prone position with the abdominal probe attached, erroneously high readings will be registered by the thermistor. The machine will respond to the high probe reading although the infant's skin temperature may be sufficiently low to require increased heat output.

For all infants, the critical temperature is higher during the first 2 days of life. Listed below are the ranges of incubator temperatures generally required by infants during the first 2 days and thereafter in relation to weight (Table 30·4).

table 30·4

DESIRABLE TEMPERATURE RANGES OF INCUBATOR

	TEMPERATURE RANGE	
INFANT'S WEIGHT	DAYS 1 AND 2	THEREAFTER
−1500 Gm	33.8–35°C (93–95°F)	32.8–33.8°C (91–93°F)
1500–2500 Gm	32.8–33.8°C (91–93°F)	31.7–32.8°C (89–91°F)
2500 Gm+	32–33°C (89.6–91.4°F)	31.1–32°C (88–89.6°F)

Humidity The relative humditiy should be approximately 85 percent during the first 2 days, and should then be reduced to about 60 percent. A *hygrometer* can be used to check humidity in the incubator. Studies indicate that a humidified atmosphere helps the baby to maintain body temperature, thus reducing oxygen consumption. When humidity is low, loss of heat through evaporation is increased.

Humidity is always administered with oxygen or when high incubator temperatures are used in order to prevent drying of the mucous membranes and dehydration. The nurse must ensure that the incubator humidifier is maintained at a high water level; that the chamber is filled with distilled water to prevent rusting; and that either a disinfectant is added to the water or sterile water is used to prevent bacterial growth. The humidified chamber should be drained, cleaned, and refilled daily.

Mist is not used because it has been found to cause maceration of the infant's skin, thereby increasing the possibility of infection.

MAINTENANCE OF ADEQUATE RESPIRATION

Respiratory Distress One of the major problems encountered by preterm infants is respiratory distress. Normally, the respiratory pattern of such infants is one of diaphragmatic breathing, fluctuations of respiratory rates, and sporadic episodes of apnea lasting up to 10 s—*periodic breathing* (7). Periodic breathing does not result in generalized cyanosis and should not be confused with true apneic episodes. Generalized cyanosis is indicative of severe distress.

The nurse must be constantly alert for indications of respiratory distress. She is in the best position to recognize that the baby is having difficulty, and is also an excellent judge of the effectiveness of therapy. A baby suffering from air hunger usually exhibits a number of the following abnormal signs. The respiratory rate is sustained in excess of 50 to 60 per minute, and cyanosis may become evident. In some cases, the infant appears ashen or pale. Flaring of the nostrils during inspiration is also indicative of difficulty.

Retraction of the chest during inspiration results from an obstruction to the flow of air into the lungs which may occur at any point in the respiratory tract. Since the lungs do not inflate adequately during inspiration, the pressure in the pleural space between the chest wall and the unexpanded lungs remain negative. The flexible chest wall is therefore pulled inward to fill the space, resulting in retraction of the chest. The thoracic wall may retract between the ribs (intercostal), below the ribs (subcostal), beneath the sternum (substernal), or above the clavicles. In severe distress, there is a simultaneous rising of the abdomen with depression of the chest—a pattern termed *see-saw* breathing.

A sigh or grunt on expiration is a clear sign of distress. By temporarily closing the glottis, the baby attempts to improve alveolar expansion by obstructing the outflow of air. The "back pressure" created increases functional residual capacity, and grunting infants are capable of significantly increasing their arterial oxygen saturation.

Suctioning In the preterm infant, obstruction of the airway often results from the accumulation of mucus and secretions in the mouth and pharynx, or from regurgitation of stomach contents. In such circumstances, suctioning becomes a lifesaving technique.

Suctioning can be accomplished with a rubber bulb syringe, but this method is limited in use since the syringe cannot be passed beyond the baby's pharynx if deeper suction is necessary, Generally, aspiration is performed with the use of a catheter attached to a suction source. The suction may be provided by the operator's mouth on a mucus trap type of apparatus or by a machine. Many pediatricians feel mechanical suction is too traumatic for the baby.

Depending upon the size of the infant, a No. 8 or 10 soft rubber French or plastic catheter is lubricated with sterile water and introduced through the infant's nose or mouth. It is advanced into the oropharynx or trachea, and then suction is applied while the catheter is slowly rotated and withdrawn.

The baby should be properly positioned during the procedure. He should be supine with the head lowered to facilitate drainage, and the neck slightly hyperextended to straighten the airway and bring the tongue forward to clear the posterior pharyngeal wall.

If suctioning is not done briefly and gently, it can result in trauma and edema of the tissues, increased production of mucus, and laryngeal spasm. It should be performed in less than 1 min, since air, as well as secretions, is aspirated, which could exaggerate the distress of the infant. There is always danger of stimulating the vagus nerve, resulting in bradycardia. If possible, suctioning should not be done after feedings, since it frequently stimulates the gag reflex. To avoid the danger of introducing infection, a new catheter must be used whenever the infant requires suctioning (Fig. 30-12).

Problems Involved in the Use of Oxygen Therapy During the 1940s, an intensive search took place to determine the cause of the high incidence of retinopathy (retrolental fibroplasia) in premature infants resulting in complete or partial blindness. By the early 1950s, valid evidence was presented showing hyperoxemia to be the primary etiologic factor. An era followed when oxygen concentrations were limited to 40 percent—even in the presence of cyanosis. Since then the restrictive policies governing the administration of oxygen have been held accountable for an increased mortality rate in infants in severe respiratory distress, as well as an increased morbidity due to brain damage and cerebral palsy. DeLeon and coworkers (8) report that because of the more liberal use of oxygen to salvage profoundly ill babies, a resurgence of retrolental fibroplasia has occurred. Obviously, the problem posed in treating infants requiring oxygen therapy is how to avoid both dangers.

In administering oxygen to sick infants, the critical factor in preventing damage to both the brain and the eyes is the partial pressure of oxygen in the arterial blood. But as yet, the exact level above which damage to the eyes will occur, or below which brain damage will result, is not known. Cavanaugh (9) suggests that it would probably be *ideal* to keep arterial oxygen concentrations between 65 to 85 mmHg. This would require a method of constantly monitoring blood gases which has not been perfected as yet.

Significance of Arterial Blood Gases In order to administer oxygen in proper dosage,

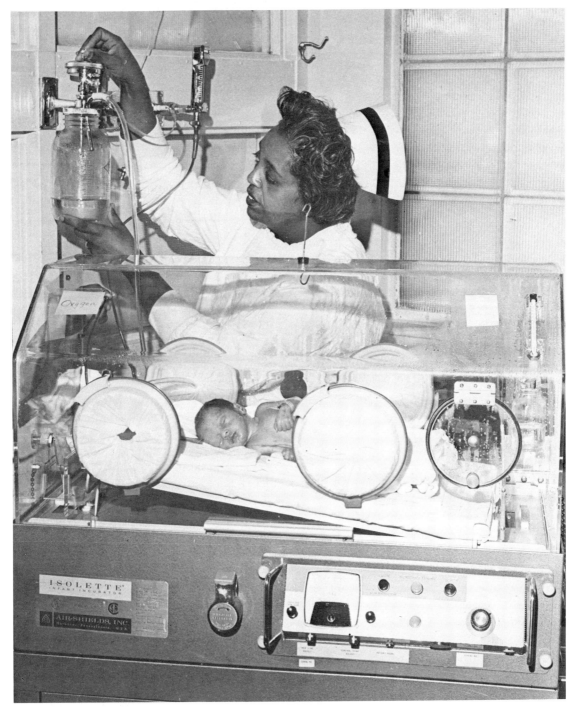

fig. 30·12 Setting up suction. Note high humidity level as indicated by condensation on the walls of the isolette. Note the infant's position. (*Photograph, courtesy of the Long Island Jewish–Hillside Medical Center, New York.*)

measurements of the infant's arterial oxygen tension must be made. The differences in the partial pressures of gases determine the direction in which these gases move—flowing from a higher pressure to a lower one. The partial pressures of oxygen and carbon dioxide are expressed as P_{O_2} and P_{CO_2} respectively. Although the P_{O_2} measures only the oxygen in solution, it generally accurately reflects the oxygen saturation of hemoglobin. In the adult, blood is almost 100 percent saturated at a P_{O_2} of between 90 to 100 mmHg, whereas in the newborn the P_{O_2} ranges between 60 to 100 mmHg.

In the infant, cyanosis does not usually occur until the P_{O_2} falls below 50 mmHg, and in the very small baby it may not appear until it falls below 32 to 42 mmHg. Therefore, difficulties often exist before cyanosis is evident, because adverse physiologic changes occur in the infant when the arterial P_{O_2} falls below 50 mmHg. Recognizing that damage occurs when the P_{O_2} falls below 50 mmHg and that levels over 100 mmHg often result in blindness and damage to the lungs, it is currently considered safe and effective to give sufficient oxygen to maintain the infant's arterial P_{O_2} between 50 to 100 mmHg. Serial determinations of arterial P_{O_2} are made to accomplish this.

LABORATORY DATA The nurse must be able to interpret the results of the blood gas determinations made on the infant. Table 30·5 outlines the normal blood gas and pH values for the infant.

In severe respiratory distress resulting from hyaline membrane disease, the characteristic biochemical abnormalities are *hypoxemia, hypercapnia,* and *acidosis.* The arterial blood gases and pH determinations found in severely ill infants are as follows:

Hypoxemia	P_{O_2} falls below 40 mmHg (normal lower limit: 50 mmHg)
Hypercapnia	P_{CO_2} *rises over 65 mm Hg (normal upper limit: 45 mmHg)*
Acidosis	pH generally below 7.15

SAMPLING SITES FOR BLOOD GAS DETERMINATIONS P_{O_2} determinations can be made only on arterial samples; capillary samples are useless for this purpose. During the first few days of life arterial blood is usually taken from an umbilical artery catheter. After the catheter is withdrawn the temporal, radial, or brachial arteries are used but separate punctures are required for each determination (Fig. 30·13).

Blood samples obtained from an indwelling umbilical *vein* catheter cannot be used to assess arterial oxygen tension but are useful for P_{CO_2} and pH determinations. The pH of

table 30·5
DEFINITIONS OF pH AND BLOOD GASES AND NORMAL VALUES

	TEST	NORMAL BLOOD GAS AND pH VALUES IN INFANT
pH	A measure of the hydrogen ion concentration	7.35–7.45
P_{CO_2}	Represents the partial pressure of carbon dioxide dissolved in plasma	30–37 mmHg
P_{O_2}	Represents the partial pressure of oxygen	60–100mmHg
HCO_3	A measure of plasma bicarbonate	20–25 mEq/l

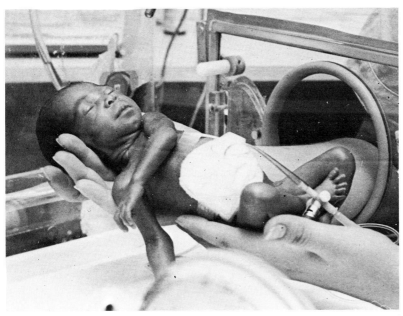

fig. 30·13 Umbilical line into one of the arteries for sequential blood gas determinations. (*Photograph by M. M. Miyato; courtesy of the Long Island Jewish–Hillside Medical Center, New York.*)

central venous blood is 0.02 to 0.03 unit lower than arterial blood; the P_{CO_2} is 5 to 6 mmHg higher.

Many centers use umbilical artery catheters for parenteral fluid administration as well as for sampling arterial blood. Complications from indwelling catheters include thromboses, emboli, hemorrhage, and infection.

Optimal Oxygen Therapy Once the need for oxygen therapy has been established, frequent blood gas determinations should be used as a guide to ambient oxygen concentrations. Infants requiring continuous oxygen therapy for protracted periods of time should be cared for in a neonatal center equipped with adequate facilities and specially trained personnel. The American Academy of Pediatrics has revised its recommendations for the use of oxygen in treating newborns (10).

Oxygen concentrations should be constantly monitored and aimed at maintaining the baby's arterial oxygen tension between 50 and 100 mmHg. The frequency of P_{O_2} determinations depends upon the condition of the infant. Samples may be required as often as every 15 min or every 6 to 8 h. Carbon dioxide tension and pH are always determined on the same blood sample.

Oxygen should always be ordered in percent concentration, not by flow rate. A variety of machines are in use which *constantly* monitor concentrations (Fig. 30·14). If such an analyzer is not available, the concentration of inspired oxygen must be measured with a conventional analyzer at least every 4 to 8 h, and at the time specimens are taken for blood gas determinations.

The nurse must keep a detailed record of the serial determinations made in reference to the percent of oxygen provided. Remember that the ultimate measure of optimal oxygen therapy is the arterial P_{O_2}.

CLINICAL GUIDE TO OXYGEN THERAPY   It is generally understood and widely practiced

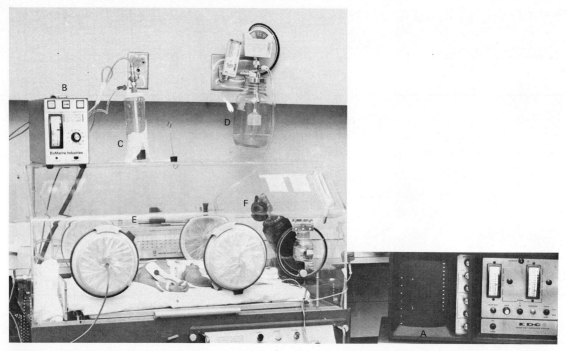

fig. 30·14 Infant with cardiac and respiratory monitoring. Attached are: A respiratory and cardiac monitor; B oxygen regulator; C oxygen humidifier (nebulizer); D wall suction; E electric infusion pump; F Ambu bag. (*Photograph, courtesy of the Long Island Jewish–Hillside Medical Center, New York.*)

that the infant who becomes cyanotic must be given enough oxygen to abolish the cyanosis. If facilities are not available for blood gas determinations, the following method has been suggested as a practical clinical guide for estimating the appropriate concentrations of inspired oxygen. The intent here is to minimize the incidence of hyperoxemia. Oxygen concentration is gradually lowered by no more than 10 percent at a time—until the infant appears slightly cyanotic. The concentration is then maintained at a 10 percent higher level. For example, if cyanosis appears at 40 percent, the concentration is kept at a 50 percent level.

REDUCING AMBIENT OXYGEN CONCENTRATION Except in cases where oxygen therapy is maintained for only a few hours, abruptly lowering concentrations is dangerous—often resulting in cyanosis and respiratory col-lapse. The longer the therapy, the longer the weaning period. Generally, a decrease of 10 percent every 3 to 4 h is well tolerated. However, a decrease of 3 to 5 percent every few hours may be necessary for infants who have received oxygen for over a week.

OXYGEN TOXICITY As previously mentioned, retrolental fibroplasia is a disease directly related to excessive exposure to oxygen. It occurs mainly in preterm infants; the shorter the infant's gestational age, the greater his vulnerability. The only change observed during the period of oxygen therapy is retinal vasospasm. Within 1 month or more following the termination of treatment with oxygen, the retinal vessels dilate and proliferate, causing edema. Until this point, the process may cease, leaving slight or no resultant visual disturbance. However, if retinal detachment and scarring develop, blindness results.

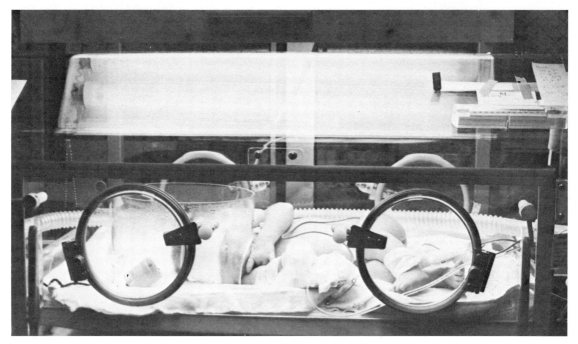

fig. 30·15 Infant with plastic hood for concentrated delivery of oxygen and humidity. The infant is under a light for treatment of bilirubin, and therefore has bandaged eyes. Note restraints and intravenous infusion into an arm vein. (*Photograph by Mary Olsen.*)

Injury to the lungs may also result from hyperoxemia. The damage is characterized by thickening of the alveolar and vascular tissues, fibrosis, and atelectasis. As a result, diffusion of oxygen across the lungs is impaired. The abnormal radiologic appearance of the lungs does not disappear until several months after oxygen therapy has been discontinued.

METHODS OF OXYGEN ADMINISTRATION

1. *Incubator:* Constant delivery of concentrations beyond 60 to 70 percent cannot be ensured in incubators. Leakage often occurs, and ambient concentrations drop rapidly when the portholes are open.
2. *Plastic head hood:* The hood should be used if concentrations must exceed 40 to 50 percent, or if the infant must be treated on an open table supplied with radiant heat from an overhead source (Fig. 30·15).

The oxygen delivered to the hood must be humidified, and should be warmed to about 34°C (93.2°F).
3. *Intermittent mask and bag therapy:* This method may be used in situations of mild distress where prolonged assistance is not required. It has also been used as an alternate approach to respiratory therapy for infants in severe respiratory distress. It is particularly appropriate for hospitals that do not have respirator programs which require special equipment and experienced personnel.

Therapy is given periodically, depending upon the needs of the infant—e.g., 10 min out of every 30. Blood gas determinations should be made before and after treatment, and are used as a guide to the frequency of baggings and oxygen requirements of the baby.

The mask must be held tightly over the

face, avoiding the eyes as well as excessive pressure to prevent trauma. Gastric distension is prevented by passing a nasogastric tube with the free end left open. Nurses should be taught the procedure with the use of an infant simulator. The major complication is pneumothorax (Fig. 30·16).

4. *Respirator therapy:* Mechanically assisted ventilation is reserved for babies in severe distress, especially those with hyaline membrane disease. Respiratory therapy is a formidable undertaking to be used only in properly manned and equipped centers. The technical problems encountered are numerous. With the exception of negative-pressure respirators, an endotracheal tube must be inserted and

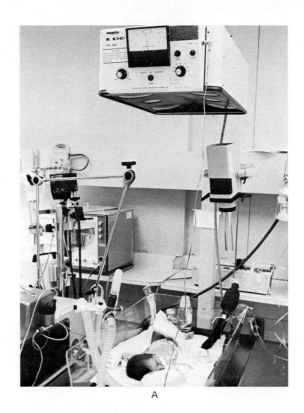

fig. 30·16 Radiant heat crib, for infant receiving frequent therapy, continuous monitoring, and close observation. (*Courtesy of the Long Island Jewish— Hillside Medical Center, N.Y. Photograph by Herbert Bennett.*)

A

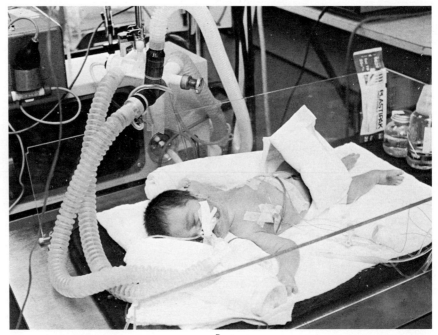

B

maintained in proper position. Should it slip forward into the trachea, it may enter the right main-stem bronchus and occlude the left one—leaving the left lung unaerated. Changes in lung compliance may necessitate adjustments in pressure and volume settings. The oxygen delivered to the baby must be humidified. It is essential that blood gases and pH be monitored at frequent intervals. Complications of respirator therapy include blockage of the endotracheal tube, pneumothorax, and infection.

The care of a baby receiving such treatment is a challenge, and nursing responsibilities consist of regulating the respirator, observing the condition of the infant, maintaining bronchial toilet, suctioning the tracheal tube hourly or as frequently as is necessary, rotating the infant's position, and assisting with the collection of blood specimens.

The two major types of respirator used are:

1. *Positive-pressure respirator.* A specific volume of tidal air is delivered to the lungs under restricted pressure via an endotracheal tube. The respirator is adjusted to permit the infant to trigger the machine even though his inspiratory efforts are very weak. If the infant fails to trigger it, automatic cycling occurs.
2. *Negative-pressure respirator* (tank respirator). The infant's body from the neck down is enclosed in a chamber intermittently surrounded by negative pressure, resulting in the movement of gas into and out of the lungs. A motor-driven vacuum connected to the body compartment produces the negative pressure. The body compartment is separated from the head compartment by an iris diaphragm that fits snugly around the baby's neck. The ambient oxygen concentration is controlled in the head chamber.

5. *Continuous Positive Airway Pressure* (CPAP): In the future, continuous positive airway pressure therapy may reduce the need for mechanical respirators. However, this method of therapy requires that the infant be able to breathe spontaneously. The intent of CPAP is to maintain pressures above zero in the lungs even at the end of expiration, thereby forcing retention of air and preventing alveolar collapse. Studies indicate that arterial P_{O_2} increases with this type of therapy.

The treatment is carried out by delivering specific concentrations of oxygen through an endotracheal tube. The gas expired by the infant passes through an outflow system that is partially occluded by a screw clamp to maintain end-expiratory pressures above zero. The pressure can be regulated by the degree of occlusion exerted by the screw clamp. An aneroid manometer continuously registers the pressure within the system. At first, the pressure may be set as high as 12 mmHg, but it is gradually lowered over a period of several days.

NUTRITIONAL REQUIREMENTS AND FEEDING

The optimal requirements of the low-birthweight infant are not known. Recent evidence indicates that there is a critical period of brain growth in the newborn, and studies suggest that early postnatal malnutrition may permanently impair this growth. Much controversy exists regarding all aspects of feeding premature infants; i.e., when to start, nutritive requirements, safest method, strength of formula, etc. At present, early feedings (oral or intravenous) are preferred by most practitioners.

Since the preterm's growth rate parallels fetal growth, both his protein and caloric needs are higher than those of the infant born at term.

The type and amount of fat to be given are also in question. Since the premature baby tends to absorb fats poorly, most formulas used have a low fat content. Yet, fatty acids are apparently essential and efficiently absorbed, and a deficiency may result in loose stools and skin lesions.

The premature's rapid growth and low antenatal storage of vitamins can result in significant deficiencies. The administration of multivitamin preparations is begun very early. These preparations usually contain vitamins A, C, D, E, and a number of the B group. Vitamins are given just before the bottle feeding. If the baby cannot suck on a dropper, or is being tube-fed, the vitamins are added to the formula. Some nurseries use formulas prepared with vitamins added so that additional supplements are not necessary. At about the third week of life, the infant is given iron to compensate for the depletion of fetal stores and to support his rapid growth.

The physician prescribes the formula and the amount according to the baby's condition. At first he is given sterile water or a glucose solution. As his condition permits, he progresses to diluted and then full-strength formula. A variety of recommended feedings include breast milk, skimmed milk, evaporated milk, and proprietary formulas.

Because of the infant's small stomach capacity, overfeeding can result in regurgitation or vomiting followed by aspiration, abdominal distension, or respiratory distress. At first, the volume of formula ordered may be as small as 2 to 3 ml. Adjustments are made in accordance with the infant's ability to tolerate larger volumes. Babies who are able to suck on the nipple are fed every 3 h, and tube-fed babies every 1 to 2 h. As the infant matures and approaches 4 lb, he is usually satisfied with feedings every 4 h. If distension is noted, the nurse should bubble the baby before the feeding.

Four basic principles which the nurse must adhere to when feeding the infant include (1) use of sterile equipment, (2) administering the correct amount of formula, (3) conserving the infant's energy, and (4) preventing aspiration of fluid. To avoid disturbing the baby after feeding, all necessary nursing care should be done beforehand.

Methods of Feeding The nipple method is usually used for babies over 1500 Gm who can suck well without tiring. Bottle feeding should not exceed 20 min. A small, soft, cross-cut nipple is generally used. If a nipple with holes is used, the milk should drop slowly when the bottle is inverted. The infant should be held in an upright position, bubbled during and after feeding, and then positioned on his abdomen. He may also be positioned on his left side since this posture facilitates bubbling and helps prevent regurgitation.

GAVAGE The infant is fed through a catheter passed via the mouth and esophagus into the cardiac end of the stomach (Fig. 30·17). Formula is passed through the barrel of a syringe attached to the catheter. Two methods are appropriate for measuring the distance the catheter should be passed. This can be accomplished by extending the tube from the tip of the ear to the tip of the nose to the xiphoid process, or simply be extending it from the bridge of the nose to the xiphoid process. The tube is then marked with tape to ensure that it will be inserted the correct distance. The procedure for gavage feeding is outlined below:

1. Collect all equipment and measure the formula.
2. Place the baby in a dorsal recumbent position.
3. Restrain the infant.
4. Measure and mark the correct distance to pass the catheter. (A No. 8 or 10 French catheter is used, depending upon the size of the infant.)
5. Lubricate the end of the catheter with sterile water.

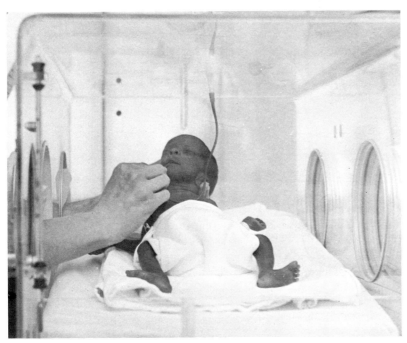

fig. 30·17 Gavage feeding of the preterm infant. (*Courtesy of the Long Island Jewish–Hillside Medical Center, New York.*)

6. Insert the catheter through the infant's mouth. Although the possibility of passing the catheter into the larynx is slight, the nurse always verifies that the tube is properly positioned in the stomach by using one of the following methods:

   a. Insert the end of the catheter into a medicine glass filled with sterile water. Watch for regular bubbling which indicates that the tube is in the trachea.

   b. Flick the baby's heel to stimulate crying. If he cries, the tube is properly positioned.

   c. Gently aspirate for gastric contents.

   d. Insert 0.5 ml air through the tube while listening with a stethoscope for the rush of air as it enters the stomach.

7. Attach the barrel of the syringe to the catheter and administer the premeasured amount of formula by slow gravity flow.

8. Pinch the tube and withdraw it quickly.

(This prevents dripping of the formula from the tube into the pharynx from where it could be easily aspirated.)

9. Hold the baby in a sitting position and bubble him. (Avoid pressure on his stomach.)

10. Position the infant on the abdomen or left side. (The baby should also be placed in a low Fowler's position for 1/2 h after feeding to encourage bubbling and hinder regurgitation.)

During the feeding, the nurse must observe the baby for rapid respirations, retractions, and cyanosis which could indicate the need for a rest period or interruption of the feeding. As the baby matures and his sucking ability improves, he may be alternately gavage- and bottle-fed. If the infant repeatedly sucks on the tube, it may indicate that he is ready for nipple feedings.

INDWELLING NASOGASTRIC TUBE A plastic

tube is passed through the nostril into the stomach, and left in place for a variable length of time. The formula is administered through a syringe attached to a catheter. The upper part of the catheter is taped to the infant's face. The tube should be changed at least every 3 to 5 days. The proximal end of the catheter is closed between feedings, either by a device fitted with a stopper or by clamping it.

The position of air in the stomachs of premature infants has been studied, resulting in the recommendation that small infants requiring tube feedings be fed while positioned on their stomachs. This is not possible if the infant is in respiratory distress; such an infant should be fed in a position halfway between his stomach and right side. A diaper roll can be used to support the infant in this position. The head of the mattress should be slightly elevated.

The nurse should open the tube for a few minutes before the feeding to permit escape of air from the stomach. Proper positioning of the tube must be assured by using the method described earlier of inserting air through the tube. Some practitioners recommend aspirating the stomach of air and fluid content before feeding. This permits expulsion of air from the stomach, and prevents overfeeding. The amount of material obtained is deducted from the total amount of feeding ordered. The substance (food and fluid) aspirated is returned to the stomach before the feeding, in order not to deplete electrolytes. The new feeding is injected at a slow, steady pace, or allowed to enter the tube by gravity flow. Afterwards 1 ml sterile water is administered to clear the tube of milk. If the baby evidences any signs of distress, the feeding is slowed or discontinued. After feeding, the infant should be placed on his abdomen. If the baby is dyspneic, he is placed on his left side.

INTRAVENOUS FEEDING This method of feeding provides the infant with fluids and calories via an umibilical venous or arterial catheter, or by peripheral intravenous routes.

PARENTERAL ALIMENTATION Infusions containing proteins and sugar are given to the infant via an umbilical venous or arterial catheter, or by peripheral intravenous routes. The catheter is attached to an infusion pump. This method is used when oral feedings must be delayed, or to supplement nipple or tube feedings which frequently cannot provide an adequate nutritive intake. Since most infants can be given a limited intake of nutrients via the oral route, supplemental alimentation is generally sufficient.

Recently, Penden (11) and Driscoll (12) reported on the use of *total* intravenous alimentation in low-birth-weight infants. All the nutrients are administered by catheter into the superior vena cava. This method of feeding is complex, requiring excellent personnel and facilities. It carries many hazards, and the use of this technique as the sole method of feeding should be reserved for very select high-risk infants.

NASOJEJUNAL FEEDING Cheek (13) has reported on feeding premature and full-term infants by passing an indwelling tube through the nose and stomach into the small intestine. Continuous feedings are then administered via an infusion pump. An isotonic solution must be used to prevent dumping. The researchers reported that this technique of feeding infants demonstrated excellent utilization of nutrients as measured by good weight gain.

DISORDERS REQUIRING INTRAVENOUS THERAPY

Biochemical equilibrium in the preterm infant is vital to his life. The infant's fluid and electrolyte balance is so delicate that it is easily upset by immaturity or illness. The speed with which a small baby can become dehydrated, hypoglycemic, or acidotic is startling. Intravenous therapy is frequently lifesaving to these infants.

Dehydration and Electrolyte Imbalance If the infant does not receive fluids, he will become dehydrated within a few hours. Vomiting and diarrhea can result in a critical loss of fluid and electrolytes.

The infant's fluid requirements are extremely high because his very large surface area in proportion to body weight necessitates great heat production to maintain life. The heat produced by the infant consumes at least twice as much water per kilogram of body weight as the adult. The baby's rapid growth results in a high production of metabolites. Therefore, he has a greater *obligatory water loss*; i.e., he needs a large amount of water to rid the body of waste materials. In addition, the kidneys are immature and do not efficiently concentrate urine.

The preterm infant may not evidence typical signs of dehydration such as fever, reduced skin turgor, sunken eyeballs and fontanels, dryness of the tongue and mucous membranes, and reduced urinary output. The most obvious and significant indication of dehydration in very small infants is *weight loss.*

Depletion of electrolytes usually accompanies dehydration. Sodium and potassium imbalances are frequently encountered. Blood tests are done to determine fluid and electrolyte replacement needs.

At first, the low-birth-weight infant is unable to take oral feedings in sufficient amounts to meet his fluid needs. In the first few days his requirements are low because of edema, but they quickly increase to approximately 150 ml/kg/day. If the baby cannot take fluids or is unable to take sufficient amounts through the gestrointestinal tract, intravenous therapy will be given.

Hypoglycemia The very small infant is susceptible to hypoglycemia because of his low stores of glycogen. In addition, the infant's metabolic response to cold stress, acidosis, and hypoxia results in the abnormal utilization of glucose. The normal range of blood sugar concentration in low-birth-weight infants is 20 to 100 mg/100 ml. Two consecutive samples indicating a blood sugar level below 20 mg/100 ml is diagnostic.

It is estimated that disturbed glucose homeostasis causes symptoms in about 5 to 10 percent of these babies. Signs and symptoms are confusing and overlapping with those of other conditions, e.g., apnea, cyanosis, dyspnea, tachypnea, tremors, irritability, upward rolling of the eyes, convulsions, coma, lethargy, weak cry, and refusal to feed. If the signs exhibited disappear within 5 min after intravenous glucose is administered, hypoglycemia is probably the etiologic factor.

In infants weighing less than 1250 Gm, low blood sugar levels are particularly common after birth and in the days following. Intravenous glucose solutions are given routinely to these small infants after birth and at variable periods thereafter. Blood sugar tests should be performed every 4 to 8 h for the first 2 days, and thereafter continued at less frequent intervals for about a week.

Early feeding of premature infants has been found in many studies to reduce the likelihood of hypoglycemic episodes. One critical factor noted by most researchers is that a sudden cessation of intravenous administration may cause marked hypoglycemia in otherwise normal infants. Intravenous fluids must be continued until oral intake is adequate.

If hypoglycemia is diagnosed, the infant is immediately treated with 25 percent glucose solution. Once blood sugar levels stabilize at normal values for a period of 24 to 48 h, the concentration of glucose infused is lowered to 10 percent and later to 5 percent. Untreated cases may result in death or brain damage.

Acid-Base Disturbances Acid-base disturbances frequently cause death in small infants. These problems occur in response to cold stress, respiratory difficulty, starvation, infection, and gastrointestinal disturbances. In order to give intelligent care and assess the patient's progress, the nurse must be able to correlate laboratory data with the infant's clinical course. This requires a basic understanding of the dynamics of acid-base balance.

The acidity of any fluid is expressed as pH—a value of 7 being considered neutral. However, the normal range of pH for arterial blood is slightly alkaline—7.35 to 7.45, and values under or over these are considered acidic or alkaline respectively. The majority of clinical deviations occur between a pH of 7.00 and 7.25, representing serious acidosis. Death ensues when the pH falls below 6.8 or rises above 7.8.

Acids—both *volatile* and *fixed*—are relentlessly produced in the body, and must be neutralized and eliminated in order to maintain the delicate pH balance.

Carbonic acid—which is volatile—is the major acid produced in the body. The carbon dioxide resulting from tissue metabolism goes into solution as carbonic acid, but the protein buffer system of the erythrocytes prevents the pH from falling below normal. The portion of carbonic acid which enters the erythrocytes is buffered by hemoglobin, where a series of chemical reactions converts it to bicarbonate. This bicarbonate is then released into plasma as sodium bicarbonate. Therefore, a large quantity of the carbon dioxide that orginates in the tissues is carried in plasma as sodium bicarbonate. The carbonic acid remaining in the blood is eliminated through the lungs as carbon dioxide.

The principal fixed acids produced by normal metabolism are lactic, sulfuric, and phosphoric. These acids are neutralized while carried in the blood by the sodium bicarbonate/carbonic acid buffer system, and finally eliminated through the kidneys. For example, lactic acid is buffered by sodium bicarbonate and converted to sodium lactate plus carbonic acid. The salt (sodium lactate) is excreted through the kidneys, and the carbonic acid exhaled as carbon dioxide.

It is evident, therefore, that three principal mechanisms function to protect the body against excessive accumulation of acids:

1. Buffering activity of the erythrocytes and plasma.
   1. Protein buffer system of hemoglobin for volatile carbonic acid
   b. Sodium bicarbonate/carbonic acid buffer system for fixed acids—lactic, sulfuric, phosphoric
2. Elimination of carbon dioxide through the lungs (Blood levels of CO_2 are controlled by the lungs.)
3. Excretion of fixed acids through the kidneys (The concentration of bicarbonate is controlled by the kidneys.)

ACIDOSIS AND ALKALOSIS Acid-base balance is primarily dependent upon the relative quantities of bicarbonate and carbonic acid present in the extracellular fluid. The normal ratio of this buffer system is 20 parts bicarbonate (HCO_3) to 1 part carbonic acid (H_2CO_3). The chart shown in Table 30·6 demonstrates how a shift in the normal ratio can result in acidosis or alkalosis. Equilibrium will be affected by changes in the concentration on either side. A decrease in bicarbonate or an increase in carbonic acid results in a lowered pH, or acidosis; an increase in bicarbonate or a decrease in carbonic acid results in a higher pH, or alkalosis.

LABORATORY TESTS FOR MEASURING ACID-BASE STATUS Table 30·5 outlines the major tests performed to assess the infant's acid-base status; whereas Table 30·6 indicates the variations in pH, P_{CO2}, and HCO_3 expected in the major disturbances.

COLLECTION OF SAMPLES The above tests

table 30·6

BLOOD GAS AND pH VARIATIONS IN THE MAJOR DISTURBANCES

TEST	METABOLIC ACIDOSIS	METABOLIC ALKALOSIS	RESPIRATORY ACIDOSIS	RESPIRATORY ALKALOSIS
pH	↓	↑	↓	↑
P_{CO_2}	Ratio to HCO_3 ↑	Ratio to HCO_3 ↓	↑	↓
HCO_3	↓	↑	Ratio to P_{CO_2}	Ratio to P_{CO_2} ↑

are performed on arterial blood samples if an indwelling umbilical artery catheter is in place. If this route is not available, samples of capillary blood for P_{CO_2} and pH determinations can be obtained from a heel prick. In order to obtain an arterialized capillary sample, the heel of the infant must be warmed with a moist pack for 5 min before the sample is taken. As mentioned previously, oxygen tension can be determined accurately only from arterial blood. Thus blood obtained from a heel prick is of no use in P_{O_2} testing.

To avoid inaccurate results, blood gas and pH determinations should be carried out immediately after the samples are collected. If necessary, the blood can be stored in the refrigerator for up to 2 h before testing without significant alterations in readings. Blood samples must never be kept at room temperature.

Etiology of Disturbances and Compensatory Mechanisms When shifts in the normal bicarbonate/carbonic acid ratio result in acid-base derangement, the body attempts to compensate for the particular shift through specific physiologic processes. If compensation is successful, a normal ratio *comparable* to 20 parts bicarbonate to 1 part carbonic acid is reestablished so that the pH remains normal. The compensatory mechanisms are described under the specific classifications of disturbances listed below.

METABOLIC ACIDOSIS This disturbance results from an increase in the concentration of nonvolatile acids. The major causes include excessive accumulation of acids from impaired metabolism and infection, excessive loss of base from diarrhea, and impaired renal functioning preventing the adequate excretion of acids.

As fixed acids accumulate in the blood, the bicarbonate level drops in order to neutralize the acids. The normal 20:1 ratio of bicarbonate to carbonic acid is altered. *Hyperventilation* is the compensatory process. Through excess excretion of carbon dioxide, it may be possible to lower the carbonic acid concentration to match the lowered bicarbonate level, thereby restoring the normal ratio. Although the pH remains normal if the infant compensates, both the serum bicarbonate concentration and the P_{CO_2} are low.

METABOLIC ALKALOSIS An increase in the concentration of bicarbonate results in metabolic alkalosis. In the infant, the primary causes are administering excessive doses of sodium bicarbonate intravenously, and the loss of large quantities of hydrochloric acid from persistent vomiting, causing an excessive accumulation of base.

In this disturbance, the infant *hypoventilates* in an effort to retain carbon dioxide and thus increase the carbonic acid concentration to match the increased level of bicarbonate. In this compensated state, the pH is normal, but both the serum bicarbonate concentration and the P_{CO_2} are elevated.

RESPIRATORY ACIDOSIS An increase in the concentration of carbonic acid due to inadequate pulmonary gas exchange produces respiratory acidosis. Asphyxia and hyaline membrane disease are the primary causes.

As carbonic acid builds up in the blood, the kidneys retain bicarbonate in an effort to bring the buffer ratio back into balance. If the baby compensates, the pH remains normal, but both the P_{CO_2} and the serum bicarbonate concentration are elevated.

The respiratory attempt to hyperventilate and eliminate the excessive carbon dioxide is generally not successful because of the underlying pulmonary disease. *Tachypnea* is the result of this extraordinary effort.

RESPIRATORY ALKALOSIS This disorder results from an increase in the concentration of base. The major cause is hyperventilation, which produces excessive elimination of carbon dioxide. In high-risk infants, it has been encountered in situations where mechanical respirators have been improperly set.

In an effort to offset the decrease in carbonic acid, the kidneys increase the excretion of bicarbonate. In this compensated condition, the pH remains normal, but the serum bicarbonate concentration and the P_{CO_2} are low.

Since most preterm infants tend to be slightly acidotic, with the pH falling as low as 7.25, pathologic problems may easily result in severe acidosis. The small infant's lungs and kidneys function with little reserve capacity to excrete excess acids, and therefore small babies are extremely liable to respiratory and metabolic acidosis.

It is possible for the infant to suffer from both metabolic and respiratory disturbances simultaneously. Such a condition is termed *mixed acidosis* or *alkalosis*. Mixed acidosis is the most common problem found in preterm infants suffering from hyaline membrane disease and asphyxia. In this condition, the combination of retained carbon dioxide and diminished bicarbonate results in a serious decrease in pH, which is frequently lethal to the infant. The treatment of acidosis is administration of sodium bicarbonate intravenously. The exact quantity is ordered by the physician, and it is always diluted to avoid damage to the blood vessels from the extremely alkaline pH.

intravenous therapy

In the first few precarious days following the premature's birth, parenteral therapy is frequently used to administer water, electrolytes, glucose, sodium bicarbonate, nutrients, and drugs.

Small infants are given minute amounts of fluid because of their small blood volume. A baby weighing 1160 Gm (2$\frac{1}{2}$ lb) has a blood volume of approximately 116 ml. It is impressive to compare this small volume with that of 5000 to 6000 ml found in the adult. Babson (14) states that in the first 3 days of life, the volume is about 70 to 80 ml/kg/24 h; then as tolerated the volume is gradually increased to 135 ml/kg/24 h. Thus, in the first few days—depending upon age and condition—the preterm infant receives approximately 3 to 8 ml intravenous fluid per hour. (There appears to be a consensus among authorities that the water requirement is approximately 150 ml/kg/24 h from about the fourth day on.) Although the physician orders the specific solution and amount to be given, it is the nurse who ensures that the required therapy is precisely carried out.

The most accessible veins in which to start an infusion are in the scalp (Fig. 30·18). A scalp vein infusion may require use of a sand bag to hold the infant's head in position. The intravenous infusion may also be started in one of the peripheral veins of the extremities. If the site is in the arm or ankle, a small armboard will be necessary to immobilize the part. Various types of restraints are often necessary on an extremity to prevent movements which might result in dislodging the needle (Fig. 30·19).

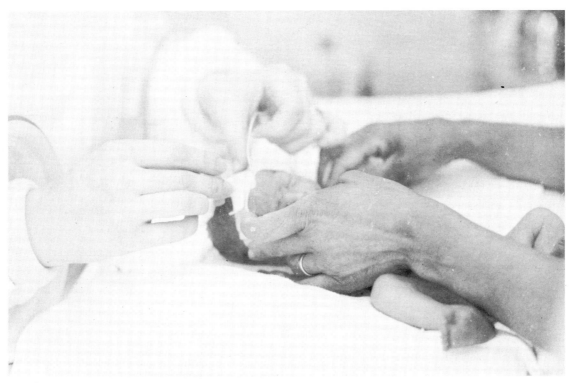

fig. 30·18 Starting an intraveneous infusion in a scalp vein.

Convenient but potentially dangerous sites of administration are the umbilical vein or artery. In intensive care units, umbilical catheterizations are now commonly performed to administer fluids to high-risk and sick infants. The catheter is marked with radiopaque material so that, after insertion, its proper position in the vessel can be assured through x-ray. The major complications include infection, thrombophlebitis, and liver damage.

The rate of administration is best controlled by using an electric infusion pump. Infusion pumps reduce the risks of dehydration and circulatory overload. However, infiltration does occur with these devices.

Infusion accidents can be prevented by careful observation and hourly charting of intake and output. Edema around the infusion site indicates infiltration; if this is noted, the nurse must immediately discontinue the infu-

sion. An infiltrated intravenous infusion may interfere with circulation in the extremity, signs of which include pallor, cyanosis, and cool skin temperature below the affected area.

During therapy, the nurse must be alert for significant physiologic changes in the infant's condition. Dehydration or circulatory overload is best diagnosed by changes in weight. Infants should be weighed at least every 12 to 24 h. In order to avoid disconnecting monitors every time the baby is weighed, all the equipment attached to the infant should be included in the initial base-line weight. All intake and output must be measured, and specific gravity and glucose tests performed on each voided specimen. The nurse keeps a record of all serial pH and blood gas determinations made.

Hypodermoclysis may be substituted for intravenous therapy if there is difficulty in

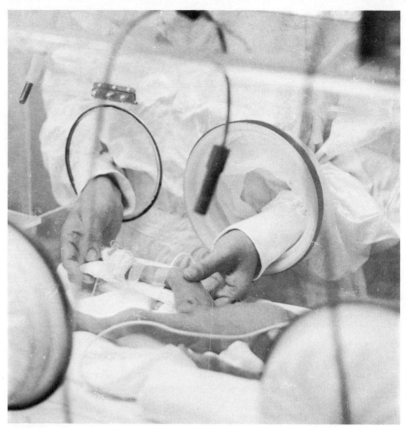

fig. 30·19 Note small board to which leg is attached for an infusion into an ankle vein.

using the veins. It is also used for fluid supplements. Small amounts of isotonic fluid are injected into the subscapular area, either by continuous drip or by injection.

prevention of infection

Postnatal infection is acquired from personnel, from equipment, and from other infants in the nursery. The preterm baby is more vulnerable to infection than the full-term infant. He has a poor defense against invasion by infectious agents because of a low level of antibodies circulating in the plasma (im-

munoglobins), immature phagocytosis, and inability to localize infection.

The *lack* of specific symptoms indicative of infection is unique in the preterm infant. Fever is often absent, and coughing is rare. Even in the presence of a fulminating infection, only vague symptoms may be observed, i.e., refusal to feed, lethargy, hyperirritability, vomiting, diarrhea, low-grade fever, cyanosis, irregular respirations, and apnea.

The three most common bacterial diseases found in premature infants are pneumonia, septicemia, and meningitis. Approximately 75 to 85 percent of these bacterial infections are caused by gram-negative rods—

principally *Escherichia coli* and *Pseudomonas aeruginosa*, in that order. Gram-positive cocci—*streptococci* being the most common—are the major cause of the remaining 15 to 24 percent of these infections.

In the late 1950s and early 1960s, *staphylococci* were the primary etiologic factor in nursery epidemics. This resulted in the enforcement of stringent isolation and medical aseptic practices in the nursery. Whether or not these rigid policies influenced the subsequent decline of epidemiologic strains of staphylococci is uncertain and unproved. Some researchers have suggested that the main reason staphylococci epidemics have diminished may be the passing of a boom phase in the long-term natural life cycle of the organisms. With the present relaxation of rigid infection control techniques in many nurseries, it remains to be seen if an upsurge of epidemics will occur.

Many studies have been published regarding the spread of staphylococcal infections in newborns. Colonization occurs when the organisms settle on the tissue of the skin, nose, and throat without producing disease. There is a much higher incidence of disease in infants who have become colonized with the organisms. These infections may occur while the infant is in the nursery or after discharge. Many infants become ill at home. In some cases, the infant remains well but spreads the infection to other family members. The practice of good hand-washing technique by nursery personnel is considered the most crucial factor in preventing the spread of staphylococci in the nursery.

Following the decline of epidemics of staphylococcal infections, nurseries have experienced a rise in the incidence of infections due to gram-negative rods—*Pseudomonas* being one of the most prevalent. These bacteria are termed "water bugs" by Wheeler (15) because they can thrive and proliferate in water alone. The introduction of a gamut of mechanical equipment in the care of infants is the principal cause of the high incidence of these infections. Gram-negative bacteria in the nursery are spread primarily by contaminated equipment, particularly those utilizing moisture of any kind, i.e., incubators, and plastic sleeves on portholes, resuscitative equipment, face masks, suction machines, wash basins, Zephiran solutions, soap dishes, etc. The surveillance and sterilization of equipment are essential in preventing spread of infection. It is the nurse's responsibility to ensure that all equipment used is appropriately cleaned and sterilized. If the equipment permits, all potentially infectious objects should be autoclaved or gas-sterilized. When oxygen is in use, the humidifier must be changed daily and the water changed every 8 h. Plastic disposable tubes should be used from oxygen outlets and discarded every 24 h. At present, the trend is to simplify infection control techniques used in the nursery, the rationale being that many of the rigid practices of the past proved useless when tested scientifically. The single most important factor in preventing spread of infection by any organism is handwashing. The principal mode of cross-infection is failure of personnel to wash hands between the handling of different infants. Personnel should perform a 2 min scrub to a level above the elbows when first entering the nursery, and wash for 30 to 60 s between caring for different babies. Both soaps and detergents are used. Heeding the warnings issued in 1971, many institutions have banned the use of hexachlorophene. However, because some nurseries have experienced a subsequent outbreak of staphylococcal infections, they have resumed limited use of hexachlorophene detergents for personnel caring for infants. Iodinated detergents are effective against gram-negative rods as well as gram-positive organisms, but such preparations are often irritating to the skin.

Personnel giving direct care to the infant in a crib or incubator should wear short-sleeved scrub dresses to facilitate washing. A long-sleeved gown should be worn by personnel when removing an infant from an incubator or bassinet, and must be changed between the handling of different infants. Some institutions do not require physicians and other personnel to wear gowns provided the infant is cared for in the incubator. The use of hairnets, caps, and masks has been discontinued.

The majority of postnatally acquired infections are preventable if sensible hygienic practices of proved value are carried out. It is neither possible nor desirable to secure a germ-free environment in the nursery, and all practices are designed to minimize the risk of spreading infection by personnel, equipment, and cross-contamination of infants. The nurse is in a better position than other staff members to ensure the success of infection control procedures, because of her close and continuous contact with the infants. The baby must be closely observed for redness at the base of the cord, discharge from the eyes, skin eruptions, changes in skin color, and signs of respiratory infection. Any suggestive symptom must be immediately reported to the physician. The nurse should be aware of the incidence of infections in the nursery, and alert to possible sources of contamination. She must accept the responsibility of appraising and regulating the hygienic demeanor of the many specialists, technicians, and ancillary personnel involved in the infants' care. Sick personnel pose a serious threat to the infant and should not enter the nursery.

Studies have shown that the incidence of infectious disease does not increase when parents are allowed into the nursery, but the precautions regarding handwashing and gowning must be enforced.

"Suspect" and isolation nurseries are no longer considered essential except for infants with diarrhea and draining infections.

routine daily care

Throughout this chapter, the nurse's responsibilities have been described in detail in relation to the infant's specific problems and needs. Routine care procedures differ at various institutions, but the basics are summarized below:

The nurse gives total care to the infant at periodic intervals in order to avoid repeatedly disturbing him. All equipment is collected beforehand, and the nurse must work efficiently—giving complete care without tiring or exhausting the baby. If the infant's vital signs are not monitored, they are taken before the baby is handled.

When a baby is admitted to the nursery, a bath should not be given until the temperature has stabilized for at least 4 h. Studies carried out by Kopelman (16) and Powell (17) indicate that small premature infants are particularly susceptible to the toxic effects of hexachlorophene. Therefore, such preparations should not be used for bathing. Despite tradition, it is not necessary to bathe infants completely on a daily basis. In fact, it is important that the complete bath be omitted for small sick infants. Even if a bath is not given, the genitals and creases of the thighs and buttocks must be kept clean.

Small babies are weighed daily before feedings; larger ones less often. The small baby may lose 10 to 20 percent of his birth weight, and the larger infants from 5 to 10 percent in the first week of life. Very small infants often take 1 month or even longer to regain their birth weights.

In order to facilitate postural drainage from the lungs, the infant's position should be changed every 1 to 2 h. The incubator can be adjusted to provide a Fowler's or Trendelenburg position. If respiratory distress is observed, the infant should be placed in a low Fowler's position. In this position, the flexed neck may cause narrowing of the trachea so that a thin diaper roll may be needed under the shoulders to slightly hyperextend the infant's neck. Flexed and abducted arms will permit greater expansion of the thorax. When the baby is placed in a Fowler's position, a diaper roll inserted under the buttocks prevents him from slipping down in the incubator (Fig. 30·20). An infant in respiratory distress must never be positioned on his abdomen.

During the entire process of caring for the baby, the nurse closely observes his respirations, skin condition, color, cry, activity, and muscle tone. It may be necessary to stimulate the infant by flicking his heel in order to test the quality of the cry. The times of the first voiding and defecation should be noted. In a study of 180 preterm infants, Mangurten (18) reported that 80 percent of the infants passed the first stool by 24 h after birth. It should be dark green and sticky. The nurse should be concerned if it appears pale and firm, since it then may be indicative of a meconium plug causing obstruction or Hirschsprung's disease. Abdominal distension must be detected immediately, since it may signify gastrointestinal disturbance, and interferes with respiration. Below are listed critical observations which can be made only by nurses, not by monitors.

1. Respiratory distress characterized by grunting, retractions, flaring nares, pallor, or cyanosis
2. Detection of regurgitation and vomiting (to prevent aspiration)
3. Sucking ability and acceptance of feedings
4. Skin condition, color, and lesions
5. Changes in activity
6. Frequency and character of urine and stools

After morning care, the baby's condition is noted and recorded every 1 to 4 h, depending upon his condition. All efforts should be made to assign one nurse to a particular infant in order to ensure consistency of approach and valid comparative observations.

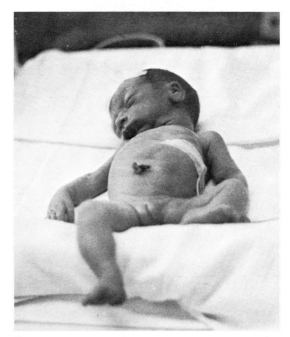

fig. 30·20 Infant in a slightly elevated position with a diaper roll to prevent slipping down.

psychologic needs of the mother of a preterm infant

In recent decades we have come to understand the adverse and often devastating effects suffered by an infant separated from its mother. It has been well established that the infant requires a warm, intimate, and continuous relationship with its mother or mother surrogate in order to ensure normal psychologic and physical development. Knowing that early maternal deprivation affects the infant, it appears reasonable to conjecture that to some degree maternal behavior may be altered by isolation from the infant. The important—and as yet unanswered—question today is whether a critical or sensitive period exists for the mother in the immediate postnatal period in which physical contact is important for the development of normal mothering behavior.

Animal studies have repeatedly demonstrated that the development of normal mothering behavior for most species requires immediate physical contact with the young in the postnatal period. If the animal mother is separated from the infant during the critical period after delivery, deviant maternal behavior usually results. Infant deprivation in many species results in the actual rejection and/or destruction of the offspring.

Researchers suggest that bonds of affection begin to form before delivery, but that they are fragile and vulnerable in the early days of life. The human studies in this area focus on observing the mother/newborn relationship. Klaus and coworkers (19) suggest that the human mother exhibits specific routine behavior patterns after delivery. They have shown through filmed observations that "touch" and "eye-to-eye" contact appear to play an important role in establishing bonds of affection between the mother and her infant. They reported that when alert mothers of full-term infants were presented their nude newborns, each mother began touching her baby's extremities with her fingertips, and within a few minutes used her entire hand to stroke the infant's body. The expression of affection and love for the baby was repeatedly evidenced by the mother assuming an *en face* position in relation to her baby; i.e., the mother rotated the position of her face in such a way that her eyes and those of the infant directly met (see Fig. 16·1). During the first hour of life the baby's reaction was observed to coincide with the mother's natural response of eye-to-eye contact. The baby was then alert, attentive, and able to meet the intense gaze of the mother. Many great artists have been able to capture on canvas this moving expression of love and tenderness.

In the future, further investigation may reveal that alterations in current hospital policies are required for the ultimate good of mother and baby. Klaus (20) contends that separation in the immediate newborn period may be a significant component in mothering

disorders connected with failure to thrive, child abuse, and emotional and behavioral problems found in both natural and adopted children.

Progressive neonatal centers are already attempting to alter procedures to decrease the effects of physical separation. The mother expects a perfect baby, and a preterm infant brings with it shock, grief, anxiety, fear, and a blow to her self-esteem as a mother. Her defenses are down and she requires support. The guilt and psychologic sense of separation felt by the mother are intense. She should be encouraged to see her infant at the earliest opportunity. It has been demonstrated that unless parents have a history of serious emotional disorders, their grief is not compounded by early and close contact with an infant who does not survive. As soon as the infant's condition permits, the mother should visit and fondle the baby while it is still in the incubator, and should repeatedly bathe and feed the baby before discharge from the hospital. The nurse should explain in detail all the equipment surrounding the infant, and all questions should be answered with simple, honest explanations and with great patience.

Throughout life, all human beings have the same basic needs and perform the same basic functions. It is the quality with which one moves through the experiences of day-to-day living that gives life meaning, value, and beauty. The need of the infant for uncompromising love, care, and affection is so crucial to his future development and life that any effort made by the professional to secure a meaningful mother/infant relationship is a significant contribution to the human condition.

references

1. *Standard and Recommendations for Hospital Care of Newborn Infants*, American

Academy of Pediatrics, Evanston, Ill., 1971, p. 11.

2. Denis Cavanagh, and M. R. Talisman, *Prematurity and the Obstetrician*, Appleton-Century-Crofts, Inc., New York, 1969, p. 29.

3. L. O. Lubchenco et al., "Sequelae of Premature Birth," *American Journal of Diseases of Children*, **106**:101, 1973.

4. G. Rawlings, et al., "Changing Prognosis for Infants of Very Low Birth Weight," *The Lancet*, **1**:516, 1971.

5. L. M. Dubowitz, V. Dubowitz, and C. Goldberg, "Clinical Assessment of Gestational Age in the Newborn Infant," *Journal of Pediatrics*, **77**:1, 1970.

6. P. H. Perlstein, N. K. Edwards, and J. M. Sutherland, "Apnea in Premature Infants and Incubator-air-temperature," *New England Journal of Medicine*, **282**:461, 1970.

7. V. Chernick, F. Heldrich, and M. E. Avery, "Periodic Breathing of Premature Infants," *Journal of Pediatrics*, **64**:330, 1964.

8. A. S. DeLeon, J. H. Elliot, and D. B. Jones, "The Resurgence of Retrolental Fibroplasia," *Pediatric Clinics of North America*, **17**:309, 1970.

9. Cavanagh, op. cit., p. 456.

10. *Standard and Recommendations for Hospital Care of Newborn Infants*, op. cit., p. 12.

11. V. H. Penden and J. T. Karpel, "Total Parenteral Nutrition in Premature Infants," *Journal of Pediatrics*, **81**:137, 1972.

12. J. M. Driscoll et al., "Total Intravenous Alimentation in Low Birth-weight Infants: A Preliminary Report," *Journal of Pediatrics*, **81**:145, 1972.

13. J. A. Cheek and G. F. Staub, "Nasojejunal Alimentation for Premature and Full-term Newborn Infants," *Journal of Pediatrics*, **82**:955, 1973.

14. S. G. Babson and R. C. Benson, *Management of the High-risk Pregnancy and Intensive Care of the Neonate*, 2d ed., The C. V. Mosby Company, St. Louis, 1971, p. 204.

15. W. E. Wheeler, "Water Bugs in the Bassinet," *American Journal of Diseases of Children*, **101**:273, 1961.

16. Arthur E. Kopelman, "Cutaneous Absorption of Hexachlorophene in Low Birth-weight Infants," *Journal of Pediatrics*, **82**:972, 1973.

17. H. Powell et al., "Hexachlorophene Myelinopathy in Premature Infants," *Journal of Pediatrics*, **82**:976, 1973.

18. H. H. Mangurten, C. I. Slade, and C. J. Reidle, "First Stool in the Preterm, Low Birth-weight Infant," *Journal of Pediatrics*, **82**:1033, 1973.

19. M. Klaus, J. Kennell, N. Plumb, et al., "Human Maternal Behavior at the First Contact with Her Young," *Pediatrics*, **46**:187, 1970.

20. M. Klaus and J. Kennell, "Mothers Separated from Their Newborn Infants," *Pediatric Clinics of North America*, **17**:1015, 1970.

bibliography

Altemeier, W. A., and R. T. Smith: "Immunologic Aspects of Resistance in Early Life," *Pediatric Clinics of North America*, **12**:663, 1965.

Auld, P. A. M.: "Oxygen Therapy for Premature Infants," *Journal of Pediatrics*, **78**:705, 1971.

Barrie, D.: "Incubator-borne *Pseudomonas pyocyanea* Infection in a Newborn Nursery," *Archives of Diseases of Children*, **40**:555, 1965.

Beard, A. F., et al.: "Neonatal Hypoglycemia: A Discussion," *Journal of Pediatrics*, **79**:314, 1971.

Bryan, M. H., et al.: "Supplemental Intravenous Alimentation in Low Birth-weight Infants," *Journal of Pediatrics*, **82**:940, 1973.

Cavanagh, Denis, and M. R. Talisman: *Prematurity and the Obstetrician,* Appleton-Century-Crofts, Inc., New York, 1969.

Davies, P. A.: "Bacterial Infection in the Fetus and Newborn," *Archives of Diseases of Children,* **46**:1, 1971.

Evans, H. E., et al.: "Bacteriologic and Clinical Evaluation of Gowning in a Premature Nursery," *Journal of Pediatrics,* **78**:883, 1971.

Fanaroff, M. B., et al.: "Controlled Trial of Continuous Negative External Pressure in the Treatment of Severe Respiratory Distress Syndrome," *Journal of Pediatrics,* **82**:921, 1973.

Gotoff, S. P., and R. E. Behrman: "Neonatal Septicemia," *Journal of Pediatrics,* **76**:142, 1970.

Gregory, G. A., et al.: "Treatment of the Idiopathic Respiratory Distress Syndrome with Continuous Positive Airway Pressure," *New England Journal of Medicine,* **284**:1333, 1971.

Gruber, H. A., and M. H. Klaus: "Intermittent Mask and Bag Therapy; an Alternative Approach to Respiratory Therapy for Infants with Severe Respiratory Distress," *Journal of Pediatrics,* **76**:194, 1970.

Harris, T. R., and M. Nugent: "Continuous Arterial Oxygen Tension Monitoring in the Newborn Infant," *Journal of Pediatrics,* **82**:929, 1973.

Heese, H. deV., et al.: "Intermittent Positive Pressure Ventilation in Hyaline Membrane Disease," *Journal of Pediatrics,* **76**:183, 1970.

Kitterman, J. A., R. H. Phibbs, and W. H. Tooley: "Catheterization of Umbilical Vessels in Newborn Infants," *Pediatrics Clinics of North America,* **17**:895, 1970.

Klaus, M., R. Jerauld, N. Kreger, et al.: "Maternal Attachment: Importance of the First Post-partum Days," *New England Journal of Medicine,* **286**:460, 1972.

Korones, Sheldon B.: *High-risk Newborn Infants,* The C. V. Mosby Company, St. Louis, 1972.

Kwong, M. S., et al.: "The Effect of Hexachlorophene on Staphylococcal Colonization Rates in the Newborn Infant: A Controlled Study Using a Single-bath Method," *Journal of Pediatrics,* **82**:982, 1973.

Lubchenco, L. O., et al.: "Long-term Follow-up Studies of Prematurely Born Infants. I. Relationship of Handicaps to Nursery Routines," *Journal of Pediatrics,* **80**:501, 1972.

————: "Long-term Follow-up Studies of Prematurely Born Infants. II. Influence of Birth Weight and Gestational Age on Sequelae," *Journal of Pediatrics,* **80**:509, 1972.

Sawyer, P. R.: "The Regional Organization of Special Care for the Neonate," *Pediatrics Clinics of North America,* **17**:761, 1970.

Schlesinger, E. R.: "Neonatal Intensive Care: Planning for Services and Outcomes Following Care," *Journal of Pediatrics,* **82**:916, 1973.

Shaw, J. C. L.: "Parenteral Nutrition in the Management of Sick Low Birthweight Infants," *Pediatrics Clinics of North America,* **20**:333, 1973.

Sinclair, J. C.: "Heat Production and Thermoregulation in the Small-for-date Infant," *Pediatrics Clinics of North America,* **17**:147, 1970.

South, M. A.: "*Escherichia coli* Disease; New Developments and Perspectives," *Journal of Pediatrics,* **79**:1, 1971.

Stahlman, M., et al.: "A Six-year Follow Up of Clinical Hyaline Membrane Disease," *Pediatrics Clinics of North America,* **20**:433, 1973.

————: "Negative Pressure Assisted Ventilation in Infants with Hyaline Membrane Disease," *Journal of Pediatrics,* **76**:174, 1970.

Stephenson, J. M., et al.: "The Effect of Cooling on Blood Gas Tensions in Newborn Infants," *Journal of Pediatrics,* **76**:848, 1970.

Winick, M.: "Fetal Malnutrition and Growth Process," *Hospital Practice,* **5**:33, 1970.

World Medical Reports: "Close Neonatal Contact Makes for Better Mothers," *Pediatric News,* **5**:27, 1971.

glossary

abortion termination of pregnancy of a fetus weighing less than 500 Gm or of a pregnancy of less than 19 completed weeks after conception

spontaneous occurring without assistance; lay term, "miscarriage"

induced brought on by external methods: D and C (dilation and curettage), vacuum aspiration, salinization

abruptio placentae tearing away of the placenta from the wall of the uterus, accompanied by pain; there may be concealed bleeding or overt, visible bleeding

acini (pl.), acinus (sing.) smallest, saccular division of a gland, occurring in grapelike clusters, as in the mammary gland

acrocyanosis cyanotic or bluish discoloration of the hands and/or feet of the newborn as a result of inadequate circulation or coldness

afterbirth the products of conception (excluding the baby) that are expelled during the delivery—placenta and membranes (sac) and umbilical cord. Syn., secundines

afterpains discomfort caused by the contraction of the uterus postpartally as it returns to its prepregnant condition; usually occurring in the multipara

amenorrhea cessation or absence of menstruation

amniocentesis removal of some of the amniotic fluid from the amniotic sac by way of a needle inserted through the abdominal wall of the mother for the purpose of examining the fluid

amnion inner layer of the fetal membranes or sac, which secretes amniotic fluid

amniotic fluid embolism a rare postpartal occurrence, in which amniotic fluid enters the maternal circulation. The cells, debris and fluid form emboli, usually in the lungs.

amniotomy rupturing of the amniotic sac by artificial means

androgenic hormone a hormone that has the property of producing male secondary sexual characteristics

anencephalus a fetus born without a brain or cranial bones

anovulatory associated with lack or absence of ovulation

anoxia lack or absence of oxygen

antenatal prenatal, before birth

antepartal occurring before labor and delivery

antibody substance produced by the body for protection against the specific antigen that triggered its production

antigen any substance, usually of protein material, which triggers the production of antibodies, such as foreign blood cells, bacteria

apnea absence or cessation of respirations

areola pigmented area surrounding the nipple

asphyxia neonatorum respiratory failure in the newborn, resulting from an insufficient oxygen–carbon dioxide exchange

ballottement rebounding movement of the fetus when uterus (or cervix) is tapped by the examiner. Syn., passive fetal movement

Bandl's ring retracted ring occurring between the lower and upper segments of the uterus and resulting from an obstructed labor; may be a sign of impending uterine rupture. Syn., pathologic retraction ring

basal body temperature (BBT) lowest usual temperature of the body taken before rising

bilirubin the red-orange pigment that results from the breakdown of hemoglobin and which can cause jaundice of the skin, when the level rises above 5 mg/100 ml in the newborn.

Braxton Hicks contractions painless, intermittent contractions of the uterus which occur throughout pregnancy; often mistaken for labor contractions

Braxton Hicks version a maneuver to change the position of the fetus by external and internal manipulation

breech buttocks
  breech presentation delivery in which the buttocks or feet of the fetus are presented at the outlet, instead of the vertex (head)
  footling one or both feet present at the opening
  frank buttocks are the presenting part
  full or complete buttocks and feet present at the pelvic brim

Candida albicans a yeastlike fungus which produces monilial infection in the vaginal canal of the woman, and may cause thrush in the infant

caput head

caput succedaneum swelling or edema on the head of the infant occurring during labor and/or delivery

cephalhematoma trauma of labor and delivery resulting in a collection of blood on the head of the fetus between the bone and the periosteum, defined by the suture lines

cephalic referring to the head

cerclage procedure procedure for the treatment of incompetent cervix

cholasma gravidarum brownish-yellow patches of pigmentation occurring during pregnancy, particularly on the face and neck. Syn., mask of pregnancy

choanal atresia congenital or genetic blockage of the posterior nares

chorion the outermost membrane of the developing fetus, which gives rise to the fetal portion of the placenta and extends to form the outer layer of the amniotic sac

chorionic pertaining to the chorion

chorionic gonadotropin hormone produced by the chorion and excreted in the urine of the pregnant woman; its presence in the urine is a possible sign of pregnancy

chorionic villi fingerlike projections of the chorion which invade the decidua basalis and form the fetal portion of the placenta

cleft lip congenital/genetic opening of the upper lip extending from the nares; may involve one or both nares

cleft palate congenital/genetic opening of the roof of the mouth

colostrum yellowish-white fluid expressed from the breast during pregnancy preceding the formation of milk; caloric and cathartic values of this substance are questioned

congenital laryngeal stridor a harsh, crowing, vibrating sound produced by the newborn or infant upon inspiration

Coombs' test blood test to determine the presence of antibodies
  direct determination of antibodies attached to blood cells, particularly maternal (anti-Rh) antibodies attached to fetal blood cells
  indirect determination of free-floating or unattached antibodies, particularly those (anti-Rh) in the maternal circulation (serum)

corpus luteum yellow body of material found in the site of the ruptured graafian follicle which persists for several months during pregnancy, secreting progesterone

crowning the appearance of the vertex, or head, at the external vaginal orifice

D and C dilatation and curettage; a surgical procedure involving dilation of the cervix and removal of the uterine contents

decidua enriched endometrial lining of pregnancy shed after pregnancy terminates
  basalis the portion of the endometrium underlying the embedded embryo and from which the maternal portion of the placenta is formed
  capsularis that outer portion of the decidua enveloping the embryo
  vera the remainder of the endometrium not containing the embedded embryo

dilation the act of stretching or opening

dilatation enlargement of an organ or orifice
  of the cervix; the state of enlargement or opening of the cervix to allow for passage of the fetus

Döderlein's bacillus common vaginal gram-negative organism producing lactic acid which tends to inhibit the growth of pathogenic organisms

Down's syndrome formerly known as mongolism; a congenital/genetic abnormality in which 47 chromosomes are present in the fetus

dystocia difficult, abnormal labor

eclampsia abnormal reaction of the body to pregnancy, resulting in convulsions and possible coma; usually preceded by hypertension, albuminuria, and edema

ectopic pregnancy pregnancy that occurs outside the uterine cavity

effacement thinning of the cervix to allow for passage of the fetus; in primigravidas, occurs prior to dilatation, and in multigravidas, occurs simultaneously with dilatation

engagement descent of the fetus into the pelvis until the presenting part reaches the level of the ischial spines

engorgement stasis of blood and lymph in the breast, causing tenderness, firmness, and discomfort prior to onset of lactation

episiotomy a surgical incision of the perineum to enlarge the external vaginal opening to prevent laceration of the vulva, perineum, and adjacent structures

Epstein's pearls tiny, white, beadlike epithelial cysts on the roof of the mouth of the newborn on either side of the median ridge; not to be confused with thrush, which is patchy

erythroblastosis fetalis hemolytic disorder of the fetus or newborn in which maternal anti-Rh antibodies destroy fetal blood cells, causing jaundice and other symptoms

estriol a metabolite produced by the placenta, found in the urine of pregnant women and measured in an attempt to determine placental function or dysfunction

estrogenic hormone a hormone which has the property of producing female secondary sexual characteristics

fetal pertaining to fetus

fetus the offspring from the moment of conception until the pregnancy is terminated

fontanel the space at the junction of three or more fetal and cranial bones, covered with a tough membrane
anterior junction of sagittal, frontal, and coronal sutures, on anterior portion of skull. Syn., "soft spot," greater fontanel
posterior junction of lambdoid and sagittal sutures. Syn., lesser fontanel

foramen ovale opening between the right and left atria of the heart in the fetus; closes after birth

fundus the upper portion of the uterus

gestation length of time necessary for intrauterine growth and development of the fetus

graafian follicle fluid-filled sac in the ovary housing the maturing ovum

gravid pregnant

gravida a pregnant woman
primigravida woman pregnant for the first time
multigravida woman pregnant for the second time or more

hemorrhage in obstetrics, loss of blood in excess of 500 ml after the third stage of labor

hyaline membrane disease see *idiopathic respiratory distress syndrome* (RDS)

hydatidiform mole grapelike, cystic masses of degenerated chorionic villi, usually benign

hydramnios "water"; excessive amniotic fluid. Syn., polyhydramnios

hyperemesis gravidarum excessive, severe vomiting during pregnancy

hypofibrinogenemia reduced amounts of fibrinogen in the blood

hypospadias congenital/genetic defect in which the urethra of the male opens on the underside of the penis

hypoxia deficient amount of oxygen

icterus jaundice

icterus gravis neonatorum see *erythroblastosis fetalis*

idiopathic respiratory distress syndrome a severe respiratory syndrome of the newborn or preterm infant resulting in the development of a hyaline membrane in the lungs; may be fatal. Syn., RDS, hyaline membrane disease

inertia (uterine) inefficient, weak, or absent uterine contractions
primary occurring early in labor
secondary occurring after labor is established. Syn., uterine dysfunction

involution returning of the pelvic organs and structures to resemble their prepregnant state or condition

ischemia reduction of blood supply to an area

jaundice yellowish color of skin, sclera, mucous membrane, and excretions. Syn., icterus

kernicterus excessive bilirubin deposits in the brain, causing neurologic changes; may cause permanent brain damage or death

lanugo soft, fine, downy hair found on preterm and newborn infants

lightening the tilting or dropping of the fetus forward and downward into the true pelvis; occurs 2 or 3 weeks before the end of gestation in the primigravida, or at the beginning of labor in many multigravidas

linea nigra the darkening of the abdominal line between the umbilicus and the symphysis pubis during pregnancy, caused by hormonal changes

lochia uterine discharge after delivery which consists of the sloughing decidua, tissue, blood, and cells; lasts 2 or 3 weeks

mastalgia pain in the breast

mastitis inflammation of the breast

menarche first menstrual flow

menorrhagia abnormally long or excessive menstrual bleeding

menses menstruation

menstruation cyclic uterine discharge of blood, tissue, and cells as a result of hormonal changes in the body. Syn., menses

mentum chin

milia tiny, white or yellow beadlike sebaceous cysts found primarily on the face of the newborn

miscarriage lay term for spontaneous abortion

mittelschmerz lower abdominal pain generally associated with ovulation

molding temporary changes in the shape of the head of the newborn, as it accommodates to the birth canal during labor and delivery

multigravida a woman who has been pregnant more than once

multipara a woman who has delivered more than once

neonatal referring to the newborn infant

nephrotoxic any substance or material which exerts a poisonous effect on the kidney

newborn infant a living infant during the first 27 days, 23 h, and 59 min of its life

nidation embedding of the fertilized ovum into the lining of the uterus

nulligravida a woman who has never been pregnant

nullipara a woman who has never delivered a viable baby

occiput back of the head; occipital bone

ophthalmia neonatorum acute, purulent conjunctivitis of the eyes of the newborn, usually caused by gonococcus

organogenesis the growth of various tissues of the fetus into organs. Period of organogenesis—first 12 weeks.

ototoxic any substance or material poisonous to the ear

ovum female reproductive cell

oxytocin synthetic or natural substance which stimulates the uterus to contract

parity the state of having given birth to one infant or more than one infant; multiple births are considered as one parous delivery

parturient a laboring woman

parturition the act of giving birth

phenylketonuria (PKU) a genetic disorder involving the deficiency of the enzyme phenylalanine hydroxylase

phlegmasia alba dolens phlebitis of the femoral or iliac vein, resulting in edema of the leg. Syn., milk leg

placenta previa abnormally low implantation of the placenta in the uterus

polyhydramnios excessive amniotic fluid. Syn., hydramnios

position the relationship of a designated point on the presenting part of the fetus to a designated point in the maternal pelvis which has been divided into four quadrants

postpartum the period of time following delivery

preeclampsia abnormal bodily reaction to pregnancy characterized by edema, hypertension, and proteinuria, and occurring after the twentieth week of pregnancy; often referred to as toxemia

premature infant an infant born up through 37 completed weeks of gestation. Syn., preterm infant

presentation relationship of the long axis of the fetus to the long axis of the mother. Syn., lie

presenting part that anatomic part of the fetus that is closest to the cervix and felt by the examiner on vaginal or rectal examination—usually the head or buttocks

primigravida woman pregnant for the first time

primipara woman who has delivered for the first time a viable infant (over 20 weeks' gestation)

pseudocyesis false pregnancy

puerperium the 42 days after delivery

quickening the first active movements of the fetus detectable by the mother, at approximately 16 to 18 weeks of gestation

respiratory distress syndrome (RDS) see *idiopathic respiratory distress syndrome*

resuscitation restoration of breathing, life, or consciousness of one who is apparently dead and whose respirations have ceased

retrolental fibroplasia (RLF) a fibrous membrane which may occur behind the lens in the eye as a result of high oxygen concentration administered to a preterm infant

rugae transverse folds of the vaginal mucous membrane

secundines placenta and fetal membranes

Shirodkar technique purse-string suturing procedure for an incompetent cervix

show blood-tinged mucous discharge occurring during labor as the cervix dilates. Syn., bloody show

souffle, fetal a blowing or whistling sound of the blood as it rushes through the fetal arteries in the umbilical cord. Syn., funic souffle, umbilical souffle, Kennedy's sign

souffle, uterine the blowing, blurred sound of the maternal blood as it rushes through the uterine arteries. Syn., Kergaradec's sign

spermatozoon male reproductive cell. Syn., sperm

spinnbarkheit changes in the stretchability of the cervical mucosa during ovulation

stillborn a fetus, over 20 weeks' gestation, born without life

subinvolution a delay in the return of the pelvic organs and structures to their prepregant state

supine hypotensive syndrome hypotension resulting from the pressure of the enlarged uterus upon the vena cava, blocking venous return

syncope fainting or light-headedness, common in early pregnancy

teratogen any agent or substance which has the capacity to alter fetal growth and development

term infant a live baby born after 38 to 42 weeks of gestation (from time of last menstrual period). Syn., full-term infant

thrush white, patchy oral lesions of the newborn caused by *Candida albicans*

toxemia see *preeclampsia, eclampsia*

tracheoesophageal fistula (TEF) congenital/genetic disorder in which the esophagus and trachea are connected, or the esophagus ends in a blind pouch and there is a lower connection in the trachea to the esophagus

Trichomonas vaginalis protozoan infection of the vagina; Skene's ducts and urinary tract may also be infected

trimester approximately one-third of the gestational period

first trimester the first day of the last normal menstrual period through 14 weeks' gestation

second trimester fifteenth through twenty-eighth week of gestation

third trimester twenty-ninth through the forty-second completed week of gestation and birth

umbilical cord life line between the fetus and placenta through which nourishment and waste pass; contains two arteries and one vein surrounded by Wharton's jelly. Syn., funis

vernix caseosa cheeselike covering on the fetus which protects the skin from the drying and wrinkling properties of the amniotic fluid

viability capability of survival, over 20 weeks' gestation

Wharton's jelly gelatinous connective tissue which surrounds the umbilical vessels giving support to the umbilical cord

zygote the fertilized ovum

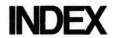
INDEX

INDEX

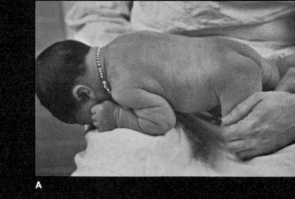

A

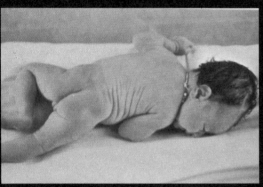

B

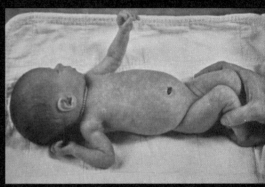

C

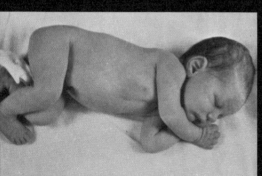

D

Plate 3 Newborn skin colors. A Variation in color over pressure areas; B pale skin color; C normal mottling; D jaundice, ripe-peach color. *(Courtesy of Mead Johnson Company.)*